THE NEURONAL CEROID LIPOFUSCINOSES (BATTEN DISEASE)

THE NEURONAL CEROID LIPOFUSCINOSES (BATTEN DISEASE)

Second Edition

Edited by

Sara E. Mole
MRC Laboratory for Molecular Cell Biology; Molecular Medicines Unit, UCL Institute of Child Health; and Department of Genetics, Evolution and Environment, University College London

Ruth E. Williams
Evelina Children's Hospital, Guy's and St Thomas' NHS Foundation Trust, London

Hans H. Goebel
Johannes Gutenberg-University Medical Center, Mainz, Germany

Editorial Assistance by
G. Machado da Silva
MRC Laboratory for Molecular Cell Biology, University College London

OXFORD
UNIVERSITY PRESS

2011

OXFORD
UNIVERSITY PRESS

Great Clarendon Street, Oxford OX2 6DP

Oxford University Press is a department of the University of Oxford.
It furthers the University's objective of excellence in research, scholarship, and education by publishing worldwide in

Oxford New York

Auckland Cape Town Dar es Salaam Hong Kong Karachi
Kuala Lumpur Madrid Melbourne Mexico City Nairobi
New Delhi Shanghai Taipei Toronto

With offices in

Argentina Austria Brazil Chile Czech Republic France Greece
Guatemala Hungary Italy Japan Poland Portugal Singapore
South Korea Switzerland Thailand Turkey Ukraine Vietnam

Oxford is a registered trade mark of Oxford University Press in the UK and in certain other countries

Published in the United States
by Oxford University Press Inc., New York

First edition published 1999
Second edition published 2011

British Library Cataloguing in Publication Data
Data available

Library of Congress Cataloging in Publication Data
Data available

Typeset in Minion by Glyph International Bangalore, India
Printed in Great Britain
on acid-free paper by
CPI Antony Rowe Chippenham, Wiltshire

ISBN 978-0-19-959001-8

10 9 8 7 6 5 4 3 2 1

Oxford University Press makes no representation, express or implied, that the drug dosages in this book are correct. Readers must therefore always check the product information and clinical procedures with the most up-to-date published product information and data sheets provided by the manufacturers and the most recent codes of conduct and safety regulations. The authors and the publishers do not accept responsibility or legal liability for any errors in the text or for the misuse or misapplication of material in this work. Except where otherwise stated, drug dosages and recommendations are for the non-pregnant adult who is not breastfeeding.

Dedication

Recent progress in understanding the neuronal ceroid lipofuscinoses (NCLs) has relied on the contribution of many individuals and laboratories, including: clinicians who first described the disease, and refined their descriptions in the light of changing knowledge; scientists who identified the genes, studied the proteins, developed models, and work towards therapeutic options; families who agreed to donate samples, raised money to help affected families and fund research, and lobbied grant awarding bodies for more money for research. These people are numerous, and without their efforts there would be little to include in this book.

This book is dedicated to two people who represent the best of such contributors:

Pirkko Santavuori (1933–2004). Pirkko was a clinician and scientist who was recognized internationally as an expert in the NCLs as well as in her chosen discipline of child neurology. In her native country, Finland, she pioneered care and support for the whole family as well as the affected child. She also advanced the scientific understanding of the NCLs, recognizing and characterizing several different NCL types even before distinct genetic types were suspected, and contributing to the identification of three of the NCL genes. Pirkko continued to pass on her knowledge and experience all over the world, even after retirement.

J. Alfred Rider (1921–2004). Al was a clinician specializing in internal medicine and gastroenterology, and awarded many honours. He was also the father of two sons, one of whom developed Batten disease. As well as providing excellent care for his son, Al successfully lobbied Congress in the USA for more money to be dedicated to the study of NCL. He emphasized the need for an easily recognizable name for the NCLs, encouraging the use of 'Batten disease' for all NCL types. Al set up the Children's Brain Diseases Foundation in the USA in 1968 to support research into Batten disease. His surviving son, Dean, continues as President of this Foundation.

Finally, to acknowledge the families who live with Batten disease every day, we reproduce the poem, 'Once', written by **Ida Bernhardsson** (1979–2009) when she was 19 years old. Ida had CLN3 disease.

Once I was like everybody else Once I was just like them

Once I could do everything as the others and everything that I enjoyed

Once I could do all that

All that you can do when you can see

Once no longer exists Once will never return

Once will never ever return

Once is no more

The Editors

Foreword

This edition of *The Neuronal Ceroid Lipofuscinoses (Batten Disease)* is welcome. It brings to our attention progress that has been made in understanding this enigmatic group of neurodegenerative disorders that present as lysosomal storage diseases. At the same time, it reminds us that, even after many years of dedicated research, there is a long way to go before they are fully understood, and before therapy is a real option.

In retrospect, research falls into eras; first the descriptive and eponymic, which led to the renaming of the main classic disorders in 1969 as the neuronal ceroid lipofuscinoses (NCL). Reasoning led to a hard-held theory that they were associated with abnormal lipid peroxidation. This held sway for 25 years until shown to be untenable by analysis of stored material, first in the ovine model, with partial extension to other forms of the disease in human patients. The critical finding that stored material was mainly made of individual chemical species such as dolichol, neutral lipids, phospholipids, and hydrophobic proteins such as the saposins and subunit c of mitochondrial ATP synthase, was a major step forward. The arrival of molecular genetic technology again changed emphasis on direction of research.

In the last 20 years, further forms have been clinically defined and great progress made in understanding their underlying molecular genetics. We are now at *CLN10* and counting! Research has shown heterogeneity at both the genetic and molecular level with at least eight genetic loci identified and multiple mutations at most of them. This knowledge could be obtained from patients themselves without the need for animal models. Unfortunately 'reverse genetics' has not provided an understanding of the biochemical pathogenesis of these entities. The relationships between perturbed gene, its putative protein, and lysosomes are not understood for most NCL syndromes; the relationship between lysosomal storage and neuronal death is not yet understood for any one of them. As stated in the preface to the 1999 monograph 'no comprehensive or unifying molecular hypothesis exists to explain the fundamental basis of NCL'. Perhaps one does not exist outside the physical attributes of stored material. Although therapy is the immediate goal, an understanding of pathogenesis and underlying biology of each perturbed process is still important. This may not only aid development of specific and ancillary therapies, but have a wider biological importance. We should not forget this aspect as we proceed towards therapies.

Robert D. Jolly
December 2009

Preface

The concept of the neuronal ceroid lipofucinoses (NCLs) has evolved over several decades and is reviewed in Chapter 1. They are a group of inherited conditions characterized by a neurodegenerative disease course (usually with core symptoms including epilepsy, cognitive decline, and often visual failure), and the lysosomal accumulation of abnormal storage material in neurons and other cells. The storage material is autofluorescent, PAS- and Sudan black B-positive at the light microscope level, and electron dense. Recent advances in molecular genetic and cell biological research have shown that the picture is complex, with genetic and allelic heterogeneity. The NCL concept can be questioned as there are rare individuals with NCL-like symptoms but in whom no abnormal storage can be identified. It is our view, however, that the NCLs are defined by these three principal features:

1. Inherited
2. Neurodegenerative
3. Abnormal lysosomal storage of autofluorescent PAS- and Sudan black B-positive electron dense material

In this book we have aimed to update a monograph that was edited by Goebel, Mole, and Lake on behalf of the European Concerted Action Group for NCL in 1999. In the 10 years since then further NCL genes have been identified, work on cell and animal models has hugely expanded our knowledge of these conditions, the clinical syndromes have been further clarified, management approaches have changed, and therapeutic trials are in progress. We hope that this latest edition will serve as a textbook to provide a comprehensive and state-of-the-art account of the science and some of the clinical issues surrounding the NCLs today. We have designed it to be of particular use to clinicians and basic scientists as a reference work, and also to diagnostic laboratories, families, those offering professional support, and to industry. Recognized experts have jointly contributed to most of the chapters. Clearly, some readers may want to target particular sections.

Two introductory chapters (Chapters 1 and 2) present the concept of the NCLs and the evolution of the current classification system, and then a background understanding of the rules of nomenclature, gene symbols, and protein names. Three chapters will be of interest to those who diagnose or care for affected families (Chapter 3 on modern diagnostics, Chapter 4 on morphological diagnostic considerations, and Chapter 5 on clinical management). The following eight chapters are devoted to the eight identified NCL genes and their associated diseases, *CLN1–3*, *CLN5–8* and *CLN10*. *CLN4* and *CLN9* are putative genes only and are therefore not included in this section. Each of these chapters (Chapters 6–13) is subdivided into sections as follows:

- Introduction
- Molecular genetics
- Cell biology
- Clinical data
- Morphology
- Disease mechanism
- Correlations
- Diagnosis
- Clinical management
- Experimental therapy

Chapter 14 describes those clinical conditions known to be NCLs, but for which the causative genes have not yet been identified, for example, adult onset NCL ('CLN4'), some of the variant late infantile and juvenile NCLs ('CLN9'), and putative NCL genes from animal NCL models.

Chapters 15–19 describe laboratory cell and animal models of the NCLs: the genetics, proteomics, and cell biology, together with genotype–phenotype correlations.

Chapter 20 summarizes current knowledge on mutations in the NCL genes. Chapter 21 examines possible therapeutic strategies, and the concluding chapter looks forward to the developments that may be expected in the future.

Finally, two Appendices contain suggestions for further reading, useful contacts and websites, the incidence and prevalence of the NCLs by country where these are known, and a set of summary tables for easy reference. There is also a full bibliography.

Sara E. Mole,
Ruth E. Williams, and
Hans H. Goebel

Acknowledgements

We are grateful to the NCL community for their encouragement and patience in the preparation of this edition, and especially to those who made extensive and outstanding contributions, including providing figures and unpublished information, a sign of their professional interest and personal dedication to Batten disease. We thank Gisela Machado da Silva for her careful and invaluable editorial assistance. We also express our thanks for support from the Batten Disease Family Association, UK; the Batten Disease Support and Research Association, USA; and the scientific editors of a special issue on the NCLs in *Biochimica et Biophysica Acta*. The cover images have been provided by a variety of sources and were chosen to represent all facets of Batten disease: clinical, diagnostic, research, and families. We are particularly grateful to Peter Griffith of All People Photography, UK, who holds the copyright for the image of the hands of his wife and daughter who was affected with Batten disease. Finally, we acknowledge Oxford University Press for their professional support in making this second edition a reality, and for IOS Press for permitting the use of figures from the monograph *Neuronal Ceroid Lipofuscinoses (Batten Disease)*, which was essentially the first edition of this book.

The Editors

Contents

List of Abbreviations

AED	anti-epileptic drug
AAV	adeno-associated virus
AMPA	α-amino-3-hydroxy-5-methyl-4-isoxazolepropionate
ARSG	arylsulphatase G
BBB	blood brain–barrier
bp	base pair
CHO	Chinese hamster ovary
CL	curvilinear
ClC	chloride channel
CNS	central nervous system
CSF	cerebrospinal fluid
CT	computed tomography
CTG	cardiotopography
CTSD	cathepsin D
CVS	chorionic villus sampling
DBS	dried blood spots
EDTA	ethylenediaminetetraacetic acid
EEG	electroencephalography/electro-encephalogram
EP	enhancer–promoter
EPMR	progressive epilepsy with mental retardation
ER	endoplasmic reticulum
ERAD	endoplasmic reticulum-associated protein degradation
ERG	electroretinogram
EST	expressed sequence tag
FP	fingerprint
GABA	gamma-aminobutyric acid.
GFAP	glial fibrillary acidic protein
GFP	green fluorescent protein
GROD	granular osmiophilic deposit
HSC	haematopoietic stem cell
INCL	infantile NCL
JNCL	juvenile NCL
kb	kilobase
kDa	kilodalton
LGNd	dorsal lateral geniculate nucleus
LINCL	late infantile NCL
M6P	mannose 6-phosphate
M6PR	mannose 6-phosphate receptor
MBP	myelin basic protein
MEB	muscle-eye-brain
MHC	major histocompatibility complex
Mn-SOD	manganese superoxide dismutase
MPS	mucopolysaccharidosis
MRS	magnetic resonance spectroscopy
NAA	N-acetylaspartate
NCL	neuronal ceroid lipofuscinosis
NE	northern epilepsy
NMDA	N-methyl-d-aspartate
NO	nitric oxide
NPC	neuroprogenitor cell
PAF	permanganate aldehyde fuchsin
PAS	periodic acid–Schiff
PME	progressive myoclonic epilepsy
PNS	peripheral nervous system
PPT1	palmitoyl protein thioesterase 1
PTA	parallel tubular array
RL	rectilinear
RNAi	ribonucleic acid interference
RT-PCR	reverse transcriptase-polymerase chain reaction
SAP	sphingolipid activator protein
SCMAS	subunit c of mitochondrial ATPase
SCT	stem cell transplantation
SNP	single nucleotide polymorphism
SSRI	selective serotonin reuptake inhibitor
TIBDC	The International Batten Disease Consortium
TNF	tumour necrosis factor
TPP1	tripeptidyl peptidase 1
UBDRS	Unified Batten Disease Rating Scale
UK	United Kingdom
USA	United States of America
UTR	untranslated region
VEP	visual evoked potential
vLINCL	variant late infantile NCL

List of Contributors

In the individual chapters, the many contributors are usually listed in alphabetical order. Here, all contributors and editors are listed, again in alphabetical order, together with their contact details at the time of writing and currently, and the chapters or sections to which they contributed. Some originally wrote for the first edition of this book, and where this writing has been incorporated into this edition and therefore still relevant, their details remain.

Laura Åberg
Clinic for the Disabled, Rehabilitation,
Health Center, City of Helsinki,
PB 6461, 00099 Helsinki, Finland.
Email: laura.aberg@fimnet.fi
Chapter 8 CLN3 (Clinical), Chapter 9 CLN5 (Clinical; Clinical management; Diagnosis)

Chiara Aiello
Molecular Medicine & Neuroscience,
Neurogenetic Laboratory,
IRCCS Children Hospital Bambino Gesù,
Piazza S. Onofrio 4 - 00165 Rome, Italy.
Email: caiello@uniroma3.it
Chapter 12 CLN8 (Clinical; Diagnosis; Clinical management; Experimental therapy)

Joseph Alroy
Departments of Pathology Tufts University Schools of Medicine, Cummings School of Veterinary Medicine and Tufts Medical Center, Boston, Massachusetts 02111, USA.
Email: joseph.alroy@tufts.edu
Chapter 10 CLN6 (Morphology)

Glenn W. Anderson
Histopathology Department, Great Ormond Street Hospital for Children, Great Ormond Street, London WC1N 3JH, UK.
Email: anderg@gosh.nhs.uk
Chapter 4 Morphological diagnostic and pathological considerations

Taina Autti
Helsinki Medical Imaging Center,
Helsinki University Central Hospital,
BOX 340, 00029 HUS, Finaldn.
Email: taina.autti@hus.fi
Chapter 6 CLN1 (Clinical; Diagnosis; Clinical management; Experimental therapy), Chapter 8 CLN3 (Clinical), Chapter 9 CLN5 (Clinical)

Rose-Mary Boustany
Neurogenetics Program, American University of Beirut, Box: 11-0236,
Riad El Solh 11072020, Beirut, Lebanon.
Email: rb50@aub.edu.lb
Chapter 2 NCL nomenclature and classification, Chapter 3 NCL diagnosis and algorithms, Chapter 14 Genetically unassigned or unusual NCLs (CLN9)

Thomas Braulke
Department of Biochemistry, Children's Hospital, University Medical Center Hamburg-Eppendorf,
Martinistrasse 52, 20246 Hamburg, Germany.
Email: braulke@uke.uni-hamburg.de
Chapter 8 CLN3 (Cell biology); Chapter 10 CLN6 (Cell biology)

Natalia Cannelli
Institute of Medical Genetics, Catholic University School of Medicine,
Largo F. Vito 1-00168 Rome, Italy.
Email: nataliacannelli@tiscali.it
Chapter 12 CLN8 (Clinical; Diagnosis; Clinical management; Experimental therapy)

Stirling Carpenter
Institute of Molecular Pathology and Immunology of the University of Porto,
Department of Anatomic Pathology,
Hospital São João, Porto, Portugal.
Email: stirling.carpentert@gmail.com
Chapter 4 Morphological diagnostic and pathological considerations (1st edition)

Chantal Ceuterick-de Groote
Laboratory of Ultrastructural Neuropathology, Institute Born-Bunge and University of Antwerpen (Faculty of Medicine), D T 0.06, Universiteitsplein 1, B-2610 Antwerpen, Belgium.
Email: chantal.degroote@ua.ac.be
Chapter 14 Genetically unassigned or unusual NCLs (Adult onset NCL: 'CLN4')

Michael Chang
Davidson Laboratory, University of Iowa, 500 Newton Rd. 200 EMRB, Iowa City, Iowa 52242, USA.
Email: michael-chang@uiowa.edu
Chapter 7 CLN2 (Experimental therapy), Chapter 21 Therapeutic strategies

Inés Adriana Cismondi
Oral Biology Department, Faculty of Odontology. National University, Cordoba. Haya de la Torre s/n, 5000 Córdoba, Argentina.
Email: icismon@odo.unc.edu.ar
CEMECO
Center for the Study of Inborn Errors of Metabolism, Children´s Hospital, Department of Clinical Pediatrics, Neonatology and Adolescents, School of Medical Sciences, National University Cordoba. Ferroviarios 1250, 5014 Cordoba, Argentina.
Email: nclcemeco@nclcemeco.com.ar
Chapter 10 CLN6

Sandra Codlin
MRC Laboratory for Molecular Cell Biology and Department of Biology, now at Department of Genetics, Evolution and Environment, University College London, London, WC1E 6BT, UK.
Email: s.codlin@ucl.ac.uk
Chapter 15 Unicellular models

Jonathan D. Cooper
Department of Neuroscience, Centre for the Cellular Basis of Behaviour and MRC Centre for Neurodegeneration Research, The James Black Centre, King's College London, The Institute of Psychiatry, 125 Coldharbour Lane, London, SE5 9NU, UK.
Email: jon.cooper@kcl.ac.uk
Chapter 6 CLN1 (Disease mechanism), Chapter 7 CLN2 (Disease mechanism), Chapter 8 CLN3 (Disease mechanism; Experimental therapy), Chapter 9 CLN5 (Disease mechanism), Chapter 10 CLN6 (Disease mechanism), Chapter 12 CLN8 (Disease mechanism), Chapter 13 CLN10 (Disease mechanism), Chapter 17 Small animal models (Mice), Chapter 21 Therapeutic strategies

David Cregeen
Formerly North East Thames Regional Molecular Genetics Laboratory, Level 6 York House, 37 Queen Square, London WC1N 3BH, UK.
Current Email david.cregeen@gsts.com
Chapter 10 CLN6 (Diagnosis)

Beverly L. Davidson
Davidson Laboratory, University of Iowa, 500 Newton Rd. 200 EMRB, Iowa City, Iowa 52242, USA.
Email: beverly-davidson@uiowa.edu
Chapter 7 CLN2 (Experimental therapy), Chapter 21 Therapeutic strategies

Gert de Voer
Formerly at Department of Human Genetics S-4-P, Center for Human and Clinical Genetics, Leiden University Medical Center, P.O. Box 9600, 2300 Leiden, The Netherlands.
Now at Genzyme Europe B.V., Gooimeer 10, 1411 Naarden, The Netherlands,
Email: gertdevoer@yahoo.com
Chapter 16 Simple animal models (C. elegans)

Otto P. van Diggelen
Department of Clinical Genetics, Erasmus MC, Ee 2402, Dr. Molewaterplein 50, 3015 Rotterdam, The Netherlands.
Email: o.vandiggelen@erasmusmc.nl
Chapter 3 NCL diagnosis and algorithms, Chapter 6 CLN1 (Correlations), Chapter 7 CLN2 (Clinical; Diagnosis; Clinical management), Chapter 8 CLN3 (Diagnosis)

Cord Drögemüller
University of Berne, Institute of Genetics, Vetsuisse Faculty, PO-Box 8466, Berne, Switzerland.
Email: cord.droegemueller@itz.unibe.ch
Chapter 18 Large animal models (Dogs)

Milan Elleder
Institute of Inherited Metabolic Disorders, Charles University of Prague, 1st Faculty of Medicine and General University Hospital, Ke Karlovu 2, CZ-121 11 Prague 2, Czech Republic.
Email: melleder@cesnet.cz
Chapter 1 The NCLs: Evolution of the concept and classification, Chapter 2 NCL nomenclature and classification; Chapter 3 NCL diagnosis and algorithms, Chapter 4 Morphological diagnostic and pathological considerations, Chapter 7 CLN2 (Morphology), Chapter 9 CLN5 (Morphology), Chapter 10 CLN6 (Morphology), Chapter 11 CLN7 (Morphology)

Hans H. Goebel
Department of Neuropathology, Mainz University Medical Center, Langenbeckstrasse 1, D-55131 Mainz, Germany.
Email: hans-hilmar.goebel@charite.de
Editor
Acknowledgements, Dedication, Preface
Chapter 1 The NCLs: Evolution of the concept and classification, Chapter 2 NCL nomenclature and classification, Chapter 3 NCL diagnosis and algorithms, Chapter 4 Morphological diagnostic and pathological considerations, Chapter 7 CLN2 (Morphology), Chapter 8 CLN3 (Morphology), Chapter 14 Genetically unassigned or unusual NCLs (Adult onset NCL: 'CLN4'), Chapter 22 Outlook into the next decade

Adam A. Golabek
Department of Developmental Neurobiology, New York State Institute for Basic Research in Developmental Disabilities, 1050 Forest Hill Road, Staten Island, New York 10314, USA.
Email: adamgolabek@gmail.com
Chapter 7 CLN2 (Correlations)

Rebecca L. Haines
MRC Laboratory for Molecular Cell Biology and Department of Biology, University College London, WC1E 6BT, UK.
Current Email: Rebecca.Haines@imb.a-star.edu.sg
Chapter 15 Unicellular models

Matti Haltia
Department of Pathology, Haartman Institute, University of Helsinki, Haartmaninkatu 3, 00014 Helsinki, Finland.
Email: matti.j.haltia@helsinki.fi
Chapter 1 The NCLs: Evolution of the concept and classification (Main author), Chapter 4 Morphological diagnostic and pathological considerations (1st edition), Chapter 6 CLN1 (Morphology), Chapter 9 CLN5 (Morphology) Chapter 12 CLN8 (Morphology)

Riitta Herva
Department of Pathology, Oulu University Hospital, P.O. Box 22, FIN-90221 Oulu, Finland.
Email: Riitta.Herva@oulu.fi
Chapter 12 CLN8 (Morphology)

Anu Jalanko
Public Health Genomics, National Institute for Health and Welfare, Biomedicum Helsinki P.O.B 104, 00251 Helsinki (Street address: Haartmaninkatu 8, 00290 Helsinki) Finland.
Email: anu.jalanko@thl.fi
Chapter 6 CLN1 (Cell biology), Chapter 8 CLN3 (Cell biology), Chapter 9 CLN5 (Molecular genetics; Cell biology)

Gary S. Johnson
Department of Veterinary Pathobiology, College of Veterinary Medicine, 322 Connaway Hall, University of Missouri, Columbia, Missouri 65211, USA.
Email: johnsongs@missouri.edu
Chapter 18 Large animal models (Dogs)

Robert D. Jolly
Institute of Veterinary, Animal and Biomedical Sciences, Massey University, Private Bag 11222, Palmerston North 4442, New Zealand.
Email: R.D.Jolly@massey.ac.nz
Foreword

Martin L. Katz
University of Missouri School of Medicine, Mason Eye Institute, Columbia, Missouri, USA.
Email: katzm@health.missouri.edu
Chapter 18 Large animal models (Dogs)

Sarah Kenrick
SeeAbility Heather House, Tadley, UK.
Email: s.kenrick@seeability.org
Chapter 8 CLN3 (Clinical management)

Elizabeth Kida
Department of Developmental Neurobiology, New York State Institute for Basic Research in Developmental Disabilities, Staten Island, New York 10314, USA.
Email: etkida@yahoo.com
Chapter 7 CLN2 (Correlations)

Claudia Kitzmüller
MRC Laboratory for Molecular Cell Biology and Department of Biology, University College London, WC1E 6BT, UK.
Email: claudia.kitzmueller@meduniwien.ac.at
Chapter 6 CLN1 (Correlations), Chapter 8 CLN3 (Correlations), Chapter 9 CLN5 (Correlations), Chapter 10 CLN6 (Correlations; Clinical management)

Romina Kohan
CEMECO - Center for the Study of Inborn Errors of Metabolism, Children's Hospital, Department of Clinical Pediatrics, Neonatology and Adolescents, School of Medical Sciences, National University Cordoba, Ferroviarios 1250, 5014 Cordoba, Argentina.
Email: nclcemeco@nclcemeco.com.ar.
Secretary of Science and Technology, National University Cordoba.
Chapter 10 CLN6

Alfried Kohlschütter
Department of Paediatrics, University Medical Centre Hamburg-Eppendorf, Martinistr. 52, D-20246 Hamburg, Germany.
Email: kohlschuetter@uke.uni-hamburg.de
Chapter 2 NCL nomenclature and classification, Chapter 3 NCL diagnosis and algorithms, Chapter 7 CLN2 (Clinical; Diagnosis; Clinical management), Chapter 8 CLN3 (Diagnosis), Chapter 10 CLN6 (Clinical; Diagnosis)

Outi Kopra
National Institute for Health and Welfare, Folkhälsan Institute of Genetics and Neuroscience Center, P.O. Box 63, FIN-00014, University of Helsinki, Biomedicum Helsinki, Finland.
Email: outi.kopra@helsinki.fi
Chapter 6 CLN1 (Cell biology), Chapter 9 CLN5 (Cell biology)

Christopher A. Korey
Department of Biology, College of Charleston, 66 George Street, Charleston, South Carolina 29424, USA.
Email: koreyc@cofc.edu
Chapter 16 Simple animal models (Drosophila)

Maria Kousi
Folkhälsan Institute of Genetics, Department of Medical Genetics and Neuroscience Center, Biomedicum Helsinki, Haartmaninkatu 8, 00014 University of Helsinki, Finland.
Email: maria.kousi@helsinki.fi
Chapter 11 CLN7

Aija Kyttälä
Public Health Genomics, National Institute for Health and Welfare, Biomedicum Helsinki P.O.B 104, 00251 Helsinki (Street address: Haartmaninkatu 8, 00290 Helsinki) Finland.
Email: aija.kyttala@thl.fi
Chapter 8 CLN3 (Cell biology)

Brian D. Lake
Formerly at Department of Histopathology, Great Ormond Street Hospital for Children, Great Ormond Street, London WC1N 3JH, UK.
Email brianlake99r@yahoo.co.uk
Chapter 1 The NCLs: Evolution of the concept and classification, Chapter 4 Morphological diagnostic and pathological considerations (1st edition)

Ulla Lahtinen
Folkhälsan Institute of Genetics and Neuroscience Center, University of Helsinki, Haartmaninkatu 8, 00290 Helsinki, Finland.
Current address: Neuroscience Center, University of Helsinki, Viikinkaari 4, 00790 Helsinki, Finland.
Email: ulla.lahtinen@helsinki.fi
Chapter 12 CLN8 (Molecular genetics; Cell biology; Correlations)

Anna-Elina Lehesjoki
Folkhälsan Institute of Genetics and Neuroscience Center, University of Helsinki, Haartmaninkatu 8, 00290 Helsinki, Finland.
Email: anna-elina.lehesjoki@helsinki.fi
Chapter 11 CLN7, Chapter 12 CLN8 (Lead author)

Frode Lingaas
Section of Genetics, Norwegian School of Veterinary Science, P.O. Box 8146 Dep, N-0033 Oslo, Norway.
Email: frode.lingaas@veths.no; Frode.Lingaas@nvh.no
Chapter 18 Large animal models (1st edition)

Peter Lobel
Center for Advanced Biotechnology and Medicine and Department of Pharmacology, University of Medicine and Dentistry of New Jersey-Robert Wood Johnson Medical School, 679 Hoes Lane, Piscataway, New Jersey 08854, USA.
Email: lobel@cabm.rutgers.edu
Chapter 7 CLN2 (Molecular genetics)

Tuula Lönnqvist
Division of Child Neurology, Helsinki University Central Hospital, PO BOX 280, 00029 HUCH, Helsinki, Finland.
Email:tuula.lonnqvist@hus.fi
Chapter 6 CLN1 (Clinical; Diagnosis; Clinical management; Experimental therapy)

Annina Lyly
Public Health Genomics, National Institute for Health and Welfare, Biomedicum Helsinki P.O.B 104, 00251 Helsinki (Street address: Haartmaninkatu 8, 00290 Helsinki) Finland.
Email: Annina.Lyly@helsinki.fi
Chapter 6 CLN1 (Cell biology)

Gisela Machado da Silva
MRC Laboratory for Molecular Cell Biology, University College London, Gower Street, London WC1E 6BT, UK.
Email: gisela.msilva@gmail.com
General editing of all chapters

Jean-Jacques Martin
Institute Born-Bunge, D T 5, Universiteitsplein 1, B-2610 Antwerpen, Belgium.
Email: jean-jacques.martin@ua.ac.be
Chapter 14 Genetically unassigned or unusual NCLs

Jonathan W. Mink
Departments of Neurology, Neurobiology & Anatomy, Brain & Cognitive Sciences, and Pediatrics; University of Rochester Medical Center, 601 Elmwood Ave., Box 631, Rochester, New York 14642, USA.
Email: Jonathan_Mink@urmc.rochester.edu
Chapter 2 NCL nomenclature and classification, Chapter 3 NCL diagnosis and algorithms

Hannah M. Mitchison
Molecular Medicine Unit, University College London (UCL) Institute of Child Health, 30 Guilford Street, London WC1N 1EH, UK.
Email: h.mitchison@ich.ucl.ac.uk
Chapter 8 CLN3 (Molecular genetics; Disease mechanism; Correlations)

Sara E. Mole
MRC Laboratory for Molecular Cell Biology; Molecular Medicines Unit, UCL Institute of Child Health; and Department of Genetics, Evolution and Environment, University College London, Gower Street, London WC1E 6BT, UK.
Email: s.mole@ucl.ac.uk
Senior editor
Acknowledgements, Dedication, Preface, Contributors, Chapter 1 The NCLs: Evolution of the concept and classification, Chapter 2 NCL nomenclature and classification, Chapter 3 NCL diagnosis and algorithms, Chapter 6 CLN1 (Molecular genetics), Chapter 7 CLN2 (Correlations), Chapter 8 CLN3 (Morphology; Correlations; Experimental therapy), Chapter 9 CLN5 (Correlations), Chapter 10 CLN6 (Molecular genetics; Correlations), Chapter 11 CLN7 (Morphology; Correlations), Chapter 12 CLN8 (Correlations), Chapter 14 Genetically unassigned or unusual NCLs (Adult onset NCL: 'CLN4'; Other NCL variants), Chapter 17 Small animal models (Mice), Chapter 20 Mutations in NCL genes, Chapter 21 Therapeutic strategies, Chapter 22 Outlook into the next decade, Chapter 24 Appendix 2: Useful information

Liisa Myllykangas
Folkhälsan Institute of Genetics and Department of Pathology, University of Helsinki, Helsinki, Finland.
Email: liisa.myllykangas@helsinki.fi
Chapter 16 Simple animal models (Drosophila)

Riet Niezen-de Boer
Bartiméus, Oude Arnhemsebovenweg 3, 3941 Doorn, The Netherlands.
Email: rniezen@bartimeus.nl
Chapter 2 NCL nomenclature and classification, Chapter 3 NCL diagnosis and algorithms, Chapter 8 CLN3 (Clinical management)

Ines Noher de Halac
CEMECO - Center for the Study of Inborn Errors of Metabolism, Children's Hospital, Department of Clinical Pediatrics, Neonatology and Adolescents, School of Medical Sciences, National University Cordoba, Ferroviarios 1250, 5014 Cordoba, Argentina.
Email: nclcemeco@nclcemeco.com.ar
CONICET-RA- National Research Council.
Chapter 10 CLN6

Auli Nuutila
Department of Paediatrics; Central Hospital of Seinäjoki; Seinäjoki, Finland.
Chapter 9 CLN5 (Clinical; Clinical management)

David N. Palmer
Faculty of Agriculture and Life Sciences, PO Box 84, Lincoln University, Lincoln 7647, New Zealand.
Email: David.Palmer@lincoln.ac.nz
Chapter 18 Large animal models (Sheep, Cows, Others)

Sanna Partanen
Formerly at Institute of Biomedicine/ Biochemistry, University of Helsinki, Finland, Folkhälsan Institute of Genetics, Department of Medical Genetics and Neuroscience Center, University of Helsinki, Finland.
Email: sanna.partanen@thermofisher.com
Chapter 13 CLN10 (Cell biology; Correlations)

Leena Peltonen (deceased)
National Institute for Health and Welfare, Biomedicum Helsinki P.O.B 104, 00251 Helsinki
Chapter 9 CLN5 (Molecular genetics)

Rolf Pfannl
Department of Pathology, Tufts Medical Center, Tufts University School of Medicine, 800 Washington St, Boston, Massachusetts 02111, USA.
Email: RPfannl@tuftsmedicalcenter.org
Chapter 10 CLN6 (Morphology)

Maria-Liisa Punkari
NCL Consultant, Finnish Federation of the Visually Impaired, P.O. Box 41, FI 00030, Finland.
Email: ml.punkari@nkl.fi
Chapter 8 CLN3 (Clinical management), Chapter 9 CLN5 (Clinical; Clinical management)

Arne Quitsch
Dept. of Biochemistry, Children's Hospital, University Medical Center Hamburg-Eppendorf, Martinistrasse 52, 20246 Hamburg, Germany.
Email: Quitsch@uke.uni-hamburg.de
Chapter 10 CLN6 (Cell biology)

Juhani Rapola
Department of Pathology, Haartman Institute, University of Helsinki and Helsinki University Central Hospital, Haartmaninkatu 3, FIN-00014 Helsinki, Finland.
Chapter 4 Morphological diagnostic and pathological considerations (1st edition), Chapter 6 CLN1 (Morphology), Chapter 9 CLN5 (Morphology)

Maria Gil Ribeiro
Faculty of Health Sciences, University Fernando Pessoa, Porto, Portugal.
Email: gribeiro@ufp.edu.pt
Chapter 3 NCL diagnosis and algorithms

Claire Russell
Department of Veterinary Basic Sciences, Royal Veterinary College, Royal College Street, London NW1 0TU, UK.
Email: crussell@rvc.ac.uk
Chapter 17 Small animal models (Fish)

Filippo M. Santorelli
Molecular Medicine & Neuroscience, Neurogenetic Laboratory, IRCCS Children Hospital Bambino Gesù, Piazza S.Onofrio 4-00165 Rome, Italy.
Email: filippo3364@gmail.com
Chapter 12 CLN8 (Clinical; Diagnosis; Clinical management; Experimental therapy)

Angela Schulz
Children's Hospital, University Medical Center Hamburg-Eppendorf, Martinistrasse 52, D-20246 Hamburg, Germany.
Email: anschulz@uke.uni-hamburg.de
Chapter 7 CLN2 (Clinical; Diagnosis; Clinical management), Chapter 8 CLN3 (Diagnosis), Chapter 10 CLN6 (Clinical; Diagnosis; Clinical management), Chapter 14 Genetically unassigned or unusual NCLs (CLN9)

Eija Siintola
Folkhälsan Institute of Genetics and Neuroscience Center, University of Helsinki, Biomedicum Helsinki, P.O. Box 63 (Haartmaninkatu 8), FIN-00014 University of Helsinki, Finland.
Email: eija.siintola@hotmail.com.
Chapter 11 CLN7, Chapter 12 CLN8 (Molecular genetics; Cell biology; Correlations), Chapter 13 CLN10 (Molecular genetics; Cell biology; Correlations)

Alessandro Simonati
University of Verona Medical School, Department of Neurological and Visual Sciences-Neurology, Child Neurology and Psychiatry Unit. Policlinico GB Rossi, P.le LA Scuro 10, 37134 Verona.
Email: alessandro.simonati@univr.it
Chapter 2 NCL nomenclature and classification, Chapter 3 NCL diagnosis and algorithms, Chapter 12 CLN8 (Clinical; Diagnosis; Clinical management; Experimental therapy)

David E. Sleat
Center for Advanced Biotechnology and Medicine and Department of Pharmacology, University of Medicine and Dentistry of New Jersey-Robert Wood Johnson Medical School, 679 Hoes Lane, Piscataway, New Jersey 08854, USA.
Email: sleat@cabm.rutgers.edu
Chapter 7 CLN2 (Molecular genetics)

Robert Steinfeld
Department of Pediatrics and Pediatric Neurology, University of Göttingen, Robert-Koch-Str. 40, 37075 Göttingen, Germany.
Email: rsteinfeld@med.uni-goettingen.de or r.steinfeld@med.uni-goettingen.de
Chapter 13 CLN10 (Diagnosis; Clinical management)

Petter Strömme
Department of Pediatrics, Oslo University Hospital and Faculty of Medicine, University of Oslo, Oslo, Norway.
Email: petter.stromme@medisin.uio.no
Chapter 13 CLN10 (Diagnosis; Clinical management)

Maria L. Talling
Department of Child Neurology and Department of Radiology.
Helsinki University Central Hospital, Finland.
Email: miatalling@gmail.com
Chapter 8 CLN3 (Clinical)

Imke Tammen
ReproGen, Faculty of Veterinary Science, University of Sydney, 425 Werombi Road, Camden NSW 2570, Australia.
Email: imke.tammen@sydney.edu.au
Chapter 18 Large animal models (Sheep, Cows, Others)

Peter E.M. Taschner
Department of Human Genetics S-4-P, Center for Human and Clinical Genetics, Leiden University Medical Center, P.O. Box 9600, 2300 Leiden, The Netherlands.
Email: P.Taschner@lumc.nl
Chapter 16 Simple animal models (C. elegans), Chapter 19 Evolutionary conservation of NCL proteins

Meral Topçu
Hacettepe Medical Faculty, İhsan Dogramacı Children's Hospital, Department of Pediatrics, Section of Child Neurology, 06100 Ankara, Turkey.
Email: mtopcu@hacettepe.edu.tr
Chapter 11 CLN7

Richard Tuxworth
MRC Centre for Developmental Neurobiology, New Hunt's House, Guy's Hospital Campus, King's College London, London, SE1 1UL, UK.
Email: richard.tuxworth@kcl.ac.uk
Chapter 16 Simple animal models (Drosophila)

Jaana Tyynelä
Institute of Biomedicine, University of Helsinki, Biomedicum Helsinki,
P.O. Box 63 (Haartmaninkatu 8),
FIN-00014 University of Helsinki, Finland.
Email: jaana.tyynela@helsinki.fi
Chapter 9 CLN5 (Diagnosis, morphological, histochemical and biochemical analyses), Chapter 13 CLN10 (lead author), Chapter 17 Small animal models (Fish)

Sanna-Leena Vanhanen
Hyvinkää Hospital, Sairaalankatu 1.
FIN-05850, Hyvinkää, Finland.
Email: sanna-leena.vanhanen@hus.fi
Chapter 6 CLN1 (Clinical; Diagnosis; Clinical management; Experimental therapy)

Michael J. Warburton
Section of Cellular Pathology,
Department of Cellular and Molecular Medicine, St George's University of London,
Cranmer Terrace, London SW17 0RE, UK.
Email: michaelwarburton@ymail.com
Chapter 7 CLN2 (Cell biology)

Ruth E. Williams
Department of Paediatric Neurology,
SKY, Evelina Childrens Hospital, Guy's and St Thomas' NHS Foundation Trust,
Westminster Bridge Road,
London SE1 7EH, UK.
Email: ruth.williams@gstt.nhs.uk
Editor, Acknowledgements, Dedication, Preface, Chapter 2 NCL nomenclature and classification (Senior author), Chapter 3 NCL diagnosis and algorithms (Senior author) Chapter 5 General principles of medical management, Chapter 8 CLN3 (Clinical management), Chapter 22 Outlook into the next decade, Chapter 23 Appendix 1: NCL incidence and prevalence data, Chapter 24 Appendix 2: Useful information

Krystyna E. Wisniewski (deceased)
Department of Developmental Neurobiology,
New York State Institute for Basic Research in Developmental Disabilities,
Staten Island, New York 10314, USA.
Chapter 7 CLN2 (Correlations)

Chapter 1

The NCLs: Evolution of the Concept and Classification

M. Haltia with M. Elleder, H. H. Goebel, B. D. Lake, and S. E. Mole

INTRODUCTION

The term neuronal ceroid lipofuscinoses (NCLs) was coined by Zeman and Dyken in 1969 to designate a group of inherited storage disorders, clinically characterized by progressive decline of mental, motor, and visual functions (Zeman and Dyken, 1969). For many decades, the NCLs had been classified among the so-called 'amaurotic family idiocies' owing to their superficial clinical resemblance to Tay–Sachs disease, the prototype of this group. Zeman and Dyken clearly separated the NCLs from Tay–Sachs disease and related conditions, essentially on the basis of neuropathological criteria. Their novel concept literally destroyed the category of the 'amaurotic family idiocies' and largely cleared the confusion that had prevailed concerning this group for over half a century. Zeman and Dyken thus paved the way for a new and fruitful wave of research into the aetiopathogenesis of these devastating brain diseases.

This chapter outlines nearly 200 years of NCL research, with a short initial comment on lipofuscin and ceroid. The early clinical, neuropathological, and biochemical studies that gradually led to the formulation of the NCL concept are described. An account is also given of the further development of this concept with emphasis on the extremely fruitful molecular genetic studies of the last decade, resulting in the cloning of eight different NCL genes with over 260 mutations identified, and leading to the present classification of more than ten genetically distinct forms of NCL in man and further forms in animals. Finally, the evolution of ideas on the pathogenesis of NCL and international collaboration in NCL research are briefly discussed.

LIPOFUSCIN AND CEROID

Postmitotic cells, such as neurons, cells of the retinal pigment epithelium, as well as heart and skeletal muscle cells, progressively accumulate granules of yellowish brown, autofluorescent, electron-dense material called lipofuscin (Brunk and Terman, 2002, Porta, 2002). The young Danish histologist Adolph Hannover first described such granules in the cytoplasm of nerve cells in 1843 (Hannover, 1843) (Figure 1.1), and in 1886 Helene Koneff, a Russian veterinary doctor, observed their relationship to ageing (Koneff, 1886). The term lipofuscin, derived from Greek *lipo* (for fat) and latin *fuscus* (for dark), was proposed by Borst and used by Hueck for *'das fetthaltige Abnutzungspigment'* in his thorough analysis of bodily pigments in 1912 (Hueck, 1912). Hueck concluded that lipofuscin might form by oxidation of fatty acids. The time-dependent accumulation of lipofuscin in lysosomes of postmitotic cells and some stable cells is today considered the most consistent and phylogenetically constant morphological change of ageing (Porta, 2002). Material with properties similar to those typical of lipofuscin may accumulate in a number of pathological conditions, such as lysosomal storage diseases, malnutrition, tumours, and radiation-induced tissue injury. Such pathological material is occasionally called ceroid or ceroid-type lipofuscin. According to some authors, the distinction between ceroid and lipofuscin may be valid in terms of aetiology but not in terms of properties and basic mechanisms of formation (Brunk and Terman, 2002).

THE FIRST CLINICAL DESCRIPTION OF NCL

Patients with probable NCL were first reported in 1826, by Dr. Otto Christian Stengel, physician

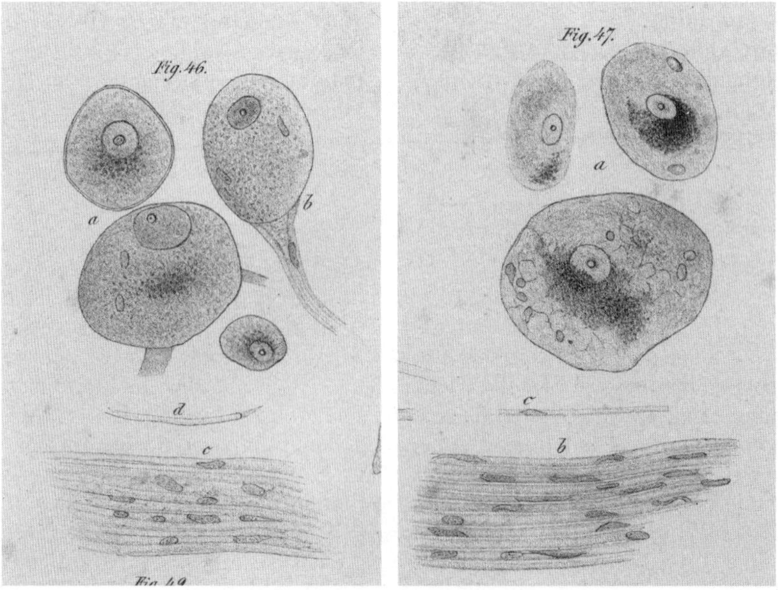

Figure 1.1 Illustration from the first description of lipofuscin granules in nerve cells, by Adolph Hannover (Hannover, 1843).

Beretning om et mærkeligt Sygdomstilfælde hos fire Sødskende i Nærheden af Røraas.

(Af C. Stengel, Læge ved Røraas Kobberverk).

Disse høist mærkværdige Sygdomstilfælde, der have viist sig her i Egnen, har jeg for en Deel været Øievidne til, og, da de vist nok baade i physiologisk og pathologisk Henseende kunde have megen Interesse, har jeg, saavidt Omstændighederne tillode det, efter Evne søgt at fremstille de Phænomener, der yttrede sig, i den Orden, de fulgte.

Figure 1.2 The title page of the first clinical description of what is now termed juvenile CLN3 disease, by Christian Stengel (Stengel, 1826a).

at the Copper Mining Company of Røraas, a small community in South-Eastern Norway (Stengel, 1826a). His report was based on four consecutive children of apparently healthy parents, two boys and two girls, whose initial development had been unremarkable. By the age of 6 years their sight began to deteriorate and, within years, the disease led to blindness, progressive mental decline, loss of speech, epileptic fits, and premature death. The clinical features are compatible with CLN3 disease, classic juvenile, although no autopsies were performed. Stengel's 'Account of a singular illness among four siblings in the vicinity of Røraas' was written in Norwegian and published in the first volume of the first Norwegian medical journal (Figure 1.2). The paper remained unnoticed until attention was focused on its historical significance by his countrymen more than a century later (Stengel, 1826b/1982).

THE NCLS AS 'AMAUROTIC FAMILY IDIOCIES'

The American neurologist Sachs presented the concept of 'amaurotic family idiocy' as part of a presidential address delivered before the New York Neurological Society in 1896. He had in 1887 reported the case of an infant with a fatal form of idiocy associated with progressive loss of vision or amaurosis. The familial character of the disease dawned on him 4 years later when a sibling of the original patient became affected with identical clinical and neuropathological changes, and he observed similarly affected siblings in two further families. Sachs considered that the ocular manifestations originally described by the British ophthalmologist Waren Tay in 1881 in the region of the yellow spot, characterized by a central brownish-red spot surrounded by a white patch, constituted an integral symptom of the new disease for which he proposed the name of 'amaurotic family idiocy' (Sachs, 1896). This disease of infantile onset subsequently became known as Tay–Sachs disease, and was later identified as GM2-gangliosidosis type A, a prototype lysosomal storage disorder.

During the first years of the 20th century a number of further familial cases of progressive loss of vision and psychomotor retardation were described, but many such cases reported by British, German, and Czech authors had a later onset. Batten (Batten, 1903, Batten, 1914, Batten and Mayou, 1915) and Vogt (Vogt, 1905, Vogt, 1909) described patients with both a late infantile and juvenile onset, Spielmeyer (Spielmeyer, 1905a, Spielmeyer, 1905b, Spielmeyer, 1908) described patients with juvenile onset, and Janský (Janský, 1908) and Bielschowsky (Bielschowsky, 1913) described patients with late infantile onset. At neuropathological autopsy, all these patients with late infantile or juvenile onset showed accumulation, within nerve cells, of granular material with lipid-like staining qualities. In their early papers both Batten and Spielmeyer had insisted that the conditions described by them were distinctly different from Tay–Sachs disease. However, inspired by the superficial clinical similarities (familial occurrence, progressive loss of vision, and psychomotor retardation) and the unifying pathological concept of intraneuronal 'thesaurismosis'(Schaffer, 1906, Schaffer, 1910) or 'storage', all these cases were gradually grouped together and considered to represent variants of 'amaurotic family idiocy' of either infantile (Tay–Sachs), late infantile (Janský–Bielschowsky), or juvenile (Spielmeyer–Sjögren) onset. In 1925 Kufs published his first report on familial adult onset intellectual deterioration with similar neuropathological features but without loss of vision (Kufs, 1925).

However, based on extensive clinical and genealogical studies, Sjögren concluded in 1931 that the juvenile type (Spielmeyer–Sjögren) is genetically separate from the infantile (Tay–Sachs) form (Sjögren, 1931). Further arguments against the unitarian view of 'amaurotic family idiocy' were provided in 1939 by the biochemical analyses of Klenk who showed an increased cerebral ganglioside concentration in the infantile form (Tay–Sachs) but not in the juvenile type (Spielmeyer–Sjögren) (Klenk, 1939). In 1962 Svennerholm confirmed Klenk's observations and identified the major storage material in the infantile form (Tay–Sachs) as GM2-ganglioside (Svennerholm, 1962).

THE CONCEPT OF THE NCLS EMERGES

Sjögren's, Klenk's, and Svennerholm's studies had already indicated that 'amaurotic family idiocy' was both genetically and biochemically heterogeneous. In the early 1960s, histochemical and electron microscopic studies showed that the intraneuronal storage cytosomes in the juvenile (Spielmeyer–Sjögren) form of 'amaurotic family idiocy' (Zeman and Donahue, 1963) radically differed from the membranous cytoplasmic bodies found in the infantile (Tay–Sachs) form (Terry and Korey, 1960). In sharp contrast to the easily extractable storage material of the infantile Tay–Sachs form, the electron-dense storage cytosomes in the late infantile (Janský–Bielschowsky) and juvenile (Spielmeyer–Sjögren) cases were largely resistant to lipid solvents and showed characteristic curvilinear (late infantile form) or predominantly fingerprint (juvenile form) patterns (Zeman and Donahue, 1963, Zeman et al., 1970). In fact, both their histochemical and ultrastructural characteristics were close to those of the autofluorescent 'lipopigments' ceroid or lipofuscin. Based on these histochemical and ultrastructural similarities, in 1969 Zeman and Dyken proposed the new term neuronal ceroid lipofuscinosis (NCL) in order to clearly distinguish the late infantile and juvenile forms of 'amaurotic family idiocy' and the histochemically similar Kufs adult onset disease from Tay–Sachs disease and other gangliosidoses (Zeman and Dyken, 1969). Somewhat later, a new infantile type of NCL was described by Haltia (Haltia et al., 1973a, Haltia et al., 1973b) and Santavuori (Santavuori et al., 1973), characterized by autofluorescent electron-dense storage cytosomes with a finely granular ultrastructure (granular osmiophilic deposits or GRODs). Furthermore, the first animal form of NCL was reported in English setter dogs by Koppang (Koppang, 1970). Subsequently, Zeman (Figure 1.3) proposed a revised classification of the NCLs, essentially based on the age of clinical onset and the ultrastructure of the storage cytosomes (Zeman, 1976). Four different types of human NCL and a canine form were distinguished. The human types included the infantile (Haltia–Santavuori), late infantile (Janský–Bielschowsky), juvenile (Spielmeyer–Sjögren), and adult (Kufs) types (Zeman, 1976). Occasional congenital cases of 'amaurotic family idiocy' had been reported since 1941 (Norman and Wood, 1941, Brown et al., 1954, Sandbank, 1968), but these were not considered in Zeman´s classification. During the subsequent decades, a number of 'atypical' or 'variant' cases were reported, mostly with a late infantile or early juvenile onset, further expanding the spectrum of human NCL. These included the 'early juvenile' or 'Indian' (Lake and Cavanagh, 1978, Elleder et al., 1997), 'Finnish' (Santavuori, 1982, Santavuori et al., 1991, Tyynelä et al., 1997), and 'Turkish' (Williams et al., 1999)

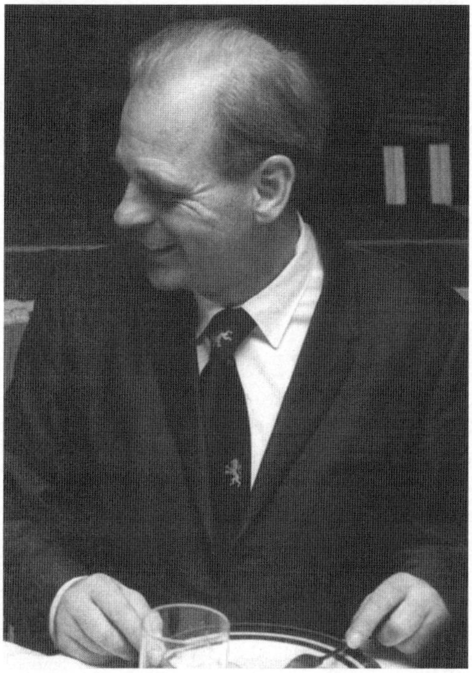

Figure 1.3 Wolfgang Zeman at the Scandinavian Neuropathological Society's 10th Anniversary Meeting, Helsinki 1975.

variant late infantile forms of NCL. Surprisingly, even 'Northern epilepsy', also known as progressive epilepsy with mental retardation (EPMR), an inherited childhood epilepsy syndrome with relatively mild mental retardation (Hirvasniemi et al., 1994), turned out to be a form of NCL on neuropathological analysis (Haltia et al., 1999, Herva et al., 2000).

While autosomal recessive inheritance is usual for the NCLs, there have been a limited number of reports of autosomal dominant adult onset NCL (Boehme et al., 1971, Nijssen et al., 2002). An increasing number of spontaneous forms of NCL have also been discovered in animals, including many breeds of dogs (Jolly et al., 1994), as well as cats (Green and Little, 1974, Nakayama et al., 1993, Bildfell et al., 1995, Weissenbock and Rossel, 1997), sheep (Jolly et al., 1980, Järplid and Haltia, 1993, Cook et al., 2002), goats (Fiske and Storts, 1988), cattle (Read and Bridges, 1969, Harper et al., 1988), horses (Url et al., 2001), and mice (Bronson et al., 1993, Bronson et al., 1998). NCL in animals is discussed in detail in Chapters 17 and 18.

BIOCHEMICAL ANALYSES OF THE STORAGE MATERIALS

For a long time, efforts at biochemical characterization of the storage materials in the NCLs were few, focused on lipids, and essentially non-contributory. However, by the end of the 1980s, analyses of the South Hampshire sheep model of NCL showed that the major component of isolated storage cytosomes was, in fact, low-molecular-weight protein rather than lipid (Palmer et al., 1986). The major 'lipopigment' protein was soon identified as subunit c of mitochondrial ATPase (Palmer et al., 1989, Fearnley et al., 1990) and this mitochondrial protein was also found as the predominant constituent of the storage bodies in most other human and animal forms of NCL, in addition to the South Hampshire ovine model (Palmer et al., 1992). In contrast, corresponding protein chemical studies of the material accumulating in the human infantile NCL established sphingolipid activator proteins (saposins) A and D as its main components (Tyynelä et al., 1993). Sphingolipid activator proteins have also been shown to accumulate in the miniature Schnauzer dog model (Palmer et al., 1997), congenital ovine NCL (Tyynelä et al., 2000), congenital human NCL (Siintola et al., 2006), and the autosomal dominant form of adult human NCL (Parry disease) (Nijssen et al., 2002). Protein chemical analyses of the principal storage material thus allow the subdivision of the various human and animal forms of NCL into two main categories: those storing subunit c of the mitochondrial ATP synthase, and those accumulating sphingolipid activator proteins A and D (see Table 1.1). The ultrastructure of the storage cytosomes seems to depend on the identity of their principal protein component. So far, storage of sphingolipid activator proteins has been invariably associated with GRODs, while accumulation of subunit c has been seen in the context of more variable ultrastructural appearances (curvilinear, rectilinear or fingerprint patterns).

THE PRIMARY GENETIC DEFECTS OF THE NCLS ARE IDENTIFIED

The modern era of NCL genetics started with studies that linked the juvenile

Spielmeyer–Sjögren type of NCL to the haptoglobin locus on the long arm of chromosome 16 (Eiberg et al., 1989). The first NCL gene, responsible for the infantile Haltia–Santavuori form of NCL, was identified by a positional candidate gene approach in 1995 in Leena Peltonen's laboratory (Vesa et al., 1995). The gene encodes palmitoyl protein thioesterase 1, a soluble lysosomal enzyme. In the very same year, the combined effort of an international consortium of five research groups led to the isolation, by positional cloning, of the gene underlying the juvenile Spielmeyer–Sjögren type (The International Batten Disease Consortium, 1995). This novel gene encodes a membrane protein (Kyttälä et al., 2006). In contrast to these first two NCL genes, the gene for the classic late infantile Janský–Bielschowsky type of NCL was identified by a biochemical approach, based on two-dimensional electrophoresis of proteins (Sleat et al., 1997). The gene product is tripeptidyl peptidase 1, another soluble lysosomal hydrolase. During the subsequent 5 years the genes underlying the 'Finnish' (Savukoski et al., 1998) and 'Indian' (Gao et al., 2002, Wheeler et al., 2002) variant late infantile forms of NCL and Northern epilepsy/EPMR (Ranta et al., 1999) were cloned. The products of all these novel genes are putative transmembrane proteins, with the exception of the CLN5 protein. While the disease of some of the patients with the 'Turkish' variant late infantile NCL was shown to be allelic to Northern epilepsy, other patients clearly had mutations in novel gene(s).

By the turn of the millennium, progress was also made concerning the primary molecular defects in the various spontaneous animal forms of NCL. The South Hampshire NCL sheep (Broom et al., 1998) and the *nclf* mice (Gao et al., 2002, Wheeler et al., 2002) turned out to be models for the 'Indian' variant late infantile NCL, and the so-called motor neuron degeneration (*mnd*) mouse (Ranta et al., 1999) and the English setter dog (Katz et al., 2005) models for disease caused by defects in the gene mutated in Northern epilepsy/EPMR. While these animal forms of NCL thus corresponded, at the molecular level, to previously established varieties of human NCL, a new NCL gene was discovered in congenital ovine NCL by a protein chemical approach (Tyynelä et al., 2000). The affected lambs had drastically reduced activity of the soluble lysosomal hydrolase cathepsin D, caused by a mutation of the *CTSD* gene. Subsequently, a cathepsin D-deficient *Drosophila* model was developed, recapitulating the key features of NCL (Myllykangas et al., 2005). Based on these observations in lambs and flies, cathepsin D deficiency was finally shown to underlie congenital human NCL (Siintola et al., 2006).

A NEW GENETIC CLASSIFICATION OF THE NCLS EVOLVES

Based on the hitherto predicted or verified gene loci, a new genetic classification of the NCLs evolved (Goebel et al., 1999, Hofmann and Peltonen, 2001, Wisniewski and Zhong, 2001, Haltia, 2003, Mole, 2004). At the moment, human NCLs are classified into ten genetic forms from *CLN1* to *CLN10* (Table 1.1), although not all these genes have been identified. The list also includes the autosomal dominant form of adult onset NCL or Parry disease. Furthermore, there are still a number of reports on atypical cases without proper genetic assignment (see Chapter 14).

A genetic classification is not always compatible with the old system, which was based on clinical and morphological phenotypes. It is important to realize that different mutations in a given gene may give rise to varying phenotypes, including different ages of onset. For example, mutations of the *CLN1* gene may result in disease with an infantile, late infantile, juvenile, or even adult onset, depending on the exact type and location of the mutation in relation to the active site of the gene product. The *CLN8* gene provides another example, one particular mutation giving rise to EPMR/Northern epilepsy and others to variant late infantile NCL. Common mutations that predominate in a given form of NCL are usually associated with the 'classic' phenotype, while rare 'private' mutations may result in a deviant or atypical clinical picture.

A NEW CLINICAL NOMENCLATURE FOR THE NCLS

Most recently, an international group of physicians and scientists with a special interest in the

Table 1.1 **Classification of human neuronal ceroid lipofuscinoses**

Disease	Eponym	OMIM number	Clinical phenotype	Former abbreviated name	Ultrastruct. phenotype	Chromosome	Gene	Gene product	Stored protein
CLN1	Haltia–Santavuori	256730	Infantile classic, late infantile, juvenile, adult	INCL	GROD	1p32	*PPT1/CLN1*	PPT1	SAPs
CLN2	Janský–Bielschowsky	204500	Late infantile classic, juvenile	LINCL	CL	11p15	*TPP1/CLN2*	TPP1	SCMAS
CLN3	Spielmeyer–Sjögren	204200	Juvenile, classic	JNCL	FP (CL, RL)	16p12	*CLN3*	CLN3	SCMAS
Kufs disease	Kufs	204300	Adult 'CLN4'	ANCL	FP, granular	?	?	?	SCMAS
CLN5	Finnish variant late infantile	256731	Late infantile variant, juvenile, adult	vLINCL	RL, CL, FP	13q22	*CLN5*	CLN5	SCMAS
CLN6	Lake–Cavanagh early juvenile variant or Indian variant late infantile	601780	Late infantile variant	vLINCL	RL, CL, FP	15q21–23	*CLN6*	CLN6	SCMAS
CLN7	Turkish variant late infantile	610951	Late infantile variant, juvenile-adult	vLINCL	RL, FP	4q28.1–28.2	*MFSD8/CLN7*	MFSD8	SCMAS
CLN8	Northern epilepsy/ EPMR	610003	EPMR, late infantile variant	vLINCL	CL-like, FP, granular	8p23	*CLN8*	CLN8	SCMAS
Juvenile variant	Juvenile variant	609055	Juvenile variant 'CLN9'	vJNCL	GROD, CL, FP	?	?	?	SCMAS
CLN10	Congenital	610127	Congenital classic, late infantile, adult	CNCL	GROD	11p15.5	*CTSD/CLN10*	Cathepsin D	SAPs
Parry	Parry	162350	Adult autosomal dominant	ANCL	GROD	?	?	?	SAPs

CNCL, INCL, LINCL, vLINCL, JNCL, vJNCL and ANCL, congenital, infantile, late infantile, variant late infantile, juvenile, variant juvenile and adult onset neuronal ceroid lipofuscinosis; EPMR, progressive epilepsy with mental retardation; GROD, granular osmiophilic deposits; CL, curvilinear profiles; FP, fingerprint bodies; RL, rectilinear profiles; SCMAS, subunit c of mitochondrial ATP synthase; SAPs, sphingolipid activator proteins.

NCLs have proposed a new nomenclature or diagnostic classification system to provide a definition for NCL subtypes that is universally understood and of value for clinicians responsible for diagnosis and treatment, diagnostic laboratories, research scientists, patients and families, and supporting health and education professionals. This is described in detail in Chapters 2 and 3, and is an axial system that derives from the genetic defect and takes into account varying phenotype, e.g. CLN1 disease, infantile or CLN1 disease, adult.

EVOLUTION OF IDEAS ON THE PATHOGENESIS OF THE NCLS

As previously mentioned, the NCLs were long conceived as 'amaurotic family idiocies' and lipidoses, along with Tay–Sachs disease. After their separation from Tay–Sachs disease and other gangliosidoses, the first aetiopathogenetic ideas were inspired by the histochemical resemblance of the storage material to the 'wear and tear lipopigments' ceroid and lipofuscin, traditionally thought to form by oxidation of fatty acids (Hueck, 1912). It was proposed, in analogy, that the basic defect in the NCLs was formation of pathological 'lipopigments', possibly due to an increased rate of peroxidation of polyunsaturated fatty acids (Zeman and Rider, 1975). However, no conclusive evidence could be presented in favour of these hypotheses, despite numerous experimental and clinical studies, including treatment of patients with various antioxidants. The final blow to the lipidosis concept came by the end of the 1980s by the demonstration of proteins, either subunit c of the mitochondrial ATP synthase (Palmer et al., 1989, Fearnley et al., 1990) or sphingolipid activator proteins (Tyynelä et al., 1993), as major components of the purified NCL storage cytosomes.

Since the discovery of the first genes causing NCL, molecular genetic and biochemical studies have led to the identification of more than 260 causative mutations in at least eight different genes underlying the various human and animal forms of NCL. Four of these genes code for soluble lysosomal proteins, whereas the products of the remaining genes are putative transmembrane proteins with still largely unknown functions (see Table 1.1). This newly discovered molecular genetic heterogeneity of the NCLs is in interesting contrast to their remarkably uniform morphological phenotype, the very basis of the whole NCL concept. All genetically separate types of NCLs share at least two of the quintessential features of NCL: 1) accumulation in the lysosomes of nerve cells and, to a lesser extent, of many other cell types, of autofluorescent, electron-dense, PAS- and Sudan black B-positive material containing subunit c of mitochondrial ATPase and/or sphingolipid activator proteins A and D, and 2) progressive and selective loss of neurons, particularly in the cerebral and cerebellar cortex and, less constantly, in the retina, leading to mental, motor, and visual problems. Any valid theory on the pathogenesis of the NCLs must account for these two phenomena and explain them at the molecular level.

The impressive set of recent molecular data now available provides a solid foundation, and the transgenic models based on them efficient tools, for studies aiming at filling the gap between the primary genetic defects and the final pathological manifestations of the NCLs. The most burning open questions include the following: 1) elucidation of the exact functions of the known NCL genes (and of novel genes yet to be identified) and the substrates and interacting partners of their products; 2) the proximate causes and mechanisms of the selective neuronal death; 3) the mechanisms of the lysosomal accumulation of subunit c of the mitochondrial ATPase and sphingolipid activator proteins and their role, if any, in the loss of neurons; 4) the links between and interactions of the various NCL gene products and the possibility of a final common pathway which might explain how numerous defects in at least eight different genes lead to a strikingly uniform pathological phenotype. Answers to these questions may not only point out molecular targets for rational therapies but also deepen our understanding of aging and neurodegenerative pathways in general.

INTERNATIONAL COLLABORATION IN NCL RESEARCH

The rapid advances made in NCL research during the past two decades would not have been possible without extensive international collaboration between clinicians, neuropathologists, paediatric pathologists, biochemists, clinical geneticists, and molecular biologists. This collaboration has been greatly facilitated by several private and public initiatives and organizations.

The Children's Brain Diseases Foundation, created in 1968 on the initiative of Dr. J. Alfred Rider (San Francisco, USA), sponsored a series of six 'round table' conferences focusing on the aetiology and pathogenesis of the NCLs in 1969–1975 (Zeman and Rider, 1975). These 'round table' conferences were followed in 1980 by the first International Symposium on Human and Animal Models of Ceroid-Lipofuscinosis in Røros, Norway, again sponsored by the Children's Brain Diseases Foundation (Armstrong et al., 1982). Since the second International Conference on the NCLs on Staten Island in 1987, international conferences/congresses on the NCLs have been held at 2–3-year intervals, usually alternating between the USA and different European countries, and have become the main scientific forum of the NCL research community.

A European Concerted Action 'Molecular, pathological and clinical investigations of neuronal ceroid-lipofuscinoses (NCL)–new strategies for prevention, diagnosis, classification and treatment' (ECA-NCL) was initiated and coordinated by Prof. Hans H. Goebel of Mainz, Germany, as part of the BIOMED 2 programme of the European Union. ECA-NCL established the 'European Clinical Registry' and the 'European Tissue Registry' and united 25 groups from different European countries to promote research in NCL. The first ECA-NCL meeting was held in Helsinki in 1996 in conjunction with the Sixth International Congress on the NCLs, with successive meetings organized in the various participating countries. ECA-NCL also produced the first edition of the book *The Neuronal Ceroid Lipofuscinoses (Batten Disease)* (Goebel et al., 1999), the forerunner to this volume.

Since the cloning of the first NCL genes in 1995, the accelerating pace of discovery of new genes and mutations underlying NCL prompted the establishment, in 1998, of an electronic NCL Mutation Database, now part of the 'NCL Resource–a gateway for Batten disease' (http://www.ucl.ac.uk/ncl/index.shtml), maintained by Dr Sara Mole at University College London. The 'NCL Resource' includes up-to-date information on the NCLs for clinicians, families, and researchers alike, and has unrestricted access. The collaboration of the patients' families and their organizations with the NCL research community has been invaluable in promoting both research and the rapid and efficient transfer of the newest scientific results to daily diagnostic and therapeutic practice for the benefit of the affected individuals.

Most recently new international efforts to identify the remaining rare NCL genes resulted in the establishment of the 'Rare NCL Gene Consortium' coordinated by Dr Sara Mole, which includes participants from Europe and the USA, and a web-based NCL Registry, initially European-based, and spear-headed by Professor Alfried Kohlschütter and Dr Angela Schulz. Clinicians contributing to this have worked together to provide up-to-date diagnostic algorithms and disease rating scales, and led to the recently proposed change in nomenclature. Similar efforts continue to take place in the USA, including the previous establishment of DNA and cell banks supported by the Batten Disease Support and Research Association.

This level of cooperation and collaboration bodes well for continued and steady progress for the NCL field at clinical, diagnostic, research, and therapeutic levels.

BIOGRAPHIES

The diseases now grouped together as the NCLs were originally described over a period of nearly 200 years, and the names of some physicians or scientists became associated with a particular type. Now, each disease can better be described according to the genetic defect. For the sake of medical history, brief biographies of the individuals who are eponymically associated with a clinical subtype, and their NCL-related work are provided. These are in alphabetical order, beginning appropriately with Batten, whose name has become the favoured colloquial term for the NCLs.

Frederick Batten (1865–1918)

Frederick Eustace Batten MA MD FRCP was born in Plymouth, Devon the son of

John Winterbotham Batten, a naval outfitter, and his wife Sarah. Frederick Batten was educated at Westminster School, and Trinity College, Cambridge where he graduated in 1887 with a degree in natural science. He qualified as MB BCh in 1891 at St Bartholomew's Hospital where he later gained his MD in 1895. After his graduation he spent time in Berlin, becoming fluent in German, then returning to England where he was appointed to the Hospital For Sick Children, Great Ormond Street. He was later also appointed as pathologist to the National Hospital for the Paralysed and Epileptic in Queen Square, London. At the time of his death in 1918 from infection following a routine prostatectomy, he was Dean of the Medical School at the National Hospital.

He was author of some 106 articles in the short time between 1892 and his untimely death in 1918. His first publication in St Bart Hospital Reports (1892) was on progressive muscular atrophy just after Werdnig (1891) but before Hoffmann (1893) had made a more complete description of what is known as Werdnig–Hoffmann disease. His other earlier works include papers on infections, but by 1900 his biological scientific approach had led to studies on neurological disorders including poliomyelitis, myasthenia, Tay–Sachs disease, encephalopathies, epilepsy, myopathies, and cerebellar syndromes, as well as studies on the muscle spindle and degenerative changes in the sensory end organs of muscle. He was co-editor (with Garrod and Thursfield) of the first edition of *Diseases of Children* published in 1913, in which he wrote chapters on organic nervous diseases and muscle disease. His inventive work in devising light celluloid splints for every form of infantile paralysis was an indication of the practical and caring physician and 'a boon to generations of childhood' (Times 1918). Higgins notes (1962) that he was enthusiastic, indefatigable, practical, and a perfectionist. He also notes that his colleagues found no trace of arrogance or egotism and that he was a tough but scrupulously fair and courteous antagonist.

His older brother, Rayner Derry Batten, had reported to the Ophthalmological Society of the UK in 1897 on macular degeneration, and he commented on his younger brother's report on cerebromacular degeneration to the same society in 1903 (Batten, 1903). In the 1897 report there was no mental defect in the two cases aged 14 and 21, unlike the two girls described by Frederick Batten, whose vision began to deteriorate between the ages of 4–6 years. He described the classic sign 'she looked out of the corners of her eyes to see an object'. This was the first then known publication on what is now CLN3 disease, juvenile although it is predated by the more recently discovered article in Norwegian by Stengel in 1826 in the journal *Eyr* (Stengel, 1826a). Mayou (1904) and others described further cases in the period to 1914 when Batten published the neuropathological findings in the *Quarterly Journal of Medicine* (Batten, 1914).

Batten was well aware of the German literature and, being fluent in German, knew of the works of Vogt (Vogt, 1905, Vogt, 1907), and Bielschowsky (Bielschowsky, 1913) as well as those of Spielmeyer (Spielmeyer, 1906) and Stock (Stock, 1908). He published in the *Proceedings of the Royal Society of Medicine* with Mayou in 1915 'Family cerebral degeneration with macular changes', a clinical and pathological description of the classic late infantile form (Batten and Mayou, 1915).

Frederick Batten was the person who described at a very early time clinical and pathological findings in two forms of NCL, although others had also described one or other of them at a similar time. The eponym 'Batten disease' is an appropriate accolade for a scientific neurologist who died prematurely in his prime, aged 52.

Max Bielschowsky (1869–1940)

Max Bielschowsky, born into a family of merchants in Breslau, now Wroclaw, Poland, attended high school/gymnasium, and commenced his medical studies at Breslau University and continued in Berlin. He graduated from the University of Munich in 1893. He then went to Frankfurt for training in anatomical pathology and worked closely with the Edinger Institute. He took over the neuropathological laboratory at the private clinic of Mendel in Berlin in 1890, from where he was recruited in 1904 to the private neurobiological laboratory of Oskar Vogt, then associated with the Charité in Berlin. When Vogt's institution became a Kaiser Wilhelm Brain Research Institute, Bielschowsky continued working there. He was dismissed from his position in 1933 and emigrated to The Netherlands where he worked at the Wilhelmina Gasthuis in Amsterdam and later in the laboratory of the Psychiatric Department at the University of Utrecht. In 1936, he returned to Germany and suffered his first stroke. The day before Great Britain declared war on Germany, he escaped with the last boat to England where he suffered a second stroke. He died in London in 1940.

Bielschowsky wrote on many aspects of neuropathology and neoplastic disease, including monographs and developed the famous Bielschowsky silver stain for axons. He wrote several papers. Two of them concerned late infantile 'amaurotic family idiocy'. First (Bielschowsky, 1913), he described three siblings who displayed nearly identical clinical symptoms and homochronism of onset of the clinical symptoms in each child. He then performed studies on their postmortem brains (Bielschowsky, 1920), again showing three similar features of NCL, i.e. lipopigment accumulation in nerve cells and loss of nerve cells, particularly in the cerebral cortex, as well as severe cerebellar atrophy in each child.

His interest in 'amaurotic family idiocy' further expanded when he examined the brain of a child who died of Niemann–Pick disease and found the same Schaffer-Spielmeyer process of neuronal storage throughout the brain. The occurrence of infantile 'amaurotic family idiocy' of Tay–Sachs in Ashkenazi Jewish children, and the same neuropathology of Niemann–Pick disease also then seen exclusively in Ashkenazi Jewish children, prompted him to consider these conditions identical (Bielschowsky, 1928). Then, while in exile in The Netherlands (Bielschowsky, 1936), he published another paper on infantile 'amaurotic family idiocy' that apparently differed from classical Tay–Sachs disease in that the retina did not appear involved. Throughout his writing on 'amaurotic family idiocy', Bielschowsky always appeared critical of Schaffer's interpretation of the so-called 'Schaffer's process of neuronal storage' or 'Schaffer–Spielmeyer process of neuronal storage' (Bielschowsky, 1932). In a small review of one of Schaffer's articles (Schaffer, 1931), Bielschowsky also extensively commented on its contents in a very critical and almost abrasive way which apparently was not unusual in those times when speculative interpretation supplemented the dearth of adequately substantiating findings.

The term Jansky–Bielschowsky was used to refer to what is now CLN2 disease, classic late infantile.

Matti Haltia (born 1939)

Matti Haltia graduated from the University of Helsinki Medical School in 1964, and defended his PhD thesis at the University of Gothenburg in 1970. After postgraduate training in pathology and neuropathology at the Universities of Helsinki, Copenhagen, and Gothenburg, he served as neuropathologist at the Helsinki University Central Laboratory of Pathology in 1978–1990, with periods of research at the Harvard University and New York University Medical Schools in 1986–1990. In 1990 he was appointed Professor of Neuropathology at the University of Helsinki, retiring in 2003.

Haltia's scientific involvement with NCL began with a diagnostic cortical biopsy of a child, suspected of GM1 gangliosidosis, submitted by his paediatric neurologist colleague Pirkko Santavuori. Neuropathological analysis of the biopsy specimen excluded, however, the possibility of any known type of gangliosidosis. In contrast, the histological, histochemical, and ultrastructural features suggested a novel type of NCL. Haltia soon diagnosed an identical disorder at neuropathological autopsy of an unrelated clinical problem case from an institution for developmental disabilities. This disease, now known as CLN1 disease, was first termed 'NCL of early onset' (Haltia et al., 1972) or 'infantile type of so-called NCL' (Haltia et al., 1973a, Haltia et al., 1973b, Santavuori et al., 1973). Haltia and collaborators later described the neuropathology (Tyynelä et al., 1997) of Finnish variant late infantile NCL (CLN5 disease), discovered by Santavuori et al. in 1982, and of 'Northern epilepsy' (Hirvasniemi et al., 1994), identifying it as a new form of NCL, now known to be one type of CLN8 disease (Haltia et al., 1999, Herva et al., 2000). Järplid and Haltia (Järplid and Haltia, 1993) reported a novel congenital ovine NCL later found to be caused by a mutation in the cathepsin D gene (Tyynelä et al., 2000). This led to the identification of a defect in cathepsin D underlying human congenital NCL (CLN10 disease) (Siintola et al., 2006) and development of the first fly model of NCL (Myllykangas et al., 2005).

Further contributions by Matti Haltia and his group include characterizations of new phenotypic and genotypic forms of Alzheimer's disease and Creutzfeldt–Jakob disease, as well as descriptions of the neuropathology of Unverricht–Lundborg disease, aspartylglucosaminuria, gelsolin amyloidosis, the PEHO syndrome, and muscle-eye-brain (MEB) disease.

Jan Janský (1873–1921)

Jan Janský was born in Prague. He studied medicine at the Charles University in Prague, where he won his medical degree on 14 May 1898. After graduation, he worked as a non-resident physician—first at the First Medical Clinic and then, from November 1899, at the Psychiatry Department, now with the rank of assistant professor. In 1907, he defended his habilitation thesis entitled 'Hematological Study of Psychotics', and in 1914 was appointed Professeur Extraordinaire and deputy head physician of the Psychiatry Department. When World War I broke out, he was sent to the front, but was released from service and sent back to Prague in 1916 after suffering a heart attack. Between 1918 and 1921 he served as head physician of the Department of Neurology and Forensic Psychiatry at the Military Hospital in Prague. Jan Janský was the first in the country to conduct practical biochemical and serological research of the cerebrospinal fluid, founding a special laboratory for such research at the Psychiatry Department. He also published a series of studies in the field of clinical psychiatry. He discovered the four known blood types (I–IV) and described them in his 1907 habilitation thesis. He published this discovery, which he based on the study of about 3000 blood samples, in the Czech journal Clinical Proceedings (Janský, 1907). He did not find what he sought—a relation between blood group types and the psychiatric disorders he studied—and so the main fruit of his efforts was the discovery of blood groups independently of Landsteiner, of whose work he was not aware. Landsteiner had described only three blood groups in 1901 (types A, B, O in current classification) and was to win a Nobel Prize in Medicine for it in 1930. However, in 1921, after Janský's death, a United States medical commission acknowledged his blood group classification.

Janský described, in 1908, a case of late infantile form of amaurotic idiocy, now CLN2 disease, late infantile. He published his observations, including autopsy results, in the Czech journal Proceedings of the Faculty of Medicine at Hradec Králové (in Czech, with an abstract in French) (Janský, 1908). The case involved a 5½-year-old boy, who was autopsied at the Czech Department of Pathological Anatomy on 28 June 1907. A copy of the paper is available, but unfortunately not the paraffin samples he used in this ground-breaking study.

The term Janský–Bielschowsky was extensively used to refer to what is now CLN2 disease, classic late infantile.

Hugo Kufs (1871–1955)

Hugo Kufs, a life-long Saxonian, was born close to Borna, from which the Borna virus and Borna-encephalitis were named. He studied medicine at the University of Leipzig. In search of a secure position as a government employee, he entered the Saxonian service of state mental hospitals and he became neuropathologist/prosector at the Saxonian mental hospital in Leipzig-Dösen in 1919 where he stayed until his retirement in 1936. He was self-taught in neuropathology, like Spielmeyer, and never trained at a neuropathological or pathological institution. After retirement, he continued at the neuropathology laboratory of the Psychiatric Department at the University of Leipzig for 2 years, until his apartment was destroyed by air raids. After the war he returned to the Brain Research Institute of Leipzig University until his death in 1955. He published on many aspects of neuropathology, especially on neurosyphilis, progressive paralysis, tuberous sclerosis, dementia, and multiple sclerosis, as well as brain tumours.

Kufs contributed four papers between 1925 and 1931 on the late-onset form of 'amaurotic family idiocy' by describing two siblings (Kufs, 1925), one with dementia and ataxia at the age of 26 years, who died at the age of 38 years, while her younger brother developed behavioural problems at the age of 10 years, followed many years later by mental deterioration and ataxia. Neither experienced seizures nor visual impairment, although their father developed retinitis pigmentosa/pigmentary retinopathy at the age of 30 years. This family constellation with visual impairment in the father but its lack in the affected children prompted Kufs to write another lengthy paper (Kufs, 1927) on the relationship of retinitis pigmentosa and 'amaurotic family idiocy'. In the absence of the known underlying genetic defect, the term Kufs disease is still used to refer to adult onset NCL without visual impairment.

Brian Lake (born 1935)

Brian Lake BSc PhD FRCPath, a 1961 chemistry graduate from Leeds University, was a histochemist and electron microscopist in the Histopathology Department at the Great Ormond Street Hospital for Children in London, later Professor, where he specialized in the diagnosis of rare metabolic disorders. His understanding of metabolic processes and scientific approach to the biopsy tissue samples presented were core to accurate diagnosis. His earlier publication in 1963 in the *British Journal of Surgery* with Martin Bodian entitled 'The rectal approach to neuropathology' had formed the basis for the diagnosis by rectal biopsy of a variety of lysosomal storage disorders and the differentiation of the various forms of Batten disease.

The diagnosis of Batten disease at Great Ormond Street Hospital for Children was achieved through the combined results of thorough neurological examination, electroencephalography (EEG), examination of lymphocytes by light microscopy, and light and electron microscopy of a rectal biopsy (later a skin biopsy was substituted for diagnosis).

The pioneering EEG studies of Ann Harden and G. Pampiglione published in 1973 (Harden et al., 1973) had shown that what was to become CLN2 disease, classic late infantile had a characteristic response to low rates of flash. As a consequence of this, a number of patients with atypical history were considered to fall into the late infantile category. However, the electron microscopy of the storage material in these patients did not have the curvilinear structure of classic late infantile CLN2 disease, but showed the fingerprint inclusions more characteristic of what was later identified as juvenile CLN3 disease.

Nicholas Cavanagh FRCP, a registrar in the neurology department with a particular interest in inherited metabolic disease, collated the notes of the 'aberrant' patients and, with Brian Lake in 1978, wrote about the new form, entitling it 'early juvenile' to reflect the ultrastructural pathology (Lake and Cavanagh, 1978). This was in contrast to the situation in Finland where Pirkko Santavuori later described, in 1982, a similar but earlier form, as variant late infantile (now CLN5 disease, late infantile variant) based on the clinical and EEG findings.

The early juvenile type (now CLN6 disease, late infantile variant) was labelled by some as the Lake–Cavanagh form of Batten disease.

Marmaduke Mayou (1876–1934)

Marmaduke Stephen Mayou FRCS, the son of George Mayou MD of Monmouth, was educated at Hereford Cathedral School and King's College Hospital where he won the Jeff Medal in 1896. He was awarded the Jacksonian prize at the Royal College of Surgeons in 1904 with an essay on the pathology and treatment of conjunctivitis. He was Hunterian Professor of surgery and pathology, pathologist and radiographer at the Central London Ophthalmic Hospital, King's Cross. His later appointments included consulting surgeon to a variety of hospitals in London and Kent.

He was an original member of the ophthalmological section of the Royal Society of Medicine, treasurer of the Council of British Ophthalmologists, and was elected as President of the Ophthalmological Society of the United Kingdom in 1933. He invented the Mayou operating lamp and the Mayou slit lamp and made many contributions to the ophthalmological literature in England and the USA. Among these contributions was an article on 'cerebral degeneration with symmetrical changes in the macula' in *Transactions of the Ophthalmological Society of the United Kingdom* in 1904. This followed a similar article in the same journal in 1903 by F.E. Batten on what is now regarded as classic juvenile CLN3 disease. Coincidentally, the 1903 paper by Batten was followed by one from Mayou describing normal fundi examined by a mercury vapour lamp, underlining his early interest in ophthalmological examination. Mayou collaborated with Batten in the 1915 article in the journal *Proceedings of the Royal Society of Medicine* entitled 'Family cerebral degeneration with macular changes' (Batten and Mayou, 1915), a follow-up of the earlier Batten paper of 1914 in the journal *Quarterly Journal of Medicine* on what is now recognized as classic late infantile CLN2 disease. Thus, Mayou was closely associated with both CLN2 and CLN3 diseases, and the eponym Batten–Mayou has been widely used.

Pirkko Santavuori (1933–2004)

Pirkko Santavuori graduated from the University of Helsinki Medical School in 1960. She subsequently worked at the Helsinki University Children's Hospital in different positions, being Physician-in-Chief of the Department of Child Neurology at her retirement in 1996. Santavuori became an internationally recognized paediatric neurologist whose scientific activity resulted in over 150 publications in international journals and books.

Pirkko Santavuori began her scientific activity by the end of the 1960s studying the epidemiology of what was then called 'juvenile amaurotic idiocy'. In this context, she encountered a patient who had developed mental retardation and visual decline at an unusually early age. On clinical grounds, she suspected GM1 gangliosidosis type II. Neuropathological analysis of a cortical biopsy excluded, however, the possibility of any known type of gangliosidosis. In contrast, the histological, histochemical, and ultrastructural features suggested a novel type of neuronal ceroid lipofuscinosis. Her neuropathologist colleague, Matti Haltia, soon diagnosed an identical disorder at neuropathological autopsy of an unrelated clinical problem case from an institution for developmental disabilities. The disease was first termed 'neuronal ceroid-lipofuscinosis of early onset' (Haltia et al., 1972) or 'infantile type of so-called neuronal ceroid-lipofuscinosis' (Haltia et al., 1973a, Haltia et al., 1973b, Santavuori et al., 1973). On the proposal of Haltia, Pirkko Santavuori now focused her research and wrote her PhD thesis on this new disorder, collecting new cases and describing their clinical neurological, ophthalmological, and electrophysiological features in detail.

Apart from her contribution to the clinical characterization of what is now CLN1 disease, infantile, Santavuori had a central role in the discovery of two further new diseases: CLN5 disease, late infantile variant, first described as Finnish variant late-infantile NCL (Santavuori et al., 1982), and muscle-eye-brain (MEB) disease (Santavuori et al., 1989), an inherited condition with striking brain and eye malformations (Haltia et al., 1997).

Torsten Sjögren (1896–1974)

Born in Södertälje, Sweden, Karl Gustaf Torsten Sjögren followed his father's example pursuing a medical career. After basic studies at the University of Uppsala, he graduated in medicine from the Karolinska Institute, Stockholm, in 1925 and defended his PhD thesis at the University of Lund in 1931. He then served as Physician-in-Chief at psychiatric hospitals in Lund and Gothenburg and from 1945–1961 as Professor of Psychiatry at the Karolinska Institutet. He was one of the pioneers of biological psychiatry in Sweden (Nilsson, 2003).

Already at an early stage of his career, Sjögren focused his research on the role of genetic factors in disorders of the nervous system. From 1926–1932 he worked at the Swedish State Institute of Racial Hygiene, Uppsala, and at the St. Lars Hospital, Lund, where he became interested in patients with 'juvenile amaurotic idiocy'. His PhD thesis consisted of careful clinical and genealogical studies of such patients and their families from Southern Sweden (Sjögren, 1931), including 39 personally examined cases. Based on statistical analyses of about 4500 members of the affected families Sjögren concluded that 'juvenile amaurotic idiocy' showed, with high probability, a 'monohybrid recessive inheritance', and was genetically distinct from 'infantile amaurotic idiocy' (Tay–Sachs disease).

Sjögren's subsequent scientific work consisted of extensive clinical, population genetic, and epidemiological studies of psychoses and dementias as well as mental retardation, particularly in certain isolated areas of northern and western Sweden. He wrote on schizophrenia, Alzheimer's disease/senile dementia, and Pick's disease, but also on Huntington's chorea, essential tremor, and dystonia musculorum deformans. In addition to what is now CLN3 disease, juvenile, Sjögren's name is associated with two further inherited forms of mental retardation: Marinesco–Sjögren syndrome (cerebellar ataxia with early onset cataracts, hypotonia, and mild to severe mental retardation) (Sjögren, 1947, Sjögren, 1950) and Sjögren–Larsson syndrome (congenital ichthyosis, spastic paraplegia or tetraplegia, pigmentary retinal degeneration, and mental retardation) (Sjögren and Larsson, 1957).

The term Spielmeyer–Sjögren–Vogt disease was used for many years to refer to what is now CLN3 disease, juvenile.

Walther Spielmeyer (1879–1935)

Walther Spielmeyer was born and grew up in Dessau. He studied medicine in Greifswald and Halle, and worked at the Institute of Pathology of the University of Halle. He then trained at the Department of Psychiatry and Neurology at the University of Freiburg where he investigated 'family amaurotic idiocy', now recognized as CLN3 disease, juvenile, in four siblings out of five with only the eldest son unaffected. While still in Freiburg, the neuropathological pattern of this disease, which he considered unique, made up the subject of his academic thesis. In 1912, he headed the pathological laboratory at the University Department of Psychiatry in Munich as the successor to Alzheimer.

Over the years, Spielmeyer attracted innumerable German and foreign investigators, some of them already renowned scientists, and became the doyen of German neuropathology. A monograph *Histopathology of the Nervous System* appeared in 1922 following *Manual Technique of Microscopic Investigation of the Nervous System* presenting the entire spectrum of non-neoplastic neuropathology. He died rather suddenly within just a week from a pulmonary disease in 1935, aged 56 years.

Spielmeyer wrote several papers on 'amaurotic family idiocy'. In 1905 (Spielmeyer, 1905a, Spielmeyer, 1905b) he presented four affected siblings who developed visual problems, dementia and motor abnormalities around the age of 6 years. He then described the siblings' condition clinically and pathologically in a separate paper (Spielmeyer, 1906) and subsequently in a major article in 1908 (Spielmeyer, 1908).

Apart from discussing 'amaurotic family idiocy' in his book *Histopathology of the Nervous System* in 1922, he wrote two review articles (Spielmeyer, 1923, Spielmeyer, 1929), mentioning additional observations only in passing and not in detail and reiterating his belief that 'family amaurotic idiocy' was a metabolic lipoidosis with different clinical forms. This belief was further reiterated in a major oral presentation in Stockholm (Spielmeyer, 1933). Finally, he used a review of a major article by Karl Schaffer (Schaffer, 1932) from Budapest, to criticize Schaffer's interpretation of the Schaffer–Spielmeyer process and stating his own opinion on this topic. Apparently, in those days, it was not unusual to seize the opportunity of criticizing the work of a colleague or an opponent by reviewing his article(s) and then stating one's own alternate view, often at greater length than the mere report on the reviewed article.

The term Spielmeyer–Vogt or Spielmeyer–Sjögren–Vogt disease was used in mainland Europe for many years to refer to what is now CLN3 disease, juvenile.

Otto Christian Stengel (1794–1890)

Otto Christian Stengel was born in Wewelsfleth close to Glückstadt in Holstein in 1794. At this time, both Schleswig–Holstein (now part of Germany) and Norway were under Danish rule. After 2 years of surgical training as a volunteer in a hospital near his home and a further 2 months of training in surgery in Copenhagen, he was regarded as qualified to work as a military surgeon, and joined the army at the age of 17. His service coincided with the Napoleonic Wars, and he practised at a military hospital in Kiel.

After the war, he was sent to Norway in 1814. Stengel became a student at the newly established Royal Fredrik University in Christiania (now Oslo), the first Norwegian university, and graduated in medicine in 1821. After completing his medical training, Stengel moved to Røros, a small mining town in the South-Eastern highlands of Norway. Here he was employed as physician at the Copper Mining Company of Røros for the subsequent 61 years.

During his exceptionally long career as a general practitioner, he was struck by a singular and tragic illness, affecting four consecutive children of a family in the vicinity of Røros, presenting by the age of 6 years with poor sight, and leading gradually to blindness, mental decline, and finally to premature death. Impressed by these observations Stengel wrote 'Account of a singular illness among four siblings in the vicinity of Røraas' which was published in the first volume of the first Norwegian medical journal *Eyr* in 1826 (Stengel, 1826a). His article was written in Norwegian and remained in the darkness of history until rediscovered by his countrymen more than a century later (Nissen, 1954, Koppang, 1966, Hansen, 1979). Stengel's article is considered to constitute the first clinical description of the typical symptoms and course of what is now known as CLN3 disease, classic juvenile.

Heinrich Vogt (1875–1957)

Heinrich Vogt was born in Regensburg/Germany. By 1957, when he died at the age of 82 years in Bad Pyrmont/Germany, Heinrich Vogt had pursued two illustrious successive careers. He studied medicine in Munich, Heidelberg, and Göttingen where he joined the University Department of Psychiatry. At the state mental hospital in Langenhagen close to Hannover, he studied neurological and mental diseases, the latter then called 'idiocy', in children. In 1909, he became associate professor and had moved to Frankfurt where he headed the neuropathological laboratory of the Neurological (Edinger) Institute until 1910. In 1911, he left the university and became chief of service of a neurological sanatorium for another 14 years. In 1926, he started his second career as a medical hydrologist/balneologist in private practice as well as at a local institute of medical hydrology. Having been asked by the Prussian Ministry to design a central national institution of balneological (science of the therapeutic use of bathing) research, in 1935, he became director of the National Institute of German Balneology in Breslau and Professor of Balneology at the University of Breslau. He was a prolific writer both in child neurology and later balneology, founded journals, and wrote several textbooks on epilepsy and balneology.

There are three papers by Vogt on 'amaurotic family idiocy', the first one in 1905 (Vogt, 1905) described eight children in three families suffering from visual impairment proceeding to blindness, motor abnormalities, behavioural problems, and final dementia. Having switched from neurology to neuropathology, he first published a review on the neuropathology of 'amaurotic family idiocy' (Vogt, 1907). Then, together with reiterated clinical findings, he published neuropathological findings of his patients, investigated earlier as a clinician, in a third paper (Vogt, 1909) in great detail. In 1908, Vogt published a paper on the diagnosis of tuberous sclerosis, establishing three pathognomonic clinical signs for the condition: epilepsy, idiocy, and adenoma sebaceum, that became known as 'Vogt's triad' and helped define this condition for the next 60 years. In 1916, he published a two-volume *Handbuch der Therapie der Nervenkrankheiten* (*Handbook on the Treatment of Nervous Diseases*).

The term Spielmeyer–Vogt or Spielmeyer–Sjögren–Vogt disease was used in mainland Europe for many years to refer to what is now CLN3 disease, juvenile.

REFERENCES

Armstrong D, Koppang N, & Rider JA (1982) *Ceroid-lipofuscinosis (Batten's disease). Proceedings of the International Symposium on Human and Animal Models of Ceroid-Lipofuscinosis*. Amsterdam, New York, Oxford, Elsevier Biomedical Press.

Batten FE (1903) Cerebral degeneration with symmetrical changes in the maculae in two members of a family. *Trans Ophthalmol Soc UK*, 23, 386–390.

Batten FE (1914) Family cerebral degeneration with macular change (so-called juvenile form of family amaurotic idiocy). *Q J Med*, 7, 444–454.

Batten FE & Mayou MS (1915) Family cerebral degeneration with macular changes. *Proc R Soc Med*, 8, 70–90.

Bielschowsky M (1913) Über spätinfantile familiäre amaurotische Idiotie mit Kleinhirnsymptonen. *Deutsche Zeitschrift für Nervenheilkunde*, 50, 7–29.

Bielschowsky M (1920) Zur Histopathologie und Pathogenese der amaurotischen Idiotie mit besonderer Berücksichtigung der zerebellaren Veränderungen. *J Psychol Neurol (Leipzig)*, 26, 123–199.

Bielschowsky M (1928) Amaurotische Idiotie und lipoidzellige Splenohepatomegalie. *J Psychol Neurol (Leipzig)*, 36, 103–123.

Bielschowsky M (1932) Review on 'Revision in der Pathobiologie und Pathogenese der Infantil-amaurotischen Idiotie' by K. Schaffer. *Zentralbl Ges Neurol Psychiatr*, 63, 367–370.

Bielschowsky M (1936) Über eine bisher unbekannte Form von infantiler amaurotischer Idiotie. *Zentralbl Ges Neurol Psychiatr*, 155, 321–329.

Bildfell R, Matwichuk C, Mitchell S, & Ward P (1995) Neuronal ceroid-lipofuscinosis in a cat. *Vet Pathol*, 32, 485–488.

Boehme DH, Cottrell JC, Leonberg SC, & Zeman W (1971) A dominant form of neuronal ceroid-lipofuscinosis. *Brain*, 94, 745–760.

Bronson RT, Donahue LR, Johnson KR, Tanner A, Lane PW, & Faust JR (1998) Neuronal ceroid lipofuscinosis (nclf), a new disorder of the mouse linked to chromosome 9. *Am J Med Genet*, 77, 289–297.

Bronson RT, Lake BD, Cook S, Taylor S, & Davisson MT (1993) Motor neuron degeneration of mice is a model of neuronal ceroid lipofuscinosis (Batten's disease). *Ann Neurol*, 33, 381–385.

Broom MF, Zhou C, Broom JE, Barwell KJ, Jolly RD, & Hill DF (1998) Ovine neuronal ceroid lipofuscinosis: a large animal model syntenic with the human neuronal ceroid lipofuscinosis variant CLN6. *J Med Genet*, 35, 717–721.

Brown NJ, Corner BD, & Dodgson MC (1954) A second case in the same family of congenital familial cerebral lipoidosis resembling amaurotic family idiocy. *Arch Dis Child*, 29, 48–54.

Brunk UT & Terman A (2002) Lipofuscin: mechanisms of age-related accumulation and influence on cell function. *Free Radic Biol Med*, 33, 611–619.

Cook RW, Jolly RD, Palmer DN, Tammen I, Broom MF, & McKinnon R (2002) Neuronal ceroid lipofuscinosis in Merino sheep. *Aust Vet J*, 80, 292–297.

Eiberg H, Gardiner RM, & Mohr J (1989) Batten disease (Spielmeyer-Sjogren disease) and haptoglobins (HP): indication of linkage and assignment to chr. 16. *Clin Genet*, 36, 217–218.

Elleder M, Franc J, Kraus J, Nevsimalova S, Sixtova K, & Zeman J (1997a) Neuronal ceroid lipofuscinosis in the Czech Republic: analysis of 57 cases. Report of the 'Prague NCL group'. *Eur J Paediatr Neurol*, 1, 109–114.

Fearnley IM, Walker JE, Martinus RD, Jolly RD, Kirkland KB, Shaw GJ, & Palmer DN (1990) The sequence of the major protein stored in ovine ceroid lipofuscinosis is identical with that of the dicyclohexylcarbodiimide-reactive proteolipid of mitochondrial ATP synthase. *Biochem J*, 268, 751–758.

Fiske RA & Storts RW (1988) Neuronal ceroid-lipofuscinosis in Nubian goats. *Vet Pathol*, 25, 171–173.

Gao H, Boustany RM, Espinola JA, Cotman SL, Srinidhi L, Antonellis KA, Gillis T, Qin X, Liu S, Donahue LR, Bronson RT, Faust JR, Stout D, Haines JL, Lerner TJ, & MacDonald ME (2002) Mutations in a novel CLN6-encoded transmembrane protein cause variant neuronal ceroid lipofuscinosis in man and mouse. *Am J Hum Genet*, 70, 324–335.

Goebel HH, Mole SE, & Lake BD (Eds.) (1999) *The Neuronal Ceroid Lipofuscinoses (Batten Disease)*. Amsterdam, IOS Press.

Green PD & Little PB (1974) Neuronal ceroid-lipofuscin storage in Siamese cats. *Can J Comp Med*, 38, 207–212.

Haltia M (2003) The neuronal ceroid-lipofuscinoses. *J Neuropathol Exp Neurol*, 62, 1–13.

Haltia M, Leivo I, Somer H, Pihko H, Paetau A, Kivela T, Tarkkanen A, Tome F, Engvall E, & Santavuori P (1997) Muscle-eye-brain disease: a neuropathological study. *Ann Neurol*, 41, 173–180.

Haltia M, Rapola J, & Santavuori P (1972) Neuronal ceroid-lipofuscinosis of early onset. A report of 6 cases. *Acta Paediatr Scand*, 61, 241–242.

Haltia M, Rapola J, & Santavuori P (1973a) Infantile type of so-called neuronal ceroid-lipofuscinosis. Histological and electron microscopic studies. *Acta Neuropathol*, 26, 157–170.

Haltia M, Rapola J, Santavuori P, & Keranen A (1973b) Infantile type of so-called neuronal ceroid-lipofuscinosis. 2. Morphological and biochemical studies. *J Neurol Sci*, 18, 269–285.

Haltia M, Tyynelä J, Hirvasniemi A, Herva R, Ranta US, & Lehesjoki AE (1999) CLN8 - Northern epilepsy. In Goebel HH, Mole SE, & Lake BD (Eds.) *The Neuronal Ceroid Lipofuscinoses (Batten Disease)*, pp. 117–124. Amsterdam, IOS Press.

Hannover A (1843) Mikroskopiske undersögelser af nervesystemet. *Det Kongelige Danske Videnskabernes Selskabs Naturvidenskabelige og Mathematiske. Afhandlinger*, 10, 1–112.

Hansen E (1979) Familial cerebro-macular degeneration (the Stengel-Batten-Mayou-Spielmeyer-Vogt-Stock disease). Evaluation of the photoreceptors. *Acta Ophthalmol (Copenh)*, 57, 382–396.

Harden A, Pampiglione G, & Picton-Robinson N (1973) Electroretinogram and visual evoked response in a form of 'neuronal lipidosis' with diagnostic EEG features. *J Neurol Neurosurg Psychiatry*, 36, 61–67.

Harper PA, Walker KH, Healy PJ, Hartley WJ, Gibson AJ, & Smith JS (1988) Neurovisceral ceroid-lipofuscinosis in blind Devon cattle. *Acta Neuropathol*, 75, 632–636.

Herva R, Tyynelä J, Hirvasniemi A, Syrjakallio-Ylitalo M, & Haltia M (2000) Northern epilepsy: a novel form of neuronal ceroid-lipofuscinosis. *Brain Pathol*, 10, 215–222.

Hirvasniemi A, Lang H, Lehesjoki AE, & Leisti J (1994) Northern epilepsy syndrome: an inherited childhood onset epilepsy with associated mental deterioration. *J Med Genet*, 31, 177–182.

Hofmann SL & Peltonen L (2001) The neuronal ceroid lipofuscinosis. In Scriver CR, Beaudet AL, Sly W, Valle D, Childs B, Kinzler KW, & Vogelstein B (Eds.) *The Metabolic and Molecular Bases of Inherited Disease*, 8th edn., pp. 3877–3894. New York, McGraw-Hill.

Hueck W (1912) Pigmentstudien. *Beitr Pathol Anat Allg Pathol*, 54, 68–232.

Janský J (1907). Haematologick studie u. psychotiku. *Sborn Klinick*, 8, 85–139.

Janský J (1908) Dosud nepopsaný pripad familiárni amaurotické idiotie komplikované s hypoplasii mozeckovou. *Sborn Lék*, 13, 165–196.

Järplid B & Haltia M (1993) An animal model of the infantile type of neuronal ceroid-lipofuscinosis. *J Inherit Metab Dis*, 16, 274–277.

Jolly RD, Janmaat A, West DM, & Morrison I (1980) Ovine ceroid-lipofuscinosis: a model of Batten's disease. *Neuropathol Appl Neurobiol*, 6, 195–209.

Jolly RD, Palmer DN, Studdert VP, Sutton RH, Kelly WR, Koppang N, Dahme G, Hartley WJ, Patterson JS, & Riis RC (1994) Canine ceroid-lipofuscinoses: A review and classification. *J Small Anim Pract*, 35, 299–306.

Katz ML, Khan S, Awano T, Shahid SA, Siakotos AN, & Johnson GS (2005a) A mutation in the CLN8 gene in English Setter dogs with neuronal ceroid-lipofuscinosis. *Biochem Biophys Res Commun*, 327, 541–547.

Klenk E (1939) Beiträge zur Chemie der Lipidosen, Niemann–Pickschen Krankheit und amaurotischen Idiotie. *Hoppe-Seyler Z Physiol Chem*, 262, 128–143.

Koneff H (1886) *Beiträge zur Kenntniss der Nervenzellen in den peripheren Ganglien*. Inaugural-Dissertation zur Erlangung der Doctorwürde. Bern, Buchdruckerei Paul Haller.

Koppang N (1966) Familiäre Glykosphingolipoidose des Hundes (Juvenile Amaurotische Idiotie). *Erg Pathol*, 47, 1–43.

Koppang N (1970) Neuronal ceroid-lipofuscinosis in English setters. *J Small Anim Pract*, 10, 639–644.

Kufs H (1925) Über eine Spätform der amaurotischen Idiotie und ihre heredofamiliären Grundlagen. *Z Ges Neurol Psychiatr*, 95, 168–188.

Kufs H (1927) Über die Bedeutung der optischen Komponente der amaurotischen Idiotie in diagnostischer und erbbiologischer Beziehung und über die Existenz 'spätester' Fälle bei dieser Krankheit. *Z Ges Neurol Psychiatr*, 109, 453–487.

Kyttälä A, Lahtinen U, Braulke T, & Hofmann SL (2006) Functional biology of the neuronal ceroid lipofuscinoses (NCL) proteins. *Biochim Biophys Acta*, 1762, 920–933.

Lake BD & Cavanagh NP (1978) Early-juvenile Batten's disease—a recognisable sub-group distinct from other forms of Batten's disease. Analysis of 5 patients. *J Neurol Sci*, 36, 265–271.

Mole SE (2004) The genetic spectrum of human neuronal ceroid-lipofuscinoses. *Brain Pathol*, 14, 70–76.

Myllykangas L, Tyynelä J, Page-McCaw A, Rubin GM, Haltia MJ, & Feany MB (2005) Cathepsin D-deficient Drosophila recapitulate the key features of neuronal ceroid lipofuscinoses. *Neurobiol Dis*, 19, 194–199.

Nakayama H, Uchida K, Shouda T, Uetsuka K, Sasaki N, & Goto N (1993) Systemic ceroid-lipofuscinosis in a Japanese domestic cat. *J Vet Med Sci*, 55, 829–831.

Nijssen PC, Brusse E, Leyten AC, Martin JJ, Teepen JL, & Roos RA (2002) Autosomal dominant adult neuronal ceroid lipofuscinosis: parkinsonism due to both striatal and nigral dysfunction. *Mov Disord*, 17, 482–487.

Nilsson I (2003) Karl Gustaf Torsten Sjögren. In Nilzén G (Ed.) *Svenskt Biografiskt Lexikon*, pp. 381–384. Stockholm.

Nissen AJ (1954) Juvenil amaurotisk idioti I Norge (Juvenile amaurotic idiocy in Norway). *Nord Med*, 52, 1542–1546.

Norman RM & Wood N (1941) Congenital form of amaurotic family idiocy. *J Neurol Psych*, 4, 175–190.

Palmer DN, Barns G, Husbands DR, & Jolly RD (1986a) Ceroid lipofuscinosis in sheep. II. The major component of the lipopigment in liver, kidney, pancreas, and brain is low molecular weight protein. *J Biol Chem*, 261, 1773–1777.

Palmer DN, Fearnley IM, Walker JE, Hall NA, Lake BD, Wolfe LS, Haltia M, Martinus RD, & Jolly RD (1992) Mitochondrial ATP synthase subunit c storage in the ceroid-lipofuscinoses (Batten disease). *Am J Med Genet*, 42, 561–567.

Palmer DN, Martinus RD, Cooper SM, Midwinter GG, Reid JC, & Jolly RD (1989b) Ovine ceroid lipofuscinosis. The major lipopigment protein and the lipid-binding subunit of mitochondrial ATP synthase have the same NH2-terminal sequence. *J Biol Chem*, 264, 5736–5740.

Palmer DN, Tyynelä J, van Mil HC, Westlake VJ, & Jolly RD (1997b) Accumulation of sphingolipid activator proteins (SAPs) A and D in granular osmiophilic deposits in miniature Schnauzer dogs with ceroid-lipofuscinosis. *J Inherit Metab Dis*, 20, 74–84.

Porta EA (2002) Pigments in aging: an overview. *Ann N Y Acad Sci*, 959, 57–65.

Ranta S, Zhang Y, Ross B, Lonka L, Takkunen E, Messer A, Sharp J, Wheeler R, Kusumi K, Mole S, Liu W, Soares MB, Bonaldo MF, Hirvasniemi A, de la Chapelle A, Gilliam TC, & Lehesjoki AE (1999) The neuronal ceroid lipofuscinoses in human EPMR and mnd mutant mice are associated with mutations in CLN8. *Nat Genet*, 23, 233–236.

Read WK & Bridges CH (1969) Neuronal lipodystrophy. Occurrence in an inbred strain of cattle. *Pathol Vet*, 6, 235–243.

Sachs B (1896) A family form of idiocy, generally fatal and associated with early blindness (amaurotic family idiocy). *NY Med J*, 63, 697–703.

Sandbank U (1968) Congenital amaurotic idiocy. *Pathol Eur*, 3, 226–229.

Santavuori P (1982) Clinical findings in 69 patients with infantile neuronal ceroid lipofuscinosis. In Armstrong D, Koppang N, & Rider A (Eds.) *Ceroid Lipofuscinoses (Batten disease)*, pp. 23–34. Amsterdam, Elsevier.

Santavuori P, Haltia M, Rapola J, & Raitta C (1973) Infantile type of so-called neuronal ceroid-lipofuscinosis. 1. A clinical study of 15 patients. *J Neurol Sci*, 18, 257–267.

Santavuori P, Rapola J, Nuutila A, Raininko R, Lappi M, Launes J, Herva R, & Sainio K (1991) The spectrum of Jansky-Bielschowsky disease. *Neuropediatrics*, 22, 92–96.

Santavuori P, Rapola J, Sainio K, & Raitta C (1982) A variant of Jansky-Bielschowsky disease. *Neuropediatrics*, 13, 135–141.

Santavuori P, Somer H, Sainio K, Rapola J, Kruus S, Nikitin T, Ketonen L, & Leisti J (1989b) Muscle-eye-brain disease (MEB). *Brain Dev*, 11, 147–153.

Savukoski M, Klockars T, Holmberg V, Santavuori P, Lander ES, & Peltonen L (1998) CLN5, a novel gene encoding a putative transmembrane protein mutated in Finnish variant late infantile neuronal ceroid lipofuscinosis. *Nat Genet*, 19, 286–288.

Schaffer K (1906) Beiträge zur Nosographie und Histopathologie der amaurotisch-paralytischen Idiotieformen. *Arch Psychiatr Nervenkr*, 42, 127–160.

Schaffer K (1910) Über die Anatomie und Klinik der Tay–Sachs'schen amaurotisch-familiären Idiotie mit Rücksicht auf verwandte Formen. *Z. Erforsch. Behandl Jugendl Schwachsinns*, 19–73, 147–186.

Schaffer K (1931) Revision in der Pathohistologie und Pathogenese der infantil-amaurotischen Idiotie. *Arch Psychiatr*, 95, 714–722.

Schaffer K (1932) Grundsätzliche Bemerkungen zur Pathogenese der amaurotischen Idiotie. *Mschr Psychiat*, 84, 117–129.

Siintola E, Partanen S, Stromme P, Haapanen A, Haltia M, Maehlen J, Lehesjoki AE, & Tyynelä J (2006b) Cathepsin D deficiency underlies congenital human neuronal ceroid-lipofuscinosis. *Brain*, 129, 1438–1445.

Sjögren T (1931) Die juvenile amaurotische Idiotie. Klinische und erblichkeitsmedizinische Untersuchungen. *Hereditas (Lund)*, 14, 197–426.

Sjögren T (1947) Hereditary congenital spinocerebellar ataxia combined with congenital cataract and oligophrenia. *Acta Psychiat Neurol Scand*, 46 (suppl), 286–289.

Sjögren T (1950) Hereditary congenital spinocerebellar ataxia accompanied by congenital cataract and oligophrenia. A genetic and clinical investigation. *Confin Neurol*, 10, 293–308.

Sjögren T & Larsson T (1957) Oligophrenia in combination with congenital ichthyosis and spastic disorders; a clinical and genetic study. *Acta Psychiat Neurol Scand*, 32 (suppl 113), 1–112.

Sleat DE, Donnelly RJ, Lackland H, Liu CG, Sohar I, Pullarkat RK, & Lobel P (1997) Association of mutations in a lysosomal protein with classical late-infantile neuronal ceroid lipofuscinosis. *Science*, 277, 1802–1805.

Spielmeyer W (1905a) Über familiäre amaurotische Idiotien. *Neurol Cbl*, 24, 620–621.

Spielmeyer W (1905b) Weitere Mitteilungen über eine besondere Form von familiärer amaurotischer Idiotie. *Neurol Cbl*, 24, 1131–1132.

Spielmeyer W (1906) Über eine besondere Form von familiärer amaurotischer Idiotie. *Neurol Cbl*, 25, 51–55.

Spielmeyer W (1908) Klinische und amaurotische Untersuchungen über eine besondere Form von familiärer amaurotischer Idiotie. *Histol und Histopathol*, 2, 193–251.

Spielmeyer W (1923) Familiäre amaurotische Idiotie. *Zentralbl Ges Ophthalmol*, 10, 161–208.

Spielmeyer W (1929) Vom Wesen des anatomischen Prozesses bei der familiären amaurotischen Idiotie. *J Psychol Neurol (Leipzig)*, 38, 120–133.

Spielmeyer W (1933) Review on 'Grundsätzliche Bemerkungen zur Pathogenese der amaurotischen Idiotie' by K. Schaffer. *Zentralbl Ges Neurol Psychiatr*, 67, 76–79.

Stengel OC (1826a) Beretning om et mærkeligt Sygdomstilfælde hos fire Sødskende I Nærheden af Röraas. *Eyr*, 1, 347–352.

Stengel OC (1826b/1982) Account of a singular illness among four siblings in the vicinity of Røraas. Reprinted in Armstrong D, Koppang N, & Rider JA (Eds.) *Ceroid-lipofuscinosis (Batten's Disease)*, pp. 17–19. Amsterdam, Elsevier/North Holland Biomedical Press.

Stock W (1908) Über eine bis jetzt noch nicht beschriebene Form der familiär auftretenden Netzhautdegeneration bei gleichzeitiger Verblödung und Über Pigmentdegeneration der Netzhaut. *Klin Mbl Augenheilk*, 5, 225–244.

Svennerholm L (1962) The chemical structure of normal human brain and Tay-Sachs gangliosides. *Biochem Biophys Res Commun*, 9, 436–441.

Terry RD & Korey SR (1960) Membranous cytoplasmic granules in infantile amaurotic idiocy. *Nature*, 188, 1000–1002.

The International Batten Disease Consortium (1995) Isolation of a novel gene underlying Batten disease, CLN3. *Cell*, 82, 949–957.

Tyynelä J, Palmer DN, Baumann M, & Haltia M (1993) Storage of saposins A and D in infantile neuronal ceroid-lipofuscinosis. *FEBS Lett*, 330, 8–12.

Tyynelä J, Sohar I, Sleat DE, Gin RM, Donnelly RJ, Baumann M, Haltia M, & Lobel P (2000) A mutation in the ovine cathepsin D gene causes a congenital lysosomal storage disease with profound neurodegeneration. *EMBO J*, 19, 2786–2792.

Tyynelä J, Suopanki J, Santavuori P, Baumann M, & Haltia M (1997) Variant late infantile neuronal ceroid-lipofuscinosis: pathology and biochemistry. *J Neuropathol Exp Neurol*, 56, 369–375.

Url A, Bauder B, Thalhammer J, Nowotny N, Kolodziejek J, Herout N, Furst S, & Weissenbock H (2001) Equine neuronal ceroid lipofuscinosis. *Acta Neuropathol*, 101, 410–414.

Vesa J, Hellsten E, Verkruyse LA, Camp LA, Rapola J, Santavuori P, Hofmann SL, & Peltonen L (1995) Mutations in the palmitoyl protein thioesterase gene causing infantile neuronal ceroid lipofuscinosis. *Nature*, 376, 584–587.

Vogt H (1905) Über familiäre amaurotische Idiotie und verwandte Krankheitsbilder. *Mschr Psychiatr Neurol*, 18, 161–171.

Vogt H (1907) Zur Pathologie und pathologischen Anatomie der verschiedenen Idiotie-Formen. *Mschr Psychiatr Neurol*, 22, 403–418.

Vogt H (1909) Familiäre amaurotische Idiotie, Histologische und histopathologische Studien. *Arch Kinderheilkd*, 51, 1–35.

Weissenbock H & Rossel C (1997) Neuronal ceroid-lipofuscinosis in a domestic cat: clinical, morphological and immunohistochemical findings. *J Comp Pathol*, 117, 17–24.

Wheeler RB, Sharp JD, Schultz RA, Joslin JM, Williams RE, & Mole SE (2002) The gene mutated in variant late-infantile neuronal ceroid lipofuscinosis (CLN6) and in nclf mutant mice encodes a novel predicted transmembrane protein. *Am J Hum Genet*, 70, 537–542.

Williams RE, Topçu M, Lake BD, Mitchell W, & Mole SE (1999) Turkish variant late infantile NCL. In Goebel HH, Mole S, & Lake BD (Eds.) *The Neuronal Ceroid Lipofuscinoses (Batten Disease)*, pp. 114–116. Amsterdam, IOS Press.

Wisniewski KE & Zhong N (2001) *Batten Disease: Diagnosis, Treatment and Research*. San Diego, CA, Academic Press.

Zeman W (1976) The neuronal ceroid lipofuscinoses. In Zimmerman HM (Ed.) *Progress in Neuropathology*, pp. 207–223. New York, Grune and Stratton.

Zeman W & Donahue S (1963) Fine structure of the lipid bodies in juvenile amaurotic idiocy. *Acta Neuropathol*, 3, 144–149.

Zeman W, Donohue S, Dyken P, & Green J (1970) The neuronal ceroid-lipofuscinoses (Batten–Vogt syndrome). In Vinken PJ, & Bruyn GW (Eds.) *Handbook of Clinical Neurology*, pp. 588–679. Amsterdam, North Holland Publ Co.

Zeman W & Dyken P (1969) Neuronal ceroid-lipofuscinosis (Batten's disease): relationship to amaurotic family idiocy? *Pediatrics*, 44, 570–583.

Zeman W & Rider JA (Eds.) (1975) The dissection of a degenerative disease. Proceedings of four round-table conferences on the pathogenesis of Batten's disease (neuroronal ceroid-lipofuscinosis). *Excerpta Medica*, p. 393. Amsterdam.

Chapter 2

NCL Nomenclature and Classification

R. E. Williams, H. H. Goebel, S. E. Mole with R.-M. Boustany, M. Elleder, A. Kohlschütter, J. W. Mink, R. Niezen-de Boer, and A. Simonati

INTRODUCTION

NCL nomenclature underwent a major change in 1969 (Zeman and Dyken, 1969) when the name 'neuronal ceroid lipofuscinosis' was used for the first time. This was proposed 25 years before the first NCL genes were identified. Since then the genes underlying most, but not all, human NCL disease have been identified, and it is clear that this group of diseases shows genetic heterogeneity (mutations in different genes may result in similar clinical disease phenotypes), allelic heterogeneity (different mutations within the same disease gene may result in very different clinical disease phenotypes), and can be phenotypically heterogeneous even within the same family (the same mutation in the same disease gene is linked with differing clinical symptoms and rates of disease progression). It is timely to review the current nomenclature, assess its accuracy and appropriateness, and, if necessary, revise it. Nomenclature is closely related to the classification of NCL diseases and has implications for NCL diagnosis.

This chapter, and the following related Chapter 3, was initially drafted by the editors, who represent clinical, molecular genetic, biological, and morphological interests, and further revised by a panel of world experts in the NCLs.

The overriding reason for classification of a disease is to provide a definition for subtypes that is universally understood. But first, a definition for the NCLs is required. A general definition of an NCL disorder is:

> A progressive degenerative disease of the brain and, in most cases, the retina, in association with intracellular storage of material that is morphologically characterized as ceroid lipofuscin or similar to it.

CURRENT NOMENCLATURE

Traditionally this group of disorders has been classified according to the age at onset of symptoms: infantile, late infantile, juvenile, and adult. These were given the common abbreviations INCL, LINCL, JNCL, and ANCL respectively, but were also known by their eponyms Haltia–Santavuori, Janský–Bielschowsky, Spielmeyer–Vogt or Batten disease, and Kufs disease (see Chapter 1). The term 'Batten disease' is used both to refer only to NCL cases of juvenile

Table 2.1 **New classification and genetic basis of NCL, based on gene defect**

	Gene symbol	Protein/cellular localization	Diseases
Soluble enzyme deficiencies	*CTSD* *CLN10*	Cathepsin D; lysosomal	CLN10 disease, congenital CLN10 disease, late infantile CLN10 disease, juvenile CLN10 disease, adult
	PPT1 *CLN1*	Palmitoyl protein thioesterase 1, PPT1; lysosomal	CLN1 disease, infantile CLN1 disease, late infantile variant CLN1 disease, juvenile CLN1 disease, adult
	TPP1 *CLN2*	Tripeptidyl peptidase 1, TPP1; lysosomal	CLN2 disease, classic late infantile CLN2 disease, juvenile
Non-enzyme deficiencies, (functions of identified proteins poorly understood at the current time)	*CLN3*	Transmembrane protein, endolysosomal membrane	CLN3 disease, classic juvenile
	(*CLN4*)	Gene not yet identified	Adult
	CLN5	Soluble forms: lysosomal	CLN5 disease, late infantile variant CLN5 disease, juvenile CLN5 disease, adult
	CLN6	Transmembrane protein; ER	(CLN6 disease, late infantile variant) CLN6 disease, early juvenile variant
	MFSD8 *CLN7*	Transmembrane protein; endolysosomal transporter	CLN7 disease, late infantile variant
	CLN8	Transmembrane protein: ER, ER-Golgi intermediate complex	CLN8 disease, EPMR CLN8 disease, late infantile variant
	(*CLN9*)	Gene not yet identified	CLN9 disease, early juvenile variant
Others: those whose classification is uncertain because of incomplete diagnostic investigations or absence of confirmed gene/mutation designation, or where NCL is a minor mutation-specific phenotype			Congenital/infantile variants Late infantile variants Juvenile variants Late onset/adult variants
	CLCN6	Transmembrane protein. *Mutations not yet found on both disease alleles in human disease*	Chloride transport defect, adult onset
	SGSH	Lysosomal. *Mutations usually cause MPSIIIA*	Adult onset

ER, endoplasmic reticulum.

onset, and to the complete collection of NCL conditions, adding further confusion. During the 1980s and 1990s it was becoming clear that for approximately 10% of cases, this was inadequate and that 'variants' exist. A late infantile variant in Finland (Santavuori et al., 1982) and early juvenile (Lake and Cavanagh, 1978) cases were described. Once disease-causing genes were identified the clinical syndromes often became associated with gene names (e.g. *CLN1* or *PPT1*) and the terms CLN1 and NCL1, for example, were used to describe infantile onset cases. That juvenile onset cases also may be due to mutations in *CLN1* is an additional difficulty for nomenclature and a system of classification. There is no universally accepted nomenclature for the NCLs in current usage.

NOMENCLATURE AND CLASSIFICATION CONSIDERATIONS

The overriding reason for the classification of a disease is to *define* a disease 'entity' undoubtedly, so that everybody associates the same meaning with each defined term. For cases where a definitive classification is not possible, a general definition of an NCL disorder will apply: 'a progressive degenerative disease of the brain and, in most cases, the retina, in association with intracellular storage of material that is morphologically characterized as ceroid lipofuscin or similar to it'.

Any disease nomenclature or diagnostic classification system should help to provide information about prognosis and guide treatment choices. It should be of value for clinicians responsible for diagnosis and treatment, diagnostic laboratories, research scientists, patients and families, and supporting health and education professionals. Therefore, where possible it must take into account:

- Clinical presentation and course—age of onset, presenting symptoms, and disease progression
- The underlying molecular and cellular pathology of the disease—full or partial deficiency in a molecular activity(ies) or gain of novel function(s)
- The precise genetic defect—mutation in a specific gene(s) and the combined effect of disease alleles when recessive or effect of one allele when dominant on gene function
- The degree of functional impairment, and
- Any additional disabilities, genetic or environmental effects which may affect disease onset and progression.

As more knowledge accumulates regarding the molecular basis of the NCLs, a complete characterization of the disease-causing mutations for affected individuals is most likely to provide prognostic information and guide therapy choices. Currently this can be achieved (at least theoretically) for many affected individuals, and together with a clinical description of the disease—as simple as congenital, infantile, late infantile, juvenile, and adult onset

Table 2.2 **Recommended gene and protein nomenclature for human and mouse using several examples**

Human		Mouse	
Gene	**Protein**	**Gene**	**Protein**
PPT1 or *CLN1*	PPT1 (or CLN1 or CLN1p)	*Ppt1*	PPT1
TPP1 or *CLN2*	TPP1 (or CLN2 or CLN2p)	*Tpp1*	TPP1
CLN3	CLN3 or CLN3p	*Cln3*	CLN3
CLN5	CLN5	*Cln5*	CLN5
CLN6	CLN6	*Cln6* (formerly *Nclf*)	CLN6
MFSD8 or *CLN7*	MFSD8 or CLN7	*Mfsd8*	MFSD8
CLN8	CLN8	*Cln8* (formerly *Mnd*)	CLN8
CTSD or *CLN10*	CTSD	*Ctsd*	CTSD

Human: http://www.genenames.org/
Mouse: http://www.informatics.jax.org/mgihome/nomen/gene.shtml
For human, gene symbols generally are italicized, with all letters in uppercase. Protein designations are the same as the gene symbol, but are not italicized; all letters are in uppercase. mRNAs and cDNAs use the same formatting conventions as the gene symbol. For mouse, gene symbols generally are italicized, with only the first letter in uppercase and the remaining letters in lowercase. Protein designations are the same as the gene symbol, but are not italicized, all letters are in uppercase. Recessive mutant phenotypes in the mouse are known by a symbol in lower cases e.g. *nclf* or *mnd*, that is later incorporated as a specific allele with the identified gene name (e.g. $Cln6^{nclf}$ or $Cln8^{mnd}$).

Table 2.3 **Former classification and genetic basis of NCL, based on age of onset**

Disease	Gene	Other names	Other recently used names
Congenital	*CTSD/CLN10*		
Infantile (INCL)	*PPT1/CLN1*	Classic infantile	
	CTSD/CLN10	Variant infantile	
Late infantile (LINCL)	*TPP1/CLN2*	Classic late infantile	
	CLN2		
Variant late infantile NCL (vLINCL)	*CLN5*	Variant late infantile	Finnish variant
	CLN6	Early juvenile	Czech or Indian variant
	MFSD8/CLN7		
	CLN8		Turkish variant
	CTSD/CLN10		
	PPT1/CLN1		
Juvenile (JNCL)	*CLN3*	Classic juvenile	
Variant juvenile	(*CLN9*)	Early juvenile	Variant juvenile with GROD
	PPT1/CLN1	Variant juvenile	
	CLN2/CLN2		
	CLN5		
Adult	*PPT1/CLN1*	Adult	Adult with GROD
	CLN5		
	CTSD/CLN10		
	SGSH		
	CLCN6+CLN7?		
Adult	(*CLN4*)	Kufs or Parry	
EPMR	*CLN8*	EPMR	Northern epilepsy

EPMR, progressive epilepsy with mental retardation; GROD, granular osmiophilic deposit.

disease—will provide the essential framework for diagnosis, ongoing management, and support.

Nomenclature must also reflect current recommended practice. For example, human gene names are always in capitals and italicized (e.g. *CLN1*), human protein names are always in capitals and non-italicized or indicated by '' or 'p' (e.g. CLN1, 'CLN1, or CLN1p), or indicated by their protein product name (e.g. palmitoyl protein thioesterase 1 or PPT1); mutations also follow a recommended nomenclature (http://www.hgvs.org/rec.html) and, when part of a mutation database, have an ID specific to that database. The terms 'NCL1', 'NCL2', etc. have no officially recommended meaning and should no longer be used.

Table 2.1 summarizes the new classification and nomenclature, and Table 2.2 recommended gene and protein nomenclature for human and mouse NCLs. For reference, the former nomenclature is summarized in Table 2.3. The complete axial system of classification is described in Chapter 3.

NCL genes were assigned '*CLN*' symbols prior to their identification. In this book, this originally assigned symbol (e.g. *CLN2*) is used in association with the currently approved or recommended symbol (e.g. *TPP1*). When the gene is identified and the encoded gene product has a specific function, then the protein symbol reflects this function (e.g. PPT1) rather than the original gene symbol (e.g. *CLN1*).

REFERENCES

Lake BD & Cavanagh NP (1978) Early-juvenile Batten's disease—a recognisable sub-group distinct from other forms of Batten's disease. Analysis of 5 patients. *J Neurol Sci*, 36, 265–271.

Santavuori P, Rapola J, Sainio K, & Raitta C (1982) A variant of Janský-Bielschowsky disease. *Neuropediatrics*, 13, 135–141.

Zeman W & Dyken P (1969) Neuronal ceroid-lipofuscinosis (Batten's disease): relationship to amaurotic family idiocy? *Pediatrics*, 44, 570–583.

Chapter 3

NCL Diagnosis and Algorithms

A. Kohlschütter, R. E. Williams, H. H. Goebel, S. E. Mole with R.-M. Boustany, O.P. van Diggelen, M. Elleder, J. Mink, R. Niezen de Boer, M.G. Ribeiro, and A. Simonati

INTRODUCTION

The aim of providing young people, carers, and professionals with a diagnosis is to provide information that leads to effective clinical management of symptoms and perhaps a cure. An accurate and complete diagnosis is also necessary for basic scientific as well as clinical research. As for Chapter 2, this chapter and the algorithms were initially drafted by the editors, who represent clinical, molecular genetic, biological, and morphological interests, and further revised by a panel of world experts in the NCLs.

THE ALGORITHMS

The algorithms have been developed as a response to many diagnostic queries from clinicians. They have been directed to support groups and laboratory scientists as well as more experienced NCL clinicians. The algorithms have not yet been audited or evaluated formally and aim only to provide a sensible logical approach to the investigation of this group of children and young adults. They may be adapted according to particular circumstances and the resources available in different countries.

Two algorithms are given.

ALGORITHM A

(Figure 3.1) should be followed for those children presenting with a history suggestive of NCL with a juvenile age of onset or CLN3 disease, classic juvenile: that is, they have isolated progressive visual impairment initially, followed by cognitive regression and seizures. The teenager with a known retinal dystrophy and absent electroretinogram who then develops seizures should also be investigated for CLN3 disease using this algorithm. Rarely, children with a similar clinical disease progression to those with CLN3 disease, classic juvenile but the ultrastructural characteristics of CLN1 disease, infantile have mutations in *CLN1*. On more detailed study, the clinical phenotype of these children does tend to be slightly different to CLN3 disease, juvenile.

ALGORITHM B

(Figure 3.2) should be followed for other children and adults presenting with features consistent with NCL. Symptoms may include any combination of refractory epilepsy, challenging behaviour, developmental slowing/regression, and visual impairment. For such children, it is likely that a battery of neurometabolic and neurogenetic investigations is planned, including electrophysiological studies, brain imaging, blood and cerebrospinal fluid (CSF) analysis. A child presenting with a possible neurodegenerative disorder: loss of previously acquired developmental skills, with or without behavioural deterioration, seizures, and visual impairment, should be investigated urgently and thoroughly in order to find an underlying diagnosis where possible. A diagnosis may have implications for treatment, further investigation of other family members, and for reproductive decisions within the affected family.

Huge advances in NCL diagnostic testing over the past decade have occurred as a result of basic scientific research. Cathepsin D (CTSD), palmitoyl protein thioesterase 1 (PPT1), and tripeptidyl peptidase 1 (TPP1) enzyme analysis in white blood cells or fibroblasts, together with testing for the common mutations or by sequencing of the whole gene in *CLN10/CTSD*, *CLN1/PPT1*, *CLN2/TPP1*, *CLN3*, *CLN5*, *CLN6*, *CLN7/MFSD8*, and *CLN8* are now available in service laboratories in many countries (complete list given at http://www.ucl.ac.uk/ncl), and are therefore accessible for more children with so far undiagnosed progressive neurological disorders.

Practical notes to accompany Algorithm B (Figure 3.2)

The preschool child with refractory seizures and plateauing of language skills, who is shown to have an occipital spike response to low flash rate photic stimulation, may have CLN2 disease, late infantile.

Most children with a history suggestive of developmental regression will be referred for further investigation. Initial investigations may include basic biochemistry, a sleep electroencephalogram (EEG), and brain imaging. Further investigations are neurometabolic tests including plasma lactate, amino acids, urine organic acids, and white cell enzymes, together with a paediatric ophthalmology assessment. If at this stage, no underlying diagnosis has been established and the possibility of NCL remains, then investigation following the algorithm is recommended.

Lithium heparin and EDTA (ethylenediaminetetraacetic acid) blood samples are collected. DNA can be extracted and stored for later use, if necessary. After discussion with the laboratory, samples can be assayed for CTSD, TPP1, and PPT1 activities, which, if reduced, will confirm CTSD deficiency (CLN10 disease), CLN2, or CLN1 disease respectively. A thick blood film can be prepared and the tail examined for the presence of vacuolated lymphocytes that, in this context, would suggest CLN3 disease, juvenile onset. A sample can be sent at the same time for preparation and later electron microscopy (EM) examination of white cells, if appropriate.

If no positive results emerge, the clinical history and all information available should be reviewed. If NCL still seems a possibility, then histological and EM examination of peripheral blood white blood cells and/or skin biopsy material should be performed. Part of the skin biopsy sample should be sent for fibroblast culture to provide a resource for further diagnostic enzyme and genetic studies without the need to re-bleed the child. Cultured fibroblasts are also a valuable research resource.

If NCL is confirmed, further enzyme and genetic tests should be requested in order to characterize the biochemical abnormality and/or gene mutation responsible in each individual case. A full list of published and recently described mutations is given at http://www.ucl.ac.uk/ncl. The most frequently encountered NCL genetic diagnoses will vary according to the family ethnic background. The order in which NCL genes are tested for mutations may need to be adjusted with this in mind.

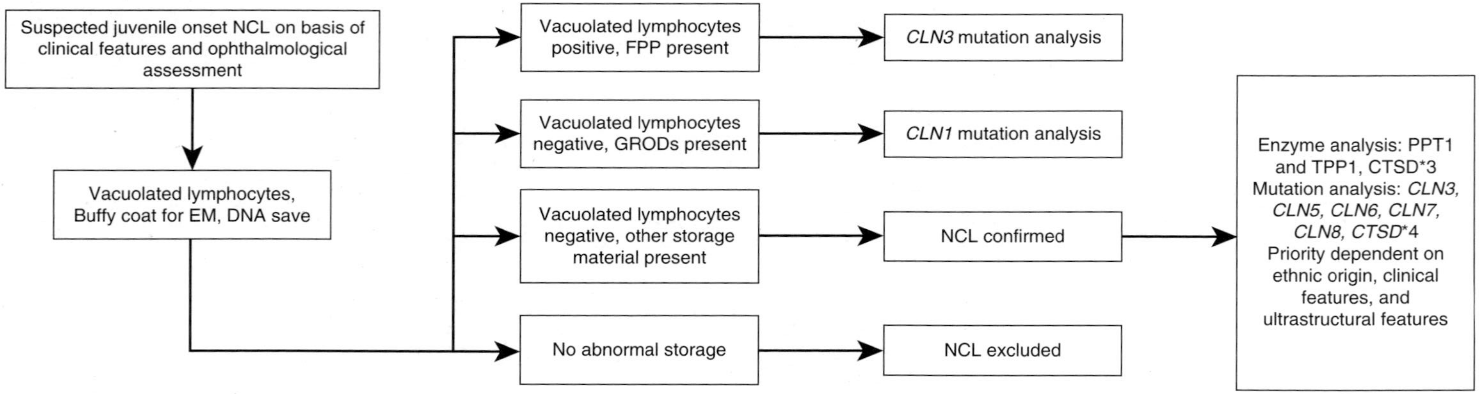

Figure 3.1 Algorithm A: suspected juvenile onset NCL.
CTSD, cathepsin D; EM, electron microscopy; FPP, fingerprint profiles; GRODs, granular osmiophilic deposits; NCL, neuronal ceroid lipofuscinoses; PPT1, palmitoyl protein thioesterase 1; TPP1, tripeptidyl peptidase 1.
*3 May have been performed earlier in the pathway.
*4 Mutation testing of additional NCL genes may become available in the future.
For up-to-date information see http://www.ucl.ac.uk/ncl

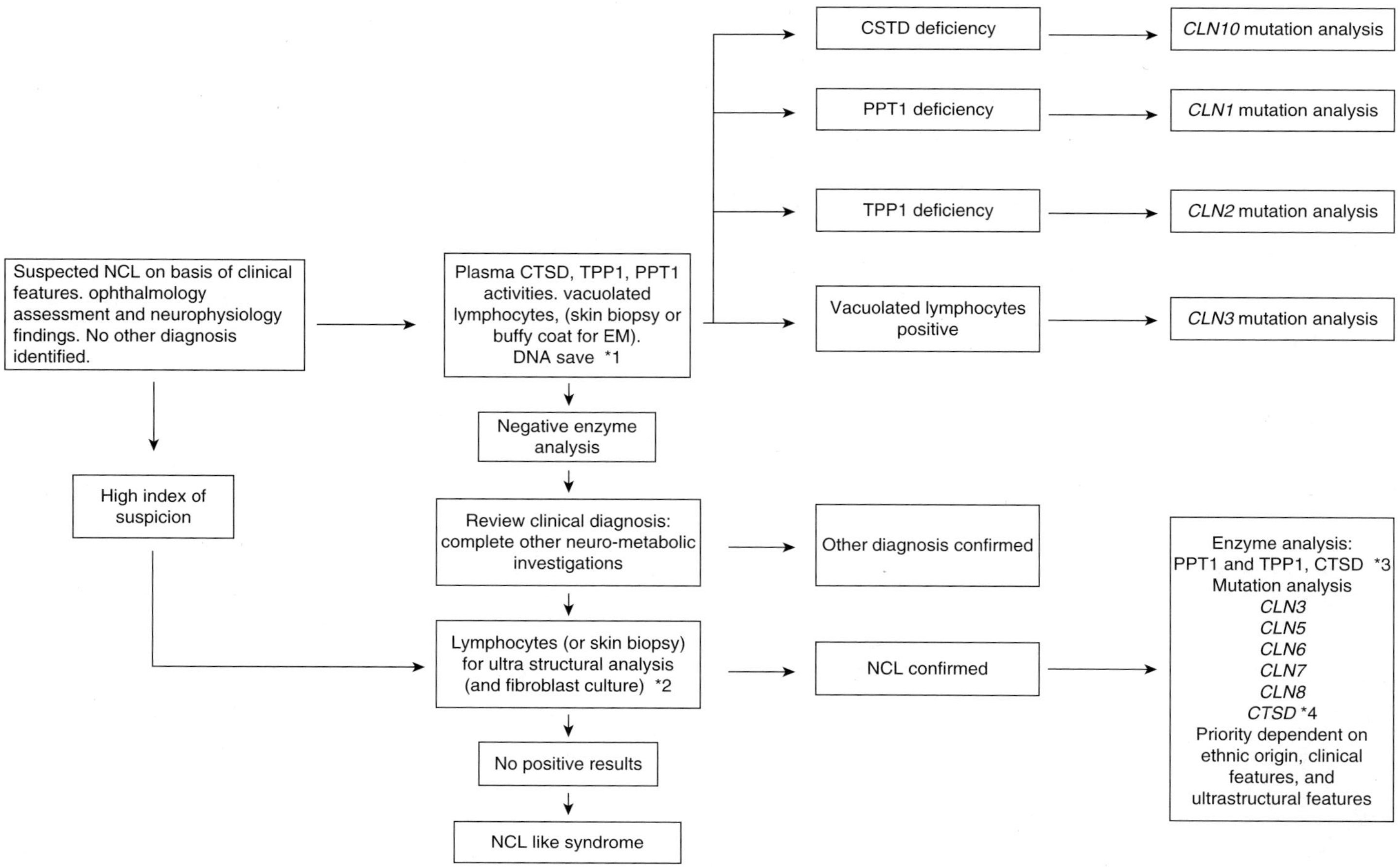

Figure 3.2 Algorithm B: suspected NCL, all types.
CTSD, cathepsin D; EM, electron microscopy; NCL, neuronal ceroid lipofuscinoses; PPT1, palmitoyl protein thioesterase 1; TPP1, tripeptidyl peptidase 1.
*1 Plasma CTSD activity may not yet be available in all diagnostic laboratories. Where there is a high level of clinical diagnostic suspicion of NCL, a blood sample should be sent for ultrastructural analysis.
*2 Samples for ultrastructural analysis should be obtained. Centres vary in sample preference and experience and therefore liaison with the examining team is essential in order that the most appropriate samples are collected and prepared adequately. Skin biopsy has the advantage over lymphocytes that the sample can be split and used also for fibroblast enzyme analysis, DNA extraction and for research purposes.
*3 May have been performed earlier in the pathway
*4 Mutation testing of additional NCL genes may become available in the future.
For up-to-date information see http://www.ucl.ac.uk/ncl

Further comments

There is, despite such investigation, a significant minority of cases for whom no diagnosis can be made despite extensive investigation including neurophysiological, biochemical, enzymatic, genetic, and imaging studies. Some of these will have an NCL-like phenotype but typical storage material in neurons is absent. The management of these children will be very similar to those having a confirmed diagnosis, requiring an integrated multidisciplinary and multi-agency approach but they cannot be given a diagnosis of an NCL disorder, which can be defined as:

> A progressive degenerative disease affecting the brain and, in most cases, the retina, in association with intracellular storage of material that is morphologically characterized as ceroid lipofuscin or similar to it.

Table 3.1 gives a summary of the early clinical features of the different classical and variant NCLs by gene.

DIFFERENTIAL DIAGNOSES

The following tables provide differential diagnoses to be considered in particular situations.

Acquired progressive visual impairment in a young child (Table 3.2)

Most children with CLN3 disease, juvenile present initially to ophthalmologists and may be first investigated in the eye clinic. Experienced paediatric ophthalmologists are able to make the diagnosis in many cases quickly, with the minimum of investigations. There are few other conditions which present with rapidly progressive visual failure over several months between the ages of 4–10 years that lead to legal blindness within 2–3 years. It has been suggested that 25% of children who are registered blind in the UK each year because of a retinal or macular cause have this condition. A review of 11 children subsequently diagnosed in one UK centre revealed that at presentation fundoscopy was normal in two children and maculopathy only evolved later. Prior to a confirmed NCL diagnosis, some children had been considered to have cone/rod dystrophy, macular dystrophy, and retinal dystrophy. Night blindness and photophobia were common symptoms (Collins et al., 2006).

Intractable epilepsy and developmental regression in a young child

The EEG may give important evidence in favour of NCL as an underlying diagnosis in young children presenting with refractory seizures, provided activation with slow rate photic stimulation is performed. In CLN2 disease, late infantile onset, early EEGs often show a paroxysmal occipital spike response to slow rate photic stimulation (Pampiglione and Harden, 1977, Binelli et al., 2000). This can alert the physician to the diagnosis. The electroretinogram (ERG) may be diminished with an unusually exaggerated visual evoked potential (VEP).

Vacuolated lymphocytes (Table 3.3)

In a child who has progressive visual impairment but is otherwise well, there should be a low threshold for *CLN3* mutation analysis for the common 1kb deletion. In one reported series, approximately 40% of samples referred for analysis because of ophthalmological concerns were positive for vacuolated lymphocytes indicative of CLN3 disease (Anderson et al., 2005).

PROPOSED AXIAL DIAGNOSTIC SYSTEM OF CLASSIFICATION

The genes underlying most, but not all, human NCL disease have now been identified and it has become clear that this group of diseases shows genetic heterogeneity (mutations in different genes may result in similar clinical disease phenotype), allelic heterogeneity (different mutations within the same disease gene may result in very different clinical disease phenotypes), and can be phenotypically heterogeneous even within the same family (the same mutation in the same disease gene may result in differing clinical symptoms and rates of disease progression). As a consequence of these research developments, we suggest that clinicians should aim to provide every child and family with detailed diagnostic information at

Table 3.1 **Early clinical features of the different classical and variant NCLs**

Disease	Usual age of onset of symptoms (years)	Early symptoms and signs	Neurophysiological findings	Ultrastructural findings	Usual survival (years)	References
CTSD: congenital	Neonatal	Neonatal epileptic encephalopathy, microcephaly, respiratory distress		GRODs		Siintola et al., 2006, Steinfeld et al., 2006
CLN1: infantile	Infancy	Regression in infancy, seizures, spasticity, and visual failure	Iso-electric EEG by 3 years old	GRODs	9–13	Santavuori et al., 1973
CLN2: late infantile	2–4	Seizures, developmental regression, visual failure, and myoclonus	Photic response. Giant VEP, SEP. ERG extinction	CL	6–12+	Sleat et al., 1997
CLN1: late infantile variant	2–4	Developmental regression, irritability, seizures, and visual failure	Vanishing EEG. Giant VEP, SEP. ERG extinction	GRODs	5–12+	Vesa et al., 1995
CLN5: late infantile variant	3–7	Behaviour difficulties, cognitive decline, seizures, visual failure, myoclonus, and motor disorder	Giant VEP, SEP, ERG extinction	Mixed	Teenage+	Santavuori et al., 1982, Santavuori et al., 1991, Holmberg et al., 2000, Pineda-Trujillo et al., 2005
CLN6: late infantile variant	1–5	Visual failure, cognitive decline, seizures, visual failure, myoclonus	ERG extinction	Mixed	Teenage+	Sharp et al., 2003
CLN7: late infantile variant	1.5–6	Visual failure, cognitive decline, seizures, myoclonus	Giant VEP, SEP. ERG extinction	Mixed	Teenage+	Topçu et al., 2004, Siintola et al., 2007, Aiello et al., 2009, Kousi et al., 2009
CLN8: late infantile variant	1.5–7	Visual failure, congnitive decline, seizures, myoclonus	Giant VEP, SEP. ERG extinction	Mixed	Childhood	Topçu et al., 2004, Siintola et al., 2005
CLN8: EPMR	5–10	Seizures, slow cognitive decline	EEG slowing and spikes, ERG unaffected	GRODs, CL	40+	Hirvasniemi and Karumo, 1994, Hirvasniemi et al., 1994, Hirvasniemi et al., 1995
CLN3: juvenile	3–8	Visual failure, seizures and cognitive decline, motor, behavioural, and language difficulties	ERG extinction	Vacuolated lymphocytes, FPP	20–40	Munroe et al., 1997, Bäckman et al., 2005
CLN1: juvenile	4–6	Visual failure, seizures, behavioural problems and cognitive decline		GRODs	10–20	Crow et al., 1997, Hofmann et al., 1999) Stephenson, 1999
Adult	Teenage–40+	Variable		Variable		

CL, curvilinear bodies; ERG, electroretinogram; FPP, fingerprint profiles; GRODs, granular osmiophilic deposits; SEP, somatosensory evoked potential; VEP, visual evoked potential. See individual chapters on each gene for more details.

Table 3.2 **Causes and investigations of acquired progressive visual impairment in children**

Retinal disorders	Optic neuropathies
CAUSES	
Choroidoretinitis	Leber's hereditary optic neuropathy
Viral encephalitis, measles, etc.	
Genetic	Bilateral optic neuritis
Laurence–Moon	Post viral
Alström–Hallgren	Multiple sclerosis
Usher	
Other isolated genetic retinopathies	
Neurodegenerative	Drug related
Peroxisomal	Isoniazid, penicillamine, etc.
Mitochondrial	
NCLs	
Abetalipoproteinaemia	
Mucopolysaccharidoses	
Cerebellar/spinocerebellar degenerations	
Norrie disease	Compressive lesions
	Optic glioma
	Pituitary/hypothalamic tumours
Fuchs' disease	Dominant hereditary optic neuropathy
Vascular disease	DIDMOAD
Vitamin E deficiency	
INVESTIGATIONS	
Paediatric ophthalmology review and fundoscopic examination	
ERG and visual evoked potentials	
Consider MRI brain imaging	
As appropriate:	As appropriate:
Viral studies	Viral studies: blood and CSF
Urine organic acids	Plasma glucose, lactate
Lactate	Paired CSF and plasma oligoclonal bands
Vacuolated lymphocytes	
BP and hearing assessment	
Renal function	
VLCFA	
Vitamin E level	
DNA save	
Genetics opinion	

CSF, cerebrospinal fluid; DIDMOAD, diabetes insipidus, diabetes mellitus, optic atrophy, and deafness; ERG, electroretinogram; MRI, magnetic resonance imaging; VLCFA, very long chain fatty acid.

clinical, biochemical, and genetic levels where possible.

We therefore propose an axial diagnostic classification system not unlike those evolved for the epilepsies and for mental health disorders in children (ICD-10; Engel, 2006). Eponyms should largely be dropped. Although clinically the term 'NCL disorders' is preferred as an overall description, families and those who support them, including fundraisers, require a term that is easy to use, and the already adopted term 'Batten disease' fits this purpose, and can be continued in this context.

The proposed axial system for NCL disorders is as follows:

Axis 1: Affected gene
For example: *CLN1*, *CLN2*, *CLN3*, etc.

Axis 2: Mutation diagnosis—this includes if possible the disease-causing mutations on both disease chromosomes, using internationally standardized notation. It may also

Table 3.3 **Diagnoses and investigations associated with vacuolated lymphocytes in the peripheral blood (after Anderson et al. 2005)**

Disease	Common presenting symptoms
CLN3 disease, juvenile	Visual impairment early school years
Pompe's disease	Hypotonia, cardiac failure, hepatomegaly, death usually within first year
Adult onset acid maltase deficiency	Progressive proximal muscle weakness
Wolman's disease	Diarrhoea and vomiting, failure to thrive, hepatosplenomegaly
GM1 gangliosidosis	Hypotonia at birth, failure to thrive, coarse facial features, hepatosplenomegaly, cardiomyopathy
Galactosialidosis	Progressive cerebellar and extrapyramidal signs, myoclonus and cognitive impairment later, hepatosplenomegaly, dysmorphic features
Mucopolysaccharidosis	Failure to thrive, early developmental delay, hepatosplenomegaly and coarse facial features, mild to severe skeletal changes
I cell disease	Early developmental regression, coarse facial features
Niemann–Pick type A	Hepatosplenomegaly in infancy, early developmental delay, failure to thrive
Fucosidosis	Early developmental delay, progressive spasticity and regression in infancy, and coarse facial features, hepatosplenomegaly.
Mannosidosis	Hepatosplenomegaly, hearing loss and coarse facial features, corneal opacities.
Salla disease	Early developmental delay, progressive cerebellar and extrapyramidal signs, late cognitive impairment. Rare outside Finland
Neuraminidase deficiency (sialidosis II)	Myoclonus, coarse facial features, hepatosplenomegaly. Rare outside Finland

Investigations
Urine amino acids
Urine organic acids
Urine glycosaminoglycans
Urine mucopolysaccharides
Plasma white cell enzymes
Skin biopsy, histopathology and enzyme analysis of cultured fibroblasts
Appropriate genetic mutation analysis once likely diagnosis made on basis of clinical features and biochemical results

include information regarding the predicted effect of the gene product, for example, a truncation mutation predicted to result in a short non-functional protein.

Axis 3: Biochemical phenotype—enzymopathy or deficiency of membrane protein etc.
For example: CTSD, PPT1, or TPP1 deficiency. Enzyme results may be included with reference ranges and type of tissue studied.

Axis 4: Clinical phenotype—gives an indication of age of onset and possible disease course.
For example: congenital, infantile, late infantile, juvenile, adult onset.

Axis 5: Ultrastructural features—particularly important for those cases where no positive diagnostic biochemical or genetic information is available. Should include the specimen type studied (e.g. skin, rectum, conjunctiva) and may include cell types affected. For example: GROD, CL, RL, FP (tissue).

Axis 6: Functionality—this may be a description of current abilities and function, and ultimately may use a universally recognized clinical scoring system, for example, the Hamburg scales (Steinfeld et al., 2002) and the Unified Batten Disease Rating Scale (UBDRS) (Marshall et al., 2005).

Axis 7: Other remarks of possible medical relevance (e.g. additional disabilities, genetic or environmental effects that may affect disease onset and progression).

The diagnostic classification is thus likely to give a 'pedigree' of information with the option to omit some of the information. In particular, Axes 5, 6, and 7 may not be necessary or useful in the majority of cases, depending on the purpose for which the information is being used.

It has been suggested that an abbreviated system would be useful in clinical practice, combining perhaps Axes 1 and 4 only. For example, CLN1 disease, infantile and CLN3 disease, juvenile could be used.

Good tests for the proposed NCL nomenclature are whether it works for all diseases caused by mutations in *CLN1*, whether it works for the very specific disease phenotypes caused by different mutations in *CLN8*, or whether it works for diseases arising from mutations in more than one allele. The following are **hypothetical examples**:

1 Infantile NCL
A child presenting in infancy who has PPT1 deficiency and mutations in *CLN1*:
Short form: CLN1 disease, infantile (alternatively: infantile CLN1 disease or CLN1 disease, classic infantile).
Axis 1: *CLN1*
Axis 2: cln1.001+cln1.001, p.[Arg122Trp]+[Arg122Trp] (p.R122W homozygote)
Axis 3: PPT1 deficiency: white blood cells level 5nmol/hr/mg protein (normal range 17–139)
Axis 4: infantile
Axis 5: GROD (rectum)
Axis 6: Hamburg LINCL score 1, gastrostomy dependent, seizures partially controlled on three anti-epileptic drugs, non-ambulant, no speech, frequent chest infections
Axis 7: younger sibling affected.

2 Juvenile NCL with GRODs
A child presents with visual failure and subsequently develops seizures and loses skills, is negative for vacuolated lymphocytes and has mutation in *CLN1*:
Short form: CLN1 disease, juvenile (alternatively: juvenile CLN1 disease).
Axis 1: *CLN1*
Axis 2: cln1.004+cln1.009, p.[Thr75Pro]+[Arg151X] (p.T75P/R151X heterozygote)
Axis 3: PPT1 deficiency: white blood cells level 12nmol/hr/mg protein (normal range 17–139)
Axis 4: juvenile
Axis 5: GROD (skin)
Axis 6: Hamburg 'JNCL' Score: 5, UBDRS score: physical 47; seizure 12; behaviour 15
Axis 7: mild asthma, no additional difficulties or major health concerns.

3 Variant late infantile NCL, normal enzymes and no mutations identified so far:
Short form: NCL, late infantile variant (alternatively: variant late infantile disease).
Axes 1 and 2: no mutations found in coding region of *CLN3*, *CLN6*, *CLN7*, *CLN8*, *CLCN6* by sequencing of genomic DNA
Axis 3: normal CTSD, PPT1 and TPP1 on blood and fibroblast samples
Axis 4: late infantile variant
Axis 5: mixed FPP, RL, and CVL (skin)
Axis 6: Hamburg 'LINCL' score: 2
Axis 7: single parent.

4 Classical juvenile NCL:
Short form: CLN3 disease, juvenile (alternatively: juvenile CLN3 disease or CLN3 disease, classic juvenile).
Axis 1: *CLN3*
Axis 2: cln3.001+cln3.001, 1kb del+1kb del (homozygous for the 1kb intragenic deletion)
Axis 3: not applicable
Axis 4: juvenile
Axis 5: FPP (skin)
Axis 6: Hamburg 'JNCL' score: 1; UBDRS score: physical 78; seizure 20; behaviour 23
Axis 7: in residential care setting.

5 Late infantile variant:
Short form: CLN8 disease, late infantile variant (alternatively: late infantile CLN8 disease).
Axis 1: *CLN8*
Axis 2: cln8.008+cln8.008, p.[Gly22fs]+[Gly22fs]
Axis 3:
Axis 4: late infantile
Axis 5:
Axis 6:
Axis 7:

6 Progressive epilepsy with mental retardation (EPMR):
Short form: CLN8 disease, EPMR (alternatively: EPMR CLN8 disease).
Axis 1: *CLN8*
Axis 2: cln8.001+cln8.001, p.[Arg24Gly]+[Arg24Gly]
Axis 3:

Axis 4: EPMR
Axis 5:
Axis 6:
Axis 7:

7 Adult onset NCL:
Short form: CLN1 disease, adult (alternatively: adult CLN1 disease).
Axis 1: *CLN1*
Axis 2: cln1.050+cln1.009, p.[Cys45Tyr]+[Arg151X]
Axis 3: PPT1 (0.09)
Axis 4: adult
Axis 5: GROD (rectum)
Axis 6:
Axis 7:

8 Adult onset NCL:
Short form: NCL, adult (alternatively: adult NCL disease).
Axis 1: *CLN5* and *CLCN6*
Axis 2: CLN5:p.[Trp224]+[Tyr374Cys]+CLCN6:p.[Thr628Arg]
Axis 3: normal CTSD, PPT1, and TPP1 on blood and fibroblast samples
Axis 4: adult
Axis 5: GROD and CL (skin)
Axis 6:
Axis 7: father is heterozygous carrier of *CLCN6* and *CLN5* mutations.

In reality the information will be gained in a different order from that above and information for some axes may not be complete. Exclusion information may be available, for example, late infantile onset disease with normal TPP1 activity and no identified mutations in *CLN5* or *CLN6*.

Some diagnostic investigations give definitive results enabling NCL classification, for example, reduced PPT1 enzyme activity and mutations in two disease *CLN1* alleles. Other diagnostic investigations give important descriptive data which guide the order of further biochemical and genetic investigations but which do not add to the definitive diagnostic NCL classification, for example, ultrastructural analysis.

ACKNOWLEDGEMENTS

R.E.W. would like to acknowledge the following colleagues for their specialist input for this chapter: Mr Luis Amaya, Consultant Paediatric Ophthalmologist, Guy's and St Thomas' NHS Foundation Trust, London; Dr Marie Jackson, Director of Supra Regional Laboratory for Genetics, Guy's and St Thomas' NHS Foundation Trust, London; Dr Glenn Anderson, Consultant Histopathologist, Great Ormond Street Hospital for Children, London; Dr Sushma Goyal, Consultant Paediatric Neurophysiologist, Guy's and St Thomas' NHS Foundation Trust, London.

REFERENCES

Aiello C, Terracciano A, Simonati A, Discepoli G, Cannelli N, Claps D, Crow YJ, Bianchi M, Kitzmüller C, Longo D, Tavoni A, Franzoni E, Tessa A, Veneselli E, Boldrini R, Filocamo M, Williams RE, Bertini ES, Biancheri R, Carrozzo R, Mole SE, Santorelli FM (2009) Mutations in MFSD8/CLN7 are a frequest cause of variant-late infantile neuronal ceroid lipofuscinosis. *Hum Mutat*, 30, E530–540.

Anderson G, Smith VV, Malone M, & Sebire NJ (2005) Blood film examination for vacuolated lymphocytes in the diagnosis of metabolic disorders; retrospective experience of more than 2,500 cases from a single centre. *J Clin Pathol*, 58, 1305–1310.

Bäckman ML, Santavuori PR, Åberg LE, & Aronen ET (2005) Psychiatric symptoms of children and adolescents with juvenile neuronal ceroid lipofuscinosis. *J Intellect Disabil Res*, 49, 25–32.

Binelli S, Canafoglia L, Panzica F, Pozzi A, & Franceschetti S (2000) Electroencephalographic features in a series of patients with neuronal ceroid lipofuscinoses. *Neurol Sci*, 21, S83–87.

Collins J, Holder GE, Herbert H, & Adams GG (2006) Batten disease: features to facilitate early diagnosis. *Br J Ophthalmol*, 90, 1119–1124.

Crow YJ, Tolmie JL, Howatson AG, Patrick WJ, & Stephenson JB (1997) Batten disease in the west of Scotland 1974-1995 including five cases of the juvenile form with granular osmiophilic deposits. *Neuropediatrics*, 28, 140–144.

Engel J (2006) *Multiaxial classification of child and adolescent psychiatric disorders: The ICD-10 classification of mental and behavioral disorders in children and adolescents*. Geneva, WHO.

Hirvasniemi A, Herrala P, & Leisti J (1995) Northern epilepsy syndrome: clinical course and the effect of medication on seizures. *Epilepsia*, 36, 792–797.

Hirvasniemi A & Karumo J (1994) Neuroradiological findings in the northern epilepsy syndrome. *Acta Neurol Scand*, 90, 388–393.

Hirvasniemi A, Lang H, Lehesjoki AE, & Leisti J (1994) Northern epilepsy syndrome: an inherited childhood onset epilepsy with associated mental deterioration. *J Med Genet*, 31, 177–182.

Hofmann SL, Das AK, Yi W, Lu JY, & Wisniewski KE (1999) Genotype-phenotype correlations in neuronal ceroid lipofuscinosis due to palmitoyl-protein thioesterase deficiency. *Mol Genet Metab*, 66, 234–239.

Holmberg V, Lauronen L, Autti T, Santavuori P, Savukoski M, Uvebrant P, Hofman I, Peltonen L, & Jarvela I (2000) Phenotype-genotype correlation in eight patients with Finnish variant late infantile NCL (CLN5). *Neurology*, 55, 579–581.

Kousi M, Siintola E, Dvorakova L, Vlaskova H, Turnbull J, Topçu M, Yuksel D, Gokben S, Minassian BA, Elleder M, Mole SE, Lehesjoki AE (2009). Mutations in CLN7/MFSD8 are a common cause of variant late-infantile neuronal ceroid lipofuscinosis. *Brain*, 132, 810–819.

Marshall FJ, de Blieck EA, Mink JW, Dure L, Adams H, Messing S, Rothberg PG, Levy E, McDonough T, DeYoung J, Wang M, Ramirez-Montealegre D, Kwon JM, & Pearce DA (2005) A clinical rating scale for Batten disease: reliable and relevant for clinical trials. *Neurology*, 65, 275–279.

Munroe PB, Mitchison HM, O'Rawe AM, Anderson JW, Boustany RM, Lerner TJ, Taschner PE, de Vos N, Breuning MH, Gardiner RM, & Mole SE (1997) Spectrum of mutations in the Batten disease gene, CLN3. *Am J Hum Genet*, 61, 310–316.

Pampiglione G & Harden A (1977) So-called neuronal ceroid lipofuscinosis. Neurophysiological studies in 60 children. *J Neurol Neurosurg Psychiatry*, 40, 323–330.

Pineda-Trujillo N, Cornejo W, Carrizosa J, Wheeler RB, Munera S, Valencia A, Agudelo-Arango J, Cogollo A, Anderson G, Bedoya G, Mole SE, & Ruiz-Linares A (2005) A CLN5 mutation causing an atypical neuronal ceroid lipofuscinosis of juvenile onset. *Neurology*, 64, 740–742.

Santavuori P, Haltia M, Rapola J, & Raitta C (1973) Infantile type of so-called neuronal ceroid-lipofuscinosis. 1. A clinical study of 15 patients. *J Neurol Sci*, 18, 257–267.

Santavuori P, Rapola J, Nuutila A, Raininko R, Lappi M, Launes J, Herva R, & Sainio K (1991) The spectrum of Janský-Bielschowsky disease. *Neuropediatrics*, 22, 92–96.

Santavuori P, Rapola J, Sainio K, & Raitta C (1982) A variant of Janský-Bielschowsky disease. *Neuropediatrics*, 13, 135–141.

Sharp JD, Wheeler RB, Parker KA, Gardiner RM, Williams RE, & Mole SE (2003) Spectrum of CLN6 mutations in variant late infantile neuronal ceroid lipofuscinosis. *Hum Mutat*, 22, 35–42.

Siintola E, Topçu M, Kohlschutter A, Salonen T, Joensuu T, Anttonen AK, & Lehesjoki AE (2005) Two novel CLN6 mutations in variant late-infantile neuronal ceroid lipofuscinosis patients of Turkish origin. *Clin Genet*, 68, 167–173.

Siintola E, Lehesjoki AE, & Mole SE (2006) Molecular genetics of the NCLs—status and perspectives. *Biochim Biophys Acta*, 1762, 857–864.

Siintola E, Topçu M, Aula N, Lohi H, Minassian BA, Paterson AD, Liu XQ, Wilson C, Lahtinen U, Anttonen AK, Lehesjoki AE (2007) The novel neuronal ceroid lipofuscinosis gene MFSD8 encodes a putative lysosomal transporter. *Am J Hum Genet*, 81, 136–146.

Sleat DE, Donnelly RJ, Lackland H, Liu CG, Sohar I, Pullarkat RK, & Lobel P (1997) Association of mutations in a lysosomal protein with classical late-infantile neuronal ceroid lipofuscinosis. *Science*, 277, 1802–1805.

Steinfeld R, Heim P, von Gregory H, Meyer K, Ullrich K, Goebel HH, & Kohlschutter A (2002) Late infantile neuronal ceroid lipofuscinosis: quantitative description of the clinical course in patients with CLN2 mutations. *Am J Med Genet*, 112, 347–354.

Steinfeld R, Reinhardt K, Schreiber K, Hillebrand M, Kraetzner R, Bruck W, Saftig P, & Gartner J (2006) Cathepsin D deficiency is associated with a human neurodegenerative disorder. *Am J Hum Genet*, 78, 988–998.

Topçu M, Tan H, Yalnizoglu D, Usubütün A, Saatci I, Aynaci M, Anlar B, Topaloglu H, Turanli G, Kose G, & Aysun S (2004) Evaluation of 36 patients from Turkey with neuronal ceroid lipofuscinosis: clinical, neurophysiological, neuroradiological and histopathologic studies. *Turk J Pediatr*, 46, 1–10.

Vesa J, Hellsten E, Verkruyse LA, Camp LA, Rapola J, Santavuori P, Hofmann SL, & Peltonen L (1995) Mutations in the palmitoyl protein thioesterase gene causing infantile neuronal ceroid lipofuscinosis. *Nature*, 376, 584–587.

Chapter 4

Morphological Diagnostic and Pathological Considerations

G. Anderson, M. Elleder, and H.H. Goebel (formerly with S. Carpenter, M. Haltia, B.D. Lake, and J. Rapola)

INTRODUCTION

Diagnosis for a patient with NCL can still require morphological diagnosis when no changes are detected by initial enzyme or mutation tests. Once morphological diagnosis has been made, and based on the results, appropriate enzyme, and/or molecular genetic studies can be recommended, along with genetic counselling. These diagnostic tests are available at a number of specialized laboratories (see http://www.ucl.ac.uk/ncl).

The morphological diagnosis of NCL rests upon the ultrastructural demonstration of NCL-specific structures. This is usually (should be exclusively) in extracerebral tissues, of which circulating lymphocytes and skin or rectal biopsy are most suitable. Other tissues which have been accessed in the past, such as conjunctiva or skeletal muscle, and rarely liver or brain, are no longer used, except, perhaps for brain biopsy in adult NCL. The results of light microscopic studies can be available within a short time-scale (hours to days), but are of limited diagnostic value. The necessary definitive electron microscope ultrastructural studies may take longer (days to weeks).

DEFINITIONS OF THE ULTRASTRUCTURAL PATTERNS FOUND IN NCL

Granular osmiophilic deposits

Granular osmiophilic deposits (GRODs) are membrane-bound, finely granular rounded bodies, measuring up to 0.5μm in diameter that may form aggregates of up to 5μm. This form is

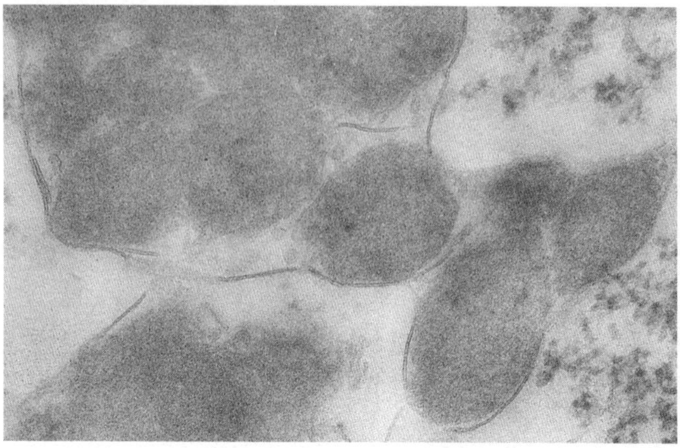

Figure 4.1 Densely packed granular lipopigments, granular osmiophilic deposits (GRODs) typical of CLN1 disease, postmortem brain, ×100,000.

found in the neurons of the central nervous system (CNS) (Figure 4.1) and peripheral nervous system (PNS). In other cell types the granularity is looser (Figure 4.2), and there may be a suggestion of a lamellar substructure. GRODs are the diagnostic feature of CLN1 and CLN10/CTSD diseases. GRODs are not found in association with any of the other inclusions listed below, except in very rare examples of so far undefined types of NCL.

The spectrum of GRODs has recently been extended to the newly identified human disease of cathepsin deficiency (Siintola et al., 2006, Steinfeld et al., 2006) described in neurons and astrocytes in autopsied CNS tissues and formerly called congenital NCL (Humphreys et al., 1985, Garborg et al., 1987) as well as in a nerve fascicle of biopsied skin (Steinfeld et al., 2006). GRODs are also associated with rare examples of so far undefined types of adult NCL (Nijssen et al., 2003). Partial GROD-like condensation may be encountered in other types of NCL (see below).

Curvilinear profiles

Curvilinear (CL) profiles are uniformly curved, short, thin lamellar stacks of alternating dark and light lines with only minor variations in the degree of bending. They usually fill the whole storage lysosome, and are membrane-bound,

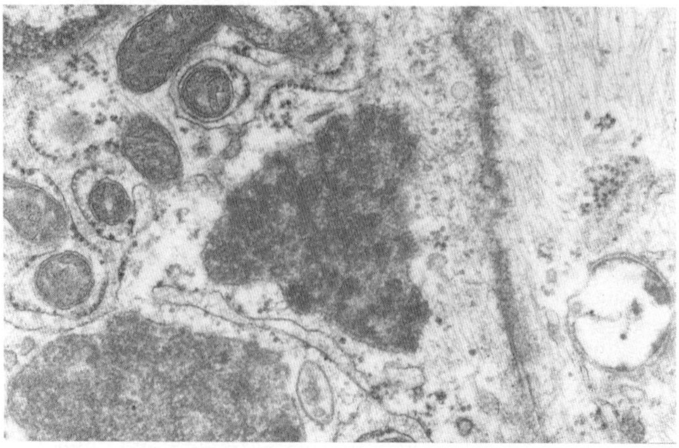

Figure 4.2 More loosely packed granular lipopigments, GRODs, in extracerebral lipopigments typical of CLN1 disease, endothelial cell, ×54,000.

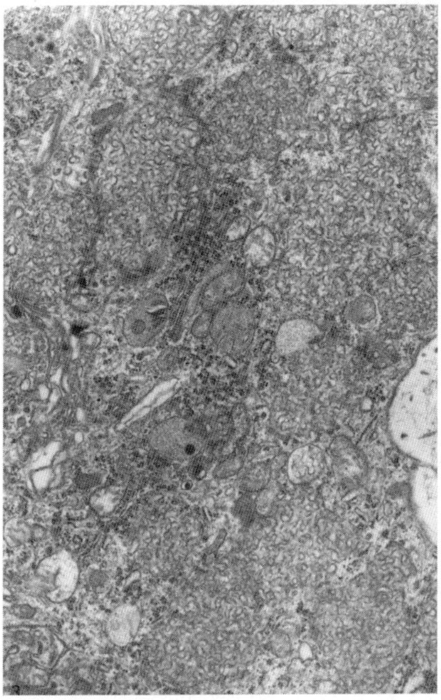

Figure 4.3 Numerous purely curvilinear bodies, typical of CLN2 disease, classic late infantile, appendiceal neuron, ×10,000.

forming CL bodies (Figure 4.3). Dimensions of the lines (light or dense) range from 1.9–2.4nm (Figure 4.4). The lamellar structure may sometimes be less distinct. The CL profiles are buried in a light intervening matrix, the amount and density of which are seldom increased. Typical CLs dominate the ultrastructure in CLN2 disease, classic late infantile. They may occur in other NCL types but as a highly variable phenomenon that should be distinguished from the whole range of curved membranous profiles of the rectilinear complex (see below).

Rectilinear complex

The typical rectilinear (RL) profile represents a short oligolamellar, often pentalaminar stack with a prevailing straight course. It differs from the CL profiles not only by the shape but also by width and distinctness of the internal lines, which range from 2.8–3.8nm. The central line may be rather prominent and dense.

Besides the classic RL profiles there are several other variants of RL that differ in shape but are identical in their internal structure. A common RL variant may strongly resemble the CLs by shape. However, the general arrangement is not so regular, their curves are somewhat flattened, and their internal lamination is wider (see above).

Other forms of the RL complex may also be found less frequently in some biopsy samples and in autopsy tissues. RL stacks of longer course may be present which may resemble loosely stacked classical membranous cytoplasmic bodies composed of polar lipids. This form is more common in the mouse and dog models

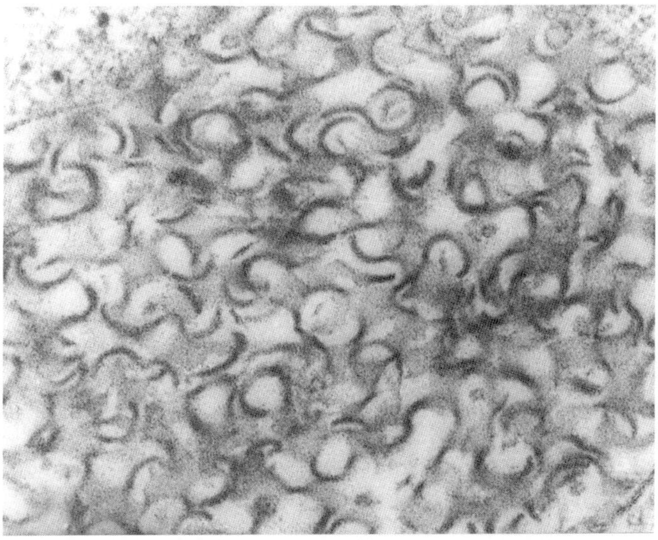

Figure 4.4 Curvilinear profiles at high magnification, typical of CLN2 disease, classic late infantile, appendiceal neuron, ×104,000.

of NCL. When short and stacked to greater extent they may resemble fragmented fingerprint bodies.

The RL complex dominates the ultrastructure of the storage material in CLN3 disease, juvenile and in CLN5, CLN6, CLN7, and CLN8 diseases, late infantile variants. Some of the RL variants may be prevalent in some tissues; i.e. the typical RL is a feature of the inclusions in the skeletal muscle of patients with CLN3, CLN5, CLN6, CLN7, and CLN8 diseases. The RL complex is very often found in association with fingerprint profiles.

NOTE

Due to the occurrence of the described RL variants in many types of NCL, it is recommended that the umbrella term 'RL complex' (Figure 4.5) be used to cover true RLs and all the other subvariants.

Fingerprint profiles

Fingerprint (FP) profiles (Figure 4.6) are composed of paired parallel lines of 7.6–9.6nm width with the central (internal) lucent line ranging between 1–3nm. In very dense FP profiles the central lucent line is barely visible, as much of the space is occupied by the flanking dense lines. The paired parallel lines are separated from each other by a lighter 3–4nm thick *intervening layer*, the origin of which is not certain. Its frequent merging with the lysosomal matrix suggests it may be derived from it and that, in turn, the matrix components might play an important role in the crystalloid arrangement seen in some planes of section. Careful inspection of these deposits shows that the width of the intervening zone may differ considerably. In such 'loosened' FPs (Figure 4.7) the basic lamellae are widely separated, but still exhibit the typical crystalloid pattern. Sometimes the crystalloid deposits are located in a mesh of unorganized single membranes resembling to some extent the basic FP lamellae. The FPs also exist in a rudimentary 'fragmented' form which makes them less distinct. FPs are found in a 'pure' form (i.e. without any CL or RL complex component) in the neurons of the PNS in CLN3 disease, classic juvenile, CLN5 disease, and CLN6 disease. FPs differ from other FP-like crystalloids which are created by complete fusion of the basic membranes in which the intervening lucent layer is missing.

Mixed fingerprint and curvilinear/ rectilinear complex profiles

Mixed FP and CL/RL complex profiles (Figure 4.8) may occur within the same storage body. This is a feature found in smooth muscle cells and endothelial cells in skin and rectal biopsies, and in the sweat gland epithelial cells of the biopsied skin from patients with CLN3 disease, classic juvenile, CLN5 disease, and CLN6 disease. This combination of FP with RL can be dominating.

Condensation of the storage compartment may be responsible for loss of or rudimentary appearance of the lamellar pattern (Figures 4.9 and 4.10). The high degree of condensation may sometimes strongly resemble the so-called GRODs, but is never seen as a dominating generalized structural pattern as GRODs are in CLN1 and CTSD diseases. The condensed fingerprint pattern may be seen particularly in the lymphocytes in cases of the CLN6 and CLN7 diseases, late infantile variants. The condensation could be regarded as a modification of the lysosomal storage material by decreased hydration with subsequent obscuring of the primary lamellar profiles.

In contrast, there are rare vacuolar changes in which the storage body contains essentially electron-lucent material with a minor FP/RL complex component, more often found in CLN3 disease, juvenile than in other NCLs. For example, extensive vacuolar transformation of the storage compartment was described in spiral neurons in CLN3 disease, juvenile (Elleder, 1989, Elleder et al., 1989).

There can also be fusion of storage lysosomes, which may be accompanied by pronounced modification of the stored material. This process is expressed in a selected population of cerebral neurons (basal ganglia and dentate nucleus, in particular). The lysosomal fusion leads to sizeable spheroid formation (Figures 4.11–4.13), localized in the neuronal perikarya. This may occur without any change of the ultrastructure or is accompanied, in many instances, by progressive densification of the

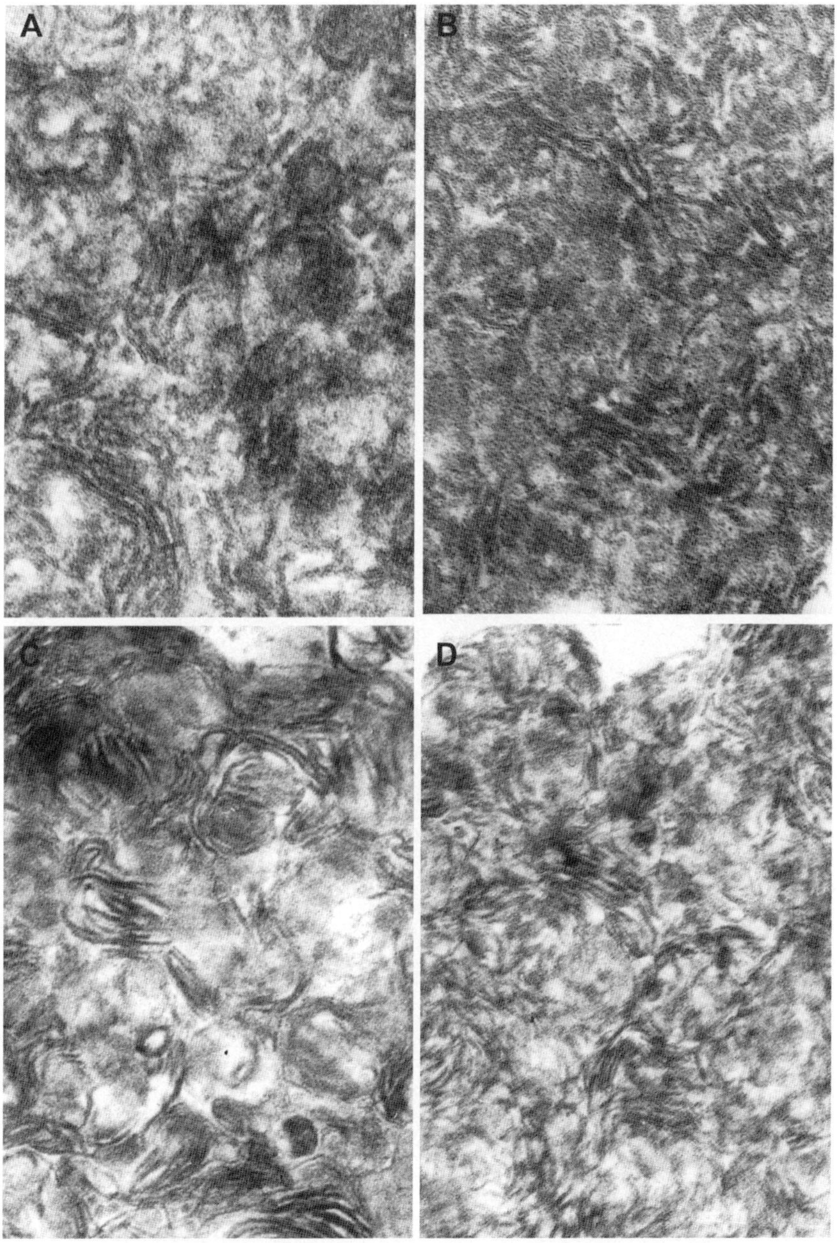

Figure 4.5 A rectilinear complex with slightly wavy course of the rectilinear profiles at various length and bending patterns, some superficially resembling curvilinear profiles, typical of CLN7 disease, late infantile variant, eccrine sweat gland epithelial cells. (A): ×104,000; (B): ×76,000; (C): ×66,000; (D): ×58,000.

stored material leading ultimately to complete obliteration of its ultrastructural details. This process occurs variably in all individual forms of NCL (Elleder, 1978, Elleder and Tyynelä, 1998). The process of densification is paralleled by a distinct change in the staining pattern and by loss of immunodetectability of the specific NCL protein deposits (saposins in CLN1 disease and SCMAS in other NCL forms). It has not been described extraneuronally. There is evidence that the densified spheroid deposits accumulate lactosylceramide that is absent from the rest of the storage compartment in the affected neurons (Hulková et al., 2005). It

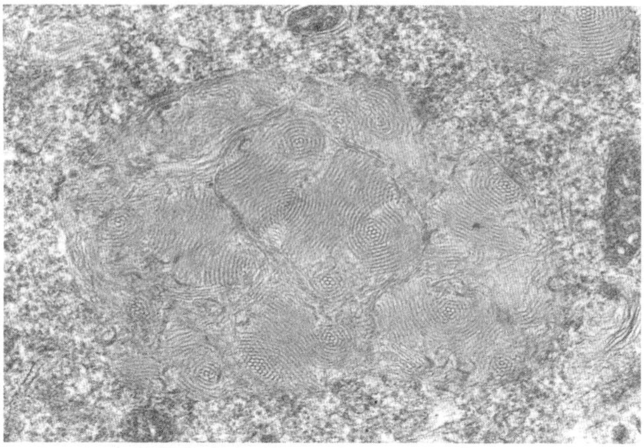

Figure 4.6 Pure fingerprint body, typical of CLN3 disease, rectal neuron, ×75,000.

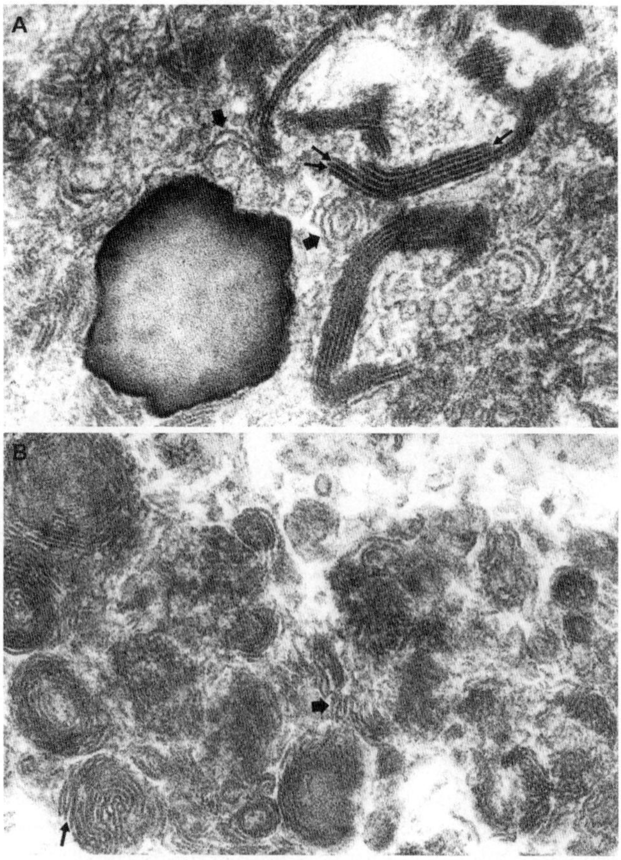

Figure 4.7 (A) Typical dense fingerprint profiles embedded in a mesh of unorganized, short, thick, single membranous profiles (thick arrows) with various degrees of bending. Thin arrows point to free communication of the light layer of the fingerprint body with the matrix, ×104,000. (B) Loose fingerprint profiles of lower density (thick arrow) with free communication of enlarged intramembranous space with matrix (thin arrows), typical of CLN7 disease, late infantile variant, eccrine sweat gland epithelial cells, ×72,000.

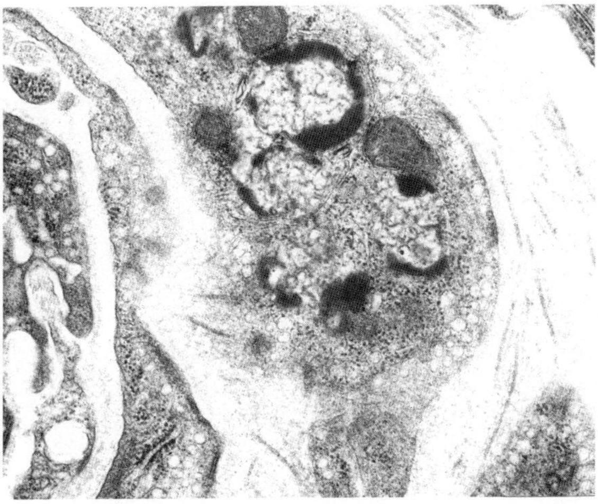

Figure 4.8 Mixed fingerprint curvilinear rectilinear lipopigment, typical of CLN3 disease, juvenile, rectal mural cell of a vessel, ×30,000.

is also worth commenting that in these modified spheroid-shaped storage lysosomes there is prominent accumulation of a lipid-bound (organic solvent extractable) concanavalin A reactive compound, most probably dolichol PP oligosaccharide (Elleder, 1989), in contrast to other storage neurolysosomes, in which the non-lipid concanavalin A reactive compound dominates. This progressive modification, which is still unexplained, differs from the rest of the NCL storage compartment that does not undergo any comparable process. It might reflect specific contact of the storage neurolysosomes with other cell compartments. It has not been described extraneuronally.

NCL LIPOPIGMENTS IN EXTRACEREBRAL TISSUES

The tissue of preference is now a skin biopsy or fresh circulating lymphocytes. However, other types are discussed below for completeness.

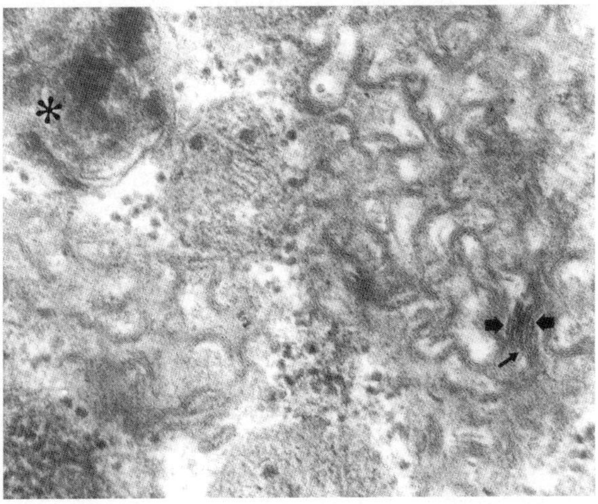

Figure 4.9 Amorphous storage lysosome of condensed type (asterisk) and lysosomal curvilinear-like deposits and small fingerprint focus (between the thick arrows), the membranes of which are in intimate contact with stacked curvilinear-like membranes (thin arrow), typical of CLN7 disease, late infantile variant, dermal endothelial cell, ×76,000.

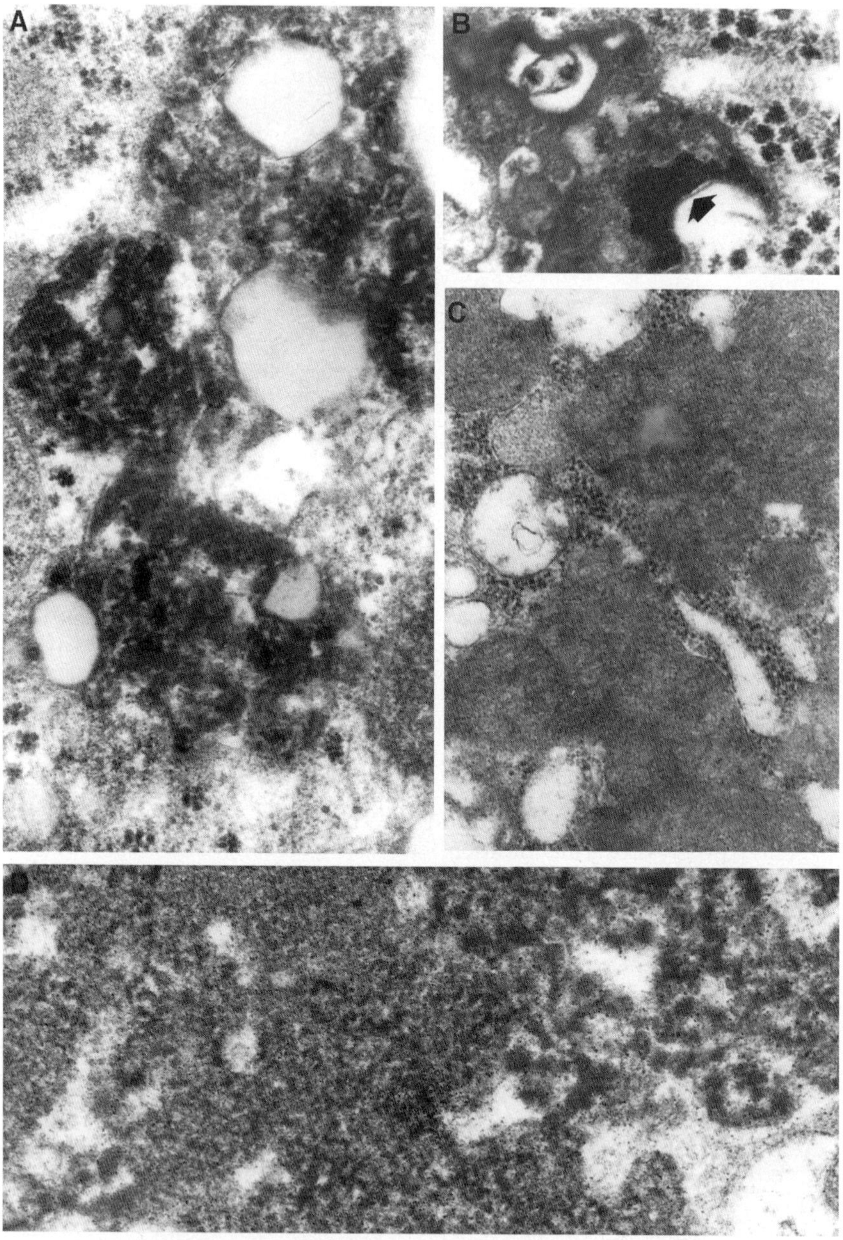

Figure 4.10 Lipopigments with condensed content and thus decreased recognizability of membranous profiles, typical of CLN7 disease, late infantile variant: (A) and (B) liver, amorphous semi-dense lipopigment mass in hepatocytic lysosomes distinct from spontaneously formed lipofuscin in various acquired liver disorders. Thick arrow in (B) points to a haemosiderin focus in the storage lysosome, ×58,000; (C) and (D) show cerebral tissue of the same patient. Condensed almost amorphous compartments (C), ×32,000 and discrete fragments of fingerprint profiles in otherwise amorphous content (D), ×52,000.

Lymphocytes

Examination of peripheral blood lymphocytes by light and electron microscopy can provide a simple, non-invasive, accurate aid to NCL diagnosis. Blood films can first be examined for vacuolated lymphocytes (Anderson et al., 2005), normally associated only with CLN3 disease, juvenile and certain other storage disorders. The remaining (fresh) blood sample is centrifuged to make a buffy coat (concentrated white cell layer), fixed in glutaraldehyde and processed

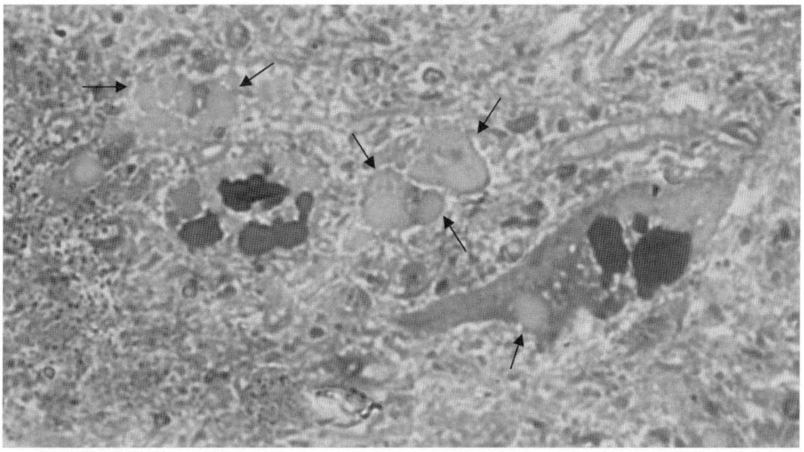

Figure 4.11 CLN2 disease: semithin plastic-embedded section stained with alkalized toluidine blue. Note neurons with lysosomal storage dominated by enlarged spheroid bodies stained either minimally (arrows) or strongly. The strongly stained deposits correspond to those displaying densification in ultrathin sections. Brain (nucleus niger) ×40 objective.

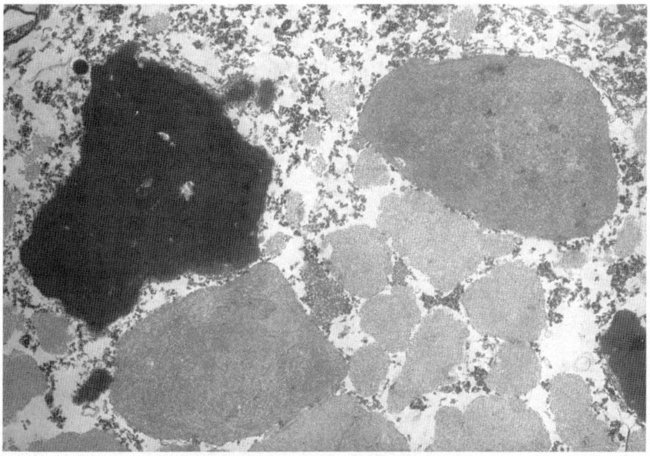

Figure 4.12 CLN2 disease: neuron with storage lysosomes (filled with curvilinear profiles) that fuse to form larger spheroid bodies. In one of them (on the left) the stored content undergoes progressive densification. Brain (nucleus niger), ×5000.

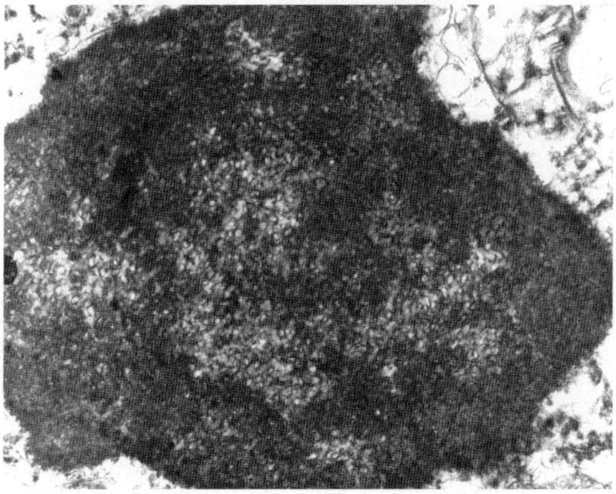

Figure 4.13 CLN2 disease: detailed spheroid inclusion in an intermediate stage of progressive densification. Brain (nucleus niger), ×30,000.

into resin for ultrathin sectioning and examination. Lack of contrast may occasionally impair recognition of NCL storage bodies, and CL or GRODs may be difficult to detect in this situation. It is important when examining a buffy coat strip, that at least 100 lymphocytes should be examined, especially in cases where a variant form of NCL may be suspected, due to the low incidence of positive cells. It should be stressed that attempts to identify the storage lysosomes in lymphocytes using autofluorescence have so far failed. Whether this reflects low sensitivity or other interfering factors is not known.

Ultrastructurally, specific NCL bodies in lymphocytes (Ikeda and Goebel, 1979) include GRODs in CLN1 disease, infantile, late infantile, juvenile, adult variants, CL bodies in CLN2 disease, classic late infantile, FPs within membrane-bound lysosomal vacuoles in CLN3 disease, classic juvenile (Kimura and Goebel, 1988), and compact, often quite large single inclusions with a condensed FP pattern frequently in association with a lipid droplet in CLN5, CLN6, CLN7, and CLN8 diseases, late infantile variants (Anderson et al., 2006) (Figure 4.14). In contrast, lymphocytic inclusions have not yet been reported in adult onset NCL. The normally occurring parallel tubular arrays (PTAs), and the tubuloreticular inclusions seen after a viral illness have been mistaken for NCL-specific inclusions, and care should be taken to recognize these as different and non-diagnostic features in peripheral lymphocytes. Lysosomal FPs may occasionally be found in mucopolysaccharidoses (MPSs) as well (Goebel et al., 1981)

The vacuolar change found in CLN3 disease, classic juvenile is readily seen by light microscopy of a stained peripheral blood film, particularly in the trails, an area not usually examined in routine haematological practice (Anderson et al., 2005). A limited number of lysosomal disorders have vacuolated lymphocytes, which allows differential diagnosis (Table 3.3) (Ikeda et al., 1982, Anderson et al., 2005). These include mucolipidoses II and III, the MPSs, sialidosis and GM1 gangliosidosis type I. Electron microscopy in these conditions is not necessary since there is no specific ultrastructural detail to be found within the vacuoles, provided that the lymphocytes have been well fixed for electron microscopy, and not given rise to sometimes considerable swelling of mitochondria and disruption of

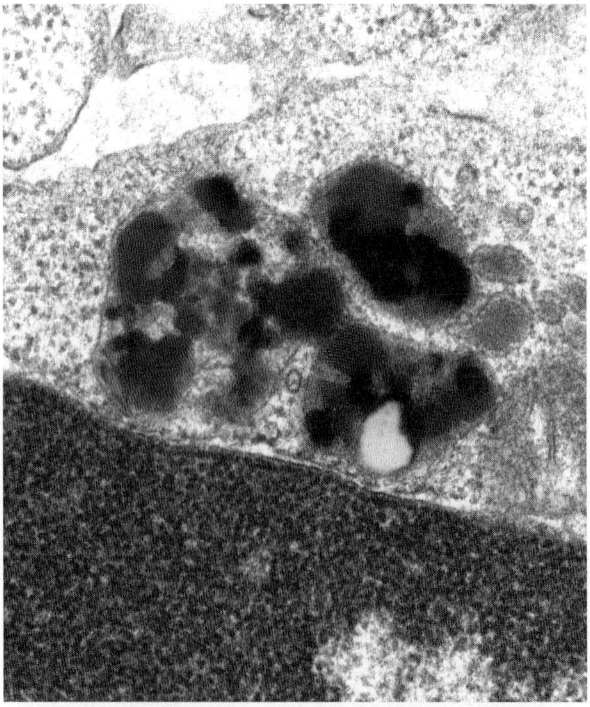

Figure 4.14 Condensed storage inclusions, with fingerprint profiles and a lipid droplet, typical of CLN5, CLN6, CLN7, CLN8 diseases, variant late infantile, lymphocyte from a buffy coat preparation, ×26,000.

their cristae resulting in artificial vacuoles. In the clinical setting of a child with deteriorating vision with no other symptoms, the light microscopic demonstration of vacuolated lymphocytes in the trails of peripheral blood film is almost confirmatory of the diagnosis of CLN3 disease, classic juvenile (see Chapter 3).

Skin biopsy

Skin biopsy is a simple procedure, and a representative sample obtained by a 3mm punch must be deep enough to include eccrine sweat glands, because epidermal cells contain very few lysosomal residual bodies, including NCL lipopigments (Kaesgen and Goebel, 1989). A biopsy from the inner side of the upper arm is ideal. The biopsy should not be taken from the axillary region since no changes typical of NCL are present in the apocrine sweat glands. A second smaller biopsy may be taken to establish a fibroblast culture for enzyme or DNA studies.

Skin contains a wealth of diverse cell types including cells of epithelial, mesenchymal, and neuroectodermal origin, and these may provide a higher diagnostic yield than lymphocytes, both for NCL types as well as for several other neurometabolic and neurodegenerative diseases (e.g. certain lysosomal and peroxisomal disorders, infantile neuroaxonal dystrophy and Lafora body disease). The most important cell type in the skin for diagnosis is the secretory eccrine sweat gland epithelial cell, which must, for an unknown reason, have a high lysosomal turnover. The diagnostic study of skin is incomplete without having examined eccrine sweat gland epithelial cells, particularly when NCL-specific lipopigment bodies have not been identified in other dermal cells. Sebaceous glands and apocrine sweat glands do not form NCL bodies.

A skin biopsy will contain GRODs in CLN1 disease, pure CL bodies in CLN2 disease, classic late infantile, and mixed FPs and profiles of the RL complex, as well as vacuolation, in CLN3 disease, classic juvenile. In CLN5 and CLN6 disease, late infantile variants the appearances are similar, if not identical, to those in CLN3 disease, classic juvenile. There can also be admixture of NCL-specific profiles. In adult NCL, FP profiles have been reported, but FP profiles within eccrine sweat gland epithelial lipopigments may not necessarily be exclusive evidence of adult NCL (Goebel et al., 1995). Thus, in adult NCL, dermal cells other than eccrine sweat gland epithelial cells should be examined for NCL-specific lipopigment bodies. The additional cells to examine in all cases of suspected NCL include smooth muscle cells and endothelial cells, particularly those of the larger blood vessels. In NCL, fibroblasts in general do not exhibit evidence of storage, except in CLN1 disease where GRODs may be found. It is usual practice to find evidence of storage in at least two of the above-mentioned cell types before a diagnosis of NCL is made. Isolated inclusions in a macrophage are not enough evidence.

It should be noted that mast cell granules are a frequent source of misdiagnosis of NCL. Another cause of confusion is membranous bodies in normal eccrine sweat gland ducts, the origin of which is not easy to interpret (Carpenter, 1988). They may represent degenerated mitochondria (Figure 4.15). Also, there are pleiomorphic inclusions in subepidermal and perivascular macrophages, composed of remnants of phagocytosed melanin mixed with lipopigment structures.

An acid phosphatase reaction will indicate the involvement of the sweat gland epithelial cells in cryostat sections of a skin biopsy, but will not differentiate NCL from other lysosomal storage disorders. Lysosomal NCL deposits display strong uniform and homogenous activity of acid phosphatase (using the azocoupling technique with naphthol ASBI phosphate and hexazonium pararosaniline). By this, they differ from distinct age pigment deposits (lipofuscin) seen almost regularly in young controls (after age 10 years) in which the activity is mostly confined to the periphery of individual lipofuscin granules. Outer root sheath epithelial cells of hair follicles in the catagen phase may be strongly autofluorescent and acid phosphatase-positive (M. Elleder, personal experience). Note that if the skin biopsy sample is delivered in the physiological solution or in the transport tissue culture medium the autofluorescence may be quenched; however, acid phosphatase activity persists and the ultrastructure is unchanged (M. Elleder, personal experience in CLN2 disease).

There are further differential diagnostic aspects to be heeded when studying skin. Non-specific enlargement of unmyelinated terminal axons with degenerative changes may be found in NCL. But since these changes can also be found in other lysosomal disorders they are

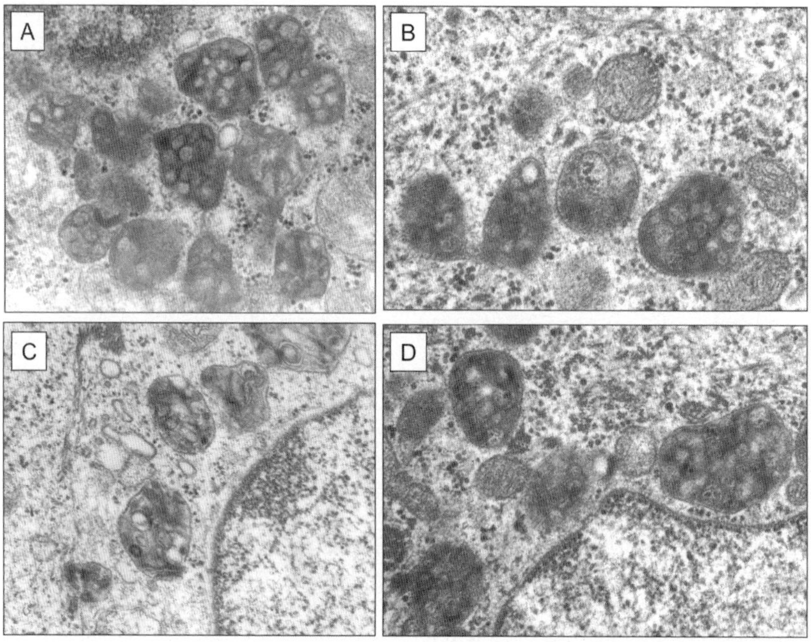

Figure 4.15 (A–D) Inclusions considered putative abnormal mitochondria in eccrine sweat gland ductal epithelial cells which might resemble normal lysosomes in NCL. The samples are from patients with unrecognized neurological disorders and Zellweger disease, ×50,000.

not diagnostic without other evidence of NCL, or other specific inclusions, in different cell types (Walter and Goebel, 1988). The neuroaxonal dystrophies are characterized by enlarged unmyelinated terminal axons among smooth muscle cells and particularly around sweat gland epithelial cells, filled with irregular cisternal profiles, mitochondria, and dense bodies with an occasional cleft identical with those seen in the brain in this group of conditions (Kimura et al., 1987). In Lafora body disease, polyglucosan bodies may be formed within ductal sweat gland epithelial cells, but these are better seen in the axillary apocrine sweat gland epithelium (Goebel, 1997).

Rectal biopsy

Rectal biopsy (preferably as cryostat sections of frozen samples) has in the past been used for light microscopical assessment of NCL to determine whether neuronal storage is present and to define which cell types are involved. This can be done using an acid phosphatase reaction, staining with Sudan black, periodic acid–Schiff (PAS), Luxol fast blue and examination, with epi-illumination or dark-ground transmitted ultraviolet light, for autofluorescence. Young children will have little or no normal lipofuscin (age pigment), but healthy adults may have striking amounts. The differentiation of age pigment from the specific NCL autofluorescence can be difficult but with a good combination of filters (excitation around 360–390nm; barrier filter with cut off at 410nm), the specific autofluorescence of NCL is towards the yellow end of the spectrum, while normal lipofuscin has a more orange colour.

In rectal tissue, the neurons of the submucosal (and myenteric) plexuses display GRODs in CLN1 disease, classic infantile, CL bodies in CLN2 disease, classic late infantile, and pure FP inclusions (without evidence of the components of the rectilinear complex) in CLN3 disease, classic juvenile, and in CLN5 and CLN6 diseases, late infantile variants.

Other tissues

Skeletal muscle fibres show ultrastructural evidence of storage that may be very difficult to identify even when the diagnosis has been confirmed by other means. In NCL caused by mutations in CLN1 disease, classic infantile GRODs are found, while CL bodies, which may be condensed, are seen in CLN2 disease, classic late infantile. No FP profiles are found in the skeletal muscle fibres of the juvenile or variant forms of NCL; instead there are profiles of the RL complex, which may be difficult to differentiate from true CL bodies. For these reasons, muscle biopsy is not a recommended procedure for diagnosis of NCL. Again, differential diagnostic considerations may be important. Long-term treatment with chloroquine may result in the formation in skeletal muscle fibres (and possibly in skin) of lysosomal inclusions similar to, or identical with CL bodies. However the clinical details of the patient should allow this finding to be put in context.

The spectrum of NCL lipopigment formation in other extracerebral tissues such as *conjunctiva* and *liver*, has been less well explored, although each of these tissues displays type-specific ultrastructural patterns of NCL.

Peripheral nerves have rarely been biopsied although mural cells of endoneurial and perineurial vessels and Schwann cells (more of unmyelinated than myelinated axons) have been found to harbour NCL-specific lipopigments. Dermal Schwann cells of unmyelinated axons have, so far, been found as the sole extracerebral cell population to carry lipopigments of the GROD type in the newly described CLN10/CTSD disease (Steinfeld et al., 2006) although sampling problems prevented sufficient scrutiny of other dermal cell types. In similar patients with congenital NCL (Humphreys et al., 1985, Garborg et al., 1987), earlier, electron microscopic studies of *postmortem cerebral* tissues had revealed paired membranous and granular lipopigments in astrocytes (Humphreys et al., 1985) and purely granular lipopigments without CL and lamellar structures in the brainstem, respectively (Garborg et al., 1987). New ultrastuctural data need to be provided of extracerebral tissues in future biopsy studies of similar cases.

OTHER PATHOLOGICAL CONSIDERATIONS

The extracerebral distribution pattern of *storage of subunit c of mitochondrial ATPase* (SCMAS) differs between CLN2, CLN3, CLN5, and CLN6 diseases (Elleder et al., 1997). In CLN2 disease the staining is strong, uniform, and generalized, i.e. present in all cell types affected by storage. In CLN3, CLN5, and CLN6 diseases, the staining of SCMAS is absent in several storage-affected cell types (typically in hepatocytes), i.e. these cells display abnormal autofluorescence, increased acid phosphatase activity, and abnormal deposits by EM. In the CNS, SCMAS immunostaining is much more uniform in CLN2 disease as there is absence of FPs, which do not stain for SCMAS (Rowan and Lake, 1995). This storage pattern is very useful for revision of autopsy cases. Relatively strong staining for SCMAS in smooth muscle cells, cardiocytes, and hepatocytes was observed in a case with increased autophagy (Sikora et al., 2007) suggesting that increased degradation of mitochondria might lead to excessive lysosomal SCMAS accumulation.

Other lipopigments, not related to the NCL, are pure finely granular lipopigments in all forms of vitamin E deficiency, hereditary and acquired ones including the Bassen–Kornzweig syndrome or Abetalipoproteinaemia. Regular lipofuscin or age/wear-and-tear lipopigments are largely composed of a coarse granular matrix and solitary or multiple lipid droplets of varying sizes. Lamellar or membrane fragments may occasionally be incorporated in the granular component. Again, the ultrastructure of lipofuscin may show considerable heterogeneity in various areas of the human brain (Boellaard and Schlote, 1986) and extracerebral tissues.

The heterogeneous ultrastructure of lipopigments in different animal models, both inside and outside of the brain, can best be learned from the individual chapters and illustrations on animal models in this book. Lipopigments accruing in the pigment variant of NCL are described in Chapter 8 on CLN3.

As regards *lysosomal storage in other lysosomal disorders*, the ultrastructure of lysosomal residual bodies can, in principle, be divided into two groups: vacuolar and non-vacuolar. Vacuolar lysosomes are rich in carbohydrate compounds, non-vacuolar ones are rich in sphingolipids and proteins. Hence, MPSs, mucolipidoses, and oligosaccharidoses chiefly show lysosomal vacuoles while type-II glycogenosis may show lysosomal vacuoles filled with remnants and ill-defined glycogen granules if tissue preservation is insufficient, but non-vacuolar lysosomes filled with crisp electron-dense glycogen granules when tissue preservation is good. Lymphocytes in certain MPSs contain vacuolar lysosomes in which occasional FP inclusions can be found (Goebel et al., 1981). The ultrastructure of lysosomal storage inclusions not only depends on their compounds, but also on the types of cells forming these lysosomal residual bodies and the disturbed metabolism of lysosome-targeted metabolites. In MPS, neurons contain Zebra bodies indicating sphingolipids rather than mucopolysaccharides. In mucolipidosis IV, non-vacuolar lamellar inclusions, sometimes resembling membranous cytoplasmic bodies of gangliosidoses, and vacuolar lysosomes occur, though in different types of cells. A similar lysosomal dichotomy is seen in GM1-gangliosidosis, sialidosis, and galactosialidosis.

Non-vacuolar lysosomal residual bodies, though different in ultrastructure to the lysosome-storing cell type in the same lysosomal disease, are seen in sphingolipidoses, both of the neuronal and the demyelinating types. Thus, membranous cytoplasmic bodies accrue in neurons of the gangliosidoses, while prismatic, tufaceous and herring-bone types of lysosomal residual bodies accumulate in metachromatic leucodystrophy, needle-like structures in Krabbe disease, mixed lamellar electron-lucent lysosomal residual bodies in Niemann–Pick disease, and needle-like structures of a different type in Gaucher disease.

PRENATAL DIAGNOSIS

Diagnostic tests can be carried out prenatally in a family that has already had an affected child. In families in whom there is no enzyme deficiency and the gene has not been identified, identification of typical inclusions by electron microscopy are performed on chorionic villus cells (CVS, chorionic villus sampling) from the placenta. The procedure is usually performed at 10–12 weeks of a pregnancy and results may take several weeks. There is a low risk of miscarriage.

It must be emphasized that a prenatal diagnosis of NCL, if followed by termination of the pregnancy, should be confirmed whenever possible by an electron microscopic examination and biochemical analysis of the fetal tissues. This is necessary for audit of the laboratory procedures, and may provide additional helpful information for family counselling, post-termination.

In CLN1 disease the biochemical assay of PPT1 activity allows an independent means of diagnosis on CVS. Ultrastructural studies of blood vessels in CVS have a similar independent confirmatory role in CLN1 disease, probably in CLN3 disease, classic juvenile, and possibly in CLN5 disease, late infantile variant. In CLN2 disease, classic late infantile amniotic fluid cells (and fetal lymphocytes and fetal skin at a later gestational age) have shown prenatal formation of CL bodies, and although in an affected pregnancy there was some minor evidence of CL body formation in placental vessels at 20 weeks, there are to date no data on CVS in pregnancies affected with CLN2 disease. In a series of chorionic villus samples examined ultrastructurally (Fowler et al., 2007) positive findings were reported in two cases of CLN2 disease of approximately 15 weeks' gestation, confirmed by enzyme assay. In other types of NCL there are no data on the electron microscopy of prenatal samples.

REFERENCES

Anderson G, Smith VV, Malone M, & Sebire NJ (2005) Blood film examination for vacuolated lymphocytes in the diagnosis of metabolic disorders; retrospective experience of more than 2,500 cases from a single centre. *J Clin Pathol*, 58, 1305–1310.

Anderson GW, Smith VV, Brooke I, Malone M, & Sebire NJ (2006) Diagnosis of neuronal ceroid lipofuscinosis (Batten disease) by electron microscopy in peripheral blood specimens. *Ultrastruct Pathol*, 30, 373–378.

Boellaard JW & Schlote W (1986) Ultrastructural heterogeneity of neuronal lipofuscin in the normal human cerebral cortex. *Acta Neuropathol*, 71, 285–294.

Carpenter S (1988) Morphological diagnosis and misdiagnosis in Batten-Kufs disease. *Am J Med Genet*, 5 Suppl, 85–91.

Elleder M (1978) A histochemical and ultrastructural study of stored material in neuronal ceroid lipofuscinosis. *Virchows Arch B Cell Pathol*, 28, 167–178.

Elleder M (1989) Lectin histochemical study of lipopigments with special regard to neuronal ceroid-lipofuscinosis. Results with concanavalin A. *Histochemistry*, 93, 197–205.

Elleder M, Goebel HH, & Koppang N (1989) Lectin histochemical study of lipopigments: results with concanavalin A. *Adv Exp Med Biol*, 266, 243–258.

Elleder M, Sokolova J, & Hrebicek M (1997) Follow-up study of subunit c of mitochondrial ATP synthase (SCMAS) in Batten disease and in unrelated lysosomal disorders. *Acta Neuropathol*, 93, 379–390.

Elleder M & Tyynelä J (1998) Incidence of neuronal perikaryal spheroids in neuronal ceroid lipofuscinoses (Batten disease). *Clin Neuropathol*, 17, 184–189.

Fowler DJ, Anderson G, Vellodi A, Malone M, & Sebire NJ (2007) Electron microscopy of chorionic villus samples for prenatal diagnosis of lysosomal storage disorders. *Ultrastruct Pathol*, 31, 15–21.

Garborg I, Torvik A, Hals J, Tangsrud SE, & Lindemann R (1987) Congenital neuronal ceroid lipofuscinosis. A case report. *Acta Pathol Microbiol Immunol Scand A*, 95, 119–125.

Goebel HH (1997) Neurodegenerative diseases: Biopsy diagnosis in children. In Garcia JH, Budka H, McKeever PE, Sarnat HB, & Sima AAF (Eds.) *Neuropathology. The Diagnostic Approach*, pp. 581–635. St. Louis, MO, Mosby.

Goebel HH, Ikeda K, Schulz F, Burck U, & Kohlschutter A (1981) Fingerprint profiles in lymphocytic vacuoles of mucopolysaccharidoses I-H, II, III-A, and III-B. *Acta Neuropathol*, 55, 247–249.

Goebel HH, Warlo I, Klockgether T, & Harzer K (1995) Significance of lipopigments with fingerprint profiles in eccrine sweat gland epithelial cells. *Am J Med Genet*, 57, 187–190.

Hulková H, Ledvinova J, Asfaw B, Koubek K, Kopriva K, & Elleder M (2005) Lactosylceramide in lysosomal storage disorders: a comparative immunohistochemical and biochemical study. *Virchows Arch*, 447, 31–44.

Humphreys S, Lake BD, & Scholtz CL (1985) Congenital amaurotic idiocy—a pathological, histochemical, biochemical and ultrastructural study. *Neuropathol Appl Neurobiol*, 11, 475–484.

Ikeda K & Goebel HH (1979) Ultrastructural pathology of lymphocytes in neuronal ceroid-lipofuscinoses. *Brain Dev*, 1, 285–292.

Ikeda K, Goebel HH, Burck U, & Kohlschutter A (1982) Ultrastructural pathology of human lymphocytes in lysosomal disorders: a contribution to their morphological diagnosis. *Eur J Pediatr*, 138, 179–185.

Kaesgen U & Goebel HH (1989) Intraepidermal morphologic manifestations in lysosomal diseases. *Brain Dev*, 11, 338–341.

Kimura S & Goebel HH (1988) Light and electron microscopic study of juvenile neuronal ceroid-lipofuscinosis lymphocytes. *Pediatr Neurol*, 4, 148–152.

Kimura S, Sasaki Y, Warlo I, & Goebel HH (1987) Axonal pathology of the skin in infantile neuroaxonal dystrophy. *Acta Neuropathol*, 75, 212–215.

Nijssen PC, Ceuterick C, van Diggelen OP, Elleder M, Martin JJ, Teepen JL, Tyynelä J, & Roos RA (2003) Autosomal dominant adult neuronal ceroid lipofuscinosis: a novel form of NCL with granular osmiophilic deposits without palmitoyl protein thioesterase 1 deficiency. *Brain Pathol*, 13, 574–581.

Rowan SA & Lake BD (1995) Tissue and cellular distribution of subunit c of ATP synthase in Batten disease (neuronal ceroid-lipofuscinosis). *Am J Med Genet*, 57, 172–176.

Siintola E, Partanen S, Stromme P, Haapanen A, Haltia M, Maehlen J, Lehesjoki AE, & Tyynelä J (2006) Cathepsin D deficiency underlies congenital human neuronal ceroid-lipofuscinosis. *Brain*, 129, 1438–1445.

Sikora J, Dvorakova L, Vlaskova H, Stolnaja L, Betlach J, Spacek J, & Elleder M (2007) A case of excessive autophagocytosis with multiorgan involvement and low clinical penetrance. *Cesk Patol*, 43, 93–103.

Steinfeld R, Reinhardt K, Schreiber K, Hillebrand M, Kraetzner R, Bruck W, Saftig P, & Gartner J (2006) Cathepsin D deficiency is associated with a human neurodegenerative disorder. *Am J Hum Genet*, 78, 988–998.

Walter S & Goebel HH (1988) Ultrastructural pathology of dermal axons and Schwann cells in lysosomal diseases. *Acta Neuropathol*, 76, 489–495.

Chapter 5

General Principles of Medical Management

R. E. Williams

INTRODUCTION

Despite the findings of extensive basic scientific and clinical research, the NCLs remain a group of neurodegenerative disorders for which there is currently no cure. They share many features with other paediatric progressive neurological disorders. They are, however, characterized by some unique and complex clinical problems. Medical management should follow general principles and good practice, but should also incorporate an appreciation of the special needs of this group. Parents and families are also often keen to explore complementary and experimental therapeutic approaches alongside traditional medicine.

Much can be done to alleviate symptoms using the approaches of traditional medicine. Clinical care aims to minimize the impact of symptoms such as seizures, maintain and promote skills, and to optimize quality of life for affected individuals and their families. Even when potentially curative therapies become available, there will still be an important place for holistic and symptomatic medical care. A multidisciplinary and multiagency (health, education, and social services) approach is essential and must be child-centred. The World Health Organization (http://www.who.int/cancer/palliative/definition/en/) has developed a definition of palliative care for children who are suffering from a life-limiting illness:

> Palliative care for children is the active total care of the child's body, mind and spirit, and also involves giving support to the family. It begins when illness is diagnosed, and continues regardless of whether or not a child receives treatment directed at the disease. Health providers must evaluate and alleviate a child's physical, psychological, and social distress. Effective palliative

care requires a broad multidisciplinary approach that includes the family and makes use of available community resources; it can be successfully implemented even if resources are limited. It can be provided in tertiary care facilities, in community health centres and even in children's homes.

In this definition of palliative care, a holistic approach of patient care is clearly described.

Much of current medical, nursing, and therapy practice in the NCLs does not have a solid evidence base. Much of what is presented here is based on personal practice and narrative or anecdotal evidence from professional colleagues both in the UK and internationally.

EPILEPSY

A symptomatic generalized epilepsy syndrome is a dominant feature of all NCLs. In some NCLs, particularly those with onset in the infantile and late infantile age ranges, the epilepsies are usually considered with the progressive myoclonic epilepsies (PMEs).

Epilepsy: CLN3 disease

Epilepsy occurs in all children with classic juvenile CLN3 disease and is a major feature from the middle school years onwards. In a Finnish series, the mean age of onset of seizures was 10 years (Åberg et al., 2000). Seizures are often generalized and initially only occasional, becoming more frequent and with the onset of other seizure types (focal onset, atypical absences, and later myoclonic) within 1–2 years. Subtle partial seizures, which may be prolonged, are often difficult to recognize and may be difficult to describe and classify.

Combination anti-epileptic drug (AED) therapy is usually but not always necessary eventually. Seizures should be managed according to usual epilepsy principles: monotherapy where possible, one drug change at a time using minimum dosages necessary to achieve reasonable seizure control. Each child is, of course, unique and not all with the same condition respond in the same way to similar drug regimens. A balance must be struck between reasonable seizure control and side effects of medication. Although at present the NCLs are progressive and incurable, worsening seizures may not be a sign of the last stages of the disease and consideration should be given to modifying drug regimens in order to improve seizure control and hence quality of life.

Practice varies throughout Europe and North America regarding which AED is used as first line. It is generally agreed that carbamazepine, vigabatrin, and gabapentin may worsen seizures in the PMEs. Sodium valproate, lamotrigine, and topiramate have been helpful individually and in combination in CLN3 disease, juvenile onset (Åberg et al., 1999, Åberg et al., 2000). More recently, levetiracetam has been shown to be effective and also improves the tremor seen in some young people (R. Niezen-de Boer, personal communication, Abstract 10th International NCL Conference 2005). Some children and young people do suffer prolonged convulsive episodes which can be treated along standard lines with rectal or buccal benzodiazepines or with rectal paraldehyde. A short course of oral clobazam has also been used to terminate clusters of seizures

Epilepsy: infantile and late infantile onset NCLs (CLN1, 2, 5, 6, 7, 8 diseases)

Children subsequently found to have either CLN2 disease, late infantile onset, or one of the variant late infantile onset NCLs may present with seizures, and epilepsy often quickly becomes the dominant feature. Seizures may be generalized tonic–clonic, atonic, or of focal onset initially. Commonly other seizure types develop and some may be difficult to classify. Seizures may or may not respond initially to medication, but usually become resistant to treatment within 12–36 months of onset. Myoclonus gradually becomes more evident in parallel with loss of mobility and communication skills, and may become a major symptom in the later stages of disease. Myoclonic status is seen occasionally.

Children with CLN1 disease, infantile onset, also have frequent seizures from an early stage together with myoclonic jerks. The clinical picture is dominated, however, by loss of skills and severe motor disability.

The earlier comments referring to general principles of epilepsy drug management in

CLN3 disease also apply here. In general, carbamazepine, vigabatrin, and gabapentin should be avoided as seizure control may worsen with these agents. Lamotrigine may exacerbate myoclonus and may be responsible for an accelerated loss of skills, especially mobility. Valproate, clobazam, and topiramate have been helpful singly or in combination. Levetiracetam shows promise and its use should be evaluated further. Piracetam may be used for myoclonus with good effect. A ketogenic diet has yet to be established as a management option in this condition, but NCL is not a contraindication to its use. Phenobarbitone, orally or via continuous subcutaneous infusion, may be of use for end-stage myoclonic status. Phenytoin may also be beneficial in the late stages (Miyahara et al., 2009).

NUTRITION AND FEEDING: ALL NCL TYPES

Progressive difficulties with chewing and swallowing are inevitable in all common NCLs of childhood onset. Alternative methods of enteral feeding are generally recommended at some stage because of any or a combination of the following problems: the increased risk of choking and aspiration; poor calorie intake and poor weight gain; excessive time taken to complete meals safely. Clearly attention to seating and posture during mealtimes is essential, along with regular review of the texture and speed of food presentation and delivery. Observation of feeding by an experienced speech and language therapist from time to time is mandatory in optimizing feeding strategies and ensuring safety. Speech and the ability to safely chew and swallow a variety of food textures often show deterioration at around the same time. Planning the placement of a nasogastric or gastrostomy tube to supplement feeding may bring clear benefits in terms of enhanced calorie intake, improved general well-being, and reliable drug administration. Parents are often initially reluctant to proceed with surgery but it should be remembered that many children may continue to have some food by mouth. The option of using a tube for drugs and supplementary fluids and nutrition usually results in improved quality of life for the entire family.

GUT AND CONSTIPATION: ALL NCL TYPES

Aggressive management of constipation with simple laxatives, bowel stimulants, and suppositories and/or enemas as necessary to ensure a regular bowel habit may help to avoid exacerbations of seizures, motor spasms, and emotional/psychiatric symptoms in older children and young adults.

ORAL SECRETIONS AND CHEST COMPLICATIONS: ALL NCL TYPES

Excessive drooling becomes a problem often when oral secretions cannot be easily controlled because of deteriorating mouth and tongue movements. Drooling may be exacerbated by benzodiazepines used to treat seizures. Hyoscine patches and regular oral glycopyrrolate have been of benefit. Botulinum toxin injections to the salivary glands may be helpful, but the effect is temporary, and repeated injections may be required.

Attention to seating, posture, adequate nutrition, and hydration is vital to maintain good chest health and respiratory function. A number of children benefit from prophylactic antibiotics through the winter months and regular chest physiotherapy performed by parents and carers following guidance from a physiotherapist. There is no evidence to suggest that children and young adults with NCL have an additional vulnerability to infections above that experienced by others with complex neurodisability. In the UK, seasonal influenza vaccination is recommended.

MOBILITY AND SPATIAL AWARENESS: TEENAGERS AND YOUNG ADULTS WITH CLN3 DISEASE

Young people with juvenile CLN3 disease develop a very characteristic stooped posture and slow shuffling gait. They have particular difficulties initiating movement, and in performing activities of daily living. They lose balance easily and early warnings include frequent trips and falls. Anxiety is often prominent and particularly related to stairs and uneven surfaces. Early mobility training before sight is lost completely is recommended.

Attention to posture and seating, lifting, and handling issues are very important from early on. Enjoyable and therapeutic activities such as swimming and walking should be encouraged in order to enhance well-being, maintain good posture, independence, and prevent injury and deformity. The role of anti-Parkinsonian drugs has been explored and practice varies. Potential drawbacks in the use of L-dopa treatment include drug interactions and the risk of long-term extrapyramidal effects together with the risk of acute neuroleptic malignant syndrome (Vercammen et al., 2003). An open study in Finland assessed the response to L-dopa of 21 young people using a modified UPDRS (United Parkinson's Disease Rating Scale) before and during treatment. There was a favourable response to levodopa at 1 year over a small control group (Åberg et al., 2001). The long-term effects in this condition have not been studied.

MOTOR DISORDER: INFANTILE AND LATE INFANTILE NCLS

Later features of these diseases include pyramidal and extrapyramidal movement disorders. Treatment will usually include attention to seating, posture management, and physiotherapy aiming to maintain range of movement and prevent joint contractures. Muscle relaxants such as baclofen and low-dose benzodiazepines have a place. Botulinum toxin injections may be considered. A choreiform movement disorder is common and high doses of trihexyphenidyl hydrochloride (benzhexol, Artane®) may be necessary.

COMMUNICATION: CLN3 DISEASE

The evolution of speech and communication difficulties in juvenile CLN3 disease has a very characteristic quality. As with movements, there is difficulty initiating a phrase or sentence resulting in dysfluency. Speech becomes pressured. Recurrent themes of conversation are common and often exasperating for carers. Understanding is preserved well beyond the ability to communicate freely with others, with consequent frustration and sometimes anger. The variability in abilities from day to day is significant and an additional challenge for teachers, therapists, and carers. Medical management includes attention to dental health, saliva control, and extrapyramidal movement disorder.

The importance of life story work and memories of important events, objects, and feelings, is well recognized amongst those professionals working closely with young people affected by juvenile CLN3 disease (see http://www.seeability.org).

EMOTIONAL AND MENTAL HEALTH: CLN3 DISEASE

Seventy-four per cent of young adults with juvenile CLN3 disease have emotional or behavioural symptoms (Bäckman et al., 2005). A familiar and safe environment with a structured but varied daily programme of activities has been found to be most helpful. Daily routines should be adapted for the individual and be flexible, depending on the mood and day-to-day variation of abilities. Life story and memory work, which are also very important, have already been mentioned earlier with regards to communication.

Hallucinations may be a prominent feature. Often these are visual, but auditory and sensory hallucinations may also occur. They may be unpleasant but this is not always the case. The pathophysiological basis of these hallucinations is unclear. It is likely that they may sometimes represent misinterpretation of visual clues and that attention to environmental lighting and shadows is therefore important. The relationship between hallucinations, sleep disturbance, epileptic activity (clinically evident and subclinical), and visual failure is not understood. Acutely, a quiet and familiar space, with minimum interference and calming reassurance from one key person, often eases the situation. Sometimes, a single dose of an antipsychotic drug such as oral risperidone is needed early in the course of a hallucination in order to terminate a distressing episode. A few young people require regular antipsychotic medication. Regular use of antipsychotics may be necessary but important side effects include weight gain and exacerbation of extrapyramidal movement disorders (Gospe and Jankovic, 1986). Increased tiredness, lowered seizure threshold, and the potential for malignant neuroleptic syndrome, are also significant concerns (Bäckman et al., 2001). Risperidone is probably most widely used in this condition, but experience using olanzapine and sulpiride also exists.

Occasionally depression is a dominant problem and treatment with a selective serotonin reuptake inhibitor (SSRI) is indicated (Åberg et al., 2001).

SLEEP DISTURBANCE: ALL NCL TYPES

Sleep disturbance is common but not invariable in juvenile CLN3 disease—sometimes before the onset of epilepsy. Melatonin was not found to be very helpful in a small group of young people in Finland with sleep disturbance (Hätönen et al., 1999).

Children with infantile and late infantile onset NCL seem almost invariably to have problems, both settling to sleep and staying asleep at night. The cause of any pain or distress should be sought with careful attention to skin, teeth, constipation, bones, and joints. Some children are helped by analgesia, including opiates, especially in the late stages of disease (Mannerkoski et al., 2001). Melatonin does not seem to be very helpful. Chloral hydrate can be used to help settle children at night and to reduce irritability by day. It also may improve myoclonic jerks.

FAMILY CARE AND SUPPORT

Families and carers also have needs which change over time: coming to terms with a new diagnosis; understanding the illness; accessing appropriate medical, educational, and social care support. Bereavement counselling during the early stages should be offered, together with written information and contact details for professionals and parent support groups. Most families will have a multitude of professional contacts and appointments. The identification of a key worker who is able to coordinate and arrange meetings and appointments between professionals and parents/carers should be encouraged.

ACKNOWLEDGEMENTS

Grateful thanks are given to families and carers, to professional multidisciplinary colleagues in the UK and elsewhere in Europe, and to the members of the UK Batten Disease Professional Group. Special thanks go to Sarah Kenrick of SeeAbility Heather House.

REFERENCES

Åberg L, Kirveskari E & Santavuori P (1999) Lamotrigine therapy in juvenile neuronal ceroid lipofuscinosis. *Epilepsia*, 40, 796–799.

Åberg LE, Bäckman M, Kirveskari E & Santavuori P (2000) Epilepsy and antiepileptic drug therapy in juvenile neuronal ceroid lipofuscinosis. *Epilepsia*, 41, 1296–1302.

Åberg LE, Rinne JO, Rajantie I & Santavuori P (2001) A favorable response to antiparkinsonian treatment in juvenile neuronal ceroid lipofuscinosis. *Neurology*, 56, 1236–1239.

Bäckman ML, Åberg LE, Aronen ET & Santavuori PR (2001) New antidepressive and antipsychotic drugs in juvenile neuronal ceroid lipofuscinoses—a pilot study. *Eur J Paediatr Neurol*, 5 Suppl A, 163–166.

Bäckman ML, Santavuori PR, Åberg LE & Aronen ET (2005) Psychiatric symptoms of children and adolescents with juvenile neuronal ceroid lipofuscinosis. *J Intellect Disabil Res*, 49, 25–32.

Gospe SM, Jr. & Jankovic J (1986) Drug-induced dystonia in neuronal ceroid-lipofuscinosis. *Pediatr Neurol*, 2, 236–237.

Hätönen T, Kirveskari E, Heiskala H, Sainio K, Laakso ML & Santavuori P (1999) Melatonin ineffective in neuronal ceroid lipofuscinosis patients with fragmented or normal motor activity rhythms recorded by wrist actigraphy. *Mol Genet Metab*, 66, 401–406.

Mannerkoski MK, Heiskala HJ, Santavuori PR & Pouttu JA (2001) Transdermal fentanyl therapy for pains in children with infantile neuronal ceroid lipofuscinosis. *Eur J Paediatr Neurol*, 5 Suppl A, 175–177.

Miyahara A, Saito Y, Sugai K, Nakagawa E, Sakuma H, Komaki H & Sasaki M (2009) Reassessment of phenytoin for treatment of late stage progressive myoclonus epilepsy complicated with status epilepticus. *Epilepsy Res*, 84, 201–209.

Vercammen L, Buyse GM, Proost JE & Van Hove JL (2003) Neuroleptic malignant syndrome in juvenile neuronal ceroid lipofuscinosis associated with low-dose risperidone therapy. *J Inherit Metab Dis*, 26, 611–612.

Chapter 6

CLN1

T. Autti, J.D. Cooper, O.P. van Diggelen, M. Haltia, A. Jalanko, C. Kitzmüller, O. Kopra, T. Lönnqvist, A. Lyly, S.E. Mole, J. Rapola, and S.-L. Vanhanen

INTRODUCTION

Mutations in the *CLN1* gene cause classic CLN1 disease, infantile, formerly known as infantile NCL (INCL) or Santavuori–Haltia disease, as well as CLN1 disease with later ages of onset. *CLN1* encodes an enzyme, palmitoyl protein thioesterase 1, making it suitable for current therapeutic development. Few other NCL types have onset in infancy.

MOLECULAR GENETICS

Identification of the *CLN1* gene

A random genome scan for the *CLN1* gene in Finnish families resulted, in 1991, in linkage to markers on 1p32 (Järvelä, 1991) Linkage disequilibrium mapping in Finnish disease alleles assigned the locus to a 300kb critical region. Fine mapping of this region revealed that the gene encoding palmitoyl protein thioesterase 1 (PPT1) was a positional candidate for the *CLN1* gene. Identification of multiple mutations in this gene in CLN1 disease, infantile patients verified that the *PPT1* gene was the *CLN1* gene (Vesa et al., 1995).

Gene structure

The *PPT1* gene consists of nine exons spanning 25kb of chromosomal DNA. A single mRNA of 2.4kb is detected on RNA blotting of a variety of human tissue, and it encodes a 306-amino acid polypeptide (Schriner et al., 1996).

Mutations

To date, 49 different mutations have been described (http://www.ucl.ac.uk/ncl/cln1.shtml) currently comprising 23 missense mutations, six mutations within conserved elements of splice junctions or which probably affect splicing, eight small deletions or insertions, one large deletion, one mutation that affects the initiation codon, nine nonsense mutations, and one undefined mutation that prevents transcription (Vesa et al., 1995, Das et al., 1998, Mitchison et al., 1998, Munroe et al., 1998, Santorelli et al., 1998, Salonen et al., 2000, Waliany et al., 2000, van Diggelen et al., 2001a, Mole et al., 2001, Mazzei et al., 2002, Bi et al., 2006, Bonsignore et al., 2006, Kalviainen et al., 2007, Ramadan et al., 2007, Kohan et al., 2009, Kousi et al., 2009, Simonati et al., 2009) (and unpublished). These include the most common mutation, accounting for about 40% of alleles in the US population, a premature stop codon at arginine 151 (p.Arg15X) that results in a severely truncated protein. Another common missense mutation (p.Thr75Pro) represents approximately 17% of US subjects and is associated with CLN1 disease, juvenile with granular osmiophilic deposits (formerly vJNCL/GROD). A cluster of these subjects has been identified in Scotland and all US subjects report Scottish or Irish ancestry (Das et al., 1998, Mitchison et al., 1998). All cases of CLN1 disease, infantile in Finland carry a common missense mutation (p.Arg122Trp) that leads to an unstable protein that is degraded in the endoplasmic reticulum (ER) (Hellsten et al., 1996). The remaining mutations are infrequent, with many being reported in one or a few families only.

Five polymorphisms are now known.

PPT2

A second lysosomal thioesterase has been described that shares 20% identity with PPT1. The second thioesterase does not complement the metabolic defect in CLN1 disease cells, and its physiological role remains to be determined. However, mice lacking this gene do get NCL-like disease (Gupta et al., 2001). The location of the *PPT2* gene is on human chromosome 6p21.3 (Soyombo and Hofmann, 1997). To date, no patients have been described with mutations in *PPT2*.

CELL BIOLOGY

Tissue distribution of PPT1

In mouse and rat, *Ppt1* mRNA and protein are expressed in most tissues, the expression being highest in spleen, lung, and testis (Salonen et al., 1998, Isosomppi et al., 1999, Suopanki et al., 1999b). In the central nervous system (CNS) the expression of *Ppt1* is under developmental control. This is in contrast to two other NCL genes, *Cln2/Tpp1* and *Cln10/Ctsd* that are expressed at relatively constant mRNA levels throughout development (Suopanki et al., 2000), suggesting a distinctive role of PPT1 in brain development. The expression of *Ppt1* mRNA in the brain increases during brain maturation reaching a peak level in early adulthood (Isosomppi et al., 1999, Suopanki et al., 1999a). *In situ* hybridization analysis shows that *Ppt1* transcripts are found widely but not homogeneously in the brain. The most intense signal is detected in the cerebral cortex (layers II, IV–V), CA1–CA3 pyramidal cells of the hippocampus, granule cells of the dentate gyrus, and the hypothalamus. The expression is mainly neuronal, although some signal can also be detected in glial cells. Also, in the embryonic human brain, *PPT1* mRNA is expressed at the beginning of cortical neurogenesis, and this expression increases as cortical development proceeds. In the developing cortical plate, expression is found in postmitotic migrating neuroblasts and neuroblasts that have completed migration. *Ppt1* mRNA is also expressed in the developing thalamus as well as in the future Purkinje cell layer of the cerebellum (Heinonen et al., 2000). These findings further support the strong significance of PPT1 for development of a wide range of maturing neurons.

Spatial and temporal expression of *Ppt1* in the rat and mouse brain resembles that of synaptophysin, a 38kDa synaptic vesicle protein that has an increasing expression corresponding to the postnatal time course of synaptogenesis (Isosomppi et al., 1999, Suopanki et al., 1999a, Suopanki et al., 2000). This expression pattern strongly suggests that *PPT1* has a general significance for the brain cells and its expression reflects the response to maturation and growth of the neural networks.

Protein structure and function

Palmitoyl protein thioesterase (PPT1; EC 3.1.2.22) is a well-characterized enzyme that was first purified from bovine brain as an enzyme that cleaves palmitate from H-Ras *in vitro* (Camp and Hofmann, 1993). The enzyme has, however, a broad substrate specificity, cleaving fatty acyl chains of lengths 14–18 carbons from cysteine residues in proteins and peptides as well as palmitoyl-CoA (Camp et al., 1994) and S-palmitoyl thioglucoside (van Diggelen et al., 1999). The specific *in vivo* substrates of the enzyme are yet to be determined. The pH optimum of PPT1 is broad and varies with the substrate. Other biochemical properties of the enzyme include instability at alkaline pH, inhibition by the histidine-active reagent diethylpyrocarbonate and insensitivity to the serine inhibitor phenylmethanesulfonyl fluoride (PMSF) (Das et al., 2000). The PPT1 polypetide consists of 306 amino acids and a signal sequence of 25 amino acids in the N-terminus that is co-translationally cleaved. PPT1 is a monomeric globular protein that migrates as a 37/35kDa doublet and is reduced to 31kDa upon deglycosylation (Verkruyse and Hofmann, 1996). PPT1 has three asparagine-linked glycosylation sites at amino acid positions 197, 212, and 232 and all of them are utilized *in vivo*. The glycans are endoH sensitive, demonstrating that PPT1 possesses only N-type glycosylation. Proper glycosylation is required for stability and activity of the enzyme (Bellizzi et al., 2000). PPT1 is not known to have any other modifications than glycosylation.

The crystal structure of bovine PPT1 reveals an α/β-hydrolase fold, typical of lipases, with a catalytic triad composed of Ser115–His289–Asp233 (Figure 6.1). The structure of the acyl-enzyme intermediate confirmed the identity of Ser115 as the nucleophile and identified the hydrophobic cleft that accommodates the fatty acid chain. Bovine PPT1 is 95% identical to human PPT1 at the amino acid level (Bellizzi et al., 2000). The crystal structure of PPT1 provides insights into the structural basis for the phenotype associated with PPT1 mutations. Kinetic properties of the mutant enzymes have been thoroughly characterized and it appears that decreased enzyme stability rather than decreased catalytic efficiency plays a role in determining the phenotype (Das et al., 2001). Structural model analysis of 11 mutant PPT1 molecules revealed that those mutations that abolished enzyme activity were located in the core region of the molecule, whereas those that retained residual activity had smaller structural effects that were localized near the surface of the enzyme (Ohno et al., 2010).

PPT2, an enzyme with weak amino acid similarity (26%) to PPT1, shows acyl thioesterase activity against palmitoyl-CoA (Soyombo and Hofmann, 1997). The three-dimensional structure of PPT2 is very similar to PPT1 (Calero et al., 2003), but it is unable to remove palmitate groups from several S-palmitoylated proteins *in vitro*. Conversely, PPT2 hydrolyses both long- and short-chain fatty acyl-CoA substrates, whereas PPT1 has a more restricted range of fatty acyl chain lengths (Soyombo and Hofmann, 1997).

Another acyl protein thioesterase, APT1, a 29kDa cytosolic protein, removes palmitate from proteins on the cytosolic surface of the membranes (Duncan and Gilman, 1998). APT1 exhibits lysophospholipase activity towards palmitoylated glycerol-3-phosphocholine and it removes palmitate from G protein α subunits, H-Ras and endothelial nitric oxide synthase *in vitro* (Sugimoto et al., 1996, Duncan and Gilman, 1998, Yeh et al., 1999). To date, human mutations in APT1 have not been reported and the role of APT1 *in vivo* is less characterized.

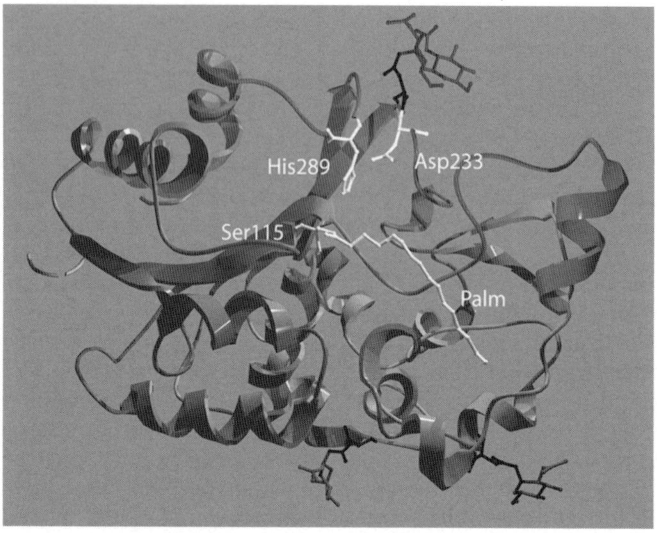

Figure 6.1 The molecular structure of PPT1. The three-dimensional structure of the native bovine palmitoyl protein thioesterase 1 (PPT1) complexed with palmitate (1EH5, Protein Data Bank, http://www.rcsb.org/pdb/). PPT1 has an α/β-hydrolase fold with a catalytic triad and it removes fatty acids, such as palmitate, from lipid-modified proteins. The polypeptide backbone structure is shown as α-helices, β-sheets, and coils. The three N-linked glycan structures (grey) on the surface of the molecule and the respective glycosylated asparagine-amino acids (black) are shown as stick models. The amino acids of the catalytic triad are labelled and drawn as white stick models. Palmitate binds in a hydrophobic groove on the surface of PPT1 and is shown here as complexed with Ser115. The image was made with DeepView/Swiss PdbViewer 3.7 (SP5) and rendered with POV-Ray.

Cellular distribution and targeting

PPT1 is routed to late-endosomes/lysosomes via the mannose-6-phosphate receptor-mediated pathway in non-neuronal cells (Hellsten et al., 1996, Verkruyse and Hofmann, 1996). Overexpression studies in different cell types show that most PPT1 polypeptides containing disease mutations are not correctly transported to lysosomes. They remain in the ER, most probably due to improper folding (Vesa et al., 1995, Salonen et al., 2000, Das et al., 2001). Several lysosomal enzymes undergo proteolytic processing in the lysosomes and PPT1 is modified by dipeptidyl aminopeptidase at the N-terminus (Camp and Hofmann, 1995).

Mannose-6-phosphorylation of PPT1 in neurons has not been experimentally characterized but two-dimensional gel electrophoresis analyses of human brain mannose-6-phosphoproteome identified PPT1 as a major mannose-6-phosphate modified protein (Sleat et al., 2005). Studies in neuronal cultures suggest additional roles for the enzyme. In brain tissue as well as in cultured neurons PPT1 is detected in the cell soma, the axonal varicosities, and presynaptic terminals (Isosomppi et al., 1999, Heinonen et al., 2000, Ahtiainen et al., 2003), which are sites of active membrane transport. Fractionation and immunoelectron microscopy studies with endogenous PPT1 from mouse brain (Lehtovirta et al., 2001) and immunohistochemical staining in rat brain (Suopanki et al., 2002) have further shown that the enzyme is distributed in synaptosomes and synaptic vesicles. Immunofluorescence analyses have also denoted lysosomal localization of endogenous PPT1 in mouse neurons (Virmani et al., 2005).

PPT1-associated molecular networks

Protein palmitoylation, the addition and removal of the fatty acid palmitate to proteins, has a crucial role in controlling and modulating protein–membrane interactions, protein stability, trafficking, and aggregation, and it can be permanent or transient. Two related palmitoyltransferases were first identified in yeast *Saccharomyces cerevisiae* (reviewed in Linder and Deschenes, 2007). Erf2 palmitoylates yeast Ras proteins, whereas Akr1 modifies yeast casein kinase, Yck2. Erf2 and Akr1 share a domain referred to as DHHC, which is cysteine-rich and contains a conserved aspartate–histidine–histidine–cysteine signature motif, suggested to be directly involved in the palmitoyl transfer reaction. Numerous genes encoding DHHC domain proteins are found in all eukaryotic genome databases (reviewed in Mitchell et al., 2006). In neurons, palmitoylation has a key role in targeting proteins for transport to nerve terminals and for regulating trafficking at synapses (El-Husseini and Bredt, 2002, Smotrys and Linder, 2004; reviewed in Huang and El-Husseini, 2005). Palmitoylated proteins are abundant in the nervous system and include synaptotagmins, the exocytic SNARE SNAP-25, GAD65, GAP-43, the neuronal scaffold PSD-95, as well as numerous ion channels and receptors. Moreover, many of these proteins can serve as substrates for various DHHC domain proteins (e.g. HIP14 (DHHC17), DHHC15, DHHC2, 3, and 7) (reviewed in (Mitchell et al., 2006). Clearly, identification of DHHC palmitoyltransferases has been a significant contributor in understanding the protein-mediated palmitoylation.

The exact physiological function and *in vivo* substrates of PPT1 still remain elusive, but PPT1 may participate in several distinct cellular processes, including apoptosis, endocytosis, vesicular trafficking and synaptic function. PPT1 might be involved in cell death signalling, because overexpression of *PPT1* protects cells against apoptosis induced by C2-ceramide or PI3 kinase inhibitor (Cho and Dawson, 2000). Reduced expression of *PPT1* by RNAi increases the susceptibility of neuroblastoma cells to induced apoptosis (Cho et al., 2000). Under basal conditions, PPT1-deficient lymphoblasts are more sensitive to apoptosis (Zhang et al., 2001). In contradiction, PPT1 was shown to modulate tumour necrosis factor (TNF) alpha-induced apoptosis, since cells from CLN1 disease, infantile patients or a CLN1 disease mouse are partially resistant to TNF-induced cell death (Tardy et al., 2009). Overexpression of Ppt1 in the developing eye of *Drosophila* resulted in increased apoptosis (Korey and MacDonald, 2003). It may be that connection between PPT1 function, depalmitoylation and apoptosis is highly dependent on the cellular context.

PPT1 deficiency in CLN1 disease, infantile patient fibroblasts results in elevation of lysosomal pH and defects in endocytosis (Holopainen et al., 2001, Ahtiainen et al., 2006). Endocytic abnormalities and transport defects along the endocytic pathway have previously been reported also in other neurodegenerative disorders including Huntington's disease (Metzler et al., 2001), Alzheimer's disease (Cataldo et al., 2000), classical lysosomal storage diseases such as Niemann–Pick type C and mucolipidosis type IV (Chen et al., 1998, Sun et al., 2001), as well as in other NCL diseases (Luiro et al., 2004). Moreover, cell biological analyses reveal that hypersecretion and abnormal processing of prosaposins are connected to PPT1 deficiency, implying that the accumulation of saposins in CLN1 disease (see later) may result from an endocytic defect (Ahtiainen et al., 2006). Further studies in neurons are needed to elucidate the detailed action of PPT1, saposins, and other vesicular proteins and the specific molecular mechanisms where the lack of PPT1 results in neurodegeneration in CLN1 disease.

Transcript and lipid profiling analyses suggest that PPT1 deficiency is connected to neuroinflammation and changes in brain lipid composition (Kakela et al., 2003, Jalanko et al., 2005). These changes are observed in the end stage of disease and may not reflect direct consequences of *PPT1* deficiency. To date, only sparse information is available from events at the early stages of the disease. Transcript profiling of the *Ppt1* knockout mouse at 10 weeks of age (Elshatory et al., 2003), suggests dysregulation of lipid metabolism, trafficking, glial activation and calcium homeostasis, all of which have been connected to the tissue pathogenesis of human CLN1 disease (Das et al., 1999, Cho et al., 2001, Haltia, 2003, Kakela et al., 2003; reviewed in Jalanko et al., 2006). Preliminary data arising from neuron cultures reveal no alterations in synaptic transmission or density in *Ppt1*-deficient neurons, whereas the number of readily releasable pool of synaptic vesicles is reduced (Virmani et al., 2005). *Ppt1* deficiency in neurons has also been linked to ER-mediated cellular stress (Kim et al., 2006, Zhang et al., 2006). Recently, gene expression profiling revealed similar changes in $Ppt1^{-/-}$ and $Cln5^{-/-}$ mice (von Schantz et al., 2008). Genes regulating neuronal growth cone stabilization, or encoding adenylate cyclase-associated protein (*Cap1*), protein tyrosine phosphatase receptor type F (*Ptprf*), and protein tyrosine phosphatase 4a2 (*Ptp4a2*), were similarly affected to *Ppt1*. Primary cortical neurons from these mice displayed abnormalities in growth cone-associated proteins GAP-43, synapsin, and Rab3, as well as in cytoskeletal-associated proteins.

Accumulating evidence from both *in vitro* and *in vivo* mouse studies have highlighted the connection of PPT1 and synaptic functions (Heinonen et al., 2000, Lehtovirta et al., 2001, Suopanki et al., 2002, Ahtiainen et al., 2003, Virmani et al., 2005, Kim et al., 2008, Kielar et al., 2009). These events occur in regulated lipid microenvironments with highly specific lipid composition and lipid–protein interaction (Piomelli, 2005, Rohrbough and Broadie, 2005). Several studies report clear alterations in the lipid composition of NCL in human autopsy material (Granier et al., 2000, Kakela et al., 2003, Hermansson et al., 2005). PPT1 localizes to the sites of active membrane traffic and lipid metabolism in the neurons (Ahtiainen et al., 2003) and the lack of enzyme activity is related to endocytic and trafficking defects in non-neuronal cells (Ahtiainen et al., 2006). However, more information is needed about the initial events that disturb neuronal function in PPT1 deficiency. Additionally, the future identification of proteins that interact with PPT1 in neurons will add to our understanding of the role of PPT1 in neuronal development or survival. It has recently been reported that CLN1, like several other NCL proteins, interacts with CLN5, and that overexpression of PPT1 facilitates the lysosomal transport of a mutated CLN5 molecule (Lyly et al., 2009). CLN1, like CLN5, also binds to F1-ATPase, and subunits of F1-ATPase on the plasma membrane are increased in mice lacking PPT1 (Lyly et al., 2008).

CLINICAL DATA

The clinical course and age of onset of CLN1 disease varies considerably and there is a genotype–phenotype correlation. Diseases caused by mutations in *CLN1* range from a devastating disease with onset in infancy (CLN1 disease, infantile) to an adult onset form with symptoms presenting in the fourth decade (Mole et al., 2005). There are also forms that present in late infancy and in the juvenile age range. Granular osmiophilic deposits (GRODs) are the morphological hallmark for all CLN1 disease, and regardless of the age of onset, all have a significantly decreased enzyme activity.

CLN1 disease, infantile, was first described in the 1970s in Finland where the disease is enriched with an estimated carrier frequency of 1:70 (Santavuori et al., 1973, Vesa et al., 1995). Over 90% of Finnish CLN1 disease, infantile patients are homozygous for a severe missense point mutation (p.Arg122Trp) leading to enzyme inactivity. In the US, half of all PPT1-deficient patients had CLN1 disease, infantile (Hofmann et al., 1999). Patients from different countries with CLN1 disease, infantile and enzyme inactivity may have slight variations in their clinical course due to varying underlying mutations (Simonati et al., 2009).

As the most common form of CLN1 disease, the clinical course of CLN1 disease, infantile will be discussed in detail in the following section.

CLN1 disease, infantile

CLINICAL FEATURES

The early development of children with CLN1 disease, infantile is normal until 6–12 months of age; even until 1.5 years in some cases (Santavuori et al., 1993). Head growth often begins to decelerate before the manifestation of the first clinical signs. Muscular hypotonia may also be noted at around the same time. The child usually starts to lose previously acquired skills from the age of 12 months. The child loses speech and is unable to understand simple phrases, and becomes clumsy and loses interest in playing. Loss of vision, hyperexcitability, and restlessness are common, especially with crying at night and poor sleep. The child may have knitting hyperkinesias of the hands and upper arms. These are usually seen during some weeks or months between the ages of 16–19 months. Rapid developmental deterioration starts on average between the ages of 15–20 months. The child has acquired microcephaly and shows truncal ataxia, dystonic features, choreoathetosis, and myoclonic jerks.

Loss of vision progresses to blindness usually by the age of 2 years (Raitta and Santavuori, 1973). Ophthalmological examinations have revealed that the perception of light can be lost as early as 18 months, but more often a few months later (Santavuori et al., 1974, Vanhanen et al., 1997). Optic atrophy, involution of retinal vessels, and brownish discoloration of the macula are typical. The pigment aggregations seen in retinitis pigmentosa or other forms of NCL are not usually seen. In most children with CLN1 disease, classic infantile the fundus is hypopigmented and the choroidal vessels are clearly visible (Santavuori, 1982, Bischof et al., 1983).

The mean age of onset of epilepsy is 30 months, but seizures may sometimes be the first sign of the disease. The most common seizure types are myoclonic, clonic, tonic, or hypomotor features, often in one part of the body lasting from a few seconds to 1–2 minutes. Generalized tonic–clonic seizures are less common (Åberg et al., 1997).

The child loses all cognitive and active motor skills before the age of 3 years. As the disease progresses he or she becomes irritable and distressed because of increasing spasticity and pain. There are two times of increased and troublesome irritability: around 2–3 years and after 7 years. Death usually occurs between of the ages 9–13 years.

NEUROPHYSIOLOGICAL FINDINGS

Neurophysiological findings in CLN1 disease, infantile are non-specific following the rapid neuronal degeneration and progression of the disease. The initial finding is decreased reactivity in the electroencephalogram (EEG) to passive eye opening and closing at around the age of 1 year. Sleep spindles are lost by the age of 2 years. By the age of 3 years, the EEG becomes iso-electric. There is extinction first, of the somatosensory evoked potentials (at about 2.5 years), then of the electroretinogram (at about 3 years), and finally the visual evoked potentials (at about 4 years) (Harden et al., 1973, Bischof et al., 1983, Vanhanen et al., 1997).

NEURORADIOLOGICAL FINDINGS

The signal intensity of the thalami compared with the putamen and caudate nuclei may show slight abnormality even before clinical symptoms are apparent and from the age of 3 months. When compared with the putamen and caudate nuclei, the thalami show lower signal intensity up to 4 years of age, equal signal intensity between the ages of 4–8 years, and higher signal intensity from the age of 8 years on T_2-weighted images. On FLAIR and proton density images the thalami first show low signal intensity in contrast to the increased signal intensity on T_1-weighted images (Figure 6.2). In addition, increased periventricular white matter signal intensity can be detected on T_2-weighted and FLAIR images from the age of 11–12 months. Cerebral atrophy is first noticed around the age of 12 months. It is very severe from the age of 4 years onwards and decreased white matter volume also shows extremely high signal intensity on T_2-weighted images, even higher than CSF. The cortex becomes very thin and can hardly be differentiated from white matter (Vanhanen et al., 1995a, Vanhanen et al., 1995b).

Proton magnetic resonance spectroscopy (^{1}H-MRS) imaging reveals the first metabolite alterations, decrease of N-acetylaspartate (NAA) and increase of choline, from the age of 3–5 months measured from the thalamus and parieto-occipital white matter. The rapid progression of the disease is reflected in reduction of all the main metabolites. By the age of 6 years

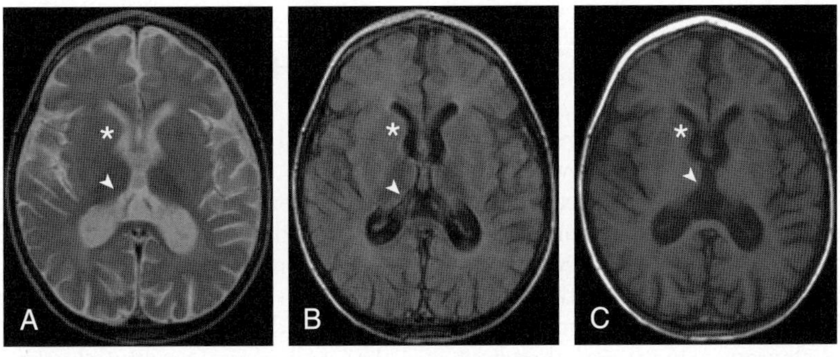

Figure 6.2 CLN1 disease, infantile: MRI of an 11-month-year old boy. Thalami (head of the arrow) show decreased signal intensity compared to caudate nuclei (star) on (A) T_2-weighted axial image (B) and FLAIR image and increased signal intensity on (C) T_1-weighted axial image.

NAA has almost completely disappeared, choline and creatine are weakly detectable but the lipid peak is high indicating almost complete neuroaxonal loss, demyelination, and gliosis (Vanhanen et al., 2004).

In CLN1 disease, infantile the most useful neuroradiological method for diagnostic purposes is magnetic resonance imaging (MRI). A combined approach using ^{1}H-MRS and MRI may be used for monitoring cases on new and experimental treatments.

CLN1 disease, late infantile

The disease starts either with cognitive decline, epilepsy, or visual loss from the age of 1.5–3.5 years. The course of the disease may resemble that of children with CLN2 disease, late infantile. Children die between the ages of 10–13 years (Wisniewski et al., 1998, Hofmann et al., 1999).

Early signs of CLN1 disease, late infantile in a group of six children from Italy with different mutations (Simonati et al., 2009) appeared by the age of 4 years at the latest, and were not homogeneous (seizures in two children, and behavioural disturbances in two). The full clinical picture appeared within 3 years after disease onset. In three children, behavioural abnormalities were the most prominent early signs, and were quickly followed by impaired motor activity with spasticity and ataxia. Decline of cognitive function occurred afterward. Severe global regression was evident in two siblings with the earliest onset. In all children, myoclonic jerks were an early, prominent feature of the disease, and they lasted longer than the sporadic tonic–clonic fits. Visual impairment was present in all patients. Patients were confined to wheelchairs by age 9 years, and were bedridden with feeding difficulties by their early teens. One of the six patients died, at age 16 years.

A common evolution of the electroencephalogram pattern was evident: traces were characterized by early alterations of background rhythms (prevalence of slow-wave component); paroxysmal activity (spikes and spike–wave complexes) was present for a relatively short period. There was a decreased amplitude of electroencephalogram activity and the disappearance of physiologic sleep spindles. No photic response was recorded in any child. Over time, the electroencephalogram flattened and became unresponsive to visual stimuli. In two children, 'giant' cortical-evoked potentials were recorded during investigations of visual pathways.

CLN1 disease, juvenile

CLN1 disease, juvenile resembles CLN3 disease, juvenile, with visual loss or learning disabilities becoming evident at the age of 5–7 years. Retinal dystrophy may be associated with pigment aggregations in the retina. Epilepsy usually develops later and motor dysfunction earlier than in classic CLN3 disease, juvenile cases (Mitchison et al., 1998, Stephenson et al., 1999).

CLN1 disease, adult

CLN1 disease, adult is rare. Two siblings with CLN1 disease, adult were originally described (van Diggelen et al., 2001a). The disease started in the third decade of life with psychiatric symptoms. This was followed by a slowly progressive cognitive decline, cerebellar ataxia, and parkinsonism. More recently a third case where disease started in the late teenage years has been reported (Ramadan et al., 2007).

One of the two sisters had decreased visual acuity with prominent optic atrophy without pigmentary changes (van Diggelen et al., 2001a). Visual evoked potentials revealed a bilateral optic neuropathy. However, despite major visual restrictions and areas of retinitis pigmentosa, there was no optic atrophy in a 24-year-old woman with CLN1 disease, adult (Ramadan et al., 2007).

MORPHOLOGY

General features

With the exception of congenital NCL (Norman and Wood, 1941, Siintola et al., 2006) CLN1 disease, infantile represents the most severe NCL. It shows the earliest age of onset and most rapid progression, and leads to a loss of almost all cortical functions by the age of 3 years (Santavuori et al., 1973, Santavuori et al., 1974). These profound functional disturbances are paralleled by rapidly evolving, drastic changes in the structural elements of the brain. Like other forms of NCL, CLN1 disease, infantile is characterized by widespread lysosomal storage, particularly involving neurons. In CLN1 disease, infantile the storage process is coupled with early and massive cortical and retinal neuronal death with pronounced glial activation. CLN1 disease, infantile belongs to the sphingolipid activator protein-storing forms of NCL along with congenital NCL, autosomal dominant NCL (Parry disease), and certain ovine and canine forms of NCL. Classic CLN1 disease, infantile, and late infantile, juvenile and adult forms of CLN1 disease are considered separately.

CLN1 disease, infantile

MACROSCOPIC AUTOPSY FINDINGS

Apart from disuse atrophy of the musculature and secondary infections, most frequently pneumonia, the macroscopic autopsy findings are limited to the brain and its coverings (Haltia et al., 1973a, Haltia, 1982). The head circumference is slightly reduced, and the calvarium is abnormally thick. On the inner aspect of the dura there is usually a thick layer of gelatinous tissue. The amount of cerebrospinal fluid is extraordinary, owing to extreme global atrophy of the brain. The brain weights are of the order of 250–450g. All cerebral gyri are narrowed and sulci widened (Figure 6.3). In patients who have died at an exceptionally early age, the medial temporal lobe structures, including the hippocampus, have been relatively spared. The cerebellum and the brain stem show commensurate reduction in size, while the spinal cord has an almost normal appearance. The optic nerves are severely atrophic and greyish, while other cranial nerves and spinal roots and nerves have a normal appearance, but may seem unduly prominent in relation to the exceedingly small brain.

The consistency of the brain is tough and rubber-like throughout. On cut surfaces the thin cerebral cortex can hardly be distinguished from the severely shrunken and greyish white matter. The basal ganglia and thalamus still retain their distinct conformation, but the globus pallidus is often unusually brownish in colour. The substantia nigra does not show any pigmentation. The inferior olivary nuclei

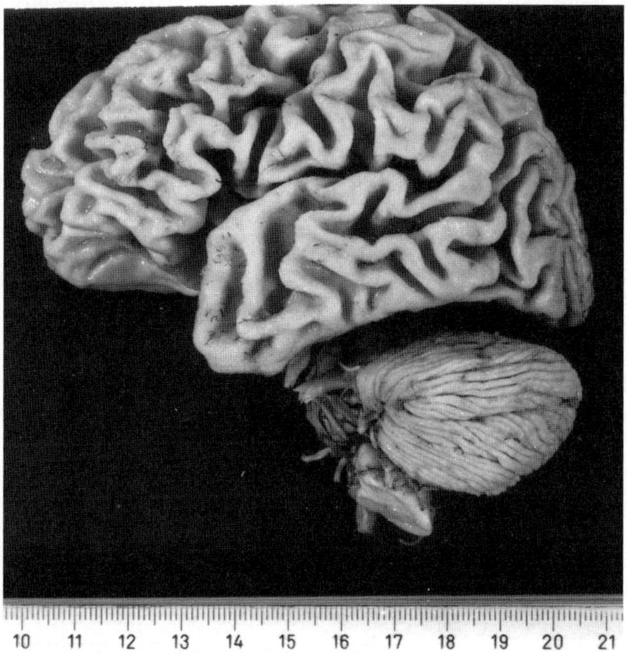

Figure 6.3 CLN1 disease, infantile: extreme generalized brain atrophy is a striking feature. This brain of a 9-year-old male patient weighed 420g. Scale in centimetres.

are prominent. The cerebellar folia are greyish and narrow with gaping sulci, but without any clear distinction between cortex and white matter. The dentate nuclei may have a brownish hue (Haltia et al., 1973a, Haltia et al., 1973b, Haltia, 1982).

POSTMORTEM MRI

In addition to extreme cerebral atrophy, postmortem MRI shows abnormal hypointensity of the grey matter structures in relation to the white matter on T_2-weighted images. The drastically altered relative intensities of the grey- and white-matter structures on the MRI scans reflect substitution of neurons with hypertrophic astrocytes and macrophages (Vanhanen et al., 1995a, Vanhanen et al., 1995b).

HISTOPATHOLOGY

The histopathological alterations in the CNS of CLN1 disease, infantile patients are dramatic, changing rapidly as a function of time. In the cerebral cortex three successive stages can be arbitrarily delineated, based on observations on a series of autopsies (Haltia et al., 1973a, Haltia, 1982) and frontal cortical brain biopsies (Haltia et al., 1973b, Santavuori et al., 1974), originally used for identifying the disease.

Stage I (up to about 2.5 years of age) is characterized by eccentric accumulation of moderate amounts of colourless or slightly yellowish storage granules in the cytoplasm of all cerebral cortical nerve cell bodies. The neuronal perikarya are not severely ballooned and axonal spindles (meganeurites) are only exceptionally seen. In occasional small neurons, the storage granules may coalesce to form dense irregular clumps or round compact inclusion bodies, surrounded by a halo. As early as the age of 1 year there is incipient neuronal loss and invasion of the cortex by scattered macrophages containing storage granules (Figure 6.4A). There is pronounced astrocytic hyperplasia and hypertrophy. Most astrocytes harbour coarse storage granules in their cytoplasm. Incipient loss of myelin and astrocytic proliferation can be seen in the subcortical white matter.

At stage II (approximately 2.5–4 years of age), the cerebral cortex shows a subtotal loss of neurons. The cortex is infiltrated by numerous macrophages containing coarse storage granules, apparently derived from destroyed neuronal perikarya (Figure 6.4B). Some of the macrophages are binucleated. There is tremendous astrocytic hyperplasia and hypertrophy. The white matter shows progressive loss of myelin and astrocytic proliferation and hypertrophy.

Stage III (after the age of 4 years) is characterized by the complete loss of cerebral cortical neurons, axons, and myelin sheaths, with few exceptions. Both the cerebral cortex and convolutional white matter essentially consist of a dense feltwork of hypertrophic astrocytes (Figure 6.4C), harbouring storage granules in their cytoplasm. The macrophages have largely disappeared. Autopsy studies at this stage show that even the granular cells and the Purkinje cells of the cerebellar cortex are entirely destroyed and replaced by a rim of hypertrophic Bergmann astrocytes. The only exceptions to this general rule of cortical neuronal destruction are the giant cells of Betz in the precentral gyrus and the neurons of the hippocampal CA1 and CA4 sectors which may be partly preserved, despite ballooning (Tyynelä et al., 2004). Prominent figures of neuronophagia can be seen around scattered dying Betz cells. The myelinated axons derived from the remaining Betz cells traverse the gliotic white matter, otherwise devoid of myelin, in isolation. In the basal ganglia and brain stem nuclei, moderate amounts of storage granules occur in virtually every nerve cell and astrocyte, with prominent infiltration by macrophages and varying degrees of neuronal loss and neuronophagia. The spinal anterior horn cells are moderately ballooned, but not decreased in number.

In the retina of most deceased patients, the photoreceptor cells, the bipolar cells, and the ganglion cells have completely disappeared, with reactive gliosis. There is loss of pigment from the retinal pigment epithelium. The atrophic optic nerve is gliotic and shows total loss of myelinated axons. Storage granules are visible in the non-pigmented ciliary epithelium of the pars plana, the pigment epithelium, as well as in the glial cells of the optic nerve (Tarkkanen et al., 1977). In a patient with CLN1 disease, infantile who had died at the unusually early age of 3 years and 2 months the fovea and macula showed significant loss of photoreceptors, inner nuclear layer neurons, and ganglion cells. The remaining cones and rods had short outer segments. The photoreceptors were better

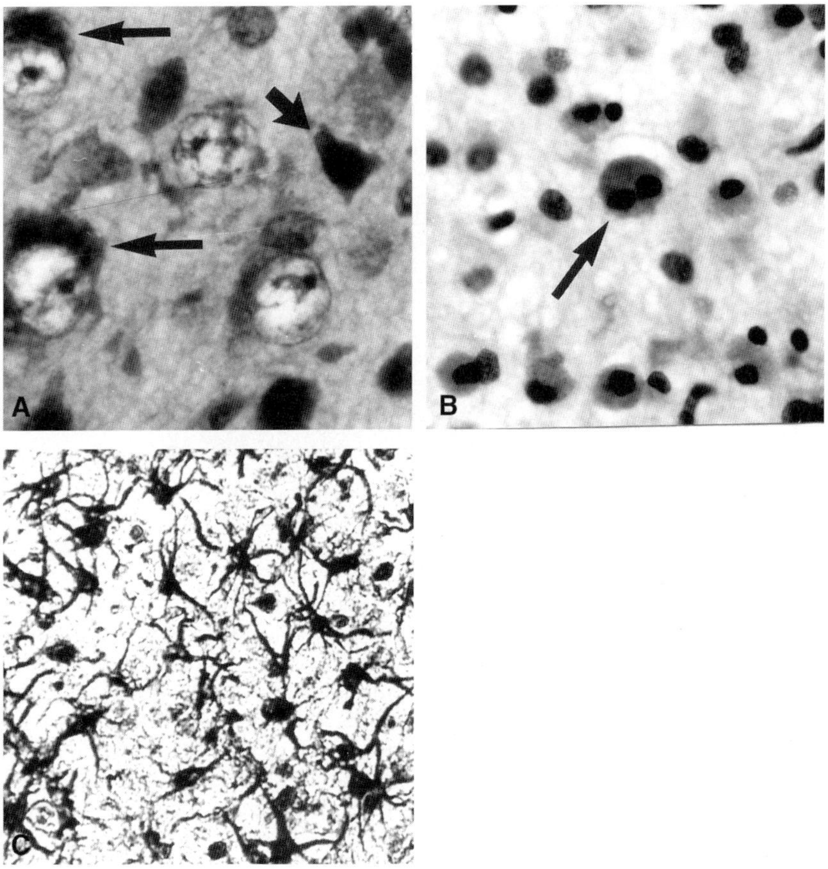

Figure 6.4 CLN1 disease, infantile. (A) At an early stage (stage I) the cortical neurons are still largely preserved, but their cytoplasm is filled with (dark) PAS-positive storage granules (thin arrows). The presence of scattered strongly PAS-positive macrophages (thick arrow) indicates incipient neuronal loss and neuronophagy. Paraffin section, PAS, ×790; (B) At the intermediate stage II almost all cortical neurons have disappeared. The cortex is infiltrated by numerous macrophages some of which are binucleated (arrow). Paraffin section, haematoxylin-eosin, ×790; (C) The late stage III is characterized by complete loss of cortical neurons and pronounced astrocytic hyperplasia and hypertrophy. Paraffin section, Cajal, ×350.

preserved in the periphery but their outer segments were short. Prominent storage deposits occurred in cone inner segments (Weleber et al., 2004).

Accumulation of typical storage granules can be seen in many tissues outside the CNS, as in neurons of the spinal ganglia and the autonomic nervous system, many epithelial cells, including eccrine sweat glands, thyroid follicles, and testes (Figure 6.5), skeletal, cardiac, and smooth muscle cells, endothelial cells, and macrophages in lymphatic tissues (Haltia et al., 1973a, Haltia, 1982). However, these peripheral deposits are usually minor and not associated with tissue destruction, but can be used for diagnostic purposes (see below). No vacuolated lymphocytes are seen in peripheral blood smears.

FLUORESCENCE MICROSCOPY AND HISTOCHEMISTRY

The storage granules are relatively resistant to various lipid solvents and can therefore be studied in paraffin sections. In unstained sections, the intraneuronal storage granules show a strong yellowish autofluorescence in ultraviolet light, while the storage granules processed by the macrophages emit a greenish light (Figure 6.6). In sections stained by the Luxol fast blue–cresylviolet method, the intraneuronal storage bodies are stained deep blue, while those within macrophages are strongly basophilic. The storage cytosomes in both neurons and macrophages are periodic acid–Schiff (PAS)- and Sudan black B-positive and show an intense acid phosphatase activity (Haltia et al., 1973a, Haltia et al., 1973b).

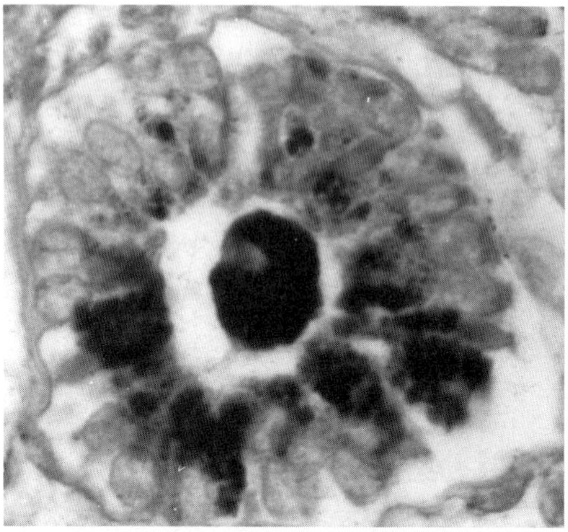

Figure 6.5 CLN1 disease, infantile: the germinal epithelium of a testicular seminiferous tubule and a macrophage (centre) contain Sudan black B-positive storage granules. Paraffin section, Sudan black B, ×790.

IMMUNOCYTOCHEMISTRY

Compositional analysis of the purified granular storage material revealed a high content of proteins (Tyynelä et al., 1993). Saposins A and D, also known as sphingolipid activator proteins (SAPs), were shown to constitute a major portion of the accumulated protein using gel electrophoresis and sequence analysis (Figure 6.7) (Tyynelä et al., 1993). Monospecific SAP antisera and an antiserum raised against storage cytosomes purified from infantile CLN1 disease brain showed strong immunoreactivity with the storage cytosomes (Figure 6.8) (Tyynelä et al., 1995), while they were not stained by an antibody against subunit c of the mitochondrial ATP synthase. The storage

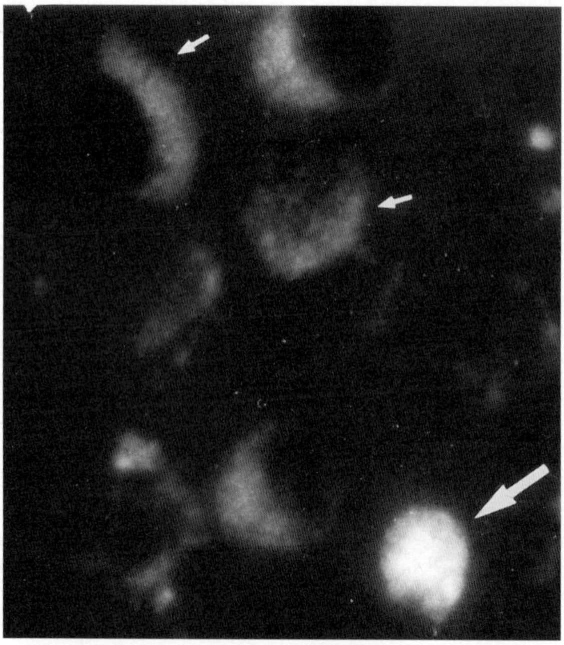

Figure 6.6 CLN1 disease, infantile: the intraneuronal storage material (thin arrows) shows autofluorescence in ultraviolet light. The macrophages (thick arrow) show a more intense autofluorescence. Unstained paraffin section, ×790.

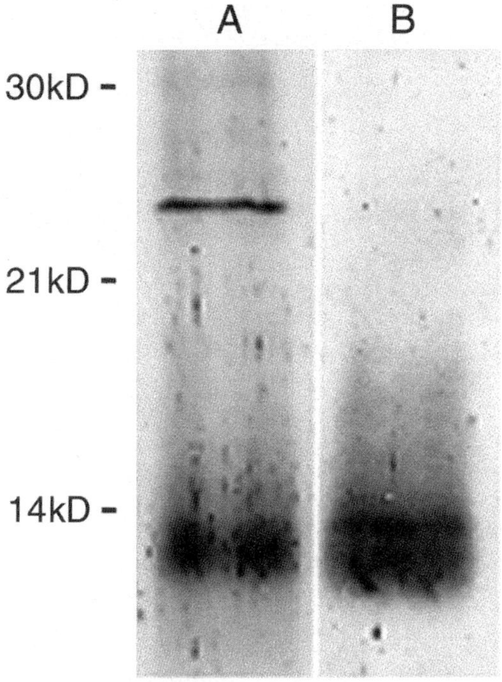

Figure 6.7 CLN1 disease, infantile: analysis of isolated CLN1 storage cytosomes. Lane A: storage cytosome proteins (5μg) fractionated on 17% SDS-PAGE, stained by Coomassie blue. Note the major protein band just below the 14kD marker. Lane B: Western blot analysis of the same sample stained using antiserum against SAP D. Molecular weight markers shown on the left.

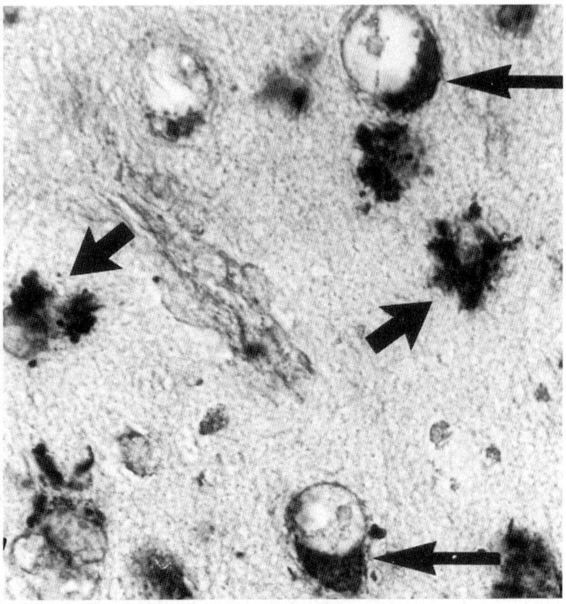

Figure 6.8 CLN1 disease, infantile: the storage material both within the neurons (thin arrows) and astrocytes (thick arrows) shows strong immunoreactivity for sphingolipid activator proteins A and D. Paraffin section, immunoperoxidase, ×500.

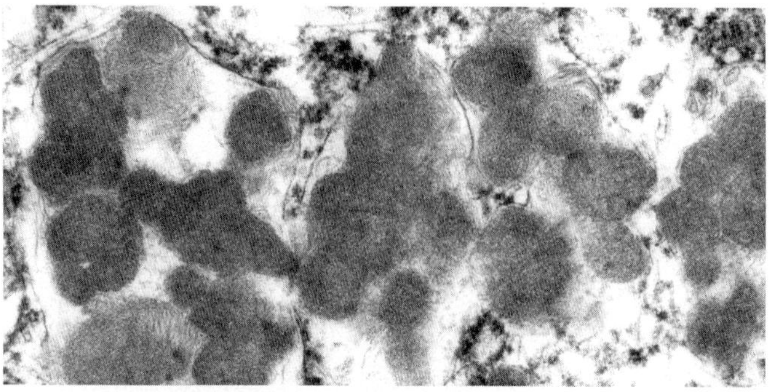

Figures 6.9 CLN1 disease, infantile: the intracytoplasmic storage cytosomes of an anterior horn neuron consist of membrane-bound aggregates of electron-dense globules ('Finnish snow balls') with a finely granular internal ultrastructure. Electron micrograph, ×34000.

cytosomes also bind a monoclonal antibody against the amyloid beta peptide (Wisniewski et al., 1990). Storage of SAPS is not limited to the brain, but occurs in many tissues (for example, pancreas, kidney, heart).

ULTRASTRUCTURE

The storage cytosomes of CLN1 disease are membrane-bound, granular cytoplasmic inclusions of 1–3μm in diameter (Haltia et al., 1973a, Haltia et al., 1973b), often called GRODs (granular osmiophilic deposits). Their ultrastructure is very different from that in most other types of NCL. Although the fine structure of GRODs is usually monotonously granular, they show some form variations which may be related to their formation, maturation, and disintegration in the cells. The different cell types harbouring GRODs may also have an effect on the form of the inclusions.

The GRODs are often composed of conglomerates of spherical globules (Figures 6.9 and 6.10). The globules are tightly or loosely bound together and, in some GRODs, the globular subunit structure is not clearly visible. However, the undulating and bulging margins of the GROD may suggest invisible globular substructure (Figure 6.11). The unit membrane encircling the GROD is sometimes tightly bound to the inclusion material (inclusions without visible subunits) or is more loosely attached (inclusions with globular substructure).

The texture of the GROD with or without globular subunits is granular and does not show obvious structural elements in contrast to other NCL types. Occasional single or paired lines or even a small stack of parallel lamellar structures within the matrix of the inclusion material is sometimes present, particularly in non-neural cells, but the overall picture in neural cells is amorphic. Lamellar structures seem to be more

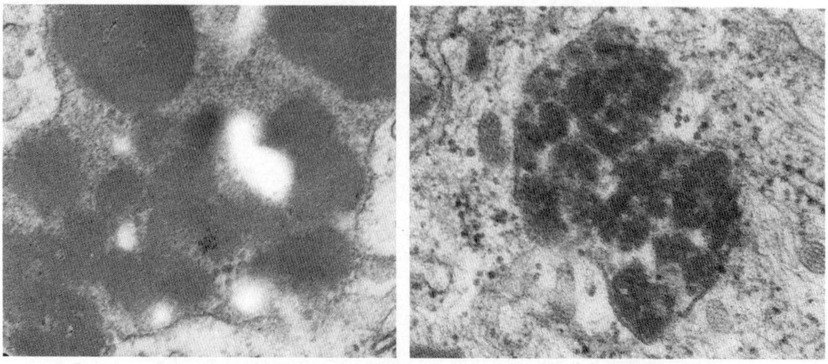

Figures 6.10 CLN1 disease, infantile: electron micrographs of GRODs showing globular subunits. Left: GRODs composed of large subunits and bound loosely together by a lysosomal membrane. Large subunits are typical for GRODs in neural cells. Autonomic ganglion cell, ×20,000. Right: GRODs in an endothelial cell showing smaller globular subunits, ×20,000.

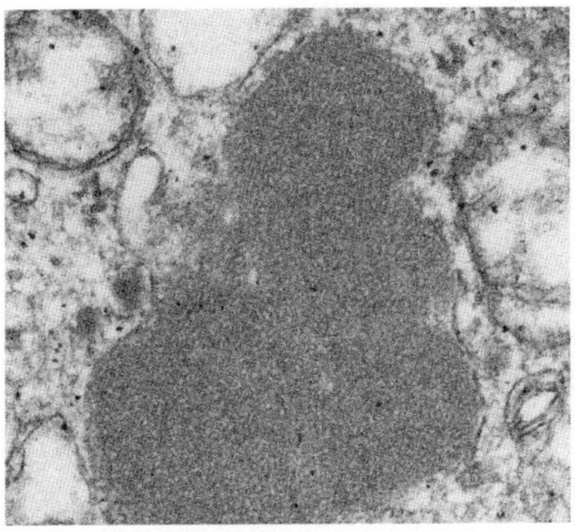

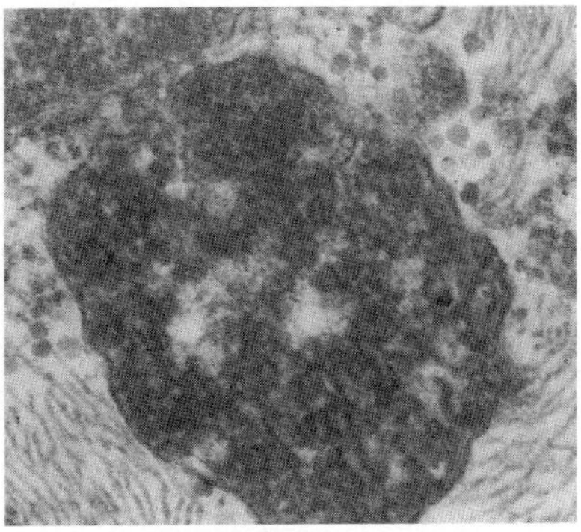

Figures 6.11 CLN1 disease, infantile. Left: GRODs in an autonomic ganglion cell showing finely granular internal texture and undulating border with tightly bound lysosomal membrane but no visible substructures, ×30,000. Right: GRODs in a perithelial cell of a chorionic villus specimen showing more loose internal texture than in the previous pictures, ×40,000.

common in patients who are over 3 years of age. Other cellular elements, such as fat globules, are very rare in GROD. The coarseness of the amorphic material varies in the inclusions (Figure 6.11). It appears to be most finely granular in inclusions not showing the globular subunits. The most loosely arranged texture is seen in the macrophages (Rapola et al., 1984), probably due to the disintegration of the inclusion material.

GRODs are present in several cell types of the nervous system, including neurons and astrocytes of the brain, retinal cells, and spinal and autonomic ganglion cells of the intestine. They are also abundant in various non-neural cells (Haltia et al., 1973a, Haltia et al., 1973b, Rapola and Haltia, 1973, Rapola et al., 1984, Goebel et al., 1988). The latter feature is of great help for electron microscopic diagnosis of CLN1 disease, infantile. Lymphocytes of the peripheral blood carry GRODs, although in variable proportions (Haynes et al., 1979, Anderson et al., 2006). The diagnosis should not be ruled out on the basis of a single negative result on lymphocytes. Conjunctiva, skin, and rectal mucosa are the most common sites for obtaining the diagnostic biopsy specimen in CLN1 disease, infantile (Ceuterick et al., 1976, Libert, 1980, Rapola et al., 1984). They all include several cell types which harbour diagnostic GRODs, usually in large numbers. We have found that endo- and perithelial cells of the blood capillaries are usually rewarding in the screening of biopsy specimens. Autonomic ganglion cells of the submucosal nerve plexus are the most reliable diagnostic cells, but they may not be present in all biopsy specimens. The epithelial and myoepithelial cells of the secretory coils of sweat glands often harbour typical inclusions. The smooth muscle cells of the intestinal muscularis mucosae and the erector pili muscle in skin show GRODs, but to a lesser extent than in other NCL types. Inclusions have been encountered in skeletal muscle and Schwann cells of the peripheral nerve. The macrophages of the lamina propria of the rectal mucosa contain large amounts of GRODs, but this shows a looser texture than that in the sessile cells (Rapola et al., 1984). Macrophages also contain lipid droplets and normal lipofuscin that may be confusing in the morphological diagnosis.

The presence of GRODs in the endo- and perithelial cells has proved to be important in the prenatal diagnosis of CLN1 disease, infantile. Chorionic villus specimens in 'risk' pregnancies contain GRODs in the capillaries of the villi in the affected fetuses (Rapola et al., 1990, Lake et al., 1998). GRODs were found as early as the 8th week of pregnancy. More than 50 correct prenatal diagnoses have been performed, with the ultrastructural findings in complete concordance with the DNA studies. In two cases where the PPT1 enzyme assay was performed at the same time the results were also concordant. Although molecular genetic investigation has made electron microscopy less necessary in prenatal diagnosis, it still has a role in cases where molecular genetic analysis is not available or gives equivocal results.

DIAGNOSTIC PROBLEMS

Diagnostic errors are not uncommon in the electron microscopic study of CLN1 disease, infantile. Blood lymphocytes have been mentioned as a source of false negative results, and sometimes it is time consuming to screen tissues, such as skin or chorionic villus specimens for GRODs, where they may be present in small numbers. However, false negative results can be overcome with repeated investigation where the clinical indications are strong. False positive findings are common and can be clinically damaging. Since the fine structure of the GROD is amorphous, there are several sources of diagnostic error: normal secretory granules of blood leucocytes and glandular tissues; so-called residual bodies in many cells; lipofuscin granules and large normal dense lysosomes appear to be the most common sources of false interpretation of the findings. The structured inclusions of different NCL types other than those caused by mutations in *CLN1* may sometimes show very condensed structures reminiscent of GROD (Åberg et al., 1998). Review of the histopathology by experienced pathologists, with investigation of different cell types, is essential in cases where there is doubt.

CLN1 disease, late infantile and juvenile

MACROSCOPY

In the limited number of cases recorded (Lake et al., 1996) there is marked atrophy of the brain, which weighed approximately 50% of normal. The cerebellum was also atrophic. In one study of CLN1 disease, late infantile cerebral and cerebellar atrophy was apparent in the early neuroradiological investigations, and was followed by rapid shrinkage of the hemispheres, increased size of the ventricular cavities, and decreased volume of the hemispheric white matter (Simonati et al., 2009).

HISTOPATHOLOGY, HISTOCHEMISTRY, AND ULTRASTRUCTURE

There is neuronal loss with the cytoplasm of the remaining neurons distended by the accumulation of a granular sudanophilic, PAS-positive, and strongly autofluorescent material. The granules are only weakly stained with Luxol fast blue (this apparent difference in the intensity of staining from CLN1 disease, infantile may be related to slight differences in technique and different dye batches). Astrocytes, smooth muscle cells, and endothelial cells of the arteriolar walls also contain granular material with the same staining characteristics. In the atrophic cerebellum there is almost complete loss of Purkinje cells and granule cells, with proliferation of Bergmann astrocytes. Immunohistochemical analysis showed no accumulation of subunit c of mitochondrial ATP synthase, but there was strong staining for saposins A and D in the sites of storage.

In rectal biopsies the neurons of the myenteric and submucosal plexuses contain the same granular material, which is also evident in the smooth muscle cells and endothelial cells. No vacuolated lymphocytes are present in peripheral blood, but electron microscopy reveals GRODs in the cytoplasm of lymphocytes. Surprisingly, however, in a small number of PPT1-deficient patients with juvenile onset disease and in one with a late infantile onset, lymphocytes were found with GRODs mixed with curvilinear or fingerprint profiles (Das et al., 1998).

Electron microscopy of tissue samples (Figure 6.12) shows the granular material to have the same ultrastructural characteristics as that in CLN1 disease, infantile, and is identical to GRODs. The neurons in the peripheral nervous system may have, associated with the GROD, a minor lipid-like component more commonly associated with normal lipofuscin. In two cases of CLN1 disease, late infantile there were also scattered fingerprint profiles (Simonati et al., 2009).

CLN1 disease, adult

In a CLN1 disease patient with adult onset, psychiatric problems, cognitive decline, progressive ataxia, extrapyramidal symptoms, and visual dysfunction led to a cutaneous biopsy that showed GRODs in sweat gland cells by electron microscopy, prompting the diagnosis of CLN1 disease, adult. Profound deficiency of PPT1 was subsequently demonstrated by fluorogenic enzyme assay both in the patient and her similarly affected sister (van Diggelen et al., 2001b). However, it is important to keep in mind that in some adult patients GRODs may occur without PPT1 or CTSD deficiency (Nijssen et al., 2003).

DISEASE MECHANISM

Despite identification of the *PPT1* gene as underlying infantile onset NCL (Vesa et al., 1995),

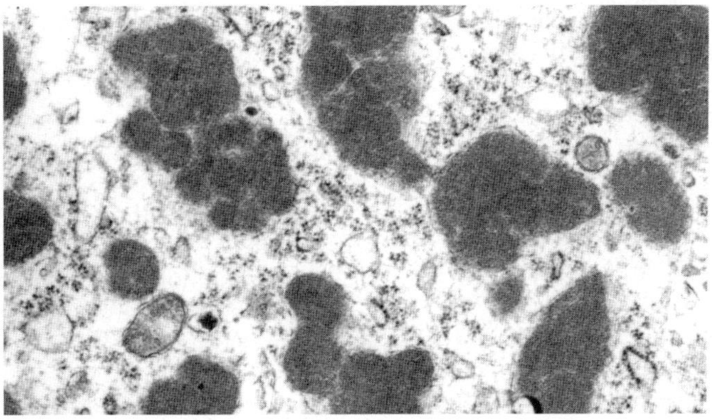

Figure 6.12 CLN1 disease, juvenile: GRODs in biopsied rectal neuron, ×15,000.

it remains unclear how mutations in this gene lead to the devastating neurodegenerative phenotype of CLN1 disease, classic infantile. However, *PPT1* mutations which leave a higher residual level of PPT1 activity result in later onset and more slowly progressing forms of NCL (Kalviainen et al., 2007), suggesting that the loss of PPT1 activity is the key event in pathogenesis. Although PPT1 is known to remove long-chain fatty acids from modified cysteine residues (Hofmann and Peltonen, 2001, Lu et al., 2002, Wei et al., 2008), the natural *in vivo* substrates and precise role of PPT1 in the CNS are still uncertain.

The generation of *Ppt1* mutant mice has provided a valuable resource to investigate these issues (Gupta et al., 2001, Jalanko et al., 2005). ER and oxidative stress and activation of the unfolded protein response (Kim et al., 2006, Zhang et al., 2006), lymphocyte recruitment due to increased levels of lysophosphatidylcholine (Zhang et al., 2007), compromised lipid metabolism and trafficking (Ahtiainen et al., 2007, Lyly et al., 2008), synaptic reorganization (Virmani et al., 2005, Kim et al., 2008, Kielar et al., 2009), excitotoxicity (Kielar and Cooper, unpublished observations), and inflammatory responses (Qiao et al., 2007, Saha et al., 2008), have all been suggested as contributing to the pathogenesis of murine CLN1 disease, but the relative importance of these events is at present unclear. As in human CLN1 disease, the CNS of *Ppt1* mutant mice displays widespread and profound neuron loss and glial activation within the cortical mantle, cerebellum and a variety of subcortical structures (Gupta et al., 2001, Bible et al., 2004, Jalanko et al., 2005). Nevertheless, both reactive and neurodegenerative changes display a high degree of regional and cellular selectivity, especially in the cortex and hippocampus (Bible et al., 2004), which is particularly apparent in the earlier stages of pathogenesis (Kielar et al., 2007). As in other forms of NCL, the thalamocortical system is a particular focus of CLN1 disease pathogenesis, with a distinctive and localized astrocytosis preceding neuron loss and subsequent microglial activation (Kielar et al., 2007). Progressive changes in the expression of proteins involved with synaptic function/stability and cell cycle regulation are also evident in *Ppt1* mutant mice, before morphologically detectable synaptic or axonal pathology (Kielar et al., 2009). It is also apparent that the cerebellum displays a progressive loss of Purkinje neurons in *Ppt1* deficient mice, although granule cells appear to be relatively spared (Gupta et al., 2001, Bible et al., 2004, Kielar et al., 2007, Macauley et al., 2009). Once again, these neurodegenerative changes were preceded by astrocytosis with evidence for primary astrocyte pathology early in disease progression (Macauley et al., 2009).

These landmarks of disease progression are being used to direct the targeting and timing of a variety of therapeutic approaches including AAV-mediated gene transfer (Griffey et al., 2004, Griffey et al., 2005, Griffey et al., 2006), and neural stem cell transplantation (NSCT) (Tamaki et al., 2009). Neonatal administration of AAV2–PPT1 results in improvements in pathological and behavioural phenotypes of *Ppt1* deficient mice, but does not prolong lifespan (Griffey et al., 2004, Griffey et al., 2005, Griffey et al., 2006). Most recently, the efficacy of neural stem cell grafts for murine CLN1 disease has been reported (Tamaki et al., 2009), resulting in behavioural improvements and protection of vulnerable neuron populations and paving the way for a phase I trial of this approach in human CLN1 disease and CLN2 disease.

CORRELATIONS

Genotype–phenotype correlation

The clinical disease caused by mutations in *CLN1/PPT1* shows the greatest phenotypic variation of the NCLs, although within families with more than one affected child the clinical presentation is consistent (Das et al., 1998). The severity of the disease seems to be related to residual enzyme activity. Total loss of the protein or expression of severely truncated protein as well as mutations that result in markedly decreased enzyme stability tend to result in earlier onset disease and more rapid disease progression (Das et al., 2001).

In Finland, almost all children with CLN1 disease, infantile are homozygous for the p.Arg122Trp missense mutation, and their clinical phenotype is relatively uniform and termed CLN1 disease, classic infantile, with an age of onset of 6–24 months. Children from more genetically heterogeneous backgrounds show slightly different disease courses and a variety of mutations. The most common mutation is p.Arg151X, which is also associated with an age of onset in the infantile age range (Das et al., 1998). However, only half of all patients with PPT1 deficiency are diagnosed as infants. Several mutations lead to a later age of onset, ranging from late infancy to adulthood. Mutations p.Met1Ile, p.Thr75Pro, p.Asp79Gly, p.Cys96Tyr, p.Gln177Glu, p.Val181Leu, p.Leu219Gln, p.Leu222Pro, p.Tyr247His, p.Gly250Val, and p.Trp296X have all been associated with variants resembling CLN2, late infantile or CLN3, juvenile disease (Das et al., 1998, Mazzei, 2002, Mitchison et al., 1998), as has the splice site mutation c.125-15T>G and the 3.6kb deletion c.124+1214-235-103del3627 (Simonati et al., 2009). PPT1 activity in these cases was significantly reduced. Missense mutation p.Gly108Arg was found in two siblings with adult disease onset in their fourth decade. PPT1 activity in these two cases was still significantly reduced, albeit in the upper part of the range for CLN1 disease, classic infantile patients (van Diggelen et al., 2001a).

Genotype–morphotype correlation

Irrespective of the mutation in *CLN1* and the severity of the resulting disease, the lipopigment accumulating in patient cells shows the ultrastructural pattern of GRODs. Only two studies (Das et al., 1998) report the occurrence of GRODs mixed with curvilinear and/or fingerprint profiles in blood lymphocytes of patients with ages of onset in the late infantile and juvenile age range. However, this seems not to be a common experience.

DIAGNOSIS

Rapid psychomotor deterioration with visual failure and epileptic seizures together with the characteristic neurophysiological and neuroradiological findings described in earlier sections strongly suggest the diagnosis of classic infantile onset CLN1 disease. In most countries the diagnosis is confirmed by enzymatic assay. A reliable enzyme diagnostic test to determine the levels of PPT1 activity in peripheral leucocytes, cultured fibroblasts, dried blot spots, or using human saliva, is available (Voznyi et al., 1999, Lukacs et al., 2003, Kohan et al., 2005) and is sensitive enough for all ages of onset of disease caused by mutations in PPT1.

Enzymatic analysis may also be used in prenatal diagnosis (van Diggelen et al., 2001b). In countries, where the common mutations are well-recognized, the diagnosis can easily be confirmed by DNA mutation analysis.

CLINICAL MANAGEMENT

Treatment of CLN1 disease is symptomatic because no specific treatment is available. The Finnish experience suggests that in infantile CLN1 disease irritability, sleeping disorders, the choreoathetotic movement disorder and late pains respond best to baclofen or tizanidine, often in combination (Table 6.1). High doses given frequently (3–5 times daily) may be necessary, especially in the later stages of

Table 6.1 **Relevant drug therapy in CLN1 disease, infantile**

Symptom	Drug
Irritability	Baclofen
Sleep problems	Baclofen, tizanidine, midazolam, levomepromazin
Athetosis	Baclofen
Dystonia	Tizanidine
Spasticity + rigidity	Baclofen, tizanidine, benzodiazepines
Epilepsy	Lamotrigine, valproate, benzodiazepines
Pains	Baclofen, tizanidine, fentanyl, MO-derivatives, buprenorphine

Adapted from Santavuori et al., 1999.

the disease. In some patients during the advanced phase of the disease, fentanyl patches and orally administered morphine derivatives have been of great help in addition to baclofen and tizanidine (Mannerkoski et al., 2001).

The antiepileptic drugs of choice are lamotrigine and valproate (Åberg et al., 1997). All children with CLN1 disease, classic infantile suffer from feeding difficulties and constipation that need to be treated appropriately and adequately. In addition, there is plenty of need for supportive physical and psychosocial therapies.

EXPERIMENTAL THERAPY

Current experimental therapeutic strategies for CLN1 disease include clinical trials that involve neural stem cells and gene therapy directed to the CNS. They focus mainly on methods that replenish PPT1 activity, or compensate for its function. The theoretical bases of these strategies, which are still being refined, are considered in detail in Chapter 21. Because PPTI is an enzyme, CLN1 disease is likely to be one of the first NCLs to be treated successfully, although for the majority of patients, its early age of onset provides only a small window of opportunity if presymptomatic treatment is required.

Enzyme replacement

Enzyme replacement therapy for CLN1 disease has not yet been addressed. Human recombinant PPT1 has been produced in Chinese hamster ovary (CHO) cells (Lu et al., 2010). The enzyme is largely mannose 6-phosphorylated and taken up rapidly by immortalized patient lymphoblasts, where clearance of PPT1 substrates was demonstrated. This recombinant human PPT1 was rapidly cleared from plasma when injected intravenously into PPT1-deficient mice. Most of the injected dose was distributed to the kidney and liver and potentially corrective levels were also observed in heart, lung, and spleen. However, brain uptake was minimal, as expected based on experience with other intravenously administered lysosomal enzymes. This approach may be useful as an adjunct to CNS-directed therapies.

Gene therapy

An AAV2 vector containing the human *PPT1* cDNA was able to produce functional and pathological improvements when injected into the brains or the eyes of newborn PPT1-deficient mice (Griffey et al., 2004, Griffey et al., 2005, Griffey et al., 2006). These results suggest that a similar gene therapy approach may provide clinical improvements for CLN1 disease.

Cell-based therapies

Three patients with CLN1, infantile disease received haematopoietic SCT (SCT) at the Hospital for Children and Adolescents at the University of Helsinki, Finland between 1996–1998. All patients were homozygous for the p.Arg122Trp missense mutation and had a sibling with CLN1 disease, classic infantile. The first patient rejected the first graft at the age of 7 months and had mild symptoms at the second transplantation at 11 months. The two other patients were asymptomatic when they received their transplants at the age of 4 months.

PPT1 enzyme activity was normalized in peripheral leucocytes, but remained low in CSF. All patients developed CLN1, infantile disease by the age of 2 or 3 years (Lonnqvist et al., 2001). On further follow-up, the course of the disease has been similar to other CLN1 disease, infantile children who did not have SCT (T. Lönnqvist, personal communication). All the patients had full donor chimerism, and the follow-up was more than 1 year (now over 5 years), the minimum time for macrophages to reach the brain. Allogeneic SCT does not offer a cure, and suggests that haematopoietic gene therapy would not be helpful for CLN1 disease, infantile. Allogeneic SCT is therefore not recommended as therapy for patients with CLN1 disease, classic infantile.

Human neural stem cells are under intense investigation as potential therapies for both CNS injury and some CNS diseases (Cummings et al., 2006). Neurodegenerative diseases, such as CLN1 disease, have been considered as targets for experimental neural stem cell treatment. Based on promising preclinical data from neural stem cell grafting in *Ppt1* deficient mice (Tamaki et al., 2009), a phase I safety trial for this approach has been conducted at Oregon Health & Science University.

Small molecule therapies

Cysteamine bitartrate is a safe drug and able to cross the blood–brain barrier (Broyer et al., 1996), and to remove ceroid from cells from infantile CLN1 disease patients (Heritable Disorder Branch, NICHD, USA). Therefore, oral cysteamine has been given to one infant homozygous for the p.Arg122Trp missense mutation and a sibling with CLN1 disease, infantile in Finland, following the established study protocol. Oral cysteamine treatment (cysteamine bitartrate 60mg/kg/day) was given from the age of 2 months to 26 months between March 2002 and May 2003. The treatment was well tolerated. However, no positive effect was detected, and a typical clinical course and MRI findings of CLN1 disease, infantile evolved (T. Lönnqvist, personal communication).

Conclusions

To summarize, several therapeutic approaches are being or have been investigated for CLN1 disease, including enzyme replacement, gene therapy, cell-based therapies, and small molecule therapies. Current evidence suggests that restoration of PPT1 in the CNS would be important for treatment of CLN1 disease. It is currently not known whether particular cell populations within the CNS must be targeted, and whether there is an optimal time along the disease course by which treatment must be initiated. There may be risks in elevating PPT1 activity above physiological levels, and peripheral disease may develop if CNS disease is treated successfully. Further experimentation is necessary to address these issues. Importantly, the molecular mechanisms underlying the pathogenesis of CLN1 disease have not been elucidated. As a more detailed understanding of the disease process emerges, so will additional insights into therapy.

REFERENCES

Åberg L, Heiskala H, Vanhanen SL, Himberg JJ, Hosking G, Yuen A, & Santavuori P (1997) Lamotrigine therapy in infantile neuronal ceroid lipofuscinosis (INCL). *Neuropediatrics*, 28, 77–79.

Åberg L, Jarvela I, Rapola J, Autti T, Kirveskari E, Lappi M, Sipila L, & Santavuori P (1998) Atypical juvenile neuronal ceroid lipofuscinosis with granular osmiophilic deposit-like inclusions in the autonomic nerve cells of the gut wall. *Acta Neuropathol*, 95, 306–312.

Ahtiainen L, Kolikova J, Mutka AL, Luiro K, Gentile M, Ikonen E, Khiroug L, Jalanko A, & Kopra O (2007) Palmitoyl protein thioesterase 1 (Ppt1)-deficient mouse neurons show alterations in cholesterol metabolism and calcium homeostasis prior to synaptic dysfunction. *Neurobiol Dis*, 28, 52–64.

Ahtiainen L, Luiro K, Kauppi M, Tyynelä J, Kopra O, & Jalanko A (2006) Palmitoyl protein thioesterase 1 (PPT1) deficiency causes endocytic defects connected to abnormal saposin processing. *Exp Cell Res*, 312, 1540–1553.

Ahtiainen L, Van Diggelen OP, Jalanko A, & Kopra O (2003) Palmitoyl protein thioesterase 1 is targeted to the axons in neurons. *J Comp Neurol*, 455, 368–377.

Anderson GW, Smith VV, Brooke I, Malone M, & Sebire NJ (2006) Diagnosis of neuronal ceroid lipofuscinosis (Batten disease) by electron microscopy in peripheral blood specimens. *Ultrastruct Pathol*, 30, 373–378.

Bellizzi JJ, 3rd, Widom J, Kemp C, Lu JY, Das AK, Hofmann SL, & Clardy J (2000) The crystal structure of palmitoyl protein thioesterase 1 and the molecular basis of infantile neuronal ceroid lipofuscinosis. *Proc Natl Acad Sci U S A*, 97, 4573–4578.

Bi HY, Yao S, Bu DF, Wang ZX, Zhang Y, Qin J, Yang YL, & Yuan Y (2006) [Two novel mutations in palmitoyl-protein thioesterase gene in 2 Chinese babies with infantile neuronal ceroid lipofuscinosis]. *Zhonghua Er Ke Za Zhi*, 44, 496–499.

Bible E, Gupta P, Hofmann SL, & Cooper JD (2004) Regional and cellular neuropathology in the palmitoyl protein thioesterase-1 null mutant mouse model of infantile neuronal ceroid lipofuscinosis. *Neurobiol Dis*, 16, 346–359.

Bischof G, Hammerstein W, & Goebel HH (1983) [Fundus dystrophy and ceroid-lipofuscinosis]. *Fortschr Ophthalmol*, 80, 97–99.

Bonsignore M, Tessa A, Di Rosa G, Piemonte F, Dionisi-Vici C, Simonati A, Calamoneri F, Tortorella G, & Santorelli FM (2006) Novel CLN1 mutation in two Italian sibs with late infantile neuronal ceroid lipofuscinosis. *Eur J Paediatr Neurol*, 10, 154–156.

Broyer M, Tete MJ, Guest G, Bertheleme JP, Labrousse F, & Poisson M (1996) Clinical polymorphism of cystinosis encephalopathy. Results of treatment with cysteamine. *J Inherit Metab Dis*, 19, 65–75.

Calero G, Gupta P, Nonato MC, Tandel S, Biehl ER, Hofmann SL, & Clardy J (2003) The crystal structure of palmitoyl protein thioesterase-2 (PPT2) reveals the basis for divergent substrate specificities of the two lysosomal thioesterases, PPT1 and PPT2. *J Biol Chem*, 278, 37957–37964.

Camp LA & Hofmann SL (1993) Purification and properties of a palmitoyl-protein thioesterase that cleaves palmitate from H-Ras. *J Biol Chem*, 268, 22566–22574.

Camp LA & Hofmann SL (1995) Assay and isolation of palmitoyl-protein thioesterase from bovine brain using palmitoylated H-Ras as substrate. *Methods Enzymol*, 250, 336–347.

Camp LA, Verkruyse LA, Afendis SJ, Slaughter CA, & Hofmann SL (1994) Molecular cloning and expression of palmitoyl-protein thioesterase. *J Biol Chem*, 269, 23212–23219.

Cataldo AM, Peterhoff CM, Troncoso JC, Gomez-Isla T, Hyman BT, & Nixon RA (2000) Endocytic pathway abnormalities precede amyloid beta deposition in sporadic Alzheimer's disease and Down syndrome: differential effects of APOE genotype and presenilin mutations. *Am J Pathol*, 157, 277–286.

Ceuterick C, Martin JJ, Casaer P, & Edgar GW (1976) The diagnosis of infantile generalized ceroidlipofuscinosis (type Hagberg-Santavuori) using skin biopsy. *Neuropadiatrie*, 7, 250–260.

Chen CS, Bach G, & Pagano RE (1998) Abnormal transport along the lysosomal pathway in mucolipidosis, type IV disease. *Proc Natl Acad Sci U S A*, 95, 6373–6378.

Cho S & Dawson G (2000) Palmitoyl protein thioesterase 1 protects against apoptosis mediated by Ras-Akt-caspase pathway in neuroblastoma cells. *J Neurochem*, 74, 1478–1488.

Cho S, Dawson PE, & Dawson G (2000) Antisense palmitoyl protein thioesterase 1 (PPT1) treatment inhibits PPT1 activity and increases cell death in LA-N-5 neuroblastoma cells. *J Neurosci Res*, 62, 234–240.

Cho S, Dawson PE, & Dawson G (2001) Role of palmitoyl-protein thioesterase in cell death: implications for infantile neuronal ceroid lipofuscinosis. *Eur J Paediatr Neurol*, 5 Suppl A, 53–55.

Cummings BJ, Uchida N, Tamaki SJ, & Anderson AJ (2006) Human neural stem cell differentiation following transplantation into spinal cord injured mice: association with recovery of locomotor function. *Neurol Res*, 28, 474–481.

Das AK, Becerra CH, Yi W, Lu JY, Siakotos AN, Wisniewski KE, & Hofmann SL (1998) Molecular genetics of palmitoyl-protein thioesterase deficiency in the U.S. *J Clin Invest*, 102, 361–370.

Das AK, Bellizzi JJ, 3rd, Tandel S, Biehl E, Clardy J, & Hofmann SL (2000) Structural basis for the insensitivity of a serine enzyme (palmitoyl-protein thioesterase) to phenylmethylsulfonyl fluoride. *J Biol Chem*, 275, 23847–23851.

Das AK, Lu JY, & Hofmann SL (2001) Biochemical analysis of mutations in palmitoyl-protein thioesterase causing infantile and late-onset forms of neuronal ceroid lipofuscinosis. *Hum Mol Genet*, 10, 1431–1439.

Das AM, Jolly RD, & Kohlschutter A (1999) Anomalies of mitochondrial ATP synthase regulation in four different types of neuronal ceroid lipofuscinosis. *Mol Genet Metab*, 66, 349–355.

van Diggelen OP, Keulemans JL, Kleijer WJ, Thobois S, Tilikete C, & Voznyi YV (2001a) Pre- and postnatal enzyme analysis for infantile, late infantile and adult neuronal ceroid lipofuscinosis (CLN1 and CLN2). *Eur J Paediatr Neurol*, 5 Suppl A, 189–192.

van Diggelen OP, Keulemans JL, Winchester B, Hofman IL, Vanhanen SL, Santavuori P, & Voznyi YV (1999) A rapid fluorogenic palmitoyl-protein thioesterase assay: pre- and postnatal diagnosis of INCL. *Mol Genet Metab*, 66, 240–244.

van Diggelen OP, Thobois S, Tilikete C, Zabot MT, Keulemans JL, van Bunderen PA, Taschner PE, Losekoot M, & Voznyi YV (2001b) Adult neuronal ceroid lipofuscinosis with palmitoyl-protein thioesterase deficiency: first adult-onset patients of a childhood disease. *Ann Neurol*, 50, 269–272.

Duncan JA & Gilman AG (1998) A cytoplasmic acyl-protein thioesterase that removes palmitate from G protein alpha subunits and p21(RAS). *J Biol Chem*, 273, 15830–15837.

El-Husseini Ael D & Bredt DS (2002) Protein palmitoylation: a regulator of neuronal development and function. *Nat Rev Neurosci*, 3, 791–802.

Elshatory Y, Brooks AI, Chattopadhyay S, Curran TM, Gupta P, Ramalingam V, Hofmann SL, & Pearce DA (2003) Early changes in gene expression in two models of Batten disease. *FEBS Lett*, 538, 207–212.

Goebel HH, Klein H, Santavuori P, & Sainio K (1988) Ultrastructural studies of the retina in infantile neuronal ceroid-lipofuscinosis. *Retina*, 8, 59–66.

Granier LA, Langley K, Leray C, & Sarlieve LL (2000) Phospholipid composition in late infantile neuronal ceroid lipofuscinosis. *Eur J Clin Invest*, 30, 1011–1017.

Griffey M, Bible E, Vogler C, Levy B, Gupta P, Cooper J, & Sands MS (2004) Adeno-associated virus 2-mediated gene therapy decreases autofluorescent storage material and increases brain mass in a murine model of infantile neuronal ceroid lipofuscinosis. *Neurobiol Dis*, 16, 360–369.

Griffey M, Macauley SL, Ogilvie JM, & Sands MS (2005) AAV2-mediated ocular gene therapy for infantile neuronal ceroid lipofuscinosis. *Mol Ther*, 12, 413–421.

Griffey MA, Wozniak D, Wong M, Bible E, Johnson K, Rothman SM, Wentz AE, Cooper JD, & Sands MS (2006) CNS-directed AAV2-mediated gene therapy ameliorates functional deficits in a murine model of infantile neuronal ceroid lipofuscinosis. *Mol Ther*, 13, 538–547.

Gupta P, Soyombo AA, Atashband A, Wisniewski KE, Shelton JM, Richardson JA, Hammer RE, & Hofmann SL (2001) Disruption of PPT1 or PPT2 causes neuronal ceroid lipofuscinosis in knockout mice. *Proc Natl Acad Sci U S A*, 98, 13566–13571.

Haltia M (1982) Infantile neuronal ceroid-lipofuscinosis: Neuropathological aspects. In Armstrong D, Koppang N, & Rider JA (Eds.) *Ceroid-lipofuscinosis (Batten's Disease)*, pp. 105–115. Amsterdam, Elsevier Biomedical Press.

Haltia M (2003) The neuronal ceroid-lipofuscinoses. *J Neuropathol Exp Neurol*, 62, 1–13.

Haltia M, Rapola J, & Santavuori P (1973a) Infantile type of so-called neuronal ceroid-lipofuscinosis. Histological and electron microscopic studies. *Acta Neuropathol*, 26, 157–170.

Haltia M, Rapola J, Santavuori P, & Keranen A (1973b) Infantile type of so-called neuronal ceroid-lipofuscinosis. 2. Morphological and biochemical studies. *J Neurol Sci*, 18, 269–285.

Harden A, Pampiglione G, & Picton-Robinson N (1973) Electroretinogram and visual evoked response in a form of 'neuronal lipidosis' with diagnostic EEG features. *J Neurol Neurosurg Psychiatry*, 36, 61–67.

Haynes ME, Manson JI, Carter RF, & Robertson E (1979) Electron microscopy of skin and peripheral blood lymphocytes in infantile (Santavuori) neuronal ceroid lipofuscinosis. *Neuropädiatrie*, 10, 245–263.

Heinonen O, Kyttala A, Lehmus E, Paunio T, Peltonen L, & Jalanko A (2000) Expression of palmitoyl protein thioesterase in neurons. *Mol Genet Metab*, 69, 123–129.

Hellsten E, Vesa J, Olkkonen VM, Jalanko A, & Peltonen L (1996) Human palmitoyl protein thioesterase: evidence for lysosomal targeting of the enzyme and disturbed cellular routing in infantile neuronal ceroid lipofuscinosis. *EMBO J*, 15, 5240–5245.

Hermansson M, Kakela R, Berghall M, Lehesjoki AE, Somerharju P, & Lahtinen U (2005) Mass spectrometric analysis reveals changes in phospholipid, neutral sphingolipid and sulfatide molecular species in progressive epilepsy with mental retardation, EPMR, brain: a case study. *J Neurochem*, 95, 609–617.

Hofmann SL, Das AK, Yi W, Lu JY, & Wisniewski KE (1999) Genotype-phenotype correlations in neuronal ceroid lipofuscinosis due to palmitoyl-protein thioesterase deficiency. *Mol Genet Metab*, 66, 234–239.

Hofmann SL & Peltonen L (2001) The neuronal ceroid lipofuscinosis. In Scriver CR, Beaudet AL, Sly W, Valle D, Childs B, Kinzler KW, & Vogelstein B (Eds.) *The Metabolic and Molecular Bases of Inherited Disease*, 8th edn., pp. 3877–3894. New York, McGraw-Hill.

Holopainen JM, Saarikoski J, Kinnunen PK, & Jarvela I (2001) Elevated lysosomal pH in neuronal ceroid lipofuscinoses (NCLs). *Eur J Biochem*, 268, 5851–5856.

Huang K & El-Husseini A (2005) Modulation of neuronal protein trafficking and function by palmitoylation. *Curr Opin Neurobiol*, 15, 527–535.

Isosomppi J, Heinonen O, Hiltunen JO, Greene ND, Vesa J, Uusitalo A, Mitchison HM, Saarma M, Jalanko A, & Peltonen L (1999) Developmental expression of palmitoyl protein thioesterase in normal mice. *Brain Res Dev Brain Res*, 118, 1–11.

Jalanko A, Tyynelä J, & Peltonen L (2006) From genes to systems: new global strategies for the characterization of NCL biology. *Biochim Biophys Acta*, 1762, 934–944.

Jalanko A, Vesa J, Manninen T, von Schantz C, Minye H, Fabritius AL, Salonen T, Rapola J, Gentile M, Kopra O, & Peltonen L (2005) Mice with Ppt1Deltaex4 mutation replicate the INCL phenotype and show an inflammation-associated loss of interneurons. *Neurobiol Dis*, 18, 226–241.

Järvelä I (1991) Infantile neuronal ceroid lipofuscinosis (CLN1): linkage disequilibrium in the Finnish population and evidence that variant late infantile form (variant CLN2) represents a nonallelic locus. *Genomics*, 10, 333–337.

Kakela R, Somerharju P, & Tyynelä J (2003) Analysis of phospholipid molecular species in brains from patients with infantile and juvenile neuronal-ceroid lipofuscinosis using liquid chromatography-electrospray ionization mass spectrometry. *J Neurochem*, 84, 1051–1065.

Kalviainen R, Eriksson K, Losekoot M, Sorri I, Harvima I, Santavuori P, Jarvela I, Autti T, Vanninen R, Salmenpera T, & van Diggelen OP (2007) Juvenile-onset neuronal ceroid lipofuscinosis with infantile CLN1 mutation and palmitoyl-protein thioesterase deficiency. *Eur J Neurol*, 14, 369–372.

Kielar C, Maddox L, Bible E, Pontikis CC, Macauley SL, Griffey MA, Wong M, Sands MS, & Cooper JD (2007) Successive neuron loss in the thalamus and cortex in a mouse model of infantile neuronal ceroid lipofuscinosis. *Neurobiol Dis*, 25, 150–162.

Kielar C, Wishart TM, Palmer A, Dihanich S, Wong AM, Macauley SL, Chan CH, Sands MS, Pearce DA, Cooper JD, & Gillingwater TH (2009) Molecular correlates of axonal and synaptic pathology in mouse models of Batten disease. *Hum Mol Genet*, 18, 4066–4080.

Kim SJ, Zhang Z, Hitomi E, Lee YC, & Mukherjee AB (2006) Endoplasmic reticulum stress-induced caspase-4 activation mediates apoptosis and neurodegeneration in INCL. *Hum Mol Genet*, 15, 1826–1834.

Kim SJ, Zhang Z, Sarkar C, Tsai PC, Lee YC, Dye L, & Mukherjee AB (2008) Palmitoyl protein thioesterase-1 deficiency impairs synaptic vesicle recycling at nerve terminals, contributing to neuropathology in humans and mice. *J Clin Invest*, 118, 3075–3086.

Kohan R, Cismondi IA, Kremer RD, Muller VJ, Guelbert N, Anzolini VT, Fietz MJ, Ramirez AM, & Halac IN (2009) An integrated strategy for the diagnosis of neuronal ceroid lipofuscinosis types 1 (CLN1) and 2 (CLN2) in eleven Latin American patients. *Clin Genet*, 76, 372–382.

Kohan R, de Halac IN, Tapia Anzolini V, Cismondi A, Oller Ramirez AM, Paschini Capra A, & de Kremer RD (2005) Palmitoyl Protein Thioesterase1 (PPT1) and Tripeptidyl Peptidase-I (TPP-I) are expressed in the human saliva. A reliable and non-invasive source for the diagnosis of infantile (CLN1) and late infantile (CLN2) neuronal ceroid lipofuscinoses. *Clin Biochem*, 38, 492–494.

Korey CA & MacDonald ME (2003) An over-expression system for characterizing Ppt1 function in Drosophila. *BMC Neurosci*, 4, 30.

Kousi M, Siintola E, Dvorakova L, Vlaskova H, Turnbull J, Topcu M, Yuksel D, Gokben S, Minassian BA, Elleder M, Mole SE, & Lehesjoki AE (2009) Mutations in CLN7/MFSD8 are a common cause of variant late-infantile neuronal ceroid lipofuscinosis. *Brain*, 132, 810–819.

Lake BD, Brett EM, & Boyd SG (1996) A form of juvenile Batten disease with granular osmiophilic deposits. *Neuropediatrics*, 27, 265–269.

Lake BD, Young EP, & Winchester BG (1998) Prenatal diagnosis of lysosomal storage diseases. *Brain Pathol*, 8, 133–149.

Lehtovirta M, Kyttala A, Eskelinen EL, Hess M, Heinonen O, & Jalanko A (2001) Palmitoyl protein thioesterase (PPT) localizes into synaptosomes and synaptic vesicles in neurons: implications for infantile neuronal ceroid lipofuscinosis (INCL). *Hum Mol Genet*, 10, 69–75.

Libert J (1980) Diagnosis of lysosomal storage diseases by the ultrastructural study of conjunctival biopsies. *Pathol Annu*, 15, 37–66.

Linder ME & Deschenes RJ (2007) Palmitoylation: policing protein stability and traffic. *Nat Rev Mol Cell Biol*, 8, 74–84.

Lonnqvist T, Vanhanen SL, Vettenranta K, Autti T, Rapola J, Santavuori P, & Saarinen-Pihkala UM (2001) Hematopoietic stem cell transplantation in infantile neuronal ceroid lipofuscinosis. *Neurology*, 57, 1411–1416.

Lu JY, Hu J, & Hofmann SL (2010) Human recombinant palmitoyl-protein thioesterase-1 (PPT1) for preclinical evaluation of enzyme replacement therapy for infantile neuronal ceroid lipofuscinosis. *Mol Genet Metab*, 99, 374–378.

Lu JY, Verkruyse LA, & Hofmann SL (2002) The effects of lysosomotropic agents on normal and INCL cells provide further evidence for the lysosomal nature of palmitoyl-protein thioesterase function. *Biochim Biophys Acta*, 1583, 35–44.

Luiro K, Yliannala K, Ahtiainen L, Maunu H, Jarvela I, Kyttala A, & Jalanko A (2004) Interconnections of CLN3, Hook1 and Rab proteins link Batten disease to defects in the endocytic pathway. *Hum Mol Genet*, 13, 3017–3027.

Lukacs Z, Santavuori P, Keil A, Steinfeld R, & Kohlschutter A (2003) Rapid and simple assay for the determination of tripeptidyl peptidase and palmitoyl protein thioesterase activities in dried blood spots. *Clin Chem*, 49, 509–511.

Lyly A, Marjavaara SK, Kyttala A, Uusi-Rauva K, Luiro K, Kopra O, Martinez LO, Tanhuanpaa K, Kalkkinen N, Suomalainen A, Jauhiainen M, & Jalanko A (2008) Deficiency of the INCL protein Ppt1 results in changes in ectopic F1-ATP synthase and altered cholesterol metabolism. *Hum Mol Genet*, 17, 1406–1417.

Lyly A, von Schantz C, Heine C, Schmiedt ML, Sipila T, Jalanko A, & Kyttala A (2009) Novel interactions of CLN5 support molecular networking between neuronal ceroid lipofuscinosis proteins. *BMC Cell Biol*, 10, 83.

Macauley SL, Wozniak DF, Kielar C, Tan Y, Cooper JD, & Sands MS (2009) Cerebellar pathology and motor deficits in the palmitoyl protein thioesterase 1-deficient mouse. *Exp Neurol*, 217, 124–135.

Mannerkoski MK, Heiskala HJ, Santavuori PR, & Pouttu JA (2001) Transdermal fentanyl therapy for pains in children with infantile neuronal ceroid lipofuscinosis. *Eur J Paediatr Neurol*, 5 Suppl A, 175–177.

Mazzei R, Conforti FL, Magariello A, Bravaccio C, Militerni R, Gabriele AL, Sampaolo S, Patitucci A, Di Iorio G, Muglia M, & Quattrone A (2002) A novel mutation in the CLN1 gene in a patient with juvenile neuronal ceroid lipofuscinosis. *J Neurol*, 249, 1398–1400.

Metzler M, Legendre-Guillemin V, Gan L, Chopra V, Kwok A, McPherson PS, & Hayden MR (2001) HIP1 functions in clathrin-mediated endocytosis through binding to clathrin and adaptor protein 2. *J Biol Chem*, 276, 39271–39276.

Mitchell DA, Vasudevan A, Linder ME, & Deschenes RJ (2006) Protein palmitoylation by a family of DHHC protein S-acyltransferases. *J Lipid Res*, 47, 1118–1127.

Mitchison HM, Hofmann SL, Becerra CH, Munroe PB, Lake BD, Crow YJ, Stephenson JB, Williams RE, Hofman IL, Taschner PE, Martin JJ, Philippart M, Andermann E, Andermann F, Mole SE, Gardiner RM, & O'Rawe AM (1998) Mutations in the palmitoyl-protein thioesterase gene (PPT; CLN1) causing juvenile neuronal ceroid lipofuscinosis with granular osmiophilic deposits. *Hum Mol Genet*, 7, 291–297.

Mole SE, Williams RE, & Goebel HH (2005) Correlations between genotype, ultrastructural morphology and clinical phenotype in the neuronal ceroid lipofuscinoses. *Neurogenetics*, 6, 107–126.

Mole SE, Zhong NA, Sarpong A, Logan WP, Hofmann S, Yi W, Franken PF, van Diggelen OP, Breuning MH, Moroziewicz D, Ju W, Salonen T, Holmberg V, Jarvela I, & Taschner PE (2001) New mutations in the neuronal ceroid lipofuscinosis genes. *Eur J Paediatr Neurol*, 5 Suppl A, 7–10.

Munroe PB, Greene ND, Leung KY, Mole SE, Gardiner RM, Mitchison HM, Stephenson JB, & Crow YJ (1998) Sharing of PPT mutations between distinct clinical forms of neuronal ceroid lipofuscinoses in patients from Scotland. *J Med Genet*, 35, 790.

Nijssen PC, Ceuterick C, van Diggelen OP, Elleder M, Martin JJ, Teepen JL, Tyynelä J, & Roos RA (2003) Autosomal dominant adult neuronal ceroid lipofuscinosis: a novel form of NCL with granular osmiophilic deposits without palmitoyl protein thioesterase 1 deficiency. *Brain Pathol*, 13, 574–581.

Norman RM & Wood N (1941) Congenital form of amaurotic family idiocy. *J Neurol Psych*, 4, 175–190.

Ohno K, Saito S, Sugawara K, Suzuki T, Togawa T, & Sakuraba H (2010) Structural basis of neuronal ceroid lipofuscinosis 1. *Brain Dev*, 32, 524–530.

Piomelli D (2005) The challenge of brain lipidomics. *Prostaglandins Other Lipid Mediat*, 77, 23–34.

Qiao X, Lu JY, & Hofmann SL (2007) Gene expression profiling in a mouse model of infantile neuronal ceroid lipofuscinosis reveals upregulation of immediate early genes and mediators of the inflammatory response. *BMC Neurosci*, 8, 95.

Raitta C & Santavuori P (1973) Ophthalmological findings in infantile type of so-called neuronal ceroid lipofuscinosis. *Acta Ophthalmol (Copenh)*, 51, 755–763.

Ramadan H, Al-Din AS, Ismail A, Balen F, Varma A, Twomey A, Watts R, Jackson M, Anderson G, Green E, & Mole SE (2007) Adult neuronal ceroid lipofuscinosis caused by deficiency in palmitoyl protein thioesterase 1. *Neurology*, 68, 387–388.

Rapola J & Haltia M (1973) Cytoplasmic inclusions in the vermiform appendix and skeletal muscle in two types of so-called neuronal ceroid-lipofuscinosis. *Brain*, 96, 833–840.

Rapola J, Salonen R, Ammala P, & Santavuori P (1990) Prenatal diagnosis of the infantile type of neuronal ceroid lipofuscinosis by electron microscopic investigation of human chorionic villi. *Prenat Diagn*, 10, 553–559.

Rapola J, Santavuori P, & Savilahti E (1984) Suction biopsy of rectal mucosa in the diagnosis of infantile and juvenile types of neuronal ceroid lipofuscinoses. *Hum Pathol*, 15, 352–360.

Rohrbough J & Broadie K (2005) Lipid regulation of the synaptic vesicle cycle. *Nat Rev Neurosci*, 6, 139–150.

Saha A, Kim SJ, Zhang Z, Lee YC, Sarkar C, Tsai PC, & Mukherjee AB (2008) RAGE signaling contributes to neuroinflammation in infantile neuronal ceroid lipofuscinosis. *FEBS Lett*, 582, 3823–3831.

Salonen T, Hellsten E, Horelli-Kuitunen N, Peltonen L, & Jalanko A (1998) Mouse palmitoyl protein thioesterase: gene structure and expression of cDNA. *Genome Res*, 8, 724–730.

Salonen T, Jarvela I, Peltonen L, & Jalanko A (2000) Detection of eight novel palmitoyl protein thioesterase (PPT) mutations underlying infantile neuronal ceroid lipofuscinosis (INCL;CLN1). *Hum Mutat*, 15, 273–279.

Santavuori P (1982) Clinical findings in 69 patients with infantile neuronal ceroid lipofuscinosis. In Armstrong D, Koppang N, & Rider A (Eds.) *Ceroid Lipofuscinoses (Batten disease)*, pp. 23–34. Amsterdam, Elsevier.

Santavuori P, Gottlob I, Haltia M, Rapola J, Lake BD, Tyynelä J, & Peltonen L (1999) CLN1, infantile and other types of NCL with GROD. In Goebel HH, Lake BD, & Mole SE (Eds.) *The Neuronal Ceroid Lipofuscinoses (Batten Disease)*, pp. 16–36, Amsterdam, IOS Press.

Santavuori P, Haltia M, & Rapola J (1974) Infantile type of so-called neuronal ceroid-lipofuscinosis. *Dev Med Child Neurol*, 16, 644–653.

Santavuori P, Haltia M, Rapola J, & Raitta C (1973) Infantile type of so-called neuronal ceroid-lipofuscinosis. 1. A clinical study of 15 patients. *J Neurol Sci*, 18, 257–267.

Santavuori P, Vanhanen SL, Sainio K, Nieminen M, Wallden T, Launes J, & Raininko R (1993) Infantile neuronal ceroid-lipofuscinosis (INCL): diagnostic criteria. *J Inherit Metab Dis*, 16, 227–229.

Santorelli FM, Bertini E, Petruzzella V, Di Capua M, Calvieri S, Gasparini P, & Zeviani M (1998) A novel insertion mutation (A169i) in the CLN1 gene is associated with infantile neuronal ceroid lipofuscinosis in an Italian patient. *Biochem Biophys Res Commun*, 245, 519–522.

Schriner JE, Yi W, & Hofmann SL (1996) cDNA and genomic cloning of human palmitoyl-protein thioesterase (PPT), the enzyme defective in infantile neuronal ceroid lipofuscinosis. *Genomics*, 34, 317–322.

Siintola E, Partanen S, Stromme P, Haapanen A, Haltia M, Maehlen J, Lehesjoki AE, & Tyynelä J (2006) Cathepsin D deficiency underlies congenital human neuronal ceroid-lipofuscinosis. *Brain*, 129, 1438–1445.

Simonati A, Tessa A, Bernardina BD, Biancheri R, Veneselli E, Tozzi G, Bonsignore M, Grosso S, Piemonte F, & Santorelli FM (2009) Variant late infantile neuronal ceroid lipofuscinosis because of CLN1 mutations. *Pediatr Neurol*, 40, 271–276.

Sleat DE, Lackland H, Wang Y, Sohar I, Xiao G, Li H, & Lobel P (2005) The human brain mannose 6-phosphate glycoproteome: a complex mixture composed of multiple isoforms of many soluble lysosomal proteins. *Proteomics*, 5, 1520–1532.

Smotrys JE & Linder ME (2004) Palmitoylation of intracellular signaling proteins: regulation and function. *Annu Rev Biochem*, 73, 559–587.

Soyombo AA & Hofmann SL (1997) Molecular cloning and expression of palmitoyl-protein thioesterase 2 (PPT2), a homolog of lysosomal palmitoyl-protein thioesterase with a distinct substrate specificity. *J Biol Chem*, 272, 27456–27463.

Stephenson JB, Greene ND, Leung KY, Munroe PB, Mole SE, Gardiner RM, Taschner PE, O'Regan M, Naismith K, Crow YJ, & Mitchison HM (1999) The molecular basis of GROD-storing neuronal ceroid lipofuscinoses in Scotland. *Mol Genet Metab*, 66, 245–247.

Sugimoto H, Hayashi H, & Yamashita S (1996) Purification, cDNA cloning, and regulation of lysophospholipase from rat liver. *J Biol Chem*, 271, 7705–7711.

Sun X, Marks DL, Park WD, Wheatley CL, Puri V, O'Brien JF, Kraft DL, Lundquist PA, Patterson MC, Pagano RE, & Snow K (2001) Niemann-Pick C variant detection by altered sphingolipid trafficking and correlation with mutations within a specific domain of NPC1. *Am J Hum Genet*, 68, 1361–1372.

Suopanki J, Lintunen M, Lahtinen H, Haltia M, Panula P, Baumann M, & Tyynelä J (2002) Status epilepticus induces changes in the expression and localization of endogenous palmitoyl-protein thioesterase 1. *Neurobiol Dis*, 10, 247–257.

Suopanki J, Partanen S, Ezaki J, Baumann M, Kominami E, & Tyynelä J (2000) Developmental changes in the expression of neuronal ceroid lipofuscinoses-linked proteins. *Mol Genet Metab*, 71, 190–194.

Suopanki J, Tyynelä J, Baumann M, & Haltia M (1999a) Palmitoyl-protein thioesterase, an enzyme implicated in neurodegeneration, is localized in neurons and is developmentally regulated in rat brain. *Neurosci Lett*, 265, 53–56.

Suopanki J, Tyynelä J, Baumann M, & Haltia M (1999b) The expression of palmitoyl-protein thioesterase is developmentally regulated in neural tissues but not in nonneural tissues. *Mol Genet Metab*, 66, 290–293.

Tamaki SJ, Jacobs Y, Dohse M, Capela A, Cooper JD, Reitsma M, He D, Tushinski R, Belichenko PV, Salehi A, Mobley W, Gage FH, Huhn S, Tsukamoto AS, Weissman IL, & Uchida N (2009) Neuroprotection of host cells by human central nervous system stem cells in a mouse model of infantile neuronal ceroid lipofuscinosis. *Cell Stem Cell*, 5, 310–319.

Tardy C, Sabourdy F, Garcia V, Jalanko A, Therville N, Levade T, & Andrieu-Abadie N (2009) Palmitoyl protein thioesterase 1 modulates tumor necrosis factor alpha-induced apoptosis. *Biochim Biophys Acta*, 1793, 1250–1258.

Tarkkanen A, Haltia M, & Merenmies L (1977) Ocular pathology in infantile type of neuronal ceroid-lipofuscinosis. *J Pediatr Ophthalmol*, 14, 235–241.

Tyynelä J, Baumann M, Henseler M, Sandhoff K, & Haltia M (1995) Sphingolipid activator proteins (SAPs) are stored together with glycosphingolipids in the infantile neuronal ceroid-lipofuscinosis (INCL). *Am J Med Genet*, 57, 294–297.

Tyynelä J, Cooper JD, Khan MN, Shemilts SJ, & Haltia M (2004) Hippocampal pathology in the human neuronal ceroid-lipofuscinoses: distinct patterns of storage deposition, neurodegeneration and glial activation. *Brain Pathol*, 14, 349–357.

Tyynelä J, Palmer DN, Baumann M, & Haltia M (1993) Storage of saposins A and D in infantile neuronal ceroid-lipofuscinosis. *FEBS Lett*, 330, 8–12.

Vanhanen SL, Puranen J, Autti T, Raininko R, Liewendahl K, Nikkinen P, Santavuori P, Suominen P, Vuori K, & Hakkinen AM (2004) Neuroradiological findings (MRS, MRI, SPECT) in infantile neuronal ceroid-lipofuscinosis (infantile CLN1) at different stages of the disease. *Neuropediatrics*, 35, 27–35.

Vanhanen SL, Raininko R, Autti T, & Santavuori P (1995a) MRI evaluation of the brain in infantile neuronal ceroid-lipofuscinosis. Part 2: MRI findings in 21 patients. *J Child Neurol*, 10, 444–450.

Vanhanen SL, Raininko R, Santavuori P, Autti T, & Haltia M (1995b) MRI evaluation of the brain in infantile neuronal ceroid-lipofuscinosis. Part 1: Postmortem MRI with histopathologic correlation. *J Child Neurol*, 10, 438–443.

Vanhanen SL, Sainio K, Lappi M, & Santavuori P (1997) EEG and evoked potentials in infantile neuronal ceroid-lipofuscinosis. *Dev Med Child Neurol*, 39, 456–463.

Verkruyse LA & Hofmann SL (1996) Lysosomal targeting of palmitoyl-protein thioesterase. *J Biol Chem*, 271, 15831–15836.

Vesa J, Hellsten E, Verkruyse LA, Camp LA, Rapola J, Santavuori P, Hofmann SL, & Peltonen L (1995) Mutations in the palmitoyl protein thioesterase gene causing infantile neuronal ceroid lipofuscinosis. *Nature*, 376, 584–587.

Virmani T, Gupta P, Liu X, Kavalali ET, & Hofmann SL (2005) Progressively reduced synaptic vesicle pool size in cultured neurons derived from neuronal ceroid lipofuscinosis-1 knockout mice. *Neurobiol Dis*, 20, 314–323.

von Schantz C, Saharinen J, Kopra O, Cooper JD, Gentile M, Hovatta I, Peltonen L, & Jalanko A (2008) Brain gene expression profiles of Cln1 and Cln5 deficient mice unravels common molecular pathways underlying neuronal degeneration in NCL diseases. *BMC Genomics*, 9, 146.

Voznyi YV, Keulemans JL, Mancini GM, Catsman-Berrevoets CE, Young E, Winchester B, Kleijer WJ, & van Diggelen OP (1999) A new simple enzyme assay for pre- and postnatal diagnosis of infantile neuronal ceroid lipofuscinosis (INCL) and its variants. *J Med Genet*, 36, 471–474.

Waliany S, Das AK, Gaben A, Wisniewski KE, & Hofmann SL (2000) Identification of three novel mutations of the palmitoyl-protein thioesterase-1 (PPT1) gene in children with neuronal ceroid-lipofuscinosis. *Hum Mutat*, 15, 206–207.

Wei H, Kim SJ, Zhang Z, Tsai PC, Wisniewski KE, & Mukherjee AB (2008) ER and oxidative stresses are common mediators of apoptosis in both neurodegenerative and non-neurodegenerative lysosomal storage disorders and are alleviated by chemical chaperones. *Hum Mol Genet*, 17, 469–477.

Weleber RG, Gupta N, Trzupek KM, Wepner MS, Kurz DE, & Milam AH (2004) Electroretinographic and clinicopathologic correlations of retinal dysfunction in infantile neuronal ceroid lipofuscinosis (infantile Batten disease). *Mol Genet Metab*, 83, 128–137.

Wisniewski KE, Connell F, Kaczmarski W, Kaczmarski A, Siakotos A, Becerra CR, & Hofmann SL (1998a) Palmitoyl-protein thioesterase deficiency in a novel granular variant of LINCL. *Pediatr Neurol*, 18, 119–123.

Wisniewski KE, Kida E, Gordon-Majszak W, & Saitoh T (1990a) Altered amyloid beta-protein precursor processing in brains of patients with neuronal ceroid lipofuscinosis. *Neurosci Lett*, 120, 94–96.

Yeh DC, Duncan JA, Yamashita S, & Michel T (1999) Depalmitoylation of endothelial nitric-oxide synthase by acyl-protein thioesterase 1 is potentiated by Ca(2+)-calmodulin. *J Biol Chem*, 274, 33148–33154.

Zhang Z, Butler JD, Levin SW, Wisniewski KE, Brooks SS, & Mukherjee AB (2001) Lysosomal ceroid depletion by drugs: therapeutic implications for a hereditary neurodegenerative disease of childhood. *Nat Med*, 7, 478–484.

Zhang Z, Lee YC, Kim SJ, Choi MS, Tsai PC, Saha A, Wei H, Xu Y, Xiao YJ, Zhang P, Heffer A, & Mukherjee AB (2007) Production of lysophosphatidylcholine by cPLA2 in the brain of mice lacking PPT1 is a signal for phagocyte infiltration. *Hum Mol Genet*, 16, 837–847.

Zhang Z, Lee YC, Kim SJ, Choi MS, Tsai PC, Xu Y, Xiao YJ, Zhang P, Heffer A, & Mukherjee AB (2006) Palmitoyl-protein thioesterase-1 deficiency mediates the activation of the unfolded protein response and neuronal apoptosis in INCL. *Hum Mol Genet*, 15, 337–346.

Chapter 7

CLN2

M. Chang, J.D. Cooper, B.L. Davidson, O.P. van Diggelen, M. Elleder, H.H. Goebel, A.A. Golabek, E. Kida, A. Kohlschütter, P. Lobel, S.E. Mole, A. Schulz, D.E. Sleat, M. Warburton, and K.E. Wisniewski

INTRODUCTION

Mutations in the *CLN2* or *TPP1* gene cause classic CLN2 disease, late infantile, formerly known as Janský–Bielschowsky disease. *CLN2* encodes an enzyme, tripeptidyl peptidase I (TPP-I or TPP1), making it particularly suitable for current therapeutic development. Many other NCL types have onset in late infancy—these are known as variant late infantile NCL diseases and are caused by mutations in other genes (*CLN5*, *CLN6*, *CLN7/MFSD8*, *CLN8*).

MOLECULAR GENETICS

Identification of *CLN2*

Early studies (Williams et al., 1993, Yan et al., 1993) excluded *CLN2*, the gene that is mutated in classic late infantile NCL, from loci associated with other forms of NCL, demonstrating that this disease was not an allelic form of infantile or juvenile NCL. *CLN2* was subsequently mapped to chromosome 11p15 (Sharp et al., 1997) by homozygosity mapping in five consanguineous families.

CLN2 (more properly *TPP1*) and its protein product were identified using a comparative proteomic approach focused on proteins containing mannose 6-phosphate (M6P) (Sleat et al., 1997), a carbohydrate modification that functions as a signal for the targeting of newly-synthesized lysosomal proteins from the Golgi to a prelysosomal compartment via specific M6P receptors (M6PRs). Brain extracts from normal and classic late infantile patients were fractionated by two-dimensional gel electrophoresis and proteins containing M6P were visualized with a radiolabelled soluble form of the cation independent M6PR. A single protein of approximately 46kDa appeared to be missing in classic late infantile patients. This protein was purified from normal human brain by affinity chromatography on immobilized M6PR and its amino terminal sequence determined by chemical sequencing. This allowed identification of cDNA clones leading to the full-length cDNA and protein sequences, as well as mapping of the gene to 11p15.2–15.5. Two lines of evidence confirmed that defects in this gene were responsible for classic CLN2 disease, late infantile NCL. First, sequence comparisons indicated that the gene product was similar to a group of bacterial proteases that had an acidic pH optima and which were not inhibited by pepstatin, and a corresponding enzymatic activity was found to be deficient in CLN2 disease, late infantile autopsy specimens. Second, *CLN2* mutations were identified in CLN2 disease, late infantile patients, but not in normal controls.

Gene structure of *CLN2/TPP1*

CLN2, now known more properly as *TPP1* (GenBank accession number AF039704), is a small gene (approximately 6.7kb) that is located on chromosome 11p15 (Liu et al., 1998). *CLN2* comprises 13 exons and 12 small introns that range from 112–984bp, all of which contain the invariant GT…AG splice junction residues.

The human *CLN2/TPP1* gene is ubiquitously expressed and, by northern blotting on a limited set of human tissues, highest levels are seen in heart and placenta (Sleat et al., 1997). Based on expression profiling by analysis of expressed sequence tag (EST) counts (see Unigene EST Profile Viewer analysis of *CLN2/TPP1* transcription; http://www.ncbi.nlm.nih.gov/UniGene/ESTProfileViewer.cgi?uglist=Hs.523454), spleen and thymus appear to have the highest expression levels of human *CLN2/TPP1* transcript. Two transcripts have been identified which are 2503 and 3487 nucleotides in length and result from the use of alternate polyadenylation sites (Liu et al., 1998). Sequence analysis of *CLN2* ESTs has identified to date approximately 20 low abundance splice variants of unknown, but probably biologically unimportant, function (see Altsplice Entry Display for TPP1; http://www.ebi.ac.uk/asd-srv/altsplicedb.cgi?method=ENSEMBL;product=ALT;specie=H;ensembl_id=ENSG00000166340). An EST clone, zu64a10 (GenBank accession number AA400442), overlaps the 5′ end of *CLN2* but is transcribed in the opposite direction to *CLN2*. This EST is not conserved in mammals and its physiological significance, if any, remains uncertain.

Mutation spectrum

To date, nearly 70 mutations in *CLN2/TPP1* have been associated with CLN2 disease (http://www.ucl.ac.uk/ncl/cln2.shtml), currently comprising 38 missense mutations, ten mutations within conserved elements of splice junctions or which probably affect splicing, ten small deletions, one large deletion, two small insertions, and eight nonsense mutations (Sleat et al., 1997, Zhong et al., 1998, Caillaud et al., 1999, Hartikainen et al., 1999, Sleat et al., 1999, Wisniewski et al., 1999, Berry-Kravis et al., 2000, Tessa et al., 2000, Zhong et al., 2000, Lam et al., 2001, Lin and Lobel, 2001a, Mole et al., 2001, Ju et al., 2002, Lavrov et al., 2002, Steinfeld et al., 2002, Koul et al., 2007, Bessa et al., 2008, Elleder et al., 2008, Goldberg-Stern et al., 2009, Kohan et al., 2009, Kousi et al., 2009) (and unpublished). In the largest survey to date of the molecular pathology of CLN2 disease, late infantile, which was conducted on patients predominantly residing in North America and Europe (Sleat et al., 1999), two mutations were found to be particularly common: an intronic G>C transversion in the invariant AG of the intron 5 3′ splice junction, found in 38 of 115 alleles (c.509-1G>C), and predicted to affect splicing with a frameshift after p.Phe169, and a C>T transition in 32 of 115 alleles, which prematurely terminates translation at amino acid 208 of 563 (c.622C>T, p.Arg208X). No translation product was detected when cDNA encoding p.Arg208X was expressed in cultured cells (Steinfeld et al., 2004). Together, these alleles accounted for 60% of the *CLN2* mutations identified in this study. Forty per cent of patients were homozygous for either of these two alleles or were compound heterozygotes for both. An additional 38% of patients were compound heterozygotes with one of two common alleles, thus a total of 78% of patients were found to have one or two of these common mutations. In a subsequent study on patients residing in Germany or Switzerland (Steinfeld et al., 2002), 91% (20/22) were found to contain one or two of these common mutations. The fact that the majority of CLN2 disease, late infantile patients have at least one pathogenic allele that corresponds to one of these common mutations greatly facilitates genetic diagnosis of this disease.

The effects of mutations on *TPP1* are summarized in the 'Correlations' section.

At least 22 polymorphisms have been reported in *CLN2/TPP1*: four are in the 5′ untranslated region (UTR), one in the 3′ UTR, four affect the coding region with two changing amino acids, and 13 are in introns. There may be an additional one close to a splice junction.

Related genes

CLN2/TPP1 is conserved in vertebrates, but there are no other similar genes in these species.

CELL BIOLOGY

Structure and function of TPP1

Tripeptidyl peptidase I (TPP-I or TPP1) belongs to the sedolisin family of serine carboxyl peptidases (Wlodawer et al., 2003a) with MEROPS designation Family (http://merops.sanger.ac.uk). At present, TPP1 is the only known eukaryotic member of this family identified in higher eukaryotes and most other members are of fungal or bacterial origin (Wlodawer et al., 2003b). These enzymes demonstrate maximum activity at acid pH and hydrolyse a variety of synthetic peptides and protein substrates in vitro, with different enzymes having endoproteolytic and/or tripeptidyl amino peptidase activities (Wlodawer et al., 2004, Reichard et al., 2006). The sedolisins are members of the SB clan of peptidases but differ from the subtilisin family (S8) by having a catalytic tetrad consisting of Ser, Glu, Asp instead of Ser, His, Asp (Wlodawer et al., 2003b).

Recently, crystal structures for the glycosylated (Pal et al., 2008) and endoglycosidase H deglycosylated (Guhaniyogi et al., 2008) pro-form of TPP1 have been reported, revealing a conserved fold and other features of the S53 family including a calcium binding site. There are also three disulfide bonds that are unique to TPP1 that stabilize the protein fold. Importantly, analysis of these structures has identified the residues that form the charge transfer complex (catalytic triad Ser475, Glu272 and Asp276 and the oxyanion hole residue Asp360). This is supported by earlier predictions based upon modeling of TPP1 on the structures of two other members of the sedolisin family, sedolisin from *Pseudomonas* sp.101 (Wlodawer et al., 2001) and kumamolisin from *Bacillus* novo sp.MN-32 (Comellas-Bigler et al., 2004), as well as chemical modification and site directed mutagenesis studies (Lin et al 2001, Oyama et al., 2005, Walus et al., 2005). The crystal structures have provided valuable insights into the activation and catalytic mechanism of TPP1 including the molecular details of the interaction between the 151 amino acid propiece and the mature enzyme that prevents activation of the protease (Guhaniyogi et al., 2009). In addition, the structural consequences of missense mutations were evaluated (Pal et al., 2009).

The majority of missense mutations are predicted to disrupt folding, leading to instability and degradation, some confirmed (Steinfeld et al., 2004, Wujek et al., 2004). p.Val277Met, p.Gln248Pro, p.Gly284Val, p.Gly473Arg, and p.Ser475Leu probably compromise the active centre, causing loss of proteolytic activity. p.Gly277Arg and p.Ser153Pro are located within the prosegment and therefore may disturb processing of TPP1. p.Asn286Ser causes loss of one glycosylation site and complete loss of protease activity (Tsiakas et al., 2004). The effects of p.Val216Met, p.Arg266Gln, and p. Lys428Asn are unclear.

TPP1 is not inhibited by most inhibitors of serine, cysteine, aspartate, and metalloproteinases. Originally considered to be a member of the pepstatin-insensitive carboxypeptidases, a more detailed comparison of sequence homologies with other proteinases identified these enzymes as related to the subtilisin family of serine proteinases (Rawlings and Barrett, 1995). TPP1 appears to be resistant to phenylmethylsulphonyl fluoride (PMSF) (Page et al., 1993), but is slowly inactivated by diisopropyl phosphorofluoridate (DFP) which specifically modifies the active site serine, Ser475 (Lin et al., 2001). The enzyme is also sensitive to reagents that modify histidine residues but a candidate histidine that might be involved in catalysis could not be identified (Page et al., 1993, Vines and Warburton, 1998).

The *CLN2/TPP1* gene codes for a 563-amino acid product from which a 19-amino acid signal peptide is cleaved to yield a 544-amino acid pro-TPP1 (67kDa) (Sleat et al., 1997). Autocatalytic processing produces the 368-amino acid mature form (46kDa) (Lin et al., 2001) (Figure 7.1). The mature form contains all five potential N-glycosylation sites (Golabek et al., 2003) of which one, Asn286, is essential for enzymatic activity (Tsiakas et al., 2004). N-glycans on both Asn210 and Asn286 have phosphomannose groups and consequently are important for routing of TPP1 to lysosomes. Individual mutations of the other glycosylation sites did not affect enzyme processing or activity (Wujek et al., 2004).

Expression studies of mutant TPP1 showed that the change p.Gln100Arg found in two

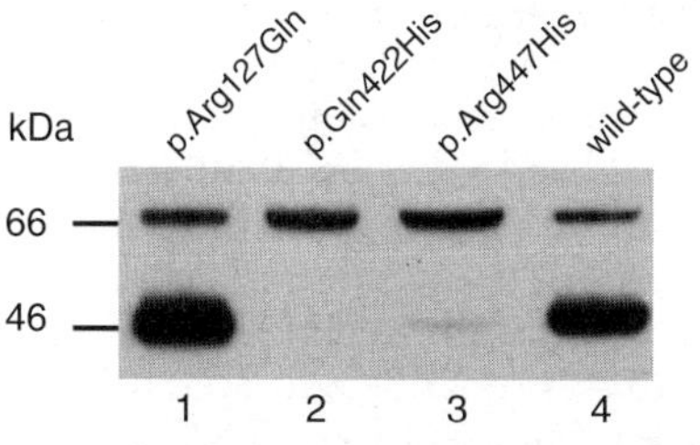

Figure 7.1 Immunoblot analysis of TPP1 mutant proteins stably expressed in Chinese hamster ovary cells. Lysates of cells expressing p.Arg127Gln (lane 1), p.Gln422His (lane 2), and p.Arg447His (lane 3) TPP1 mutants. Lane 4 shows wild-type TPP1. 20 μg protein of cell lysates per lane. Upper band represents the pro-enzyme, the lower band the processed enzyme. There is a small amount of mature TPP1 in cells expressing p.Arg447His-TPP1 mutant. Blot developed with monoclonal antibody 8C4 to TPP1 by using enhanced chemiluminescence method.

patients in association with p.Gly389Glu did not affect TPP1 activity, and was therefore likely to be a polymorphism, whereas both p. Gly389Glu and p.Arg447His reduced TPP1 activity (Lin and Lobel, 2001a). In addition, it was also postulated that p.Gly389Glu and p.Arg447His mutations may adversely affect TPP1 structure and stability. A study of four missense mutations that are located in conserved protein regions of TPP1 (p.Asn286Ser, p.Ile287Asn, p.Thr353Pro and p.Gln422His), showed that these significantly decreased enzymatic activity, blocked processing to the mature size peptidase, and led to protein retention in the endoplasmic reticulum and rapid degradation in non-lysosomal compartments (Steinfeld et al., 2004). In contrast, p.Arg127Gln, located within a non-conserved protein region did not significantly affect enzymatic activity, stability, processing, and lysosomal targeting of TPP1.

Substrate specificity and function of TPP1

Several peptide hormones have been shown to be substrates for TPP1 *in vitro*, these include cholecystokinin, neuromedin B, neuropeptide Y, glucagon, PTH-(1-34), angiotensins II and III, substance P, and the individual A and B chains of insulin (Vines and Warburton, 1998, Junaid et al., 2000, Bernardini and Warburton, 2001, Warburton and Bernardini, 2002, Kopan et al., 2004, Oyama et al., 2005). It was originally proposed that the N-termini of small unstructured polypeptides could enter the active site whereas larger globular peptides were unable to do so. Clearly, the hydrolysis of small synthetic peptides based on the N-terminal sequence of larger peptides gives little information on the susceptibility of the larger peptide to degradation by TPP1 (Bernardini and Warburton, 2001). TPP1 only appears to degrade peptides with a Mr below approximately 5kDa and has an absolute requirement for an unblocked N-terminus (Warburton and Bernardini, 2001). TPP1 has also been reported to initiate the degradation of subunit c of mitochondrial ATPase, a small (Mr 7.5kDa), extremely hydrophobic protein which is a major component of the lysosomal storage material (autofluorescent ceroid lipofuscin) in CLN2 disease, late infantile and several other forms of NCL (Ezaki et al., 2000a).

Once initiated, the degradation of subunit c is completed by cathepsin D (Ezaki et al., 1999).

Initial studies on the specificity of TPP1 towards synthetic substrates demonstrated the requirement for a hydrophobic amino acid in the P1 position and failure to hydrolyse peptides with a proline at P1 or P1′ (Warburton and Bernardini, 2001, Oyama et al., 2005). A more systematic approach using combinatorial peptide libraries of 7200 different peptide substrates to identify favoured residues at the P3, P2, P1, P1′ and P2′ sites has been carried out (Tian et al., 2006). The positively charged amino acid arginine was favoured at the P3 position and proline and a variety of hydrophobic residues at P2. Proline was the least favoured amino acid at the other four sites. Hydrophobic amino acids with bulky side chains were largely favoured at the P1 and P1′ sites and a variety of hydrophobic residues at P2′. However, the enzyme demonstrated a broad specificity with the relative substrate specificities (k_{cat}/k_M) for the majority of peptides varying over only a 100-fold range.

These observations suggest that TPP1 may function in the later stages of general protein catabolism or it may have a more specific role in the degradation of peptide hormones, possibly in specific cell types. The final stages of lysosomal protein catabolism are probably carried out by dipeptidyl (DPP) and tripeptidyl peptidases (TPP). Activities of lysosomal aminopeptidases are extremely low in major tissues such as liver and brain (M. Warburton, unpublished observation). Tripeptides released by TPP1 may act as substrates for DPP2 which shows major activity against tripeptides whereas DPP1 shows little specificity with regard to substrate length (McDonald, 1998, Turk et al., 1998). Cathepsin B (whose absence causes NCL-like disease in mice that are also lacking cathepsin L) also acts as a dipeptidyl peptidase. These observations suggest that di- and tripeptides may represent the end stages of lysosomal protein catabolism and that these products are transported into the cytoplasm for further degradation by cytoplasmic aminopeptidases. Alternatively, failure to degrade peptide hormones entering the cell by receptor-mediated endocytosis might prolong cell signalling events or, if it delays ligand-receptor dissociation, might prolong receptor downtime. Clearly, TPP1 must have a non-redundant role in some cell types since its absence has lethal consequences. At present, this probably favours the second explanation, as the major effects of the absence of TPP1 activity are observed predominantly in neuronal cells, although the role of TPP1 may differ in functionally diverse cells. There is some difficulty in explaining the cell specific pathology of the effects of absence of TPP1 activity. Although TPP1 has a ubiquitous distribution, the effects of inactivating TPP1 mutations are mostly observed in neuronal cells although some storage material is observed in other cell types. DPP1 may be able to partially compensate for TPP1 as it demonstrates a similar lack of specificity. However, DPP1 is not expressed in the brain (Pham et al., 1997, Rao et al., 1997), perhaps leaving this organ specifically vulnerable to pathological processes resulting from TPP1 deficiency (Bernardini and Warburton, 2002). However, subsequent experiments using TPP1-deficient mice that either lack or overexpress DPP1 indicated that DPP1 cannot functionally compensate for the loss of TPPI (Kim et al., 2008). TPP1 has also been shown to possess endoproteolytic activity against synthetic substrates and proteins in keeping with its proposed role in autoactivation (Ezaki et al., 2000b). Earlier studies suggesting that a tripeptidyl peptidase was involved in the degradation of collagen (McDonald et al., 1985, Andersen and McDonald, 1987) have not been confirmed and the failure of TPP1 to hydrolyse most substrates with a proline in the P1 position suggests that any action of TPP1 on intact collagen or its large degradation products may be restricted. However, as Pro is a preferred amino acid in the P2 position, it is not surprising that tripeptides of the type, Gly–Pro–X, are readily released from synthetic substrates (McDonald et al., 1985, Page et al., 1993) and such tripeptides are substrates for dipeptidyl peptidase II (McDonald and Schwabe, 1980).

Recently, the role of TPP1 in apoptosis was investigated. Apoptotic pathways requiring p53 or Bcl-2 were not involved (Kim et al., 2009). However, TPP1 appeared to contribute to tumour necrosis factor (TNF)-induced cell death (Autefage et al., 2009). Cells isolated from patients were resistant to the toxic effect of TNF, with specific TNF-induced effects being prevented. In addition, overexpression of TPP1 could induce these same effects, and correction of the lysosomal enzyme defect using a medium enriched in TPP1 enabled restoration of the TNF-induced effects.

Gene expression, cellular and tissue distribution

TPP1 has a purely lysosomal localization (Figure 7.2), unlike TPP2, which is predominantly located in the cytoplasm where it is probably involved in the degradation of peptides exiting the proteasome and in antigen presentation (Tomkinson, 1999). In some cell types, a proportion of TPP2 is localized through a GPI-anchor to the external face of the cell surface where it may regulate extracellular levels of peptide hormones (Rose et al., 1996). TPP1 is expressed in all mammals so far investigated, and genes homologous to *TPP1* have been identified in zebrafish and *Fugu* (although expression of TPP1 is much lower in some adult fish than in mammals, unpublished observations) (Wlodawer et al., 2003a). TPP1 is expressed in most mammalian tissues with high levels of expression observed in, for example, brain, liver, kidney, and testis in both humans and rodents (Kida et al., 2001, Kurachi et al., 2001). High levels of staining for TPP1 have been noted in endocrine cells and tissues which synthesize peptide hormones including neuropeptides. In the brain, neurons and glial cells demonstrate high immunoreactivity and many other cell types show some staining (Kida et al., 2001). Studies on human brain suggest that TPP1 levels increase during gestation and do not reach adult levels for about 24 months (Kida et al., 2001). In developing rat brains, TPP1 levels remained relatively constant (Suopanki et al., 2000). In retina, a tissue which also suffers pathological damage in CLN2 disease, neurons in the ganglion and inner nuclear layer were intensely stained. Results from 'quantitative' immunocytochemistry may be subject to various experimental problems, but at least give an indication of relative amounts of antigen (Taylor and Levenson, 2006).

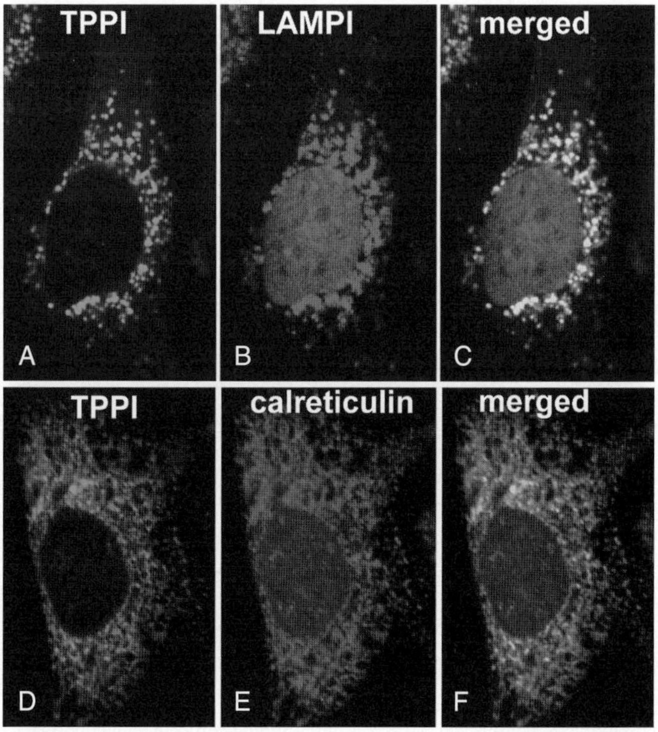

Figure 7.2 Subcellular localization of expressed wild-type TPP1 and mutant TPP1 protein (p.Gln422His) expressed in Chinese hamster ovary cells and visualized by laser-scanning confocal microscope. Wild-type TPP1 (A–C): vesicular structures visualized with polyclonal antibody to TPP1 (A) and LAMP1, a lysosomal marker (B), colocalize on the merged image (C), indicating lysosomal localization of wild-type TPP1. Mutant TPP1 (D–F): subcellular structures visualized with monoclonal antibody to TPP1 (D) and polyclonal antibodies to calreticulin (E), a marker of the endoplasmic reticulum, colocalize on the merged image (F), indicating retention of the p.Gln422His TPP1 mutant in the endoplasmic reticulum. Secondary antibodies conjugated to Alexa Fluor 488 (A, D) and Alexa Fluor 555 (B, E). Nuclei counterstained with propidium iodide. Magnification ×1000.

Whenever such experiments have been accompanied by other methods of detection such as Western blotting or assays of enzyme activity, conflicting results have been obtained for unknown reasons (Koike et al., 2002). The ubiquitous occurrence of TPP1 creates some problems in attempting to explain the specificity of CLN2 disease, late infantile with regard to the restricted types of cell affected.

In normal brain, TPP1 visualized by immunocytochemistry in all types of cells, including neurons, shows a granular pattern of stain typical for lysosomes, reaching adult distribution in early childhood (Figure 7.3) (Kida et al., 2001, Kurachi et al., 2001). Mutant proteins may not reach the lysosome (Figure 7.2). In paraffin sections of brain tissues from ten CLN2 disease patients carrying various mutations (both common and missense), either no TPP1 immunoreactivity (Figure 7.3) or residual stain confined to reactive astrocytes and some blood vessel walls could be found.

CLINICAL DATA

Clinical features

First symptoms of classic late infantile CLN2 disease occur generally between the ages of 2–4 years. Until the onset of symptoms, children are healthy and may have completely normal psychomotor development.

First symptoms include motor decline with clumsiness and ataxia, and deterioration of speech (Table 7.1). Initially these symptoms might be interpreted as delayed speech or general psychomotor development. Children may be referred for speech and language therapy before diagnosis. As the disease progresses, it becomes apparent that not only developmental delay, but regression is present. In the majority of patients loss of motor function and language ability occur in parallel, starting with a rapid decline of function around 3 years of age. Children usually are completely

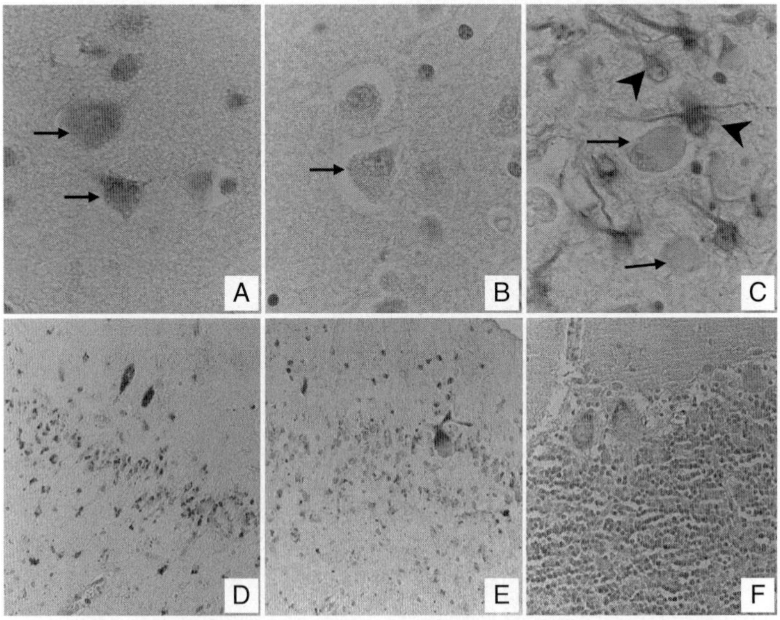

Figure 7.3 Immunoreactivity to TPP1 and subunit c of mitochondrial ATP synthase in brain tissue sections. (A) Granular pattern of TPP1 immunostaining in neurons and astrocytes in the frontal cortex of young, normal control subject. (B) Lack of TPP1 immunoreactivity in the brain tissue of an individual with CLN2 disease, homozygous for p.Arg208X. (C) Uniform staining of reactive astrocytes in CLN2 disease subject homozygous for missense mutation p.Gln422His. Note the absence of staining in the distended neurons. Arrows in (A–C) depict neurons; arrowheads indicate reactive astrocytes. (D) Lack of granule cells and Purkinje cells in the cerebellum of a CLN2 disease subject, compound heterozygous for p.Arg208X and c.509-1G>C. (E) Lack of granule cells and preserved Purkinje cell in a compound heterozygote for p.Gln422His and c.509-1G>C. (F) Preserved granule cells and Purkinje cells in the cerebellar cortex of a subject with a protracted form of CLN2 disease, a compound heterozygote for p.Arg447His and c.509-1G>C. (A–C) Monoclonal antibody 8C4 to TPP1. (D–F) Polyclonal antibody RAS138 to subunit c of mitochondrial ATP synthase. (A–C) ×600; (D–F) ×200.

Table 7.1 **Age at onset of symptoms in 17 children registered with the European NCL Case Registry, with classic CLN2 disease, late infantile**

	Number of children	Range of age of onset (years)	Median age of onset (years)
Speech delay	16	1–3.5	2.3
Seizures	16	2.5–4.5	3.0
Ataxia	17	2.5–4.6	3.5
Myoclonus	16	3–5	3.5
Regression	15	2.6–4.5	3.5
Visual failure	8	4–6	5
Chair bound	9	4–6	5.1

dependent at the age of 5 years (Steinfeld et al., 2002).

Epileptic seizures usually begin towards the end of the third year of life. They may be partial, generalized tonic–clonic, secondarily generalized, or sometimes absences. It is important to distinguish epileptic seizures from myoclonus which may coexist but should be treated differently. Myoclonus presents a major problem in many children as it is difficult to treat, and often prevents the children from resting and interrupts sleep.

From 4 years of age a gradual decline in visual ability is observed leading to complete blindness within about 3 years. In some patients, however, blindness may not become very apparent before the age of 10 years. Between the ages of 4–6 years, limb spasticity, truncal hypotonia, and loss of head control lead to complete loss of independent mobility.

Children lose the ability to swallow and many receive nutritional support using a nasogastric or gastrostomy tube. Even though this may prolong life, death usually occurs around middle teenage years.

The clinical course of classic CLN2 disease, late infantile can show some degree of variability when assessed using a clinical scoring system (Table 7.2). A clinical performance score ranging from 0–3 entailing motor function, visual function, language, and seizures has been developed (Figure 7.4) (Steinfeld

Table 7.2 **Clinical scoring system for CLN2 disease (from Steinfeld et al. 2002)**

Functional category	Performance	Score
Motor function	Walks normally*	3
	Frequent falls, clumsiness obvious	2
	No unaided walking or crawling only	1
	Immobile, mostly bedridden	0
Seizures (grand mal)	No seizure per 3-month period	3
	1–2 seizures per 3-month period	2
	1 seizure per month	1
	>1 seizure per month	0
Visual function	Recognizes desirable object, grabs at it	3
	Grabbing for objects uncoordinated	2
	Reacts to light	1
	No reaction to visual stimuli	0
Language	Normal (individual maximum)**	3
	Has become recognizably abnormal	2
	Hardly understandable	1
	Unintelligible or no language	0

*In some children, motor development was never really normal.

**In some children, normal language development was never present. In such cases, the best performance ever achieved was taken as a starting point and rated 3; when language then became recognizably worse, it was rated 2.

et al., 2002). Children with uncommon mutations in the *CLN2* gene may present with delayed disease onset, milder symptoms, and slower disease progression. Two patients have been described with disease onset at age 8 years and death in the fourth and fifth decades of life. Both were compound heterozygous for either of the common mutations p.Arg208X or c.509-1G>C and a rare missense mutation p.Arg447His (Sleat et al., 1999). One patient, who was compound heterozygous for the common p.Arg208X mutation and a rare p. Arg127Gln missense mutation, had loss of vision preceding other symptoms, similar to patients with juvenile NCL.

Children who are homozygous for the common p.Arg208X mutation can show variable onset and disease progression. The inter- and even intrafamilial variation in disease severity in CLN2 disease is considerable. A further refined clinical scoring system, which also includes neuroradiological data, has been developed for describing the neurological deterioration of CLN2 disease patients (Worgall et al., 2007).

Neurophysiology

Neurophysiological findings are very characteristic in classic CLN2 disease, late infantile patients.

The *electroencephalogram* (EEG) of classic CLN2 disease patients shows typical occipital spikes in response to slow photic (1–2Hz) stimulation (Figure 7.5). These responses may be detected even before the onset of clinical seizures and they become more exaggerated as symptoms progress.

The *electroretinogram* (ERG) of CLN2 disease, late infantile patients may be diminished even before any visual impairment is detected upon clinical examination (Figure 7.6). With progress of the disease the ERG soon becomes extinguished.

Visual evoked potentials (VEPs) are unusually enhanced in CLN2 disease, late infantile patients (Figure 7.6). Abnormally enhanced VEPs persist until late into the disease course and diminish during the final stage of the disease.

In summary, the triad of (1) abnormal EEG discharges to slow photic stimulation, (2) a giant VEP, and (3) an early diminuation or extinction of the ERG is highly characteristic of CLN2 disease, late infantile (Pampiglione and Harden, 1977).

Neuroradiology

Magnetic resonance imaging (MRI) in CLN2 disease, late infantile patients shows progressive cerebral atrophy (Figure 7.7). The atrophy is most obvious in the infratentorial region due to severe and early cerebellar involvement. MRI studies also show some white matter changes: hyperintense signals on T_2-weighted MRI scans are typically seen in the periventricular white matter (Petersen et al., 1996, Autti et al., 1997). Hypointense thalami have been reported on T_2-weighted imaging (Seitz et al., 1998).

There are few reports on magnetic resonance spectroscopy (MRS) findings in CLN2 disease, late infantile patients. A reduction of N-acetylaspartate (NAA) and an increase of *myo*-inositol and glutamate/glutamine in white matter has been reported (Seitz et al., 1998), as has a reduction of NAA and a slight increase of lactate in grey matter (Brockmann et al., 1996).

MORPHOLOGY

Gross pathology

Macroscopically, the brain may be severely atrophic with a reduced weight of 500–700g (normal >1350g). The sulci gape widely and the gyri are thin. The cerebellum is also markedly atrophic with small and firm folia. The leptomeninges overlying the brain may be thickened and the skull increased in thickness. On slicing, the cortical ribbon is thinned, with apparently normal underlying white matter. There is also thinning of the corpus callosum and enlargement of the ventricles. In the substantia nigra, neuromelanin pigmentation may be faint or absent (Elleder and Tyynelä, 1998). Visceral organs appear normal.

Light microscopy

The degree of tissue damage in CLN2 disease patients is similar. The structural damage is most

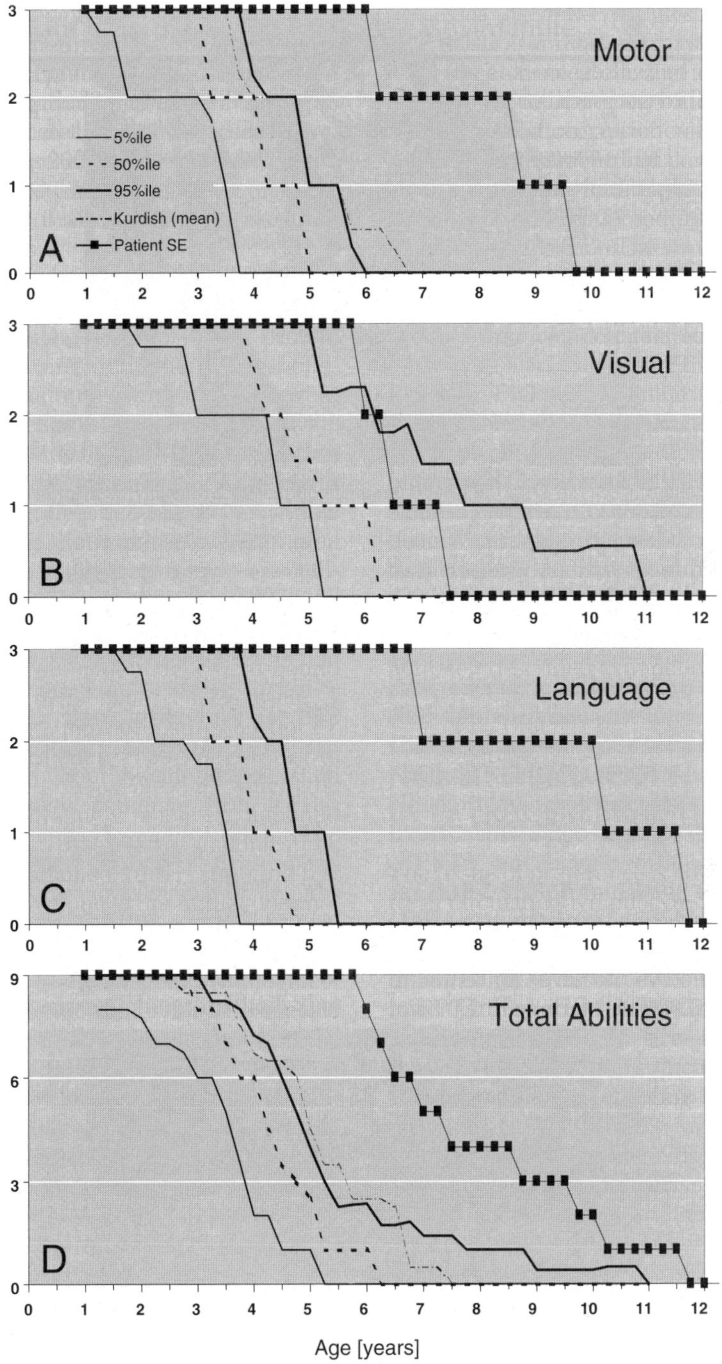

Figure 7.4 Quantitative description of the clinical course in 22 patients with *CLN2* mutations (median and confidence interval). (A–C) Scores for motor, visual, and language function according to Table 7.2. (D) Total ability score (sum of motor, visual, and language scores). Patient SE has an unusually mild (compound heterozygous) mutation. (Data from Steinfeld et al. 2002.)

prominent in the cerebellum, where granule cells are usually completely absent and only a few Purkinje cells survive, and there is prominent proliferation of Bergmann glia. All other brain areas show pronounced neuronal loss with gliosis and the presence of scattered macrophages.

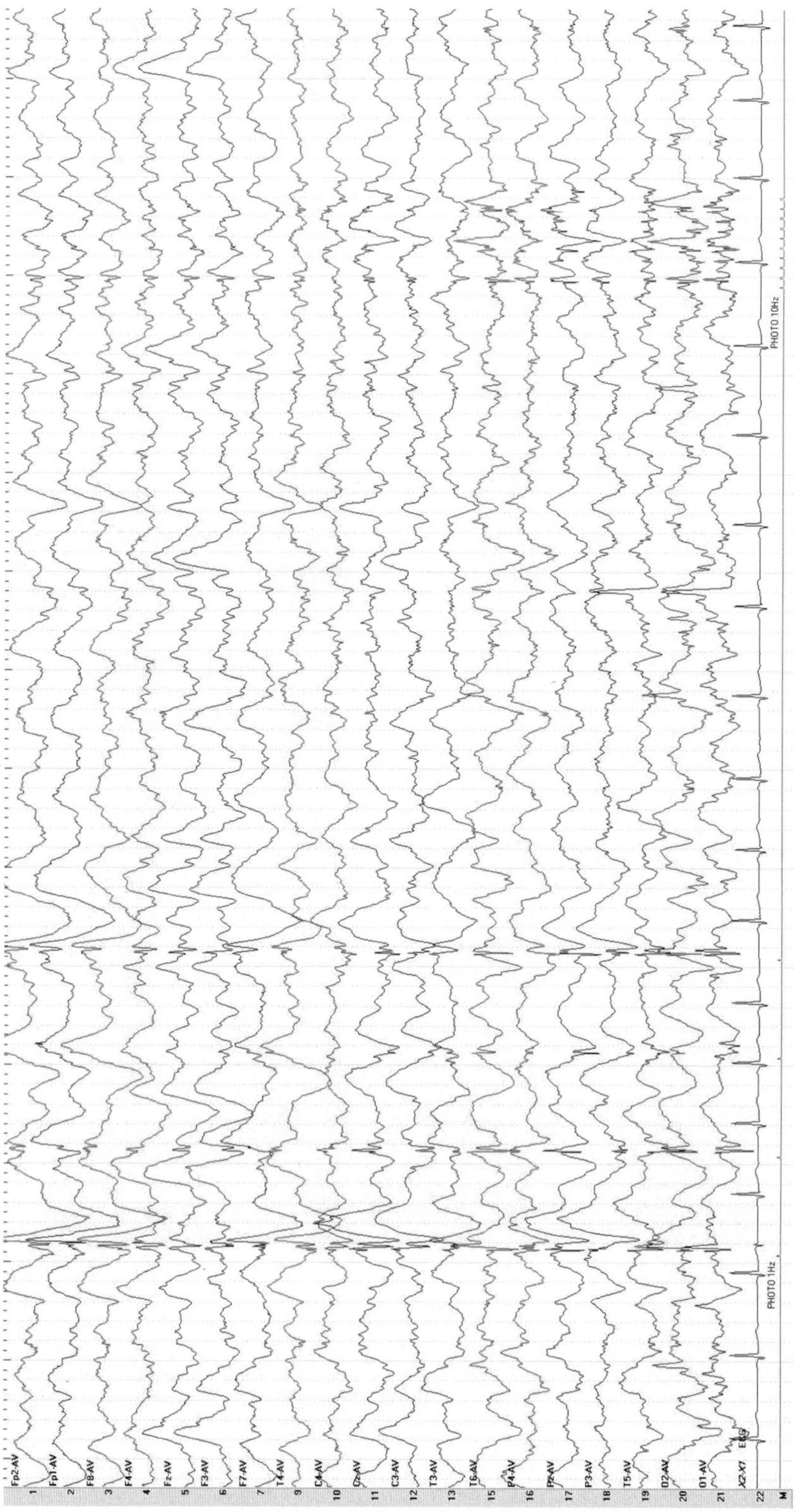

Figure 7.5 EEG of a child, age 6, with classic late infantile CLN2 disease showing photoparaoxysmal response. Spikes, particularly over the posterior half of the head, are elicited on slow photic stimulation at 1Hz (1/s), and at 10Hz, 150πV. (Illustration provided by Dr Sushma Goyal, The Evelina Children's Hospital, St. Thomas Hospital, London.)

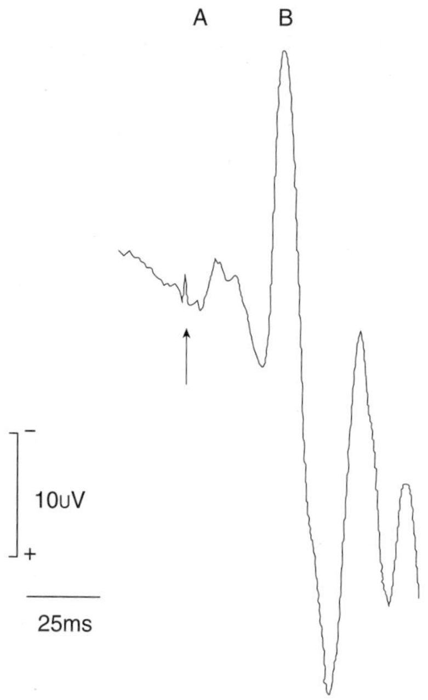

Figure 7.6 CLN2 disease, classic late infantile: recording of a flash electroretinogram from a 4-year-old. The arrow indicates the time of the flash stimulus. This is followed by a small ERG (the normal ERG should be at least 10μV), and is followed in turn by the abnormally enlarged components of the visual evoked potential derived from the vertex reference site. (Illustration provided by Dr. S. Boyd, Great Ormond Street Hospital, London.)

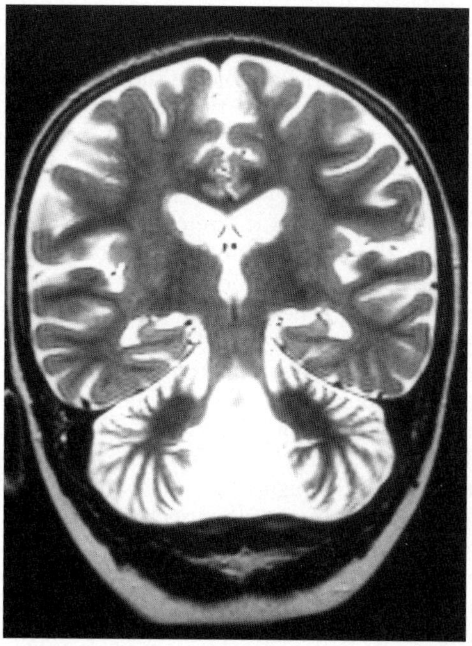

Figure 7.7 CLN2 disease, classic late infantile: magnetic resonance T_2-weighted image of a 4-year-old child showing cortical and cerebellar atrophy. There is some movement artefact. This child presented with seizures, ataxia, developmental regression, and behavioural disturbance at 3.5–4 years. There was a high amplitude spike response to photic stimulation at 1Hz on EEG and electron microscopy studies of a muscle biopsy revealed curvilinear bodies only.

Histopathologically, cortical atrophy of the brain and the cerebellum is due to severe depletion of neurons imparting an occasional sponginess to the cerebral cortex (Figure 7.8). Laminar necrosis is often present. At the end stage of the disorder, loss of neurons is usually so severe that it may be impossible to identify the normal neuronal layers, although lamina IV appears to be affected initially (R.D. Jolly and S.U. Walkley, personal communication). Immunohistochemical studies show increased BCL-2 and TUNEL staining, suggesting that neurons may disappear by apoptosis (Puranam et al., 1997), although TUNEL staining is not specific and does not differentiate between necrosis, autolytic cell death and apoptosis (Grasl-Kraupp et al., 1995). The destruction of nerve cells results in activation of microglia expressing MHC-II molecules, whereas monocyte-derived macrophages seen in acute or chronic inflammatory processes are conspicuously absent (Brück and Goebel, 1998). To a lesser extent, this activation of microglia, suggesting preservation of the blood–brain barrier,

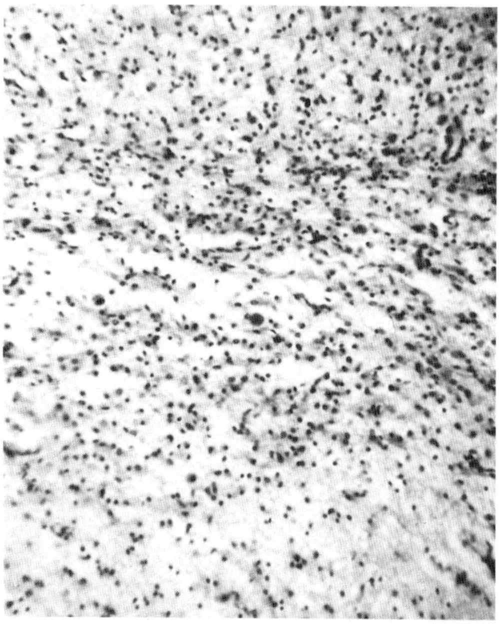

Figure 7.8 CLN2 disease, classic late infantile: loss of neurons and sponginess of cerebral cortex, haematoxylin-PAS, ×200.

may also be observed in subcortical grey and white matter indicating tissue damage and neuronal loss less obvious than in the cerebral and cerebellar cortices. In the cerebellum, both Purkinje and granular neurons are conspicuously reduced in number (Figure 7.9). Marked astrocytosis may be present (Figure 7.10).

The cytoplasm of the remaining neurons is slightly distended, with the proximal axonal segments often transformed into spindles or meganeurites. The neuronal distension, however, is less marked than that seen in the gangliosidoses. The neuronal cytoplasm contains a granular component—faintly yellowish in haematoxylin and eosin preparations. The granules share basic staining properties with ceroid and lipofuscin lipopigments (autofluorescence, sudanophilia in paraffin sections) and are strongly stained with antibody against subunit c of mitochondrial ATPase (SCMAS). The storage granules display (in frozen sections) strong acid phosphatase activity which is enhanced in those cells normally having some activity (neurons, Figure 7.11), and also in cells which do not normally have discernible activity (astrocytes, endothelial cells). The strong acid phosphatase activity at sites of storage indicates that classic CLN2 disease, late infantile is a lysosomal storage disorder. Accordingly, the granules display a strong signal for cathepsin D, a marker for the lysosome lumen, which can be easily detected even in paraffin embedded samples. Similar material is also present in astrocytes,

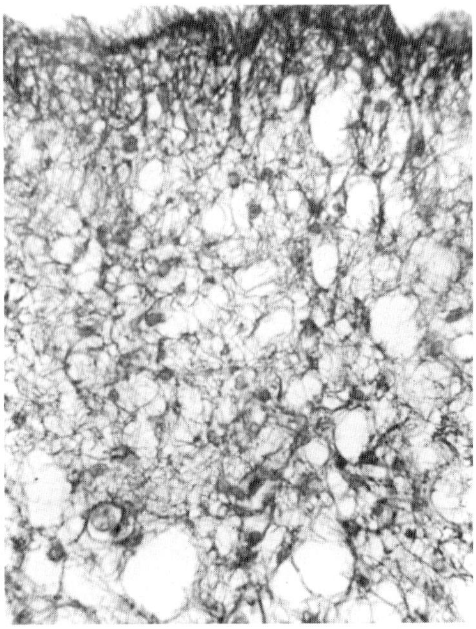

Figure 7.10 CLN2 disease, classic late infantile: dense fibrillar astrocytosis in cerebral cortex, Holzer stain, ×500.

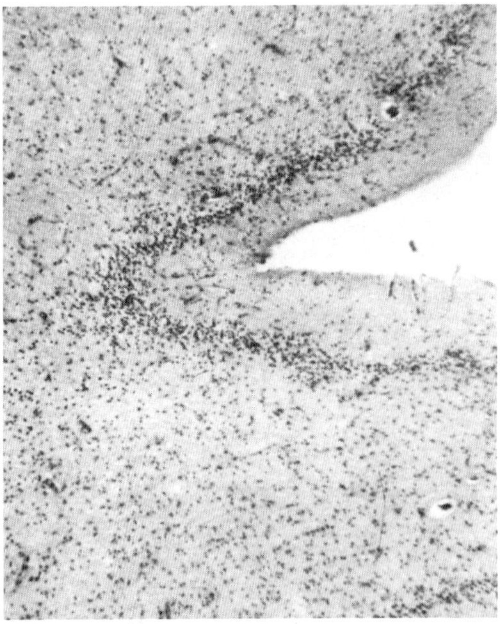

Figure 7.9 CLN2 disease, classic late infantile: severe loss of Purkinje and granular cells with proliferation of Bergmann glia, haematoxylin-eosin, ×80.

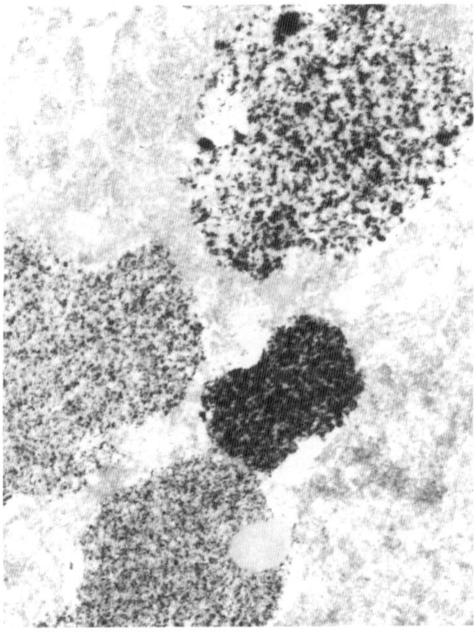

Figure 7.11 CLN2 disease, classic late infantile: acid phophatase is active in lipopigments of curvilinear type in a cerebral neuron, brain biopsy, Gömöri technique, ×16,000.

and in many other cell types throughout the body (see 'Disease mechanism' section).

Another feature of the neuronal storage process in CLN2 disease, late infantile is primary storage granule fusion ultimately leading to formation of rounded spheroids situated in the neuronal perikarya. The process of fusion is often accompanied by gradual modification of the stored material. There is gradual loss of periodic acid–Schiff (PAS) and permanganate aldehyde fuchsin (PAF) staining, reduction of both sudanophilia and autofluorescence, all well expressed in the primary storage granules. In contrast, there is an increase in Spielmeyer's myelin staining (ferriphilia). The signal for SCMAS is strongly diminished or abolished. At the ultrastructural level, there is gradual densification and loss of the curvilinear (CL) profile pattern. The processes of fusion and modification are independent. That means that there are spheroid-like inclusions composed of the unmodified storage material next to those in which the storage process has undergone the above mentioned modification (for further information, see Chapter 4).

The myelin in the white matter appears normal.

Immunohistochemistry

Immunohistochemical studies have shown that the neuronal storage material in CLN2 disease, late infantile, gives strong immunostaining for SCMAS (Figure 7.12) (Hall et al., 1991, Lake and Hall, 1993, Elleder et al., 1997), as in the South Hampshire sheep model (Palmer et al., 1989). This immunoreactivity is preserved in routinely prepared tissue blocks. The original tissues studied by Bielschowsky in 1913, when re-examined (Goebel et al., 1996), were shown to also be positive with SCMAS antibodies (Figure 7.13). Immunohistochemical studies give evidence of increased amounts of saposins A and D (Figure 7.14) (Tyynelä et al., 1995), some amyloid precursor protein (Wisniewski et al., 1990) in small and inconstant amounts (Rowan and Lake, unpublished) and no evidence of ubiquitin. The degree of subunit c accumulation in all cell types in the brain tissue is similar.

When an antibody against TPP1 became available, absence of this protein could be documented in CLN2 disease tissue by immunohistochemistry (Goebel et al., 2001), although this

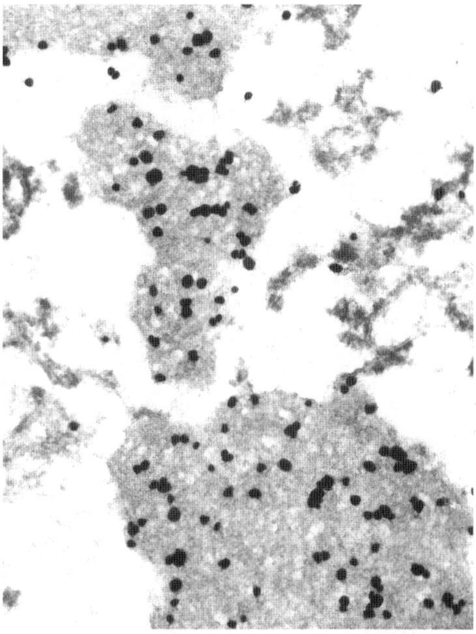

Figure 7.12 CLN2 disease, classic late infantile: immunogold-silver labelling of SCMAS over curvilinear bodies in a postmortem cerebral neuron, ×2000.

may not be a consistent finding in all cases as it will depend on the effect of the disease-causing mutation on protein stability. Using CLN1 disease, infantile as a positive control, absence of

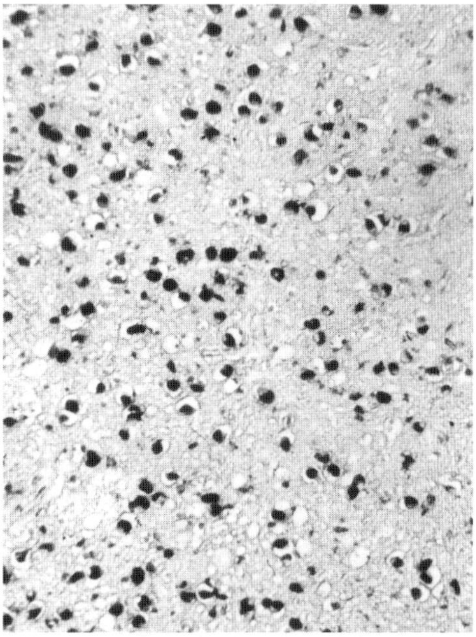

Figure 7.13 CLN2 disease, classic late infantile: M. Bielschowsky's original patient—remaining neurons are loaded with SCMAS, immunohistochemistry, ×200.

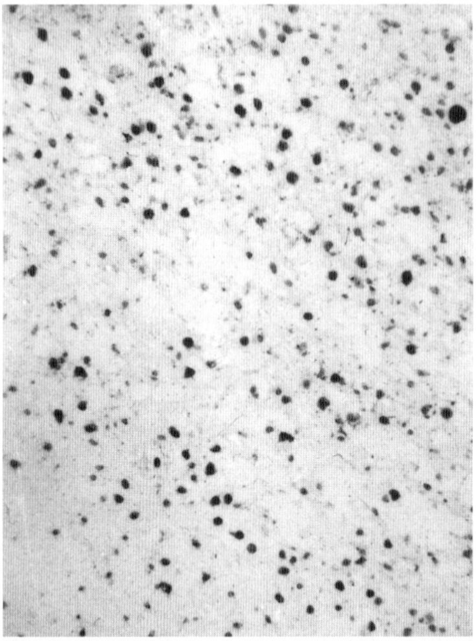

Figure 7.14 CLN2 disease, classic late infantile: M. Bielschowsky's original patient—cortical neurons also contain saposins, by courtesy of M. Haltia, immunohistochemistry, ×200.

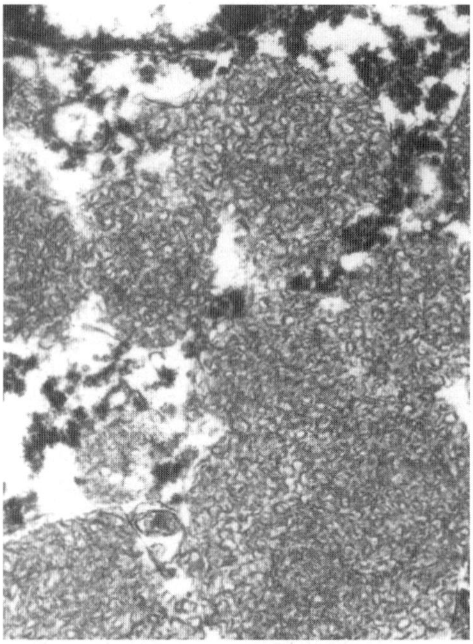

Figure 7.15 CLN2 disease, classic late infantile: pure curvilinear body in cerebral neuron, ×17,330.

the TPP1 protein could also be demonstrated in archival brain tissue originally described by Max Bielschowsky (Bielschowsky, 1920), later demonstrated to be true NCL (Goebel et al., 1996) and, subsequently by molecular analysis that identified heterozygosity for two mutations, as CLN2 disease (Wheeler et al., 2001).

Electron microscopy

Ultrastructural studies in classic CLN2 disease, late infantile (Figure 7.15) display ubiquitous CL storage body formation in all cells involved in the storage. The storage bodies are enclosed by a single unit membrane further indicating the lysosomal nature of the disease. In some areas the membrane may not be clearly discernible. The CL bodies are 'pure', do not contain granular or fingerprint (FP) components, and are not associated with the normal lipofuscin found in neurons. The CL bodies are associated with SCMAS and with acid phosphatase activity at the ultrastructural level (Figures 7.11 and 7.12).

In addition to marked CL body accumulation within the subcortical area, there may be formation of 'myoclonus bodies' or spheroids which display neither a curvilinear substructure nor have immunohistochemical reactions for SCMAS or saposins A and D (Elleder and Tyynelä, 1998). These spheroids develop in neurons of the basal ganglia as well as in those of the dentate nucleus (Elleder and Tyynelä, 1998), but they do not seem to be a consistent finding in every CLN2 disease, late infantile brain (see Chapter 4). Such spheroids can be observed in each of the NCL types caused by mutations in *CLN1*, *CLN2*, *CLN3*, and *CLN6* (Elleder and Tyynelä, 1998) (see Chapters 6, 8, and 10). The presence of such spheroids even in CLN1 disease, infantile tissues suggests that they may be an epiphenomenon; however, they do appear to be NCL-specific as they were not observed in other biochemically well-defined lysosomal disorders such as mucopolysaccharidoses and gangliosidoses and in which there may be additional SCMAS accumulation (Elleder and Tyynelä, 1998). The spheroids in NCL are different from those encountered in axons in a genetically undefined pigment variant of NCL (Goebel et al., 1995), vitamin E deficiency and other disorders where they are intra-axonal and consist of accumulated mitochondria and dense bodies. They also differ from the spheroids in the neuroaxonal dystrophies.

CL bodies of a very similar though not identical fine structure, i.e. composed of CL profiles, are a hallmark of chloroquine intoxication, usually after long-standing chloroquine treatment. As CL bodies, both in CLN2 disease and in chloroquine intoxication, are lysosomal residual bodies, they not only are high in acid phosphatase activity, but also contain the SCMAS protein as demonstrated by immunoelectron microscopy in biopsied skeletal muscle of a patient treated with chloroquine (Goebel et al., 2001). The demonstration of granular osmiophilic deposits (GRODs) in patients clinically resembling CLN2 disease, late infantile (Wisniewski et al., 1997, Wisniewski et al., 1998) suggests such patients may have mutations in the *CLN1* (Mitchison et al., 1998) gene, rather than in the *CLN2* gene, in which case PPT1 activity should be measured.

Retinal pathology

Atrophy of the retina is variable (Figure 7.16), being more severe in the peripheral than central part and commencing at the photoreceptor layer. It may proceed inward, occasionally resulting in a complete loss of neurons with a band of gliotic scarring at the end stage of the disease. Retinal pigment epithelial cells containing mixed lipopigment melanin inclusions (Figure 7.17) may migrate into the subretinal space, often reduced to a small slit, and beyond the external limiting membrane which has been re-established by Müller cells after the drop-out of the photoreceptors.

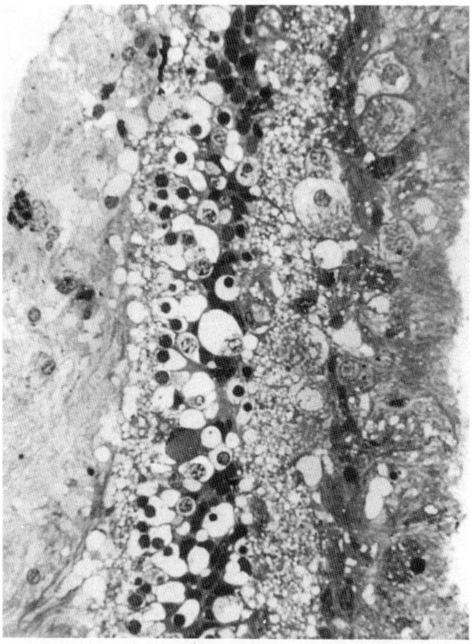

Figure 7.16 CLN2 disease, classic late infantile: presence of atrophy owing to complete loss of photoreceptors, 1µm-thick epon-embedded toluidine blue-stained section, ×500.

Although retinal cell loss by apoptosis has yet to be shown, apoptosis has been shown in primary retinal degeneration, i.e. retinitis pigmentosa (Portera-Cailliau et al., 1994, Gregory and Bird, 1995), and has been suggested as a mechanism for neuronal loss in the brain in NCL (Puranam et al., 1997). Retinal degeneration in CLN2 disease, late infantile may also occur by the same route.

Storage in extracerebral tissues

Although there is no evidence of visceral storage at light microscopic level on routine histological examination, accumulation of a sudanophilic, autofluorescent material associated with acid phosphatase activity can be readily demonstrated in many visceral tissues and cells in CLN2 disease. The accumulation is confirmed by electron microscopy when the characteristic CL body found within cerebral cells is also

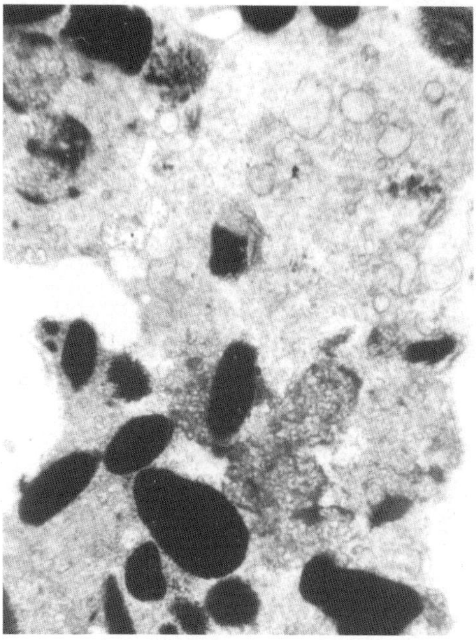

Figure 7.17 CLN2 disease, classic late infantile: retinal pigment epithelial cell contains a mixture of melanin granules and lipopigments, ×8000.

present in visceral tissues at the sites indicated by the staining reactions. Storage material in all these affected cells exhibits strong staining for SCMAS, pointing to generalized uniform storage pattern. By this it differs from other NCL types associated with SCMAS storage (see Chapter 4). Rectal neurons, smooth muscle cells, endothelial cells, cells of the exocrine and endocrine pancreas, other endocrine cells, and adipose cells all contain readily detectable CL bodies. CL bodies are particularly prominent in secretory eccrine sweat gland epithelial cells (Figure 7.18) and smooth muscle cells (Figure 7.19) providing a simple diagnostic route (skin biopsy), which is less traumatic and more laboratory-friendly than the occasionally preferred rectal or conjunctival biopsies. Fibroblasts are rarely involved in storing CL bodies, in contrast with the CLN1 disease, infantile, form where fibroblast storage of GROD may be present. In skeletal muscle there are collections of CL bodies which are present in the paranuclear regions as well as between the myofibrils. These collections may be in a condensed form and are not always easy to find, and may be difficult to differentiate from the profiles of the rectilinear (RL) complex found in the CLN3 disease, juvenile, and early juvenile/variant late infantile CLN6 disease forms. Lymphocytes, prepared from peripheral blood as a buffy coat or by Ficoll separation, also provide a diagnostically useful site for the detection of CL bodies (Figure 7.20). In the extracerebral cells, CL

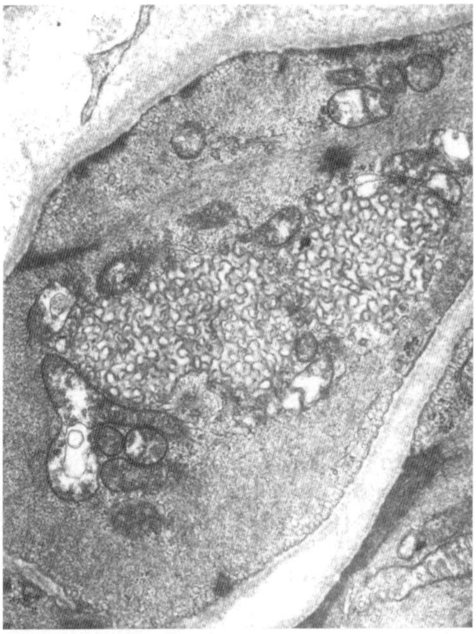

Figure 7.19 CLN2 disease, classic late infantile: a dermal smooth muscle cell contains a large purely curvilinear body, ×14,500.

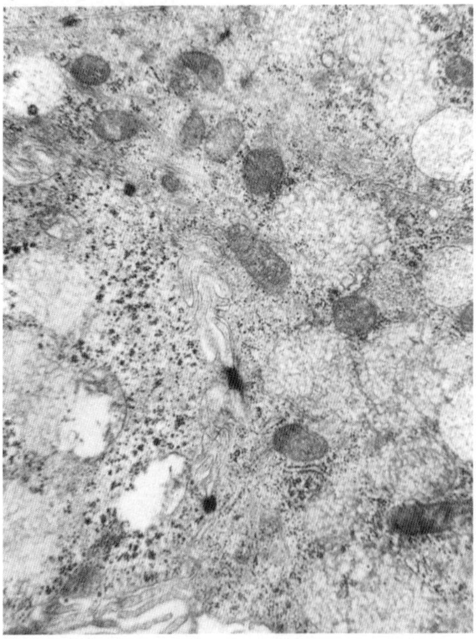

Figure 7.18 CLN2 disease, classic late infantile: pure curvilinear bodies in a secretory eccrine sweat gland epithelial cell, ×3668.

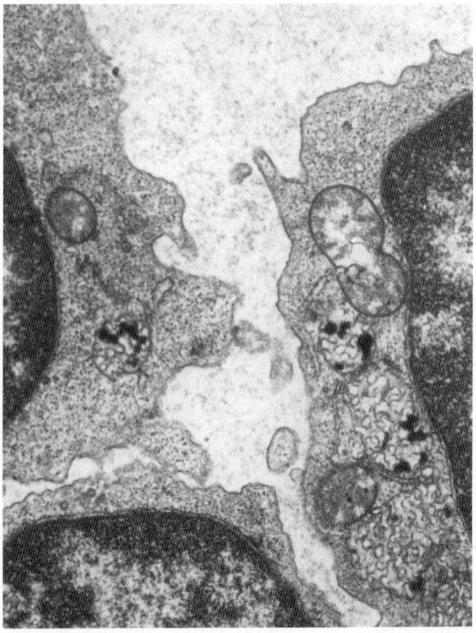

Figure 7.20 CLN2 disease, classic late infantile: two adjacent lymphocytes contain curvilinear bodies, several ones with a few dense deposits, ×15,300.

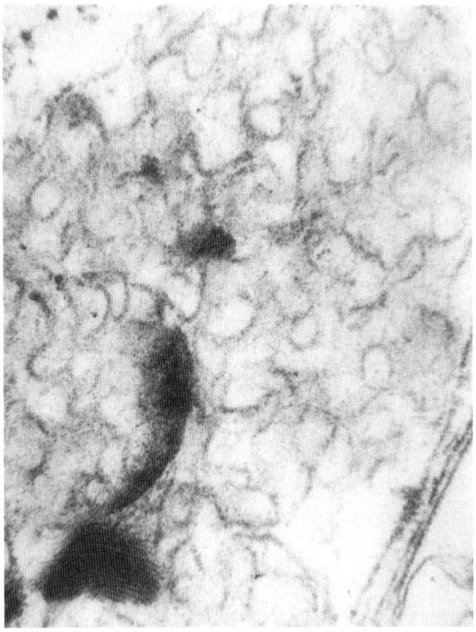

Figure 7.21 CLN2 disease, classic late infantile: an extracerebral curvilinear body contains small stacks of fingerprint lamellae, ×63,000.

bodies may be associated with occasional very rare minor FP profiles (Figure 7.21), making, where present, around 0.1–0.5% of the area. This minor component is quite different to the much greater amount (up to 50%) of FP profiles seen in association with CL or RL complex profiles found in the juvenile and variant late infantile forms (see Chapters 8–12).

CL bodies wherever they appear, have immunoreactivity to SCMAS antibodies (Figure 7.22).

In spite of the observed lysosomal accumulation of subunit c in fibroblasts in a skin biopsy from patients with CLN2 disease, late infantile (Ezaki et al., 1997), detected by immunoblotting after preparation of a lysosomal fraction, no convincing immunohistochemical or electron microscopical evidence of subunit c could be obtained after culturing these cells (Kida et al., 1993, Lake and Rowan, 1997). This is in contrast with other reported findings (Hosain et al., 1995) in which subunit c was detected.

Prenatal diagnosis

Prenatal diagnosis of CLN2 disease, late infantile is possible using uncultured amniotic fluid cells taken at amniocentesis at around 16 weeks' gestation and, prior to enzyme assay and mutation analysis becoming available, was the only available strategy. CL bodies are found in the shed peridermal cells (Figure 7.23), which constitute a small proportion of the total cell contents, but have not been found in biopsied chorion tissue (there are no reports of CVS findings from affected pregnancies). Since CL profiles have also been seen in fetal skin and fetal lymphocytes (Chow et al., 1993) these tissues or cells, respectively, may be obtained (at 20 weeks) in case amniotic fluid cells fail to contain CL bodies. However, prenatal diagnosis by enzyme assay and mutation analysis (Berry-Kravis et al., 2000, van Diggelen et al., 2001, Young et al., 2001) should now be performed as the preferred diagnostic alternative. It is important to confirm the diagnosis on fetal

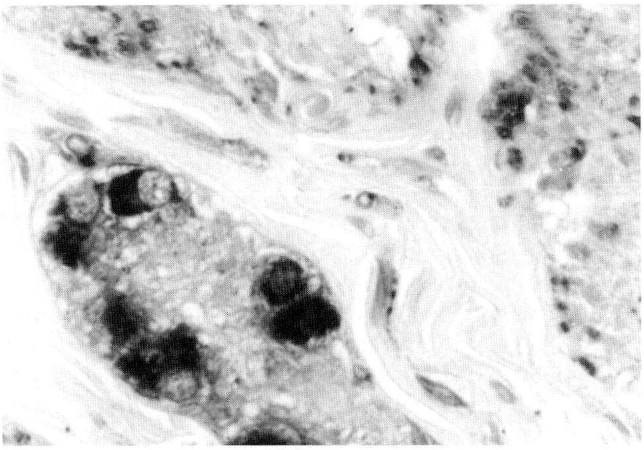

Figure 7.22 CLN2 disease, classic late infantile: SCMAS is labelled by immunoperoxidase technique in neurons and smooth muscle cells of biopsied rectum, ×570.

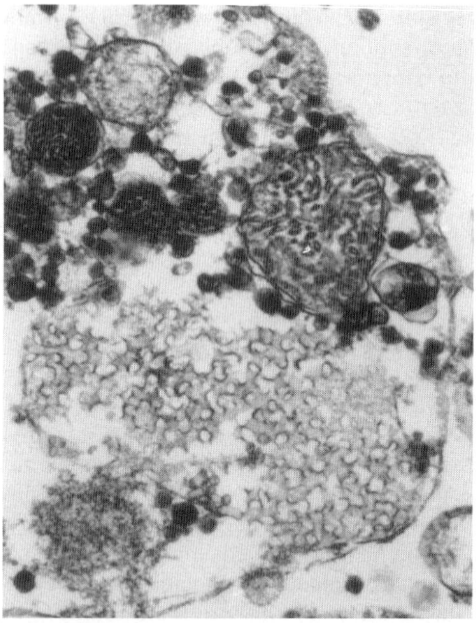

Figure 7.23 CLN2 disease, classic late infantile: a large curvilinear body in an amniotic fluid cell, ×26,800.

tissues obtained at termination of pregnancy after prenatal diagnosis of CLN2 disease, late infantile (Chow et al., 1993).

DISEASE MECHANISM

The events that lie downstream of mutations in the *CLN2* gene are poorly understood. The usual *in vivo* substrates of TPP1 remain unidentified, although details of the transport, processing and glycosylation of this enzyme and the residues critical for its activity are now emerging (Golabek et al., 2003, Wujek et al., 2004, Golabek et al., 2005, Walus et al., 2005, Guhaniyogi et al., 2009, Pal et al., 2009). Whatever mechanisms are involved, loss of TPP1 activity clearly has a profound impact upon the CNS. At autopsy, neurodegenerative changes are less pronounced than the near complete loss of neurons evident in CLN1 disease, infantile, with regional and cell-type specific effects upon neuron survival and astrocytosis apparent within hippocampal subfields (Tyynelä et al., 2004), the cortical mantle and cerebellum (Chang et al., 2008) (J. Cooper et al. unpublished observations). *Tpp1*-deficient mice display many of the same features, with a progressive neurodegenerative and reactive phenotype (Sleat et al., 2004, Chang et al., 2008). This again is pronounced within the thalamocortical system and cerebellum, with progressive waves of astroctyosis, microglial activation and synaptic loss evident (Chang et al., 2008) (J. Cooper et al. unpublished observations). The relatively early onset behavioural and neurological consequences of *Tpp1* deficiency have been described in more detail and are being used to judge the efficacy of gene transfer and enzyme replacement approaches (Passini et al., 2006, Cabrera-Salazar et al., 2007, Sondhi et al., 2007, Chang et al., 2008, Chen et al., 2009).

CORRELATIONS

Genotype–phenotype correlation

Like mutations in enzymes encoded by *CLN1/PPT1* and *CLN10/CTSD*, there is variation in the clinical phenotype of disease caused by mutations in *CLN2* (Table 7.3), including some intra-familial variability. Two patients with disease onset at 8 years, and survival to 30 and 43 years, were originally diagnosed with CLN3 disease, a juvenile form, but were later found to be compound heterozygotes for the *CLN2* missense mutation p.Arg447His (Sleat et al., 1999) and either of the two common mutations (p.Arg208X or c.509-1G > C). This amino acid change diminishes TPP1 levels and activity (Lin and Lobel, 2001a) with little processing of the proenzyme, and retention in the endoplasmic reticulum (Golabek and Kida, 2006). Patients with this mutation must produce a level of enzymatic activity that is sufficient to result in the late onset and protracted disease phenotype, perhaps with altering processing of the mutant protein in brain tissue compared to cultured cells. Distinct intra-familial clinical heterogeneity is evident in a family with three affected siblings carrying this missense mutation (Wisniewski et al., 1999). The children showed different ages at onset of the disease (ranging from 2–11 years of age) and various presenting symptoms (seizures in the child with the earliest onset, and coordination deficits in the child with the latest onset). Unusually, visual impairment was present only in the sibling with the latest onset of the disease.

Compound heterozygosity for c.380G>A, predicted to cause missense mutation p. Arg127Gln with p.Arg208X, also results in a protracted disease. A patient carrying these

Table 7.3 **Details on patients with different mutations in CLN2 from the Institute for Basic Research, Staten Island, Batten Disease Registry**

	Age at onset (years)	Presenting symptoms	Lifespan (years)	EM	TPP1 activity*
Mutations introducing frameshift/premature stop codon	Median 2.95 (n=52) Range 0.4–4.0	ES (n=29) CD (n=20) IC (n=2) VD/CD (n=1)	Median 8.4 (n=40) Range 5–15	CV*	Deficient (Sleat et al., 1997, 1999; Wisniewski et al., 2001a; Steinfeld et al., 2002)
Missense mutations	Median 3.0(n=25) Range 0.1–3.5	ES (n=17) CD (n=6) VD/CD (n=1) VD (n=1)	Median 9.5 (n=11) Range 6–16	CV*	Deficient (Sleat et al., 1997, 1999; Wisniewski et al., 2001a; Steinfeld et al., 2002)
Genotypes associated with atypical phenotype (protracted form)					
R127Q/R208X	4	VD	21	CV	5% (F) (Steinfeld et al., 2004)
R127Q/IVS5-1G>C	4	VD	?	CV/FP	ND (Zhong et al., 2000)
R447H/IVS5-1G>C (3 sibs)	2 8 11	ES CD IC	24 30 >38	CV/FP CV/FP CV/FP	ND 2–3% (B); ND (F) (Wisniewski et al., 1999); Deficient (B) (Sleat et al. 1999)
R447H/R208X	8	CD, VD	43	CV/FP	Deficient (B) (Sleat et al., 1999)
Q66X/IVS2+4A>G (3 sibs)	9 9 9	ES,CS,CD,VD ES,CS,CD,VD ES,CS,CD,VD	27 >28 >27	ND ND CV/FP	0.7–2.8% (L) 0.2–0.8% (L) (Noher de Halac et al., 2005, Bessa et al., 2008)
	3				
V480G/R208X		IC	15	CV	ND (Elleder et al., 2008)
	7				
IVS5-G>A/Insertion of intronic sequences		VD	>20	C/FP	ND

B, frozen brain tissue; CD, cognitive dysfunction; CV, curvilinear profiles; EM, electron microscopy; ES, epileptic seizures; F, fibroblasts; FP, fingerprint profiles; IC, in-coordination; L, lymphoblasts; ND, not determined; VD, visual deterioration. Asterisk by CV denotes that mixed inclusions were reported in some cases. *TPP1 activity, when available, is presented as a per cent of control values.

mutations survived until 21 years of age and had delayed onset of clinical manifestations (Steinfeld et al., 2002). Engineering of this mutation in a recombinant TPP1 had no effect on enzyme synthesis, stability, or activity. However, analysis of the native transcript bearing this mutation revealed that most but not all *CLN2* mRNAs were misspliced (Steinfeld et al., 2004). c.380G>A should therefore be regarded as a splicing rather than a missense mutation, and enough transcripts must escape aberrant splicing to provide some TPP1 activity.

Another splice-site mutation, c.89+4A>G, is associated with a protracted disease course (Noher de Halac et al., 2005). This mutation may also lead to correct splicing of some transcripts and generation of small amounts of functional TPP1. Three affected siblings carrying this mutation demonstrated similar clinical presentations with onset at 9 years of age and dependence on a wheelchair at 15–19 years of age. Two siblings were still alive at 27 and 28 years of age. Residual TPP1 activity was detected in saliva and leukocytes.

A protracted form of CLN2 disease was also reported in a child who was a compound heterozygote for c.509-1G>A and insertion of intronic sequences (nucleotides from positions 278–303 and from 709–732). This patient presented with visual deterioration at 7 years of age, followed by behavioural changes at 12 and seizures at 20 years (Hartikainen et al., 1999). The biological consequences of insertion of intronic sequences at this location must be determined. Recently, another missense mutation, p.Val480Gly, has also been reported to be associated with an attenuated CLN2 disease phenotype (Elleder et al., 2008).

One patient who was homozygous for the p. Arg208X mutation was observed to have very early onset of disease (Simonati et al., 2000), with symptoms of hypotonia and developmental delay detectable in the fourth month of life. Given that other patients with the same genotype appear to have a typical CLN2 disease, late infantile course, this early onset probably reflects other factors (for example, genetic background) rather than *CLN2* genotype *per se*. Other examples exist of aypical, early onset of clinical symptoms before the age of 1 year, including two children presenting with developmental delay (c.509-1G>C homozygote and compound heterozygote p.[Gly284Val]+[p.Phe481Cys]) (Ju et al., 2002), and three American children: two siblings presenting with seizures (compound heterozygotes c.509-1G>C with p.Arg208X) and one child presenting with speech arrest (who never spoke) (p.Arg208X homozygote) (unpublished data).

Two patients homozygous for p.Asn86Ser mutation showed slightly better performance in clinical tests than other typical CLN2 disease patients (Steinfeld et al., 2002). This mutation cancels one of five N-glycosylation sites in TPP1 (Tsiakas et al., 2004, Wujek et al., 2004) and also leads to a grossly misfolded protein (Golabek et al., 2004, Steinfeld et al., 2004, Golabek and Kida, 2006).

Several missense TPP1 mutations have been studied in heterologous expression systems—p.Arg447His, p.Arg127Gln (see above), p.Asn286Ser, p.Ile287Asn, p.Thr353Pro, p.Gln422His (Steinfeld et al., 2004, Tsiakas et al., 2004), p. Gly389Glu (Lin and Lobel, 2001a), as well as p.Gly77Arg, p.Pro202Leu, p.Arg206Cys, p.Val277Met, p.Gly284Val, p.Glu343Lys, p.Cys365Arg, p.Gln422His, and p.Ser475Leu (Golabek and Kida, 2006, Walus et al., 2010). The majority of missense mutations lead to non-functional TPP1 by affecting folding of the proenzyme in the endoplasmic reticulum, resulting in a reduction of processing of the proenzyme to the mature form, oligomerization of some of the mutated proenzymes, and their lack of specific TPP1 activity. Some improperly folded mutated TPP1 proenzymes exit the endoplasmic reticulum and appear in the conditioned media of expressing cells. However, immunoblot analysis of patients' cells (cultured fibroblasts and lymphoblasts) or postmortem brain tissues revealed a lack of detectable TPP1 in most patients examined (Kurachi et al., 2000, Kurachi et al., 2001, Wisniewski et al., 2001). Normal TPP1 levels and processing demonstrated cultured fibroblasts from a patient with missense mutation p.Ser475Leu (Golabek et al., 2003). This mutation, affecting the active-site nucleophile of TPP1 (Lin et al., 2001), produces an inactive enzyme. That inactive p.Ser475Leu-TPP1 proenzyme was processed to the mature, approximately 46kDa polypeptide in cultured cells, suggests that apart from autoactivation, human TPP1 also can be processed *in vivo* with the help of another protease (Golabek et al., 2003, Golabek et al., 2004).

Genotype–morphotype correlation

Neuropathology of one variant protracted case of CLN2 disease, characterized by the frequent null mutation (p.Arg208X) combined with the novel mutation (p.Val480Gly) showed significantly different sensitivity of various neuronal populations to TPP1 deficiency, which may be responsible for the variation in disease course (Elleder et al., 2008).

In CLN2 disease, late infantile CL profiles usually predominate in the lysosomal storage material. However in some, particularly the protracted form, FP may also be found. For example, FP and CL were detected in the brain tissue or biopsy material of one patient carrying p.Arg447His (Wisniewski et al., 1999), and postmortem study of the brain tissue of the sibling with the earliest onset of disease had markedly less severe structural damage in all brain areas than that typically observed in those affected by CLN2 disease, including the cerebellum (Figure 7.3F). Neuronal loss and glial cell proliferation were less prominent than in other CLN2 disease patients.

Another protracted CLN2 disease patient carrying c.89+4A>G (I. Noher de Halac, personal communication) had both CL and FP profiles in a skin biopsy, as had one who was a compound heterozygote for c.509-1G>C and insertion of intronic sequences (nucleotides from 278–303 and from 709–732) mixed ultrastructural pattern was also seen in one Czech patient with protracted course c.[622C>T] c.[1439T>G] (M. Elleder unpublished).

The most prominent immunostaining of reactive astrocytes was present in the brain tissue of a patient homozygous for p.Gly422His mutation (Figure 7.3C). However, the stain in reactive astrocytes was never granular, as in control subjects, but was uniform, in some cells focused in the perinuclear region, suggesting mistargeting of the mutated protein. Neuronal staining was absent, and TPP1 activity in the brain tissue of this individual was only residual (less than 1.5% of control values) (Wisniewski et al., 2001).

DIAGNOSIS

The diagnosis of CLN2 can be suspected in a previously healthy and normally developed child who shows a standstill of psychomotor development or the onset of an unexplained seizure disorder at the age of around 3 years. In this situation, testing for the enzymatic deficiency caused by a defective *CLN2* gene becomes mandatory.

The most convenient substrate for monitoring TPP1 assay, uses the fluorogenic tripeptide Ala–Ala–Phe–AMC (Vines and Warburton, 1999). In a study of 16 CLN2 disease patients, a profound deficiency of TPP1 activity was found in patients' fibroblasts, with very low residual activity (less than 2%) (van Diggelen et al., 2001). However, the residual activity in leukocytes of some of these patients, was substantially higher (van Diggelen et al., 2001). Presently, leukocytes from eight out of 20 CLN2 disease patients had considerable residual TPP1 activity (i.e. greater than 10%, but below the control range) whereas the PPT1 activity in fibroblasts from 31 CLN1 disease patients was invariably less than 2% (O. van Diggelen unpublished data). Recently, genuine CLN2 patients with clear-cut TPP1 deficiency in fibroblasts were found with apparently normal TPP1 activity in leukocytes (Drs A.H. Fensom and R. Williams, London, and Dr C. Caillaud, Paris, personal communication). The additional use of the protease inhibitors E64 and leupeptin (van Diggelen et al., 2001), may be an important factor to detect the TPP1 deficiency in leukocytes from these unusual CLN2 disease patients. Whether the method of isolating leukocytes from peripheral blood is also a determining factor is presently under investigation.

TPP1 activity (as well as the activity of PPT1, the enzyme deficient in CLN1) can also be measured in dried blood spots (DBS) with the advantage of easy handling and shipment of samples (Lukacs et al., 2003). The authors recommend the use of DBS as a screening procedure only and to confirm the diagnosis by mutation analysis or determination of the enzyme activity in fibroblasts in the case of a very low activity in dried blood. After continuous use of the DBS procedure for 4 years after publication, they have found it to be robust, but it cannot yet be excluded that some unusual CLN2 patients also have normal TPP1 activity in DBS.

Following confirmation of TPP1 deficiency by enzyme assay, mutation analysis of the *CLN2* gene should be performed to complete the clinical, biochemical and genetic NCL diagnosis.

Differential diagnosis

All progressive brain disorders in childhood deserve intensive diagnostic work-up to exclude such causes as inflammation, tumours, hydrocephalus, and toxic or metabolic disturbances. Among the degenerative disorders, those affecting mainly cerebral grey matter and clinically associated with epilepsy and dementia, include other rare NCL variants with late infantile age of onset. Those variants are variant late infantile CLN5, CLN6, CLN7 and CLN8 diseases. Diagnosis of these variants is based on clinicopathological findings and DNA study. Other diseases to be considered are the gangliosidoses and certain forms of mucopolysaccharidosis with no or minimal bodily stigmata, e.g. Sanfilippo disease. Degenerative diseases mainly affecting cerebral white matter (leukodystrophies and leukoencephalopathies) are clinically associated with early motor disturbances and are easily recognized neuroradiologically.

The diagnosis of the specific type of late infantile NCL is of great importance in order to provide genetic counselling for the affected families. Nevertheless, in rare cases clinical and histological signs support the diagnosis of NCL without identification of mutations in any of the known NCL genes. This has been reported in about 10% of NCL cases. Therefore, it is very likely that more genes causing NCL will be discovered in the future (Mole, 2004).

CLINICAL MANAGEMENT

To date there is no cure for CLN2 disease. Nevertheless, specialized palliative treatment and care can help to reduce suffering and to improve quality of life of these children and families.

Epilepsy is difficult to treat in CLN2 disease, late infantile, and complete control of seizures is not always achieved. Anticonvulsants like valproic acid are recommended whereas phenytoin, carbamazepine, and vigabatrin should be avoided. Myoclonic jerks are frequent in CLN2 disease, late infantile patients and should not be confused with epileptic seizures. They are very troublesome for the patients as they interfere with rest and sleep. Levetiracetam shows a good combined action against myoclonus and seizures. Piracetam and zonisamide are also used to treat myoclonus in CLN2 disease, late infantile. Spasticity in CLN2 disease, late infantile patients should be controlled with baclofen. It is important to know that sufficient dosages might be higher in CLN2 disease, late infantile patients than in others. Spastic crises should be avoided as they are painful. The application of delta 9-tetrahydrocannabinol (THC, dronabinol) has been reported to be beneficial in reducing pain and agitation during such crises (Lorenz, 2002), and has also been helpful in reducing discomfort in children with CLN2 disease, late infantile.

Not only paediatricians and paediatric neurologists, but also physiotherapists and occupational therapists, should be involved in treatment of CLN2 disease, late infantile. Collaboration and communication between family, medical doctors, and all other therapists are essential for providing optimal care at all levels.

New therapeutic strategies are currently being evaluated for their ability to alter the disease course of CLN2 disease, late infantile and these are discussed in the following section.

EXPERIMENTAL THERAPY

Current therapeutic strategies for CLN2 disease are experimental. They focus mainly on methods that replenish TPP1 activity, or compensate for its function. The theoretical bases of these strategies, which are still being refined, are considered in detail in Chapter 21. Because TPP1 is an enzyme, CLN2 disease is likely to be one of the first NCLs to be treated successfully.

Enzyme replacement

Production of recombinant human TPP1 has been achieved by overexpression in Chinese hamster ovary (CHO) cells, and enzyme produced in this manner can be endocytosed by cultured fibroblasts and cerebellar granule cells, largely via the M6PR. Importantly, recombinant TPP1 can reduce levels of subunit c when applied exogenously to cultured patient fibroblasts (Lin and Lobel, 2001b). Enzyme replacement studies in CLN2 disease, late infantile patients have not yet been attempted.

One strategy to deliver enzymes to the CNS is to bypass the blood–brain barrier and deliver the desired enzymes directly to the brain parenchyma or ventricular space. Recently, the intracerebroventricular delivery of TPP1 in mice has demonstrated positive effects on many disease features, with improvements in resting tremor, levels of storage material and glial activation (Chang et al., 2008), although the issues of immunotolerance and delivery to a larger brain still need to be resolved.

Activity of microglial lysosomes can degrade the amyloid fibrils in Alzheimer's disease (Majumdar et al., 2007), raising the possibility that administration of TTP1 may also help.

Gene therapy

Gene therapy studies in a CLN2 disease animal model have so far used adeno-associated viral (AAV) vectors, and expression of TPP1 in the rodent brain has been successfully achieved. AAV5-TPP1, when injected into the mouse striatum, transduces primarily neurons, including neurons in the hippocampus, increasing TPP1 activity 3–7-fold (Haskell et al., 2003). AAV2-CLN2 injected into the rat striatum led to TPP1-positive striatal neurons for the duration of the study. TPP1 was also secreted and spread along CNS white matter tracts to the substantia nigra, thalamus, and cerebral cortex. This same vector, when injected into the CNS of non-human primates, led to TPP1 expression in neurons at 13 weeks post-injection (Sondhi et al., 2005). In this study TPP1 was not detected in glial cells, suggesting that cross correction did not occur, or that it occurred at an undetectable level. Together, these studies demonstrate the feasibility of expressing TPP1 in the mammalian brain.

The therapeutic efficacy of gene transfer in CLN2 disease was tested by injecting AAV vectors expressing TPP1 into the brain of TPP1-deficient mice (Passini et al., 2006). TPP1 expressed from AAV2 or 5, when injected into the motor cortex, thalamus, and cerebellum, led to a reduction of autofluorescent storage near the injection sites. This finding was supported by electron microscopy data showing a decrease in the number of CL bodies characteristic of CLN2 disease, late infantile. In this particular study, no increase in survival of the mice was reported. In contrast, intracranial injection of human TPP1 expressed from AAV1 resulted in a widespread increase in human TPP1 activity in the brain, and injections before disease onset prevented storage, spared neurons from axonal degeneration allowing preservation of motor function, and increased life span, indicating the probable importance of early intervention (Cabrera-Salazar et al., 2007).

A gene transfer vector derived from a rhesus macaque AAV serotype has also been tested for its ability to deliver TPP1 to the TPP1-deficient mouse (Sondhi et al., 2007). AAVrh.10-TPP1 injected into four locations in each brain hemisphere of 7-week-old *Tpp1*$^{-/-}$ mice increased TPP1 activity in the brain. Treated mice displayed a histological decrease in lysosomal storage, an improvement in several measures of motor function—gait, balance beam, and grip strength, and an increase in survival. This vector was functional in naïve mice, as well as in mice pre-immunized with human serotypes of AAV, suggesting that using AAV serotypes derived from non-human primates may be advantageous in avoiding immune responses. Subsequent studies with this viral vector again suggest that treatment in the neonatal period results in increased survival rates (Sondhi et al., 2008). Further evidence for the potential of gene transfer in CLN2 disease has been provided using a systemically injected AAV2 vector with a modified capsid to target it to the vascular endothelium and cross the BBB (Chen et al., 2009). This vascular targeting was achieved by phage panning to identify a series of peptides enriched on the vascular endothelium, which were inserted into the capsid of the AAV2 vector and shown to deliver enzyme widely within the CNS and improve the disease phenotypes of mouse models of both CLN2 disease and another lysosomal storage disorder (MPSVII) (Chen et al., 2009). This study suggested that the molecular signature of the vascular endothelium was disease-specific. These are exciting studies in that they demonstrate that TPP1 can rescue the phenotype of the TPP1-deficient mice.

Although few animal studies for *CLN2* gene therapy have been completed, a human gene therapy trial for CLN2 disease commenced in 2004 (Crystal et al., 2004). Two groups of patients, one with severe disease, the other with moderate disease, received AAV2 vectors expressing human *CLN2/TPP1* by direct injection into 12 sites in the brain, six sites per hemisphere. The outcome measures of the study are based on the evolving late infantile NCL clinical rating scale, and magnetic resonance imaging of the brain regions that received injections. Treated patients trended towards a reduced rate of decline based on MRI parameters and the neurological rating scale, although the study was not large enough for statistical significance (Worgall et al., 2008). Based on their relative efficacy in TPP1-deficient mice (Sondhi et al., 2007, Sondhi et al., 2008), a second clinical trial using the newer generation of AAVrh.10-*CLN2* vectors is anticipated.

Cell-based therapies

There are several reports of CLN2 disease patients receiving bone marrow transplants as an experimental therapy. Two CLN2 disease patients received bone marrow transplants in 1997 (Lake et al., 1997), and another similar report was made in 2005 (Yuza et al., 2005). In each case the treatment did not appear to be beneficial for the CNS deficits of the patients. The reason for the lack of efficacy is not clear, but may be due to either poor donor cell engraftment, or inefficient cell migration to the CNS.

Recent efforts have focused on *ex vivo* gene therapy of haematopoietic stem cells, the precursors to numerous types of cells of the immune system, prior to transplant. The rationale is that if bone marrow-derived macrophages repopulate the brain at a relatively slow rate, perhaps overexpressing the desired enzyme in these cells would enable the few cells that do migrate to the brain to express and secrete a therapeutic level of enzyme. Recently, grafts of neuroprogenitor cells, which are largely undifferentiated cells that retain the potential to develop into neurons or glia, have demonstrated partial efficacy in improving rotarod performance, clearing storage material and protecting populations of host PPT1-deficient mice (Tamaki et al., 2009). Following these studies, a phase I clinical trial has been undertaken to determine the safety and effects of neuroprogenitor cell implantation in CLN1 disease and CLN2 disease patients.

Small molecule therapies

A significant percentage of alleles associated with CLN2 disease contain premature stop codons. In a survey of mutations in 58 CLN2 disease families, the p.Arg208X mutation accounted for approximately 28% of the mutant alleles (Sleat et al., 1999). The prevalence of stop codon mutations indicates that strategies that correct readthrough may have legitimate clinical utility for CLN2 disease. In CLN2 disease, late infantile patient fibroblasts with a nonsense mutation, treatment with gentamicin restored TPP1 activity up to 7% of normal (Sleat et al., 2001).

Conclusions

To summarize, several promising therapeutic approaches are being investigated for CLN2 disease, including enzyme replacement, gene therapy, cell-based therapies, and small molecule therapies. Current evidence suggests that restoration of TPP1 in the central nervous system would be important for treatment of CLN2 disease, but numerous important questions remain unanswered or only partially answered. Are there particular cell populations within the CNS that must be targeted? At what point along the disease course must treatment be initiated before it becomes irreversible? What are the risks of elevating TPP1 activity above physiological levels? Will peripheral disease develop if CNS disease is treated? Further experimentation is necessary to address these and other unanswered questions. Importantly, the molecular mechanisms underlying the pathogenesis of CLN2 disease have not been elucidated. As a more detailed understanding of the disease process emerges, so will additional insights into therapy.

REFERENCES

Andersen KJ & McDonald JK (1987) Subcellular distribution of renal tripeptide-releasing exopeptidases active on collagen-like sequences. *Am J Physiol*, 252, F890–8.

Autefage H, Albinet V, Garcia V, Berges H, Nicolau ML, Therville N, Altie MF, Caillaud C, Levade T & Andrieu-Abadie N (2009) Lysosomal serine protease CLN2 regulates tumor necrosis factor-alpha-mediated apoptosis in a Bid-dependent manner. *J Biol Chem*, 284, 11507–16.

Autti T, Raininko R, Santavuori P, Vanhanen SL, Poutanen VP & Haltia M (1997) MRI of neuronal ceroid lipofuscinosis. II. Postmortem MRI and histopathological study of the brain in 16 cases of neuronal ceroid lipofuscinosis of juvenile or late infantile type. *Neuroradiology*, 39, 371–7.

Bernardini F & Warburton MJ (2001) The substrate range of tripeptidyl-peptidase I. *Eur J Paediatr Neurol*, 5 Suppl A, 69–72.

Bernardini F & Warburton MJ (2002) Lysosomal degradation of cholecystokinin-(29-33)-amide in mouse brain is dependent on tripeptidyl peptidase-I: implications for the degradation and storage of peptides in classical late-infantile neuronal ceroid lipofuscinosis. *Biochem J*, 366, 521–9.

Berry-Kravis E, Sleat DE, Sohar I, Meyer P, Donnelly R & Lobel P (2000) Prenatal testing for late infantile neuronal ceroid lipofuscinosis. *Ann Neurol*, 47, 254–7.

Bessa C, Teixeira CA, Dias A, Alves M, Rocha S, Lacerda L, Loureiro L, Guimaraes A & Ribeiro MG (2008) CLN2/TPP1 deficiency: the novel mutation IVS7-10A>G causes intron retention and is associated with a mild disease phenotype. *Mol Genet Metab*, 93, 66–73.

Bielschowsky M (1920) Zur Histopathologie und Pathogenese der amaurotischen Idiotie mit besonderer Berücksichtigung der zerebellaren Veränderungen. *J Psychol Neurol (Leipzig)*, 26, 123–99.

Brockmann K, Pouwels PJ, Christen HJ, Frahm J & Hanefeld F (1996) Localized proton magnetic resonance spectroscopy of cerebral metabolic disturbances in children with neuronal ceroid lipofuscinosis. *Neuropediatrics*, 27, 242–8.

Brück W & Goebel HH (1998) Microglia activation in neuronal ceroid-lipofuscinosis. *Clin Neuropathol*, 5, 276 (poster P29).

Cabrera-Salazar MA, Roskelley EM, Bu J, Hodges BL, Yew N, Dodge JC, Shihabuddin LS, Sohar I, Sleat DE, Scheule RK, Davidson BL, Cheng SH, Lobel P & Passini MA (2007) Timing of therapeutic intervention determines functional and survival outcomes in a mouse model of late infantile batten disease. *Mol Ther*, 15, 1782–8.

Caillaud C, Manicom J, Puech JP, Lobel P & Poenaru L (1999) Enzymatic and molecular pre and postnatal diagnosis of ceroid lipofuscinoses in France. *Am J Hum Genet*, 65 (Suppl), A232.

Chang M, Cooper JD, Sleat DE, Cheng SH, Dodge JC, Passini MA, Lobel P & Davidson BL (2008) Intraventricular enzyme replacement improves disease phenotypes in a mouse model of late infantile neuronal ceroid lipofuscinosis. *Mol Ther*, 16, 649–56.

Chen YH, Chang M & Davidson BL (2009) Molecular signatures of disease brain endothelia provide new sites for CNS-directed enzyme therapy. *Nat Med*, 15, 1215–8.

Chow CW, Borg J, Billson VR & Lake BD (1993) Fetal tissue involvement in the late infantile type of neuronal ceroid lipofuscinosis. *Prenat Diagn*, 13, 833–41.

Comellas-Bigler M, Maskos K, Huber R, Oyama H, Oda K & Bode W (2004) 1.2 A crystal structure of the serine carboxyl proteinase pro-kumamolisin; structure of an intact pro-subtilase. *Structure*, 12, 1313–23.

Crystal RG, Sondhi D, Hackett NR, Kaminsky SM, Worgall S, Stieg P, Souweidane M, Hosain S, Heier L, Ballon D, Dinner M, Wisniewski K, Kaplitt M, Greenwald BM, Howell JD, Strybing K, Dyke J & Voss H (2004) Clinical protocol. Administration of a replication-deficient adeno-associated virus gene transfer vector expressing the human CLN2 cDNA to the brain of children with late infantile neuronal ceroid lipofuscinosis. *Hum Gene Ther*, 15, 1131–54.

Elleder M, Dvorakova L, Stolnaja L, Vlaskova H, Hulkova H, Druga R, Poupetova H, Kostalova E & Mikulastik J (2008) Atypical CLN2 with later onset and prolonged course: a neuropathologic study showing different sensitivity of neuronal subpopulations to TPP1 deficiency. *Acta Neuropathol*, 116, 119–24.

Elleder M, Sokolova J & Hrebicek M (1997) Follow-up study of subunit c of mitochondrial ATP synthase (SCMAS) in Batten disease and in unrelated lysosomal disorders. *Acta Neuropathol*, 93, 379–90.

Elleder M & Tyynelä J (1998) Incidence of neuronal perikaryal spheroids in neuronal ceroid lipofuscinoses (Batten disease). *Clin Neuropathol*, 17, 184–9.

Ezaki J, Takeda-Ezaki M & Kominami E (2000a) Tripeptidyl peptidase I, the late infantile neuronal ceroid lipofuscinosis gene product, initiates the lysosomal degradation of subunit c of ATP synthase. *J Biochem*, 128, 509–16.

Ezaki J, Takeda-Ezaki M, Oda K & Kominami E (2000b) Characterization of endopeptidase activity of tripeptidyl peptidase-I/CLN2 protein which is deficient in classical late infantile neuronal ceroid lipofuscinosis. *Biochem Biophys Res Commun*, 268, 904–8.

Ezaki J, Tanida I, Kanehagi N & Kominami E (1999) A lysosomal proteinase, the late infantile neuronal ceroid lipofuscinosis gene (CLN2) product, is essential for degradation of a hydrophobic protein, the subunit c of ATP synthase. *J Neurochem*, 72, 2573–82.

Ezaki J, Wolfe LS & Kominami E (1997) Decreased lysosomal subunit c-degrading activity in fibroblasts from patients with late infantile neuronal ceroid lipofuscinosis. *Neuropediatrics*, 28, 53–5.

Goebel HH, Gerhard L, Kominami E & Haltia M (1996) Neuronal ceroid-lipofuscinosis–late-infantile or Janský-Bielschowsky type–revisited. *Brain Pathol*, 6, 225–8.

Goebel HH, Gullotta F, Bajanowski T, Hansen FJ & Braak H (1995) Pigment variant of neuronal ceroid-lipofuscinosis. *Am J Med Genet*, 57, 155–9.

Goebel HH, Kominami E, Neuen-Jacob E & Wheeler RB (2001) Morphological studies on CLN2. *Eur J Paediatr Neurol*, 5 Suppl A, 203–7.

Golabek AA & Kida E (2006) Tripeptidyl-peptidase I in health and disease. *Biol Chem*, 387, 1091–9.

Golabek AA, Kida E, Walus M, Wujek P, Mehta P & Wisniewski KE (2003) Biosynthesis, glycosylation, and enzymatic processing in vivo of human tripeptidyl-peptidase I. *J Biol Chem*, 278, 7135–45.

Golabek AA, Walus M, Wisniewski KE & Kida E (2005) Glycosaminoglycans modulate activation, activity, and stability of tripeptidyl-peptidase I in vitro and in vivo. *J Biol Chem*, 280, 7550–61.

Golabek AA, Wujek P, Walus M, Bieler S, Soto C, Wisniewski KE & Kida E (2004) Maturation of human tripeptidyl-peptidase I in vitro. *J Biol Chem*, 279, 31058–67.

Goldberg-Stern H, Halevi A, Marom D, Straussberg R & Mimouni-Bloch A (2009) Late infantile neuronal ceroid lipofuscinosis: a new mutation in Arabs. *Pediatr Neurol*, 41, 297–300.

Grasl-Kraupp B, Ruttkay-Nedecky B, Koudelka H, Bukowska K, Bursch W & Schulte-Hermann R (1995) In situ detection of fragmented DNA (TUNEL assay) fails to discriminate among apoptosis, necrosis, and autolytic cell death: a cautionary note. *Hepatology*, 21, 1465–8.

Gregory CY & Bird AC (1995) Cell loss in retinal dystrophies by apoptosis–death by informed consent!. *Br J Ophthalmol*, 79, 186–90.

Guhaniyogi J, Sohar I, Das K, Stock AM & Lobel P (2009) Crystal structure and autoactivation pathway of the precursor form of human tripeptidyl-peptidase 1, the enzyme deficient in late infantile ceroid lipofuscinosis. *J Biol Chem*, 284, 3985-97

Hall NA, Lake BD, Dewji NN & Patrick AD (1991) Lysosomal storage of subunit c of mitochondrial ATP synthase in Batten's disease (ceroid-lipofuscinosis). *Biochem J*, 275 (Pt 1), 269–72.

Hartikainen JM, Ju W, Wisniewski KE, Moroziewicz DN, Kaczmarski AL, McLendon L, Zhong D, Suarez CT, Brown WT & Zhong N (1999) Late infantile neuronal ceroid lipofuscinosis is due to splicing mutations in the CLN2 gene. *Mol Genet Metab*, 67, 162–8.

Haskell RE, Hughes SM, Chiorini JA, Alisky JM & Davidson BL (2003) Viral-mediated delivery of the late-infantile neuronal ceroid lipofuscinosis gene, TPP-I to the mouse central nervous system. *Gene Ther*, 10, 34–42.

Hosain S, Kaufmann WE, Negrin G, Watkins PA, Siakotos AN, Palmer DN & Naidu S (1995) Diagnoses of neuronal ceroid-lipofuscinosis by immunochemical methods. *Am J Med Genet*, 57, 239–45.

Ju W, Zhong R, Moore S, Moroziewicz D, Currie JR, Parfrey P, Brown WT & Zhong N (2002) Identification of novel CLN2 mutations shows Canadian specific NCL2 alleles. *J Med Genet*, 39, 822–5.

Junaid MA, Wu G & Pullarkat RK (2000) Purification and characterization of bovine brain lysosomal pepstatin-insensitive proteinase, the gene product deficient in the human late-infantile neuronal ceroid lipofuscinosis. *J Neurochem*, 74, 287–94.

Kida E, Golabek AA, Walus M, Wujek P, Kaczmarski W & Wisniewski KE (2001) Distribution of tripeptidyl peptidase I in human tissues under normal and pathological conditions. *J Neuropathol Exp Neurol*, 60, 280–92.

Kida E, Wisniewski KE & Golabek AA (1993) Increased expression of subunit c of mitochondrial ATP synthase in brain tissue from neuronal ceroid lipofuscinoses and mucopolysaccharidosis cases but not in long-term fibroblast cultures. *Neurosci Lett*, 164, 121–4.

Kim KH, Sleat DE, Bernard O & Lobel P (2009) Genetic modulation of apoptotic pathways fails to alter disease course in tripeptidyl-peptidase 1 deficient mice. *Neurosci Lett*, 453, 27-30.

Kim KH, Pham CT, Sleat DE & Lobel P (2008) Dipeptidyl-peptidase I does not functionally compensate for the loss of tripeptidyl-peptidase I in the neurodegenerative disease late-infantile neuronal ceroid lipofuscinosis. *Biochem J*, 415, 225-32.

Kohan R, Cismondi IA, Kremer RD, Muller VJ, Guelbert N, Anzolini VT, Fietz MJ, Ramirez AM & Halac IN (2009) An integrated strategy for the diagnosis of neuronal ceroid lipofuscinosis types 1 (CLN1) and 2 (CLN2) in eleven Latin American patients. *Clin Genet*, 76, 372–82.

Koike M, Shibata M, Ohsawa Y, Kametaka S, Waguri S, Kominami E & Uchiyama Y (2002) The expression of tripeptidyl peptidase I in various tissues of rats and mice. *Arch Histol Cytol*, 65, 219–32.

Kopan S, Sivasubramaniam U & Warburton MJ (2004) The lysosomal degradation of neuromedin B is dependent on tripeptidyl peptidase-I: evidence for the impairment of neuropeptide degradation in late-infantile neuronal ceroid lipofuscinosis. *Biochem Biophys Res Commun*, 319, 58–65.

Koul R, Al-Futaisi A, Ganesh A & Rangnath Bushnarmuth S (2007) Late-infantile neuronal ceroid lipofuscinosis (CLN2/Janský-Bielschowsky type) in Oman. *J Child Neurol*, 22, 555–9.

Kousi M, Siintola E, Dvorakova L, Vlaskova H, Turnbull J, Topcu M, Yuksel D, Gokben S, Minassian BA, Elleder M, Mole SE & Lehesjoki AE (2009) Mutations in CLN7/MFSD8 are a common cause of variant late-infantile neuronal ceroid lipofuscinosis. *Brain*, 132, 810–9.

Kurachi Y, Oka A, Itoh M, Mizuguchi M, Hayashi M & Takashima S (2001) Distribution and development of CLN2 protein, the late-infantile neuronal ceroid lipofuscinosis gene product. *Acta Neuropathol*, 102, 20–6.

Kurachi Y, Oka A, Mizuguchi M, Ohkoshi Y, Sasaki M, Itoh M, Hayashi M, Goto Y & Takashima S (2000) Rapid immunologic diagnosis of classic late infantile neuronal ceroid lipofuscinosis. *Neurology*, 54, 1676–80.

Lake BD & Hall NA (1993) Immunolocalization studies of subunit c in late-infantile and juvenile Batten disease. *J Inherit Metab Dis*, 16, 263–6.

Lake BD & Rowan SA (1997) Light and electron microscopic studies on subunit c in cultured fibroblasts in late infantile and juvenile Batten disease. *Neuropediatrics*, 28, 56–9.

Lake BD, Steward CG, Oakhill A, Wilson J & Perham TG (1997) Bone marrow transplantation in late infantile Batten disease and juvenile Batten disease. *Neuropediatrics*, 28, 80–1.

Lam CW, Poon PM, Tong SF & Ko CH (2001) Two novel CLN2 gene mutations in a Chinese patient with classical late-infantile neuronal ceroid lipofuscinosis. *Am J Med Genet*, 99, 161–3.

Lavrov AY, Ilyna ES, Zakharova EY, Boukina AM & Tishkanina SV (2002) The first three Russian cases of classical, late-infantile, neuronal ceroid lipofuscinosis. *Eur J Paediatr Neurol*, 6, 161–4.

Lin L & Lobel P (2001a) Expression and analysis of CLN2 variants in CHO cells: Q100R represents a polymorphism, and G389E and R447H represent loss-of-function mutations. *Hum Mutat*, 18, 165.

Lin L & Lobel P (2001b) Production and characterization of recombinant human CLN2 protein for enzyme-replacement therapy in late infantile neuronal ceroid lipofuscinosis. *Biochem J*, 357, 49–55.

Lin L, Sohar I, Lackland H & Lobel P (2001) The human CLN2 protein/tripeptidyl-peptidase I is a serine protease that autoactivates at acidic pH. *J Biol Chem*, 276, 2249–55.

Liu CG, Sleat DE, Donnelly RJ & Lobel P (1998) Structural organization and sequence of CLN2, the defective gene in classical late infantile neuronal ceroid lipofuscinosis. *Genomics*, 50, 206–12.

Lorenz R (2002) A casuistic rationale for the treatment of spastic and myocloni in a childhood neurodegenerative disease: neuronal ceroid lipofuscinosis of the type Janský-Bielschowsky. *Neuro Endocrinol Lett*, 23, 387–90.

Lukacs Z, Santavuori P, Keil A, Steinfeld R & Kohlschutter A (2003) Rapid and simple assay for the determination of tripeptidyl peptidase and palmitoyl protein thioesterase activities in dried blood spots. *Clin Chem*, 49, 509–11.

McDonald JK (1998) Dipeptidyl peptidase II. In A.J. Barrett, N.D. Rawlings & J.F. Woessner (Eds.) *Handbook of proteolytic enzymes*. pp. 408–411, London, Academic Press.

McDonald JK, Hoisington AR & Eisenhauer DA (1985) Partial purification and characterization of an ovarian tripeptidyl peptidase: a lysosomal exopeptidase that sequentially releases collagen-related (Gly-Pro-X) triplets. *Biochem Biophys Res Commun*, 126, 63–71.

McDonald JK & Schwabe C (1980) Dipeptidyl peptidase II of bovine dental pulp. Initial demonstration and characterization as a fibroblastic, lysosomal peptidase of the serine class active on collagen-related peptides. *Biochim Biophys Acta*, 616, 68–81.

Mitchison HM, Hofmann SL, Becerra CH, Munroe PB, Lake BD, Crow YJ, Stephenson JB, Williams RE, Hofman IL, Taschner PE, Martin JJ, Philippart M, Andermann E, Andermann F, Mole SE, Gardiner RM & O'Rawe AM (1998) Mutations in the palmitoyl-protein thioesterase gene (PPT; CLN1) causing juvenile neuronal ceroid lipofuscinosis with granular osmiophilic deposits. *Hum Mol Genet*, 7, 291–7.

Mole SE (2004) The genetic spectrum of human neuronal ceroid-lipofuscinoses. *Brain Pathol*, 14, 70–6.

Mole SE, Zhong NA, Sarpong A, Logan WP, Hofmann S, Yi W, Franken PF, van Diggelen OP, Breuning MH, Moroziewicz D, Ju W, Salonen T, Holmberg V, Jarvela I & Taschner PE (2001) New mutations in the neuronal ceroid lipofuscinosis genes. *Eur J Paediatr Neurol*, **5** Suppl A, 7–10.

Noher de Halac N, Dodelson de Kremer R, Kohan R, et al. (2005) *Clinical, morphological, biochemical and molecular study of atypical forms of neuronal ceroid lipofuscinoses in Argentina*. pp. 103–116, Cordoba, Publicaciones Universitarias.

Oyama H, Fujisawa T, Suzuki T, Dunn BM, Wlodawer A & Oda K (2005) Catalytic residues and substrate specificity of recombinant human tripeptidyl peptidase I (CLN2). *J Biochem*, 138, 127–34.

Page AE, Fuller K, Chambers TJ & Warburton MJ (1993) Purification and characterization of a tripeptidyl peptidase I from human osteoclastomas: evidence for its role in bone resorption. *Arch Biochem Biophys*, 306, 354–9.

Pal A, Kraetzner R, Gruene T, Grapp M, Schreiber K, Grønborg M, Urlaub H, Becker S, Asif AR, Gärtner J, Sheldrick GM, & Steinfeld R (2009) Structure of tripeptidyl-peptidase I provides insight into the molecular basis of late infantile neuronal ceroid lipofuscinosis. *J Biol Chem*, 284, 3976-84.

Palmer DN, Martinus RD, Cooper SM, Midwinter GG, Reid JC & Jolly RD (1989) Ovine ceroid lipofuscinosis. The major lipopigment protein and the lipid-binding subunit of mitochondrial ATP synthase have the same NH2-terminal sequence. *J Biol Chem*, 264, 5736–40.

Pampiglione G & Harden A (1977) So-called neuronal ceroid lipofuscinosis. Neurophysiological studies in 60 children. *J Neurol Neurosurg Psychiatry*, 40, 323–30.

Passini MA, Dodge JC, Bu J, Yang W, Zhao Q, Sondhi D, Hackett NR, Kaminsky SM, Mao Q, Shihabuddin LS, Cheng SH, Sleat DE, Stewart GR, Davidson BL, Lobel P & Crystal RG (2006) Intracranial delivery of CLN2 reduces brain pathology in a mouse model of classical late infantile neuronal ceroid lipofuscinosis. *J Neurosci*, 26, 1334–42.

Petersen B, Handwerker M & Huppertz HI (1996) Neuroradiological findings in classical late infantile neuronal ceroid-lipofuscinosis. *Pediatr Neurol*, 15, 344–7.

Pham CT, Armstrong RJ, Zimonjic DB, Popescu NC, Payan DG & Ley TJ (1997) Molecular cloning, chromosomal localization, and expression of murine dipeptidyl peptidase I. *J Biol Chem*, 272, 10695–703.

Portera-Cailliau C, Sung CH, Nathans J & Adler R (1994) Apoptotic photoreceptor cell death in mouse models of retinitis pigmentosa. *Proc Natl Acad Sci U S A*, 91, 974–8.

Puranam K, Qian WH, Nikbakht K, Venable M, Obeid L, Hannun Y & Boustany RM (1997) Upregulation of Bcl-2 and elevation of ceramide in Batten disease. *Neuropediatrics*, 28, 37–41.

Rao NV, Rao GV & Hoidal JR (1997) Human dipeptidyl-peptidase I. Gene characterization, localization, and expression. *J Biol Chem*, 272, 10260–5.

Rawlings ND & Barrett AJ (1995) Families of aspartic peptidases, and those of unknown catalytic mechanism. *Methods Enzymol*, 248, 105–20.

Reichard U, Lechenne B, Asif AR, Streit F, Grouzmann E, Jousson O & Monod M (2006) Sedolisins, a new class of secreted proteases from Aspergillus fumigatus with endoprotease or tripeptidyl-peptidase activity at acidic pHs. *Appl Environ Microbiol*, 72, 1739–48.

Rose C, Vargas F, Facchinetti P, Bourgeat P, Bambal RB, Bishop PB, Chan SM, Moore AN, Ganellin CR & Schwartz JC (1996) Characterization and inhibition of a cholecystokinin-inactivating serine peptidase. *Nature*, 380, 403–9.

Seitz D, Grodd W, Schwab A, Seeger U, Klose U & Nagele T (1998) MR imaging and localized proton MR spectroscopy in late infantile neuronal ceroid lipofuscinosis. *Am J Neuroradiol*, 19, 1373–7.

Sharp JD, Wheeler RB, Lake BD, Savukoski M, Jarvela IE, Peltonen L, Gardiner RM & Williams RE (1997) Loci for classical and a variant late infantile neuronal ceroid lipofuscinosis map to chromosomes 11p15 and 15q21-23. *Hum Mol Genet*, 6, 591–5.

Simonati A, Santorum E, Tessa A, Polo A, Simonetti F, Bernardina BD, Santorelli FM & Rizzuto N (2000) A CLN2 gene nonsense mutation is associated with severe caudate atrophy and dystonia in LINCL. *Neuropediatrics*, 31, 199–201.

Sleat DE, Donnelly RJ, Lackland H, Liu CG, Sohar I, Pullarkat RK & Lobel P (1997) Association of mutations in a lysosomal protein with classical late-infantile neuronal ceroid lipofuscinosis. *Science*, 277, 1802–5.

Sleat DE, Gin RM, Sohar I, Wisniewski K, Sklower-Brooks S, Pullarkat RK, Palmer DN, Lerner TJ, Boustany RM, Uldall P, Siakotos AN, Donnelly RJ & Lobel P (1999) Mutational analysis of the defective protease in classic late-infantile neuronal ceroid lipofuscinosis, a neurodegenerative lysosomal storage disorder. *Am J Hum Genet*, 64, 1511–23.

Sleat DE, Sohar I, Gin RM & Lobel P (2001) Aminoglycoside-mediated suppression of nonsense mutations in late infantile neuronal ceroid lipofuscinosis. *Eur J Paediatr Neurol*, 5 Suppl A, 57–62.

Sleat DE, Wiseman JA, El-Banna M, Kim KH, Mao Q, Price S, Macauley SL, Sidman RL, Shen MM, Zhao Q, Passini MA, Davidson BL, Stewart GR & Lobel P (2004) A mouse model of classical late-infantile neuronal ceroid lipofuscinosis based on targeted disruption of the CLN2 gene results in a loss of tripeptidyl-peptidase I activity and progressive neurodegeneration. *J Neurosci*, 24, 9117–26.

Sondhi D, Hackett NR, Peterson DA, Stratton J, Baad M, Travis KM, Wilson JM & Crystal RG (2007) Enhanced survival of the LINCL mouse following CLN2 gene transfer using the rh.10 rhesus macaque-derived adeno-associated virus vector. *Mol Ther*, 15, 481–91.

Sondhi D, Peterson DA, Edelstein AM, del Fierro K, Hackett NR & Crystal RG (2008) Survival advantage of neonatal CNS gene transfer for late infantile neuronal ceroid lipofuscinosis. *Exp Neurol*, 213, 18–27.

Sondhi D, Peterson DA, Giannaris EL, Sanders CT, Mendez BS, De B, Rostkowski AB, Blanchard B, Bjugstad K, Sladek JR, Jr., Redmond DE, Jr., Leopold PL, Kaminsky SM, Hackett NR & Crystal RG (2005) AAV2-mediated CLN2 gene transfer to rodent and non-human primate brain results in long-term TPP-I expression compatible with therapy for LINCL. *Gene Ther*, 12, 1618–32.

Steinfeld R, Heim P, von Gregory H, Meyer K, Ullrich K, Goebel HH & Kohlschutter A (2002) Late infantile neuronal ceroid lipofuscinosis: quantitative description of the clinical course in patients with CLN2 mutations. *Am J Med Genet*, 112, 347–54.

Steinfeld R, Steinke HB, Isbrandt D, Kohlschutter A & Gartner J (2004) Mutations in classical late infantile neuronal ceroid lipofuscinosis disrupt transport of tripeptidyl-peptidase I to lysosomes. *Hum Mol Genet*, 13, 2483–91.

Suopanki J, Partanen S, Ezaki J, Baumann M, Kominami E & Tyynela J (2000) Developmental changes in the expression of neuronal ceroid lipofuscinoses-linked proteins. *Mol Genet Metab*, 71, 190–4.

Tamaki SJ, Jacobs Y, Dohse M, Capela A, Cooper JD, Reitsma M, He D, Tushinski R, Belichenko PV, Salehi A, Mobley W, Gage FH, Huhn S, Tsukamoto AS, Weissman IL & Uchida N (2009) Neuroprotection of host cells by human central nervous system stem cells in a mouse model of infantile neuronal ceroid lipofuscinosis. *Cell Stem Cell*, 5, 310–9.

Taylor CR & Levenson RM (2006) Quantification of immunohistochemistry–issues concerning methods, utility and semiquantitative assessment II. *Histopathology*, 49, 411–24.

Tessa A, Simonati A, Tavoni A, Bertini E & Santorelli FM (2000) A novel nonsense mutation (Q509X) in three Italian late-infantile neuronal ceroid-lipofuscinosis children. *Hum Mutat*, 15, 577.

Tian Y, Sohar I, Taylor JW & Lobel P (2006) Determination of the substrate specificity of tripeptidyl-peptidase I using combinatorial peptide libraries and development of improved fluorogenic substrates. *J Biol Chem*, 281, 6559–72.

Tomkinson B (1999) Tripeptidyl peptidases: enzymes that count. *Trends Biochem Sci*, 24, 355–9.

Tsiakas K, Steinfeld R, Storch S, Ezaki J, Lukacs Z, Kominami E, Kohlschutter A, Ullrich K & Braulke T (2004) Mutation of the glycosylated asparagine residue 286 in human CLN2 protein results in loss of enzymatic activity. *Glycobiology*, 14, 1C–5C.

Turk B, Dolenc I & Turk V (1998) Dipeptidyl peptidase I. In Barrett AJ, Rawlings ND & Woessner JF (Eds.) *Handbook of proteolytic enzymes*. pp. 631–34, London, Academic Press.

Tyynelä J, Baumann M, Henseler M, Sandhoff K & Haltia M (1995) Sphingolipid activator proteins (SAPs) are stored together with glycosphingolipids in the infantile neuronal ceroid-lipofuscinosis (INCL). *Am J Med Genet*, 57, 294–7.

Tyynelä J, Cooper JD, Khan MN, Shemilts SJ & Haltia M (2004) Hippocampal pathology in the human neuronal ceroid-lipofuscinoses: distinct patterns of storage deposition, neurodegeneration and glial activation. *Brain Pathol*, 14, 349–57.

van Diggelen OP, Keulemans JL, Kleijer WJ, Thobois S, Tilikete C & Voznyi YV (2001) Pre- and postnatal enzyme analysis for infantile, late infantile and adult neuronal ceroid lipofuscinosis (CLN1 and CLN2). *Eur J Paediatr Neurol*, 5 Suppl A, 189–92.

Vines D & Warburton MJ (1998) Purification and characterisation of a tripeptidyl aminopeptidase I from rat spleen. *Biochim Biophys Acta*, 1384, 233–42.

Vines DJ & Warburton MJ (1999) Classical late infantile neuronal ceroid lipofuscinosis fibroblasts are deficient in lysosomal tripeptidyl peptidase I. *FEBS Lett*, 443, 131–5.

Walus M, Kida E & Golabek AA (2010) Functional consequences and rescue potential of pathogenic missense mutations in tripeptidyl peptidase I. *Hum Mutat*, 31, 710–21.

Walus M, Kida E, Wisniewski KE & Golabek AA (2005) Ser475, Glu272, Asp276, Asp327, and Asp360 are involved in catalytic activity of human tripeptidyl-peptidase I. *FEBS Lett*, 579, 1383–8.

Warburton MJ & Bernardini F (2001) The specificity of lysosomal tripeptidyl peptidase-I determined by its action on angiotensin-II analogues. *FEBS Lett*, 500, 145–8.

Warburton MJ & Bernardini F (2002) Tripeptidyl peptidase-I is essential for the degradation of sulphated cholecystokinin-8 (CCK-8S) by mouse brain lysosomes. *Neurosci Lett*, 331, 99–102.

Wheeler RB, Schlie M, Kominami E, Gerhard L & Goebel HH (2001) Neuronal ceroid lipofuscinosis: late infantile or Janský Bielschowsky type–re-revisited. *Acta Neuropathol*, 102, 485–8.

Williams R, Vesa J, Jarvela I, McKay T, Mitchison H, Hellsten E, Thompson A, Callen D, Sutherland G, Luna-Battadano D & et al. (1993) Genetic heterogeneity in neuronal ceroid lipofuscinosis (NCL): evidence that the late-infantile subtype (Janský-Bielschowsky disease; CLN2) is not an allelic form of the juvenile or infantile subtypes. *Am J Hum Genet*, 53, 931–5.

Wisniewski KE, Becerra CR & Hofmann SL (1997) A novel granular variant (GROD) form of late infantile neuronal ceroid lipofuscinosis (CLN2) is an infantile form of NCL (CLN1) when biochemically studied. *J Neuropathol Exp Neurol*, 56, 594.

Wisniewski KE, Connell F, Kaczmarski W, Kaczmarski A, Siakotos A, Becerra CR & Hofmann SL (1998) Palmitoyl-protein thioesterase deficiency in a novel granular variant of LINCL. *Pediatr Neurol*, 18, 119–23.

Wisniewski KE, Kaczmarski A, Kida E, Connell F, Kaczmarski W, Michalewski MP, Moroziewicz DN & Zhong N (1999) Reevaluation of neuronal ceroid lipofuscinoses: atypical juvenile onset may be the result of CLN2 mutations. *Mol Genet Metab*, 66, 248–52.

Wisniewski KE, Kida E, Gordon-Majszak W & Saitoh T (1990) Altered amyloid beta-protein precursor processing in brains of patients with neuronal ceroid lipofuscinosis. *Neurosci Lett*, 120, 94–6.

Wisniewski KE, Kida E, Walus M, Wujek P, Kaczmarski W & Golabek AA (2001) Tripeptidyl-peptidase I in neuronal ceroid lipofuscinoses and other lysosomal storage disorders. *Eur J Paediatr Neurol*, 5 Suppl A, 73–9.

Wlodawer A, Durell SR, Li M, Oyama H, Oda K & Dunn BM (2003a) A model of tripeptidyl-peptidase I (CLN2), a ubiquitous and highly conserved member of the sedolisin family of serine-carboxyl peptidases. *BMC Struct Biol*, 3, 8.

Wlodawer A, Li M, Dauter Z, Gustchina A, Uchida K, Oyama H, Dunn BM & Oda K (2001) Carboxyl proteinase from Pseudomonas defines a novel family of subtilisin-like enzymes. *Nat Struct Biol*, 8, 442–6.

Wlodawer A, Li M, Gustchina A, Oyama H, Dunn BM & Oda K (2003b) Structural and enzymatic properties of the sedolisin family of serine-carboxyl peptidases. *Acta Biochim Pol*, 50, 81–102.

Wlodawer A, Li M, Gustchina A, Tsuruoka N, Ashida M, Minakata H, Oyama H, Oda K, Nishino T & Nakayama T (2004) Crystallographic and biochemical investigations of kumamolisin-As, a serine-carboxyl peptidase with collagenase activity. *J Biol Chem*, 279, 21500–10.

Worgall S, Kekatpure MV, Heier L, Ballon D, Dyke JP, Shungu D, Mao X, Kosofsky B, Kaplitt MG, Souweidane MM, Sondhi D, Hackett NR, Hollmann C & Crystal RG (2007) Neurological deterioration in late infantile neuronal ceroid lipofuscinosis. *Neurology*, 69, 521–35.

Worgall S, Sondhi D, Hackett NR, Kosofsky B, Kekatpure MV, Neyzi N, Dyke JP, Ballon D, Heier L, Greenwald BM, Christos P, Mazumdar M, Souweidane MM, Kaplitt MG & Crystal RG (2008) Treatment of late infantile neuronal ceroid lipofuscinosis by CNS administration of a serotype 2 adeno-associated virus expressing CLN2 cDNA. *Hum Gene Ther*, 19, 463–74.

Wujek P, Kida E, Walus M, Wisniewski KE & Golabek AA (2004) N-glycosylation is crucial for folding, trafficking, and stability of human tripeptidyl-peptidase I. *J Biol Chem*, 279, 12827–39.

Yan W, Boustany RM, Konradi C, Ozelius L, Lerner T, Trofatter JA, Julier C, Breakefield XO, Gusella JF & Haines JL (1993) Localization of juvenile, but not late-infantile, neuronal ceroid lipofuscinosis on chromosome 16. *Am J Hum Genet*, 52, 89–95.

Young EP, Worthington VC, Jackson M & Winchester BG (2001) Pre- and postnatal diagnosis of patients with CLN1 and CLN2 by assay of palmitoyl-protein thioesterase and tripeptidyl-peptidase I activities. *Eur J Paediatr Neurol*, 5 Suppl A, 193–6.

Yuza Y, Yokoi K, Sakurai K, Ariga M, Yanagisawa T, Ohashi T, Hoshi Y & Eto Y (2005) Allogenic bone marrow transplantation for late-infantile neuronal ceroid lipofuscinosis. *Pediatr Int*, 47, 681–3.

Zhong N, Moroziewicz DN, Ju W, Jurkiewicz A, Johnston L, Wisniewski KE & Brown WT (2000) Heterogeneity of late-infantile neuronal ceroid lipofuscinosis. *Genet Med*, 2, 312–8.

Zhong N, Wisniewski KE, Hartikainen J, Ju W, Moroziewicz DN, McLendon L, Sklower Brooks SS & Brown WT (1998) Two common mutations in the CLN2 gene underlie late infantile neuronal ceroid lipofuscinosis. *Clin Genet*, 54, 234–8.

Chapter 8

CLN3

L. Åberg, T. Autti, T. Braulke, J.D. Cooper, O.P. van Diggelen, A. Jalanko, S. Kenrick, C. Kitzmüller, A. Kohlschütter, A. Kyttälä, H.M. Mitchison, S.E. Mole, R. Niezen-de Boer, M.-L. Punkari, A. Schulz, M. Talling, and R.E. Williams

INTRODUCTION

Mutations in the *CLN3* gene cause CLN3 disease, classic juvenile formerly known as Spielmeyer–Sjögren disease. This is one of the most prevalent types of NCL worldwide, with almost all patients carrying the same disease allele. There is a possibility that mutations in *CLN3* also cause other disease phenotypes that are not currently classified with the NCLs, or are not yet recognized. *CLN3* encodes a conserved transmembrane protein whose function, to date, is unknown.

MOLECULAR GENETICS

Isolation of the *CLN3* gene

A positional cloning approach was adopted to isolate the *CLN3* gene. Genetic linkage initially mapped *CLN3* to the haptoglobin locus on chromosome 16 (Eiberg et al., 1989) and the chromosome location was subsequently refined to a region of 8cM at 16p11.2–12.1 (Mitchison et al., 1993). Three microsatellite markers in this region, *D16S288*, *D16S299*, and *D16S298*, were in strong linkage disequilibrium with *CLN3* (Mitchison et al., 1993, Lerner et al., 1994). Genotyping in a larger family collection (n=143) by The International Batten Disease (TIBD) Consortium localized *CLN3* to a smaller region of 2.1cM between markers *D16S288* and *D16S383*. Haplotype analysis indicated the presence of a founder mutation suggesting *CLN3* to be in close proximity to marker loci *D16S299* and *D16S298*. The degree of linkage disequilibrium was most striking at locus *D16S298*. The availability of linkage disequilibrium mapping data from the isolated Finnish population allowed the physical distance of *CLN3* from the closest-linked markers to be calculated, placing the gene within 8.8kb of *D16S298*. Allele '6' of marker *D16S298* was present on 96% of Finnish and 92% of European *CLN3* chromosomes, and this implied that a single common mutation was present in most patients (Mitchison et al., 1995).

Concurrent physical mapping across the *CLN3* region established a contig of cloned genomic DNA fragments that encompassed the closest genetic markers (Järvelä et al., 1995). Several genes were mapped within the *CLN3* critical region and a number were excluded following mutation analysis. A variety of different methods were then used to isolate additional gene sequences in the region, including bioinformatics, exon amplification, cDNA selection, and direct sequencing of genomic DNA clones. One 35 kilobase (kb) cosmid clone, 11A, contained the microsatellite marker *D16S298* and therefore became the focus of efforts to isolate new transcripts. A 180 basepair (bp) exon was isolated which detected a 1.7kb transcript in a fetal brain cDNA library. When the cDNA was mapped back to the *CLN3* region it was found to span the *D16S298* locus and to overlap with the region deleted in a Moroccan patient, previously shown to be missing *D16S298*. Screening of patients for mutations using the cDNA as a probe revealed a genomic deletion of 1kb in several patients but not in controls. Characterization of additional mutations subsequently confirmed that this cDNA corresponded to the juvenile NCL gene, *CLN3* (TIBD Consortium, 1995).

Gene structure

Genomic sequencing and restriction mapping of the 11A cosmid that contained the entire *CLN3* open reading frame and surrounding sequences allowed determination of the genomic structure and the complete intron–exon nucleotide sequence (Mitchison et al., 1997b). *CLN3* consists of 15 exons, spanning 15kb of the genome, which range in size from 47–356bp, with 14 introns that range from 80–4227bp. The cDNA comprises 1689bp followed by a 47bp poly (A) tail, with a predicted open reading frame of 1314bp. The microsatellite marker *D16S298* is located in intron 13.

Screening of DNA databases detected no homologies to any gene sequences of known function. However, the *CLN3* gene is highly conserved down to yeast, but is not present in plants. Exon sizes and the position and sequence of splice sites are also remarkably conserved between species.

Mutations in *CLN3*

More than 40 different disease-causing mutations have been reported in the *CLN3* gene, and full information is maintained at the NCL Mutation Database website (http://www.ucl.ac.uk/ncl) (TIBD Consortium, 1995, Munroe et al., 1997, Lauronen et al., 1999, Bensaoula et al., 2000, Kwon et al., 2005, Leman et al., 2005, Sarpong et al., 2009; and unpublished). The most common mutation is the 1kb deletion (actually 96bp; c.461–280–677+382del966), which is found in 85–90% of all CLN3 disease, classic juvenile cases in different populations, either in homozygous or heterozygous form. Patients with *CLN3* mutations are found worldwide but sharing of this common ancestral mutation represents the major founder effect in CLN3 disease, juvenile and reflects the European ancestry of the majority of CLN3 disease patients (TIBD Consortium, 1995). This preponderance of one mutation in almost all patients is unique amongst the NCLs, and is likely to be genetically significant and therefore probably also biologically (Kitzmüller et al., 2008). The breakpoints of the 1kb deletion lie in introns 6 and 8, resulting in loss of exons 7 and 8 (totalling 217bp) from the *CLN3* mRNA transcript. Repetitive *Alu* sequences at the breakpoints of the 1kb deletion suggest a possible mutation mechanism due to misalignment and recombination during DNA replication (TIBD Consortium, 1995). The 1kb deletion results in at least two mutant transcripts—one causes both a frameshift and premature termination of the remaining protein after amino acid 153, and the other arises from alternative splicing bringing the 3′ end of the transcript back into frame at residue 264 (Kitzmüller et al., 2008).

A spectrum of other *CLN3* mutations has been detected using a combination of methods. In total (44), these comprise 13 small insertions or deletions (including a 27bp and a 34bp deletion), ten missense mutations, ten nonsense mutations, six splice site mutations, four large deletions, and one intron change. The majority of known *CLN3* mutations are 'private', restricted to a single CLN3 disease, juvenile family; however, certain mutations occur with relatively higher frequency. These more common mutations often occur on a haplotype background that is shared between families and therefore these mutations are likely to represent minor founder effects (Munroe et al., 1997). These include the c.424delG and c.944–945insA splicing mutations. In addition, the arginine residue at position 334 has the highest frequency of missense mutation since p. Arg334Cys and p.Arg334Cys mutations are both relatively prevalent.

All known disease-causing missense mutations are located either in or immediately adjacent to a predicted transmembrane helix (Leu101, Glu295, Gln295) or in the conserved luminal loops (Ala158, Leu170, Gly187) or the amphipathic helix (Val330, and Arg334 which is mutated twice) or the C-terminus (Asp416) (Nugent et al., 2008) (see later).

Three non-coding and two coding single nucleotide polymorphisms have been detected in intron 4 (2), intron 13, exon 10 (p.Val277Val) and exon 15 (p.His404Arg) (Mitchison et al., 1997a, Zhong et al., 1998, Eksandh et al., 2000, Mole et al., 2001).

Expression pattern

Northern blot analysis showed that *CLN3* is expressed in a wide variety of human tissues including muscle, brain, placenta, lung, liver, skeletal muscle, kidney, and pancreas (TIBD Consortium, 1995). Expression in 64 different human tissues indicated that mRNA levels for *CLN3* are highest in gastrointestinal tissue and are also high in glandular/secretory tissue (Chattopadhyay and Pearce, 2000). Expression levels in the central nervous system (CNS) are not particularly high. In the rat brain, expression levels are highest around birth (Pane et al., 1999). The expression pattern of the *CLN3* transcript and analysis of the promoter region indicates that *CLN3* is constitutively expressed and serves a 'housekeeping' function in the cell. There are several alternative spliced transcripts, and further analysis of the expression of these different isoforms is required to determine their significance with respect to regulation of *CLN3* function in the cell.

CELL BIOLOGY

Protein structure and modifications

The *CLN3* gene encodes a hydrophobic integral membrane protein of 438 amino acids (Janes et al., 1996, Kaczmarski et al., 1999). The first empirical evidence on the topology of CLN3 was obtained by utilizing Flag-tagged CLN3 and glycosylation mutagenesis suggesting that CLN3 has five membrane-spanning domains, an extracellular/intraluminal N-terminus, and a cytoplasmic C-terminus (Mao et al., 2003). Selective cell permeabilization assays further indicated that the N-terminus is located in the cytoplasm, therefore suggesting that CLN3 is a type III transmembrane protein consisting of six membrane-spanning domains with both the N- and C-termini facing the cytoplasm (Kyttälä et al., 2004). The cytoplasmic orientation of the N-terminus was also reported by Ezaki and colleagues (Ezaki et al., 2003). The six-transmembrane domain model, with cytosolic N- and C-termini, is currently favoured due to the stronger evidence obtained from the *in vivo* studies (Kyttälä et al., 2004) and by using a highly specific CLN3 antibody (Ezaki et al., 2003). In addition, more recent computational models support this topology, with the additional inclusion of a conserved luminal amphipathic helix and changes to the position of the transmembrane domains

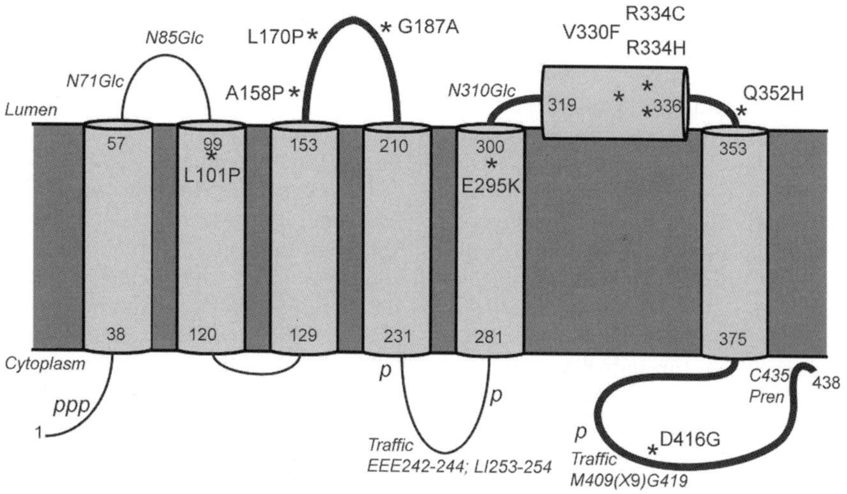

Figure 8.1 CLN3 topology. Diagrammatic representation of CLN3, which is predicted to have six membrane-spanning segments and one amphipathic segment (residues indicated), with N- and C-termini projecting into the cytoplasm. Glycosylation sites are indicated with Glc, resides important for lysosomal targeting with 'traffic' and the C-farnesylation domain with 'Pren'. Six potential cytoplasmic phosphorylation sites (p) are Ser12, Ser14, Thr19, Thr232, Ser270, Thr400. The location of known missense mutations are indicated with*. All transmembrane helices and the amphipathic helix are conserved, as are those domains represented by a bold line.

(Nugent et al., 2008). The transmembrane topology of CLN3 is presented in Figure 8.1. What may be significant is the position of conserved residues facing into the lumen of the organelle in which CLN3 is located, and thus free to interact with luminal molecular species or transduce changes in the luminal environment (e.g. pH). There is also significant conservation in the cytoplasmic C-terminal tail. Helices that interact with the lipid bilayer may modulate the activity of other membrane proteins, such as ion channels, and this activity may be influenced by the local composition of the lipid membrane.

Sequence analysis of human CLN3 predicts several potential sites for post-translational modifications. These include four putative N-glycosylation sites, and consensus sequences for phosphorylation, farnesylation, and myristoylation. Experimental studies utilizing overexpressed CLN3 have demonstrated that CLN3 synthesized in mammalian cells is detected in two different forms; the non-glycosylated 43kDa and an N-glycosylated 45kDa form (Järvelä et al., 1998). The apparent molecular weight of the glycosylated CLN3 seems to vary depending on the cell type used (Golabek et al., 1999) and mass spectrometric analyses indicate that the glycosylation of CLN3 indeed varies in different tissues (Ezaki et al., 2003). The N-glycosylated CLN3 is sensitive to endoglycosidase H indicating that the glycan structure is of high mannose type (Järvelä et al., 1998). Recently, it was demonstrated by mutational analysis that CLN3 utilizes two glycosylation sites, at Asn71 and Asn85 (Storch et al., 2007), and Asn310 may also be glycosylated (Mao et al., 2003) (Figure 8.1). Interestingly, the mouse protein possesses complex-type N-linked sugar chains different from the human CLN3 (Ezaki et al., 2003). CLN3 may also be phosphorylated, as suggested by initial analyses of Michalewski et al. (Michalewski et al., 1998, Michalewski et al., 1999); however, more exact analyses of the phosphorylation sites and the kinases involved are yet to be carried out. Six potential cytoplasmic phosphorylation sites (Ser12, Ser14, Thr19, Thr232, Ser270, Thr400) exist within the latest topological model (Nugent et al., 2008).

Membrane proteins implicated in neuronal functions often possess lipid modifications. The sequence analysis of CLN3 predicts a putative N-myristoylation site at the N-terminus and a prenylation/farnesylation motif at the C-terminus (Pullarkat and Morris, 1997, Kaczmarski et al., 1999). To date no experimental evidence exists for the presence of the N-terminal myristoylation site, whereas the CaaX farnesylation motif at the C-terminus of CLN3 (435CQLS438) is modified by a farnesyl group (Kaczmarski et al., 1999).

Localization and targeting

CLN3 has been reported to be located in many intracellular compartments. Variable results obtained by different research groups probably result from the low abundance of CLN3 in mammalian cells, the very hydrophobic nature of the protein and existence of very few good antibodies, and the use of expression systems that may saturate or interfere with its normal intracellular location. Recent opinion favoured an endosomal/lysosomal localization of CLN3 protein with trafficking through the endoplasmic reticulum (ER) and Golgi (Järvelä et al., 1998, Kida et al., 1999, Haskell et al., 2000, Kyttälä et al., 2004). Additional localization sites are suggested for neuronal CLN3 as it has been detected in the synaptosomal fraction of mouse brain and in early endosomes of neuronal cells (Luiro et al., 2001, Kyttälä et al., 2004, Storch et al., 2007). A small portions (about 10%) of the CLN3 protein can be detected at the plasma membrane (Mao et al., 2003, Persaud-Sawin et al., 2004, Storch et al., 2007) and the protein has also been discovered in a membrane lipid raft preparation (Rakheja et al., 2004). Recent work on the CLN3 orthologue in two yeast species indicates a significant localization in the Golgi apparatus (Codlin and Mole, 2009; and J. Gerst unpublished, see Chapter 15), also previously reported for CLN3 (Kremmidiotis et al., 1999), and this should be considered further for the human protein.

Two lysosomal targeting motifs mediate sorting of CLN3 in transfected non-neuronal and neuronal cells (Kyttälä et al., 2004). The first targeting motif is localized in the large cytosolic loop of CLN3 comprising a dileucine motif, LI (aa253–254) with an upstream acidic patch also contributing to lysosomal targeting (Kyttälä et al., 2004, Storch et al., 2004) (Figure 8.1). AP1 and AP3 are the main adaptor proteins facilitating the trafficking of lysosomal membrane proteins from the trans-Golgi network to the lysosomes but controversial data about binding of the dileucine signal of CLN3 to these adaptors has been presented (Storch et al., 2004, Kyttalä et al., 2005). The second lysosomal targeting motif of CLN3 is localized in the C-terminal cytoplasmic domain. This unconventional motif consists of methionine and glycine residues separated by nine amino acids [M(X)9G] (Kyttälä et al., 2004) (Figure 8.1).

Although mutations in the C-terminal prenylation site of CLN3 seem to have no effect ion lysosomal localization of CLN3 (Haskell et al., 2000), it was recently demonstrated that prenylation is involved in the endosomal sorting of the protein (Storch et al., 2007) since mutation of Cys435 impaired trafficking of CLN3 to the lysosome. Farnesylation deficient CLN3 has also been shown to be functionally impaired in complementing the defects resulting from BTN1 deficiency (yeast homologue of CLN3) in *Saccharomyces cerevisiae* (Haskell et al., 2000). Most of the substitutions and deletions of the C-terminal cytoplasmic domain of CLN3 result in accumulation of the protein in the ER, suggesting that the length of the cytoplasmic domain of CLN3 and the capability to form a prenylation-mediated loop structure might be important for intracellular trafficking of CLN3. Glycosylation however, is not important for the transport of CLN3 to lysosomes (Storch et al., 2007).

None of the so far reported CLN3 disease mutations directly affect the lysosomal targeting motifs of CLN3 (Kyttälä et al., 2004; http://www.ucl.ac.uk/ncl), although p.Asp416Gly is located between two residues important for trafficking. Disease-causing mutations usually prevent exit of the mutated protein from the ER and induce degradation of CLN3 (Järvelä et al., 1999). Mutant proteins that model these CLN3 disease mutations in fission yeast are also retained in the ER (Haines et al., 2009). However, some disease mutations, particularly those correlating to milder phenotypes of CLN3 disease, juvenile (e.g. p.Gln295Lys, p. Lys101Pro, p.Lys170Pro, p.Val330Phe, or p.Arg334His), allow at least some mutated CLN3 to leave the ER (Järvelä et al., 1999, Haskell et al., 2000). Mutant proteins modelling these same mutations in fission yeast were also able to traffic to the vacuole (Haines et al., 2009). In addition, p.Asp41Gly, when modelled in yeast slowed down trafficking of the mutant protein to the vacuole. Two yeast mutant proteins modelling p.Cys435Ser also reached the vacuole, and, in contrast to wild-type protein, were internalized.

Possible function

Despite the identification of the CLN3 gene and protein in 1995, the function of this highly conserved integral membrane protein remains elusive. CLN3 is not homologous to any known protein but the six-transmembrane domain topology of CLN3 is suggestive of a transporter function. Consistently, a distant, but potentially significant relationship between CLN3 and an equilibrative nucleoside transporter family SLC29 has been illustrated (Baldwin et al., 2004).

So far, proposed functions of CLN3 include lysosomal acidification, lysosomal arginine import, membrane fusion, vesicular transport, cytoskeletal linked function, autophagy, apoptosis, and proteolipid modification. CLN3 may have multiple functional roles affecting several pathways, or exert a primary role that affects multiple pathways, as demonstrated for the orthologous *Schizosaccharomyces pombe* yeast protein. The CLN3 protein is expressed ubiquitously but its defective function affects the CNS specifically, resulting in selective death of neuronal subpopulations (Cooper et al., 2006). Neurons may be more sensitive to the storage material, the subunit c of the mitochondrial ATP synthase (SCMAS), than other cell populations. The function of CLN3 may be linked to the maintenance of subpopulations of neurons during development or involved in, so far, unresolved metabolic pathways specific to neurons.

MAINTENANCE OF PH AND OSMOREGULATION

The first functional studies utilized the *S. cerevisiae* homologue of CLN3, Btn1p, which is 30% identical and 59% similar to human CLN3 (Croopnick et al., 1998, Pearce et al., 1999b) (see Chapter 15). A yeast strain with deleted *BTN1* (*btn1*-Δ) has a lower vacuolar pH at early growth phase compared to the wild-type strain implicating that Btn1p participates in the maintenance of vacuolar pH (Pearce and Sherman, 1998, Pearce et al., 1999a, Pearce et al., 1999b). Expression of human CLN3 complements the defect in *btn1*-Δ strain indicating that Btn1p and CLN3 have similar functions (Pearce and Sherman, 1998). In contrast, the fission yeast *S. pombe*, lacking Btn1p, shows elevated vacuolar pH (Gachet et al., 2005). Elevated lysosomal pH is also reported in human CLN3 disease, juvenile fibroblasts harbouring the major 1kb mutation of CLN3 (Holopainen et al., 2001). Simultaneous removal of Btn1p and v-ATPase in *S. pombe* results in conditional synthethic lethality in yeast, suggesting a link between Btn1p and v-ATPase functions (Gachet et al., 2005) and events that affect the cell wall (Codlin et al., 2008a). Additionally, the *S. cerevisiae btn1*-Δ strain modulates v-ATPase activity, further strengthening the connection of CLN3 to vacuolar pH homeostasis (Padilla-Lopez and Pearce, 2006), and there seems to be a connection between the protein SBDS, the ribosome maturation pathway, CLN3 and v-ATPase function (Vitiello et al., 2010). However, CLN3 disease is more than a pH-related disorder, as shown by other work in both yeast and mouse models and mammalian cells. Work in mice has suggested an osmoregulated role for CLN3p in renal control of water and potassium balance (Stein et al., 2010).

LINKS TO MEMBRANE TRAFFICKING EVENTS

Transcript profiling of the *S. cerevisiae btn1*-Δ strain revealed gross upregulation of two genes, *HSP30* (encoding Hsp30p, a down-regulator of plasma membrane H^+-ATPase) and *BTN2* encoding Btn2p (Pearce et al., 1999b). The function of both Btn2p and its mammalian homologue, Hook1, is not well understood, but is often linked to membrane trafficking (Walenta et al., 2001, Kama et al., 2007). Although no interaction between Btn1p and Btn2p proteins is detected in yeast, CLN3 interacts with mammalian Hook1 (Luiro et al., 2004). Simultaneous overexpression of CLN3 and Hook1 in COS-1 and HeLa cells resulted in aggregation of Hook1, thus supporting a functional link between the two proteins (Luiro et al., 2004).

Membrane trafficking may be affected by abnormal fusion or release of vesicles. There is some suggestion that membrane lipid content is affected when CLN3 is mutated (Rusyn et al., 2008), including the synthesis of bis(monoacylglycerol)phosphate (BMP) (Hobert and Dawson, 2007) found in lipid rafts, to which CLN3 may locate (Rakheja et al., 2004). Sterol-rich domains and sites of polarized growth on the plasma membrane are also affected when the fission yeast *CLN3* homologue *BTN1* is deleted (Codlin et al., 2008a, Codlin et al., 2008b). The function of Hook1 (and Btn2p) is tightly linked to membrane fusion events (Richardson et al., 2004) since Hook1 interacts with several Rab GTPases (Luiro et al., 2004) and Btn2p with SNARE proteins in yeast (Kama et al., 2007). Therefore, the function of CLN3 (via Hook1 interaction) may also contribute to membrane fusion. This is supported by the data showing that endocytic trafficking is impaired in CLN3-deficient cells (Fossale et al., 2004, Luiro et al., 2004), and in fission yeast cells deleted for *btn1* (Codlin et al., 2008b). Furthermore, the trafficking of *S. pombe* Btn1p, was recently connected to the Ras GTPase Ypt7p, the protein needed for vacuole fusion in yeasts. Additionally, *S. pombe* Btn1p is able to modify vacuole size (Gachet et al., 2005). Vesicular fusion events are also connected to the maturation of autophagic vesicles and recent work demonstrated that CLN3 may indeed be involved in the maturation of autophagic vacuoles (Cao et al., 2006). Autophagy is a pathway that regulates among others, mitochondrial turnover. Mitochondria can be engulfed by autophagosomes that can subsequently fuse with lysosomes. Mitochondrial function of the brain is not markedly affected *per se* in *Cln3* deficient mice, but the size of mitochondria is reported to be enlarged (Luiro et al., 2006). There is a delay in post-TGN trafficking of the mannose 6-phophate receptor in mammalian cells depleted for CLN3 (Metcalfe et al., 2008) that appears to be caused by defective release of vesicles. This defect may affect delivery of lysosomal enzymes. It is possible that many CLN3 disease phenotypes are a result of defects in multiple post-Golgi trafficking pathways, proposed as the primary defect in yeast cells from work in the fission yeast model that showed Golgi morphology was aberrant when Btn1p was deleted (Codlin and Mole, 2009).

LINKS TO ARGININE TRANSPORT

Deletion of *BTN1* in *S. cerevisiae* (*btn1*-Δ) results in depletion of endogenous vacuolar arginine levels (Kim et al., 2003) indicating that CLN3 may be involved in regulation of inward transport of basic amino acids across the vacuolar membrane. Furthermore, Btn2p is reported to genetically interact with Rsg1p, a negative regulator of arginine and lysine permease Can1p (Chattopadhyay and Pearce, 2002). The function of CLN3 in arginine transport is further supported by the data indicating that the isolated lysosomes of CLN3 disease, juvenile fibroblasts also show defective arginine transport. Arginine levels are also decreased in the serum of *Cln3* deficient mice (Pearce et al., 2003, Ramirez-Montealegre and Pearce, 2005), and subtle, but significant, changes in the activities of enzymes involved in the citrulline-nitric oxide recycling pathway altered regulation of neuronal nitric oxide synthase in the cortex and cerebellum of these *Cln3* deficient mice, with a significant decrease in arginine transport into cerebellar granule cells (Chan et al., 2009). In mammalian cells, arginine and lysine are transported by the same transport system (Pisoni et al., 1987a, Pisoni et al., 1987b) and it is currently unknown why only arginine transport is misregulated in CLN3 disease, juvenile. However, arginine levels can be dysregulated by several factors, such as cationic imbalance, suggesting that the observed phenomenon may be secondary to CLN3 deficiency. Further studies are needed to expose the possible channel function of CLN3 or its interaction with some yet unknown channel/transporter.

LINKS TO THE CYTOSKELETON

The mammalian Hook1 proteins interact with microtubules (Walenta et al., 2001) and the connection between CLN3 and Hook1 suggests that CLN3 function may be linked to the cytoskeleton (Luiro et al., 2004). The yeast Hook1 homologue, Btn2p, also interacts with ankyrin G, a multifunctional adaptor protein involved in connecting integral membrane proteins with the spectrin cytoskeleton (Weimer et al., 2005). Deletion of the fission yeast *CLN3* homologue *Btn1* affects actin patch formation and polarization (Codlin and Mole, 2009). The cytoskeletal link is further stressed by the impaired axonal transport of amino acids in the optic nerve in *Cln3* deficient mice (Weimer et al., 2005). Other links between CLN3 and cytoskeleton are provided by transcript profiling assays of *Cln3* deficient mice, indicating a defect in cytoskeletal function (Brooks et al., 2003, Elshatory et al., 2003, Luiro et al., 2006). Interestingly, the dynactin multiprotein complex, implicated also in fast axonal transport, is downregulated both at mRNA and protein levels (Luiro et al., 2006). Furthermore, movement along microtubules is essential for lysosomal function and disturbed positioning of lysosomes is reported in *Cln3* deficient mouse cerebellar neurons (Fossale et al., 2004). These observations suggest that CLN3 functions in several transport processes along actin filaments and microtubles.

Many of the processes regulated by multifunctional fodrin and Na^+, K^+ ATPase are affected in juvenile CLN3 disease and *Cln3* deficient mice. CLN3 has been shown to interact with the plasma membrane-associated fodrin and the associated Na^+, K^+ ATPase. Although the ion pumping activity of Na^+, K^+ ATPase was unchanged in *Cln3*-deficient mouse primary neurons, the immunostaining pattern of fodrin appeared abnormal in both juvenile CLN3 disease patient fibroblasts and *Cln3*-deficient mouse brains, suggesting disturbances in the fodrin cytoskeleton. Furthermore, the basal subcellular distribution, as well as ouabain-induced endocytosis, of neuron-specific Na^+, K^+ ATPase were affected (Uusi-Rauva et al., 2008).

LINKS TO APOPTOSIS AND PROTEOLIPID MODIFICATION

CLN3 is proposed to protect cells from induced apoptosis by regulation of intracellular ceramide levels. Additionally, gene targeting or RNAi-mediated downregulation of CLN3 are associated with an increased rate of apoptosis (Puranam et al., 1999, Persaud-Sawin and Boustany, 2005, Narayan et al., 2006). This might be in line with recent observations that elevated level of the calcium-binding protein, calsenilin, interacting with the C-terminal domain of CLN3, contributes to cell death in *Cln3*-deficient mouse cells (Chang et al., 2007). Cells from CLN3 disease, juvenile patients, like all the NCL disorders, show accumulation of proteolipid compounds and recent work showed a decrease in palmitoyl protein Δ-9 desaturase activity in *Cln3* deficient mice (Narayan et al., 2008), even suggesting that CLN3 itself may exert this activity (Narayan et al., 2006).

LINKS TO SIGNALLING

An interaction between CLN3 and the Notch and Jun N-terminal kinase signalling pathways has been discovered in *Drosophila* which uncovers a potential role for the RNA splicing and localization machinery in regulating CLN3 function (Tuxworth et al., 2009).

To reveal the primary functions of CLN3, all interaction partners need to be identified, the intracellular locations from which CLN3 acts need to be clarified, and the role of conserved transmembrane, cytoplasmic, and luminal domains investigated. Genome-wide strategies aiming to understand the disease at the level of the organism will also help to resolve the functional roles of CLN3.

CLINICAL DATA

Clinical features

EPIDEMIOLOGY

The incidence of CLN3 disease, juvenile in Scandinavia varies from 2.0–7.0 per 100,000 births (Uvebrant and Hagberg, 1997). In Central Europe, the reported incidence varies from 0.2–1.5 per 100,000 births (Claussen et al., 1992, Cardona and Rosati, 1995). In Canada, the incidence was estimated to be 0.6 per 100,000 births (MacLeod et al., 1976). Overall, CLN3 disease, juvenile is one of the most common types of NCL (see Chapter 23).

AGE OF ONSET AND FIRST SYMPTOMS

The leading symptom of CLN3 disease, juvenile is visual failure, first noticed usually between the ages of 4–7 years. The visual failure leads to blindness within 2–4 years of onset, but light perception may be preserved for years.

PROGRESSION OF SYMPTOMS

After visual failure, learning difficulties become evident in the early school years. Epilepsy often develops around the age of 10 years. Motor symptoms evolve around puberty and clinically manifest as extrapyramidal signs, and, to a lesser degree, pyramidal signs. The progression of motor symptoms gradually leads to loss of independent mobility. Speech difficulties usually accompany the motor problems. Indeed it is likely that the dysarthria is a manifestation of the extrapyramidal movement disorder. Psychiatric problems and sleep problems may be observed at any phase of the disease. The disease leads to premature death at a mean age of 24 years (range 10–28) in patients homozygous for the major 1kb deletion (Järvelä et al., 1997). In compound heterozygous patients, the life expectancy is more variable.

OPHTHALMOLOGIC FINDINGS

At the onset of visual failure, children often show 'overlooking' with or without head turning, in order to optimize the use of their peripheral retina. Ophthalmological examination may show typical findings: macular degeneration sometimes including a 'bull's eye' macular configuration, optic atrophy giving a pale waxy optic disc, thinning of the vessels, and accumulation of pigment in the peripheral retina (Spalton et al., 1980). These findings can resemble retinitis pigmentosa. The diffuse atrophy of the retinal pigment epithelium can be detected by angiography (Hainsworth et al., 2009). Visual evoked potentials (VEPs) and the electroretinogram (ERG) are abolished early (Raitta and Santavuori, 1981).

EPILEPSY SYNDROME

The first epileptic seizure often occurs around the age of 10 years. The symptomatic epilepsy syndrome may be refractory to medication (Åberg et al., 2000b). The predominant seizure type is generalized tonic–clonic, but complex partial seizures are also seen frequently. Typical absence seizures have not been reported. The epilepsy in CLN3 disease, juvenile is regarded as myoclonic, and enhanced somatosensory evoked potentials support the presence of a myoclonic component even though myoclonia may be not be apparent until the late stages of the disease (Lauronen et al., 1997). With increasing age and disease progression, the seizure frequency tends to increase. A progressive slowing of the background activity and increase in paroxysmal activity are typically seen in the electroencephalogram (EEG) (Larsen et al., 2001).

DEMENTIA

A mild cognitive impairment can be detected at an early stage of the disease (Lamminranta et al., 2001). At the time of diagnosis the mean verbal IQ in 14 patients with juvenile NCL was within the low average range, and subsequently fell during the 5-year-long follow-up to the borderline range. The best performed task throughout the study was 'similarities', whereas digit memory span was found to deteriorate most rapidly.

MOTOR DISTURBANCES AND SPEECH

Extrapyramidal (parkinsonian) signs were recorded in about half of the patients at the age of 12–14 years (Järvelä et al., 1997). In the remainder, these symptoms evolve later. Typical extrapyramidal signs in CLN3 disease, juvenile include rigidity, hypokinesia, stooped posture, shuffling gait, and impaired balance. Tremor is not so common.

PSYCHIATRIC AND BEHAVIOURAL DISTURBANCES

Children with CLN3 disease, juvenile suffer from a great diversity of psychiatric symptoms and the individual variability of symptoms is wide. Anxiety, aggressive behaviour, depression, and hallucinations are described (Hofman, 1990). The most commonly reported symptoms by parents and teachers are social, thought and attention problems, somatic complaints, aggressive behaviour, sleep disturbances, and speech problems (Bäckman et al., 2005, Adams et al., 2006). The young person's mood may change abruptly and angry emotional outbursts are common. Some children and young adults, however, are quiet and reserved. Others are moody and easily upset. Siblings can have quite different neuropsychiatric symptoms (Lee et al., 2010), although for these two cases the genetic basis of this disease was not established (T.S. Lee, personal communication).

Hallucinations, especially visual ones, are commonly seen in CLN3 disease, juvenile and these are often, but not always of a frightening nature. Hallucinations may cause anxiety, unrest, emotional outbursts, and sleep disturbance.

The impact of the emotional and behavioural problems on the young person and their family cannot be underestimated. The cognitive decline and loss of communication skills make the recognition, diagnosis, and treatment of these symptoms difficult. Altogether, these problems form a complex psycho-organic syndrome, which should be regarded both as a response to disease progression and as a part of the organic process.

SLEEP DISTURBANCES AND UNREST

Sleep difficulties, such as settling problems, nocturnal awakenings, nightmares, and disturbances in the respiratory pattern, are common in CLN3 disease, juvenile. These may result in daytime sleepiness, irritability, hyperactivity, and worsen other behavioural problems (Kirveskari et al., 2000). Disturbances in the respiratory pattern (without apnoea) increase with age (Telakivi et al., 1985) whereas the sleep disturbances tend to become less frequent during the later stages of the disease. Sleep problems are partly caused by the loss of the circadian rhythm in the mid-teens (Heikkilä et al., 1995), but may also be due to epileptic activity (Kirveskari et al., 2000) or may be regarded as a symptom of depression (Boustany, 1992).

FEEDING

Feeding problems are common in the late stages of the disease. Meal-times become very time-consuming and assistance may be needed. With progression of the disease, swallowing becomes impaired and may necessitate gastrostomy placement.

PUBERTY

Girls with CLN3 disease, juvenile often have an early menarche (Lou and Kristensen, 1973, Åberg et al., 2002). Menstrual cycles may be irregular or short. In addition, acne, obesity, and hirsutism are seen. These may reflect hyperandrogenism and/or polycystic ovaries associated with valproate therapy, a common anti-epileptic drug used in CLN3 disease, juvenile.

CARDIAC PROBLEMS

The heart is also affected by the disease. Progressive cardiac involvement, starting around 14 years of age with heart rate disturbance, leads to cardiomyopathy in the early twenties (Østergaard et al., 2005). Electrocardiogram (ECG) findings include bradycardia, conduction disorders, atrial flutter, sinus arrest, inverted T-waves, and depressed ST-segments. The fitting of pacemakers has improved some patients (A. Schulz personal communication).

Brain imaging

Before the age of 10 years, brain magnetic resonance imaging (MRI) is usually normal. From the age of 11 years, the thalami may show significantly decreased signal intensity on T_2-weighted images (Autti et al., 1996, Autti et al., 1997). In addition to the signal intensity abnormalities of the thalami, voxel-based morphometry, which is a neuroimaging analysis technique that allows investigation of even small focal differences in brain volumes between two groups of subjects, has shown that thalamic volumes decrease disproportionately with other parts of the brain. From the age of 14 years, slight to moderate cerebral and cerebellar atrophy appear. Magnetic resonance spectroscopy has not shown significant abnormalities (Brockmann et al., 1996), though the thalami may show slightly decreased N-acetyl-aspartate (Lauronen et al., 1999). Computed tomography (CT), single photon emission CT (SPECT), and positron emission tomography (PET) imaging methods are not useful for clinical purposes. D1 receptors on PET studies as well as striatal transporter density on SPECT studies appear to be decreased (Åberg et al., 2000a, Rinne et al., 2002).

Clinical biochemistry

In routine laboratory tests, vacuolated lymphocytes are noticed. These, in combination with the ophthalmologic findings, are in fact strongly suggestive of CLN3 disease, juvenile. Autoantibodies to glutamic acid decarboxylase (GAD65-antibodies) have been reported in patients with CLN3 disease, juvenile (Chattopadhyay et al., 2002b). However, antibodies to GAD65 may be just one of the CNS directed autoantibodies in CLN3 disease, juvenile (Lim et al., 2006).

Neurophysiology

The EEG is usually normal until the age of 9 years. Thereafter, a progressive slowing of the background activity and an increase in both generalized and focal paroxysmal activity may be noticed (Larsen et al., 2001).

MORPHOLOGY

Gross pathology

Macroscopically, the brain appears smaller than normal, having a weight reduced to 800–1000g, largely due to mild cortical atrophy, which appears to be proportional to the length of the neurological symptoms. Atrophy of the cerebellum may be more advanced, largely affecting the folia, which may appear thin and firm. On slicing, the lateral ventricles may be enlarged and the cortical ribbon, somewhat reduced in thickness, may display a brownish hue due to lipopigment formation. The substantia nigra, by contrast, may contain very little pigment. Calcification of the inner and outer cerebral surfaces as well as intracerebral vessels has been noted in some cases (Bruun et al., 1991). The white matter appears normal. Visceral organs appear normal.

Histopathology

Microscopically, there is variable neuronal depletion, which may not be very obvious. This apparent preservation of nerve cell bodies allows identification of any selective nerve cell loss. The qualitative technique of Braak and Braak (Braak and Braak, 1993) reveals selective loss of small stellate neurons in the cerebral cortical layer II (Braak and Goebel, 1978) and loss of nerve cells in cortical layer V (Braak and Goebel, 1979), while layer IV was the first affected in the ovine model for CLN6 disease (R. Jolly and S. Walkley, personal communication), perhaps due to excitotoxicity. Similarly, a selective loss of nerve cells has been demonstrated in the corpus striatum and the amygdaloid nucleus. The qualitative technique does not provide precise quantitative data, and additional morphometric and quantifying studies have yet to be performed on CLN3 disease, classic juvenile tissues. In the cerebellum there may be preservation of Purkinje cells, but reduction of their dendritic tree may be conspicuous. The granular layer is severely depleted.

As is usual, loss of neurons results in reactive cellular and fibrillar gliosis, detectable by immunostaining for glial fibrillary acidic protein (GFAP). In addition, immunohistochemical studies (Brück and Goebel, 1998) show there is activation of resident rather than monocyte-derived microglial cells. However, this microglial activation is present not only in the cerebral and cerebellar cortex and retinal tissues, but also in subcortical grey matter (Brück and Goebel, 1998) where loss of nerve cells appears to be negligible (Walkley, 1998). This latter observation may indicate that microglial activation takes place not only when neurons disappear completely, but when there may be damage to their processes leaving neuronal perikarya intact.

The cytoplasm of neurons of the CNS as well as those of the peripheral nervous system (PNS) wherever they occur contains a granular material that has a pale yellow brown colour in unstained sections. The cytoplasm is slightly distended, but less than is seen in the gangliosidoses, and in routine sections the granular material stains with periodic acid–Schiff (PAS), Sudan black, Luxol fast blue and is strongly autofluorescent (Figure 8.2). In cryostat sections of frozen tissue there is strong staining

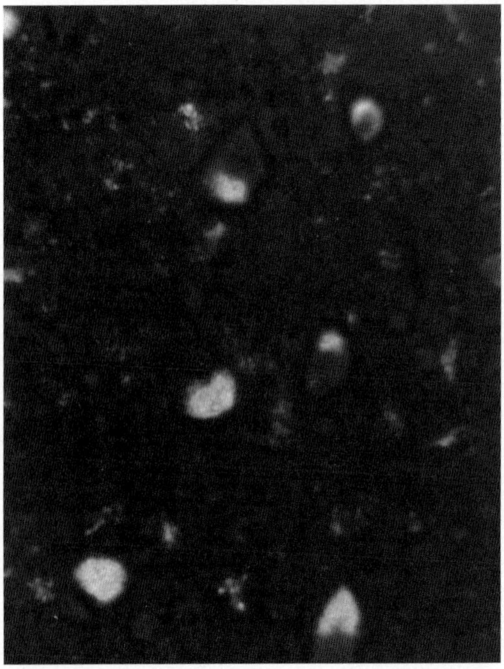

Figure 8.2 CLN3 disease, classic juvenile: intraneuronal lipopigments display strong autofluorescence, ×576.

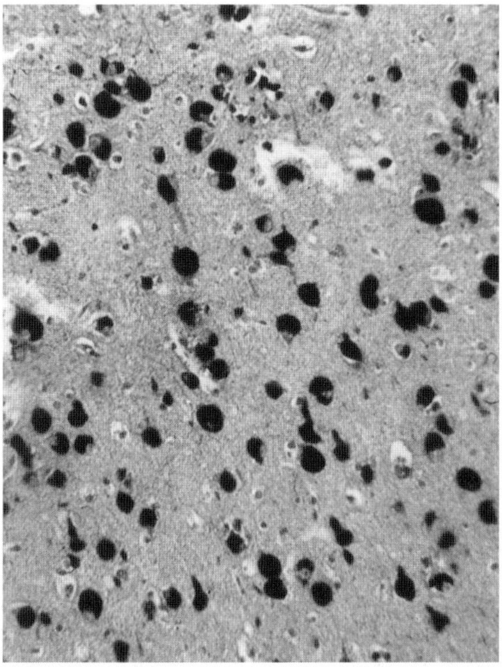

Figure 8.3 CLN3 disease, classic juvenile: SCMAS is abundantly present in cerebrocortical neurons, immunohistochemistry, ×350.

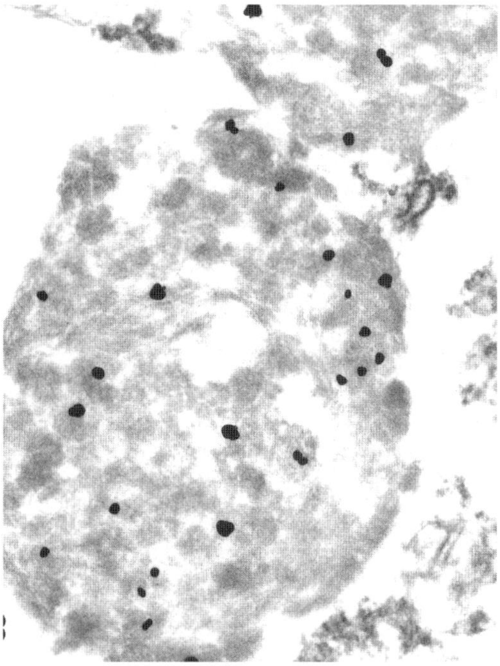

Figure 8.4 CLN3 disease, classic juvenile: immunogold-silver labelling of SCMAS over a rectilinear complex in a postmortem cerebral neuron, ×30,000.

for acid phosphatase activity. Differential extraction techniques show the PAS reaction is due to the increased dolichyl pyrophosphate oligosaccharide content (Hall et al., 1990). Similar staining patterns are found in astrocytes, endothelial cells and smooth muscle cells of the larger vessels, but in these the Luxol fast blue staining is weak or absent. Immunohistochemistry shows the storage bodies to contain SCMAS (Figures 8.3 and 8.4), but to a lesser degree than in CLN2 disease, classic late infantile, as well as saposins A and D (Tyynelä et al., 1997), and β-A4 amyloid and amyloid precursor protein (Elleder et al., 1989, Wisniewski et al., 1990a, Wisniewski et al., 1993) that is probably part of the oligosaccharide moiety of the dolichyl compounds revealed by the PAS reaction.

It should be noted that the presence of storage material does not necessarily result in neuronal dysfunction. In other cells, such as those of the exocrine pancreas, smooth, skeletal, and cardiac muscle cells, the pituitary and the neurons of the gastrointestinal tract, marked storage seems to have little or no effect on function.

Why neurons die in NCL is not well understood. A hypothesis, largely based on morphological studies on canine, ovine, and murine NCL as models of different types of human NCL, has been put forward (March et al., 1995, Walkley et al., 1995, Walkley, 1998). The hypothesis suggests excitotoxicity as a detrimental force, following loss of GABAergic neurons and mitochondrial dysfunction. Their studies indicate there is selective loss of GABAergic neurons in layer IV, an area in which there is enhanced mitochondrial cytochrome-c-oxidase activity as well as the presence of abnormally structured mitochondria.

Retinal pathology

Retinopathy, an early clinical and ophthalmological feature of CLN3 disease, classic juvenile, is the result of profound neuronal loss in the retina. Eyes early in the disease course have not been studied. At the time of death, the retina is usually highly atrophic throughout, resembling advanced retinitis pigmentosa. There is loss of neurons from all retinal layers—almost complete loss of photoreceptor cells, loss of cells in the outer nuclear layer and the outer plexiform layer, and marked atrophy of the nerve fibre layer, ganglion cell layer, and optic nerve. Proliferated Müller cells and other astrocytes rich in GFAP form a scar as the remnant of the former retina. There is migration of retinal pigment epithelial cells through the subretinal space into the inner layers of the retina. These retinal pigment epithelium cells, which are carrying lipopigments and melanin granules, possibly with macrophages, make up the characteristic bony spicular pigmented appearance observed by fundoscopy, especially when aggregated around attenuated retinal vessels. Much autofluorescent material is found in the ganglion cell layers, in some cells in the inner nuclear layer but not in the photoreceptor layer, reflecting their severe loss. There is less autofluorescent material than normal in retinal pigment epithelial cells that remain *in situ*, again reflecting their loss (Bensaoula et al., 2000). Some photoreceptors remain in the far periphery, where they have short outer segments.

The choroid and Bruch's membrane are not much affected, nor are the cornea, conjunctiva, and ciliary body.

Whether the mechanism of neuronal death in the retina of CLN3 disease, classic juvenile patients is identical to that in the brain has not been determined. However, photoreceptor cell death by apoptosis in mouse models of retinitis pigmentosa has been well established (Portera-Cailliau et al., 1994, Gregory and Bird, 1995). Although apoptosis is a widespread phenomenon of cell disappearance occurring during embryogenesis, tumour formation, and in human neurodegenerative diseases, an apoptotic process in cerebral and retinal neurons in NCL should not be inferred without appropriate evidence.

Extracerebral storage

Many cell types throughout the body contain evidence of storage on light microscopy. The staining characteristics differ slightly from those in the brain. Storage is detected by an enhanced (often from no reaction in the normal) reaction for acid phosphatase activity (Figure 8.5), by sudanophilia and by autofluorescence. The Luxol fast blue reaction is generally absent except in the neurons of the gastrointestinal tract. The cells which consistently demonstrate these characteristics are the endothelial cells, the sweat gland epithelial cells, smooth muscle cells, and skeletal muscle cells.

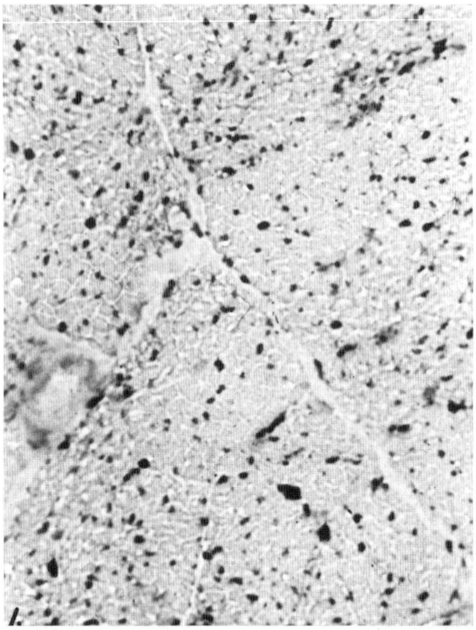

Figure 8.5 CLN3 disease, classic juvenile: pronounced punctuate histochemical activity of acid phosphatase indicates lipopigment formation in skeletal muscle fibres, ×330.

Immunohistochemically the storage bodies contain a wide range of compounds. In particular, SCMAS is found in all storage sites, although in contrast to CLN2 disease there is no immunohistochemical evidence of SCMAS in the liver, adrenal, or endocrine pancreas (Elleder et al., 1997). The exocrine pancreas has weaker staining than that observed in CLN2 disease, classic late infantile. Adipose cells and macrophages in the lamina propria of the gut, and tingible body macrophages in lymphoreticular aggregates also express SCMAS. Sphingolipid activator proteins (saposins A and D) (Tyynelä et al., 1997), certain lectins (Wisniewski and Maslinska, 1990), β-A4 amyloid, and amyloid precursor protein (Wisniewski et al., 1990a, Wisniewski et al., 1990b) have also been found.

Ultrastructurally, the lipopigments may form solid inclusions (Figures 8.6 and 8.7) or they may be found within membrane-bound vacuoles (Figure 8.8). This latter process of vacuolation appears to be unique to CLN3 disease, juvenile. This vacuolation is best known in the circulating lymphocytes (Figures 8.9–8.11),

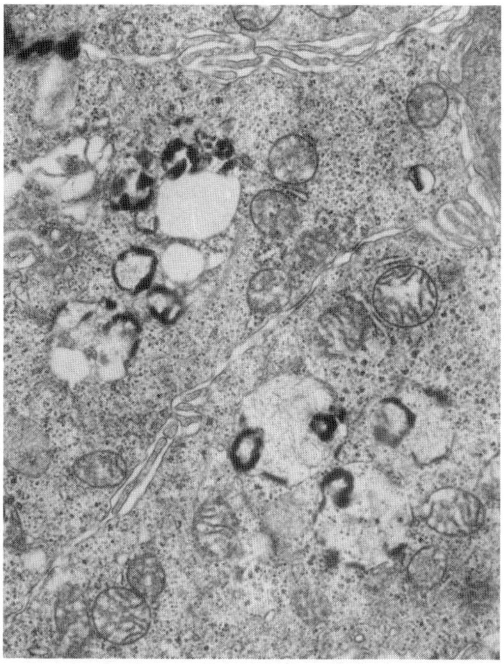

Figure 8.6 CLN3 disease, classic juvenile: solid lipopigments containing fingerprint profiles in secretory eccrine sweat gland epithelial cells, ×10,890.

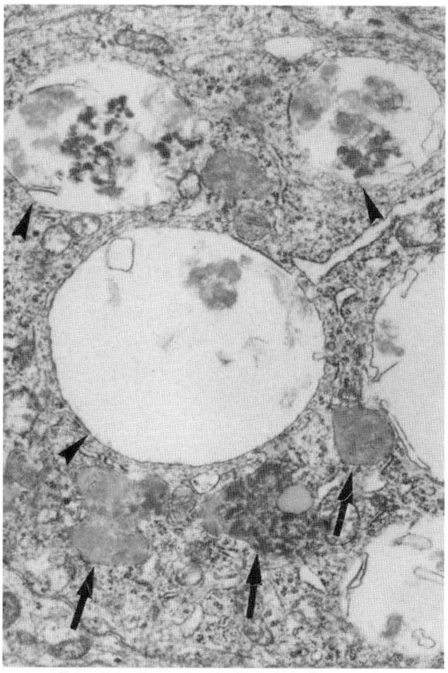

Figure 8.8 CLN3 disease, classic juvenile: a rectal neuron contains both solid lipopigments (arrows), filled with fingerprint profiles, and large membrane-bound vacuoles (arrow heads), also containing fingerprint profiles, ×12,300.

but is also often encountered in secretory eccrine sweat gland epithelial cells (Figure 8.12). It does not seem to exacerbate the disease process. However, in the inner ear spiral neurons of a case of CLN3 disease, juvenile the 'lucent type' lysosomal distension was of enormous degree, interfered with the cell vitality and caused cell death (Elleder et al., 1988). The vacuoles contain some lamellar material and some finely granular amorphous rather electron-lucent unidentified material. The degree of vacuole formation in CLN3 disease, juvenile cells might be so great that encased lamellar material may not be present in the

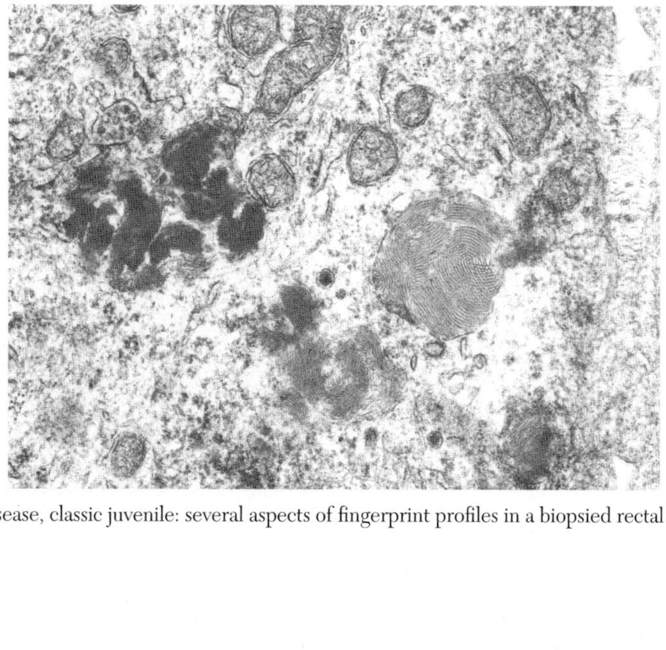

Figure 8.7 CLN3 disease, classic juvenile: several aspects of fingerprint profiles in a biopsied rectal neuron, ×50,000.

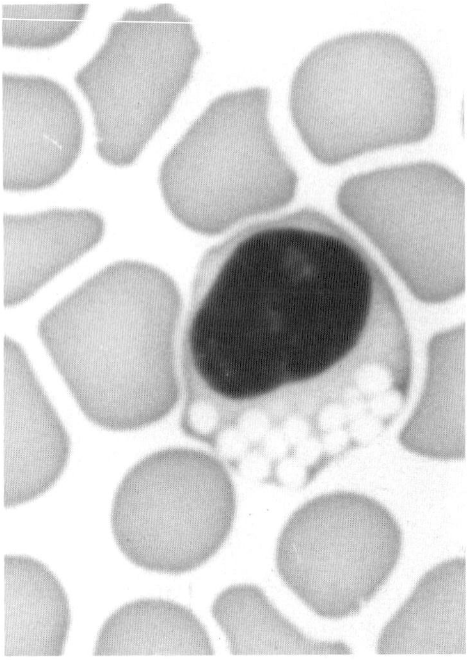

Figure 8.9 CLN3 disease, classic juvenile: distinctly vacuolated circulating lymphocyte from a routine blood smear, ×2150.

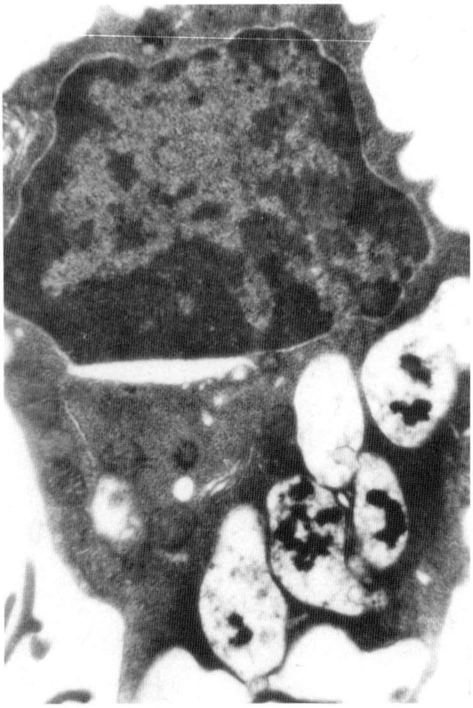

Figure 8.10 CLN3 disease, classic juvenile: a vacuolated lymphocyte contains dense inclusions, ×4800.

plane of sections. The significance of these vacuoles which are of lysosomal origin and limited by a unit membrane is as obscure as are their contents, apart from lipopigments. Fingerprint profiles may be found both within the vacuolar (Figure 8.10) and non-vacuolar lysosomes, but occasionally curvilinear or rectilinear components (Figure 8.11) are also admixed (Wisniewski and al., 1992). Neurons of the gastrointestinal tract contain pure fingerprint profiles (Figure 8.7), but in other sites mixed fingerprint/rectilinear complex/curvilinear inclusions occur. Granular components are rarely, if ever, seen in CLN3 disease, juvenile, but may be an indication of an unusual presentation of CLN1 disease. Electron-lucent droplets resembling lipid deposits may form part of the storage material in neurons but are more usually absent. In nerve cells of the PNS, lamellar inclusions with their fine structure being quite unlike that of typical CLN3 disease, juvenile have also been observed (Goebel et al., 1979). Whether these peculiar membranous inclusions actually represent storage material and whether they have a different composition is not known. In rare examples, occasional neurons of the gastrointestinal tract contain

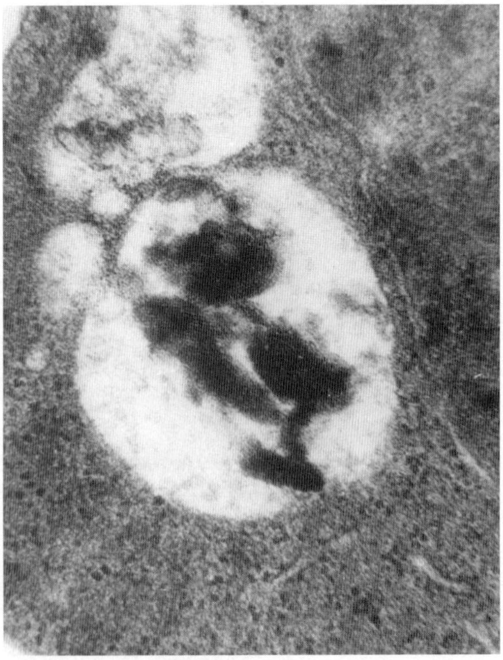

Figure 8.11 CLN3 disease, classic juvenile: at higher magnification a membrane-bound lysosomal vacuole contains fingerprint profiles, ×116,000.

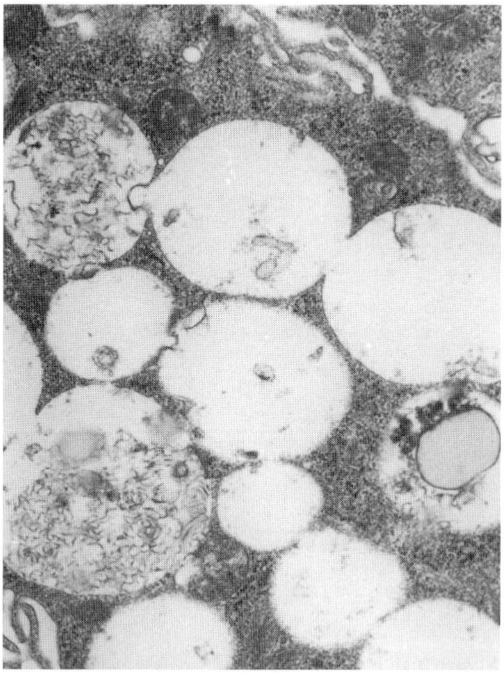

Figure 8.12 CLN3 disease, classic juvenile: membrane-bound vacuoles, empty or filled with lipopigments are present in a secretory eccrine sweat gland epithelial cell, ×13,000.

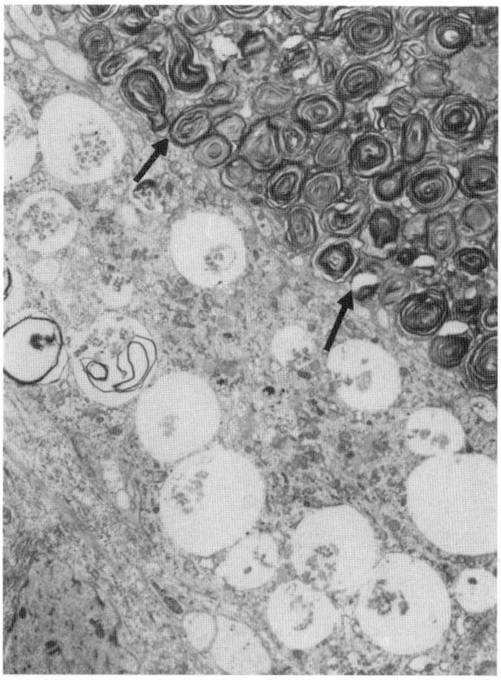

Figure 8.13 CLN3 disease, classic juvenile: an appendiceal neuron contains densely packed membranous cytoplasmic bodies (arrows), ×4300.

membranous cytoplasmic bodies (Figure 8.13) (which have the staining characteristics of ganglioside and are not autofluorescent) adjacent to neurons with pure fingerprint bodies.

No fingerprint profiles are encountered within skeletal muscle fibres in CLN3 disease, juvenile (Figure 8.14), but instead the storage material displays profiles of the rectilinear complex, which may be difficult to differentiate from curvilinear bodies (Carpenter et al., 1972, Carpenter et al., 1977). Elsewhere in the muscle sample the mixed fingerprint/rectilinear/curvilinear pattern may be found in endothelial cells.

Immunoelectron microscopy shows that SCMAS colocalizes with curvilinear/rectilinear profiles, but is not found in fingerprint profiles (Rowan and Lake, 1995). This may be due to steric factors or because no SCMAS is present in the fingerprint inclusions

While in certain instances curvilinear and fingerprint profiles may appear separately or combined within the same lysosomal residual body, the relationship between these two types of profiles has not clearly been elucidated. They may occur side by side. They may, however, also

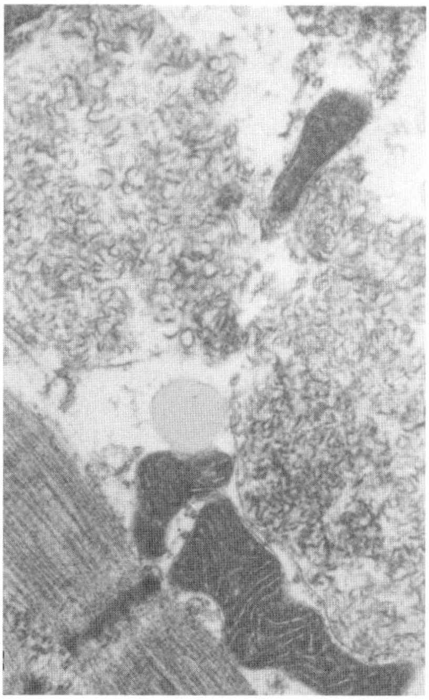

Figure 8.14 CLN3 disease, classic juvenile: curved, straight, and rectilinear profiles make up the membrane-bound lipopigment in skeletal muscle fibres, ×36,000.

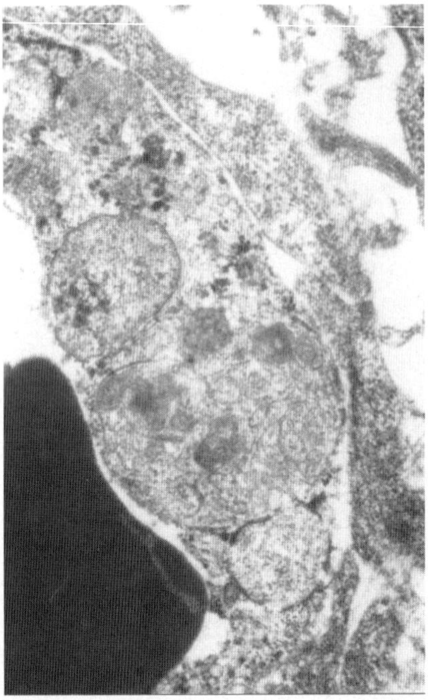

Figure 8.15 Fetal CLN3 disease: membrane-bound inclusions in an endothelial cell of a chorionic stromal vessel, ×20, 286.

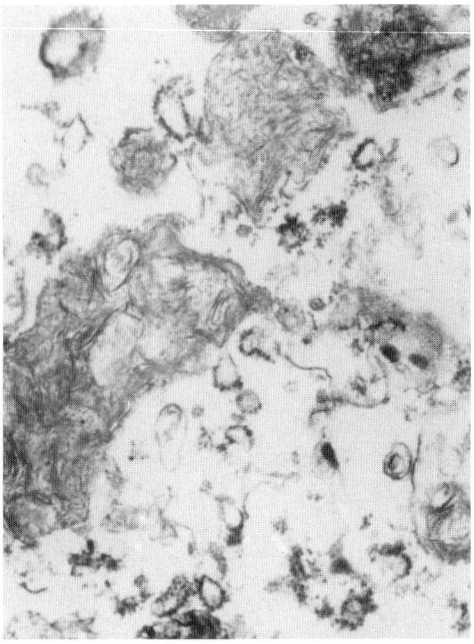

Figure 8.16 Fetal CLN3 disease: lamellar inclusion in the spinal cord of an aborted fetus, ×20, 286.

occur during developmental evolution and, if so, might possibly evolve from curvilinear profiles into fingerprint profiles. This has never been documented experimentally. However study of chorionic villi in two affected pregnancies, and of both abortuses, revealed the presence of membrane-bound inclusions in the endothelial cells (Figure 8.15) and neurons of the brain stem and spinal cord. The inclusions contained neither curvilinear nor fingerprint bodies, but membranous fragments and loose membranous whorls (Figure 8.16). Transition from curvilinear to fingerprint was not observed, and indeed no classic fingerprint inclusions were present. These two independent observations (Munroe et al., 1996, Lake et al., 1998) at least give evidence that fetal disease-specific inclusions in true CLN3 disease, juvenile seem to differ in ultrastructure from their postnatal counterparts.

DISEASE MECHANISM

Although *CLN3* was the first gene underlying a human NCL to be cloned (TIBD Consortium, 1995), the normal function of its gene product and how this is compromised by mutation has proved elusive. The lack of specific antisera that recognize the hydrophobic CLN3 protein and its low level of ubiquitous expression have made it difficult to arrive at a consensus view of its intracellular location and topography (Haskell et al., 2000, Mao et al., 2003) or to determine its normal interaction partners. As for other NCLs, analysis of the storage material has not proven useful in providing a hypothesis for the protein's function. However, studies in yeast models deficient for the CLN3 homologue Btn1p have implicated this protein in regulating the environment within the vacuole, the lysosomal equivalent in yeast (Pearce et al., 1999c, Kim et al., 2003, Gachet et al., 2005, Padilla-Lopez and Pearce, 2006). Some of these findings have been replicated in human CLN3 disease, juvenile cell lines (Ramirez-Montealegre and Pearce, 2005), although the mechanisms by which these events may lead to the neurological and neurodegenerative phenotype of CLN3 disease, juvenile remains poorly understood. Furthermore, it has been proposed that a complete lack of protein function would have even more severe cellular consequences than those characterized in classic juvenile CLN3 disease (Kitzmüller et al., 2008), although this suggestion has been questioned (Chan et al., 2008).

As might be predicted, the impact of *CLN3* mutations upon the CNS is less pronounced than in earlier onset types of NCL. As such, a greater range of regional and cell type-specific selectivity is apparent in CLN3 disease, juvenile autopsy material, with graded effects upon neuron survival according to their CNS location and cellular phenotype in the hippocampus (Tyynelä et al., 2004), and more widely in the cortex (J. Cooper et al., unpublished observations). As in several other forms of human NCL, persisting neurons are frequently encircled by GFAP positive processes (Tyynelä et al., 2004, J. Cooper et al., unpublished observations), a distinctive feature that is not evident in other storage disorders. One phenotype that is specific to both human and murine CLN3 disease, juvenile and not seen in other NCLs is the presence of an autoimmune response early in pathogenesis (Chattopadhyay et al., 2002a, Chattopadhyay et al., 2002b). It remains to be determined whether the entry and deposition of autoantibodies within the CLN3 disease, juvenile CNS is directly pathogenic (Lim et al., 2007), but immunosuppression strategies alter disease progression in these mice (Seehafer et al., 2010, see also Chapter 21). An early and low level glial response which precedes neuron loss is evident in CLN3 disease, juvenile mouse models (Pontikis et al., 2004, Pontikis et al., 2005, Weimer et al., 2009). However, this glial response appears to be atypical with incomplete morphological transformation of both astrocytes and microglia (Pontikis et al., 2004, Pontikis et al., 2005), suggesting the *Cln3* mutation may compromise the biology of these cell types (J. Cooper et al., unpublished observations). In common with several other mouse models of NCL, *Cln3* mutant mice display an early loss of thalamic relay neurons (Pontikis et al., 2005, Weimer et al., 2006), selective effects upon the survival of cortical and hippocampal interneuron populations (Mitchison et al., 1999, Pontikis et al., 2004), and characteristic cerebellar defects (Kovács et al., 2006, Weimer et al., 2009). The build up of toxic metabolites of dopamine may also contribute to the vulnerability of substantia nigra neurons and the onset of motor abnormalities in these mice (Weimer et al., 2007). There is also a mounting body of evidence for developmental delay in *Cln3*-deficient mice (Herrmann et al., 2008, Osório et al., 2009, J. Cooper et al., unpublished observations).

Currently there is debate over the mechanism of neuronal cell death in CLN3 disease, juvenile (Mitchison et al., 2004). In common with the *Cathepsin D* mutant mouse model, degenerating CNS neurons in *Cln3*-deficient mice become crowded with autophagic vacuoles and do not present any sign of apoptosis (Mitchison et al., 2004, Cao et al., 2006). Cerebellar cell cultures from *Cln3*-mutant mouse brains display basic disturbances in the autophagic pathway and its regulation (Cao et al., 2006). Evidence for altered glutamate/glutamine cycling, reduced levels of GABA, and elevated glutamate within brain of *Cln3*-mutant mice (Chattopadhyay et al., 2002a, Pears et al., 2005) suggests that excitotoxicity may play a contributory role in neuron loss in CLN3 disease, juvenile. Cultures from these mice reveal an increased vulnerability to α-amino-3-hydroxy-5-methyl-4-isoxazolepropionate (AMPA) type, but not to N-methyl-d-aspartate (NMDA) type glutamate receptor overactivation (Kovács et al., 2006), leading to the therapeutic testing in these animals of a non-competitive AMPA antagonist EGIS-8332 (Kovács and Pearce, 2008, Kovács et al., 2010). In addition to presynaptic accumulation of glutamate in *Cln3*-mutant mice (Chattopadhyay et al., 2002a), there is evidence for axonal and synaptic reorganization in murine CLN3 disease (Song et al., 2008) (Kielar and Cooper, unpublished observations). Taken together, the loss of colocalization of mutated *Cln3* with synaptic markers (Järvelä et al., 1999) and evidence for membrane trafficking defects point to abnormal intracellular trafficking as key events in CLN3 disease, juvenile pathogenesis. Indeed, this suggestion is consistent with recent evidence for interactions of CLN3 with the cytoskeleton (Uusi-Rauva et al., 2008).

CORRELATIONS

Genotype–phenotype correlation

Most CLN3 disease, juvenile patients are homozygous for the common 1kb deletion and show a classic juvenile CLN3 disease progression. However, amongst both 1kb deletion homozygotes and compound heterozygotes for the 1kb deletion and another mutation, there is inter- and intrafamilial variability in symptoms (Järvelä et al., 1997, Munroe et al., 1997). Compound heterozygotes tend to be more extremely variable. One unusual case of CLN3 disease, infantile with onset of symptoms at 5 months, has been reported (de los Reyes et al., 2004). The patient was heterozygous for the 1kb deletion but the second mutation in *CLN3* was not identified. Modifier genes and environmental factors are likely to have an influence on disease progression.

In 1kb heterozygote patients, the spectrum of disease severity is greatly influenced by the mutation on the second allele. This needs to be considered in conjunction with the proposal that the 1kb mutation does not completely abolish CLN3 function, but rather causes a mutation-specific phenotype (Kitzmüller et al., 2008; and see below). If the second mutation affects CLN3 protein structure (e.g. frameshift and nonsense mutations) and thus abolishes CLN3 function, a classic juvenile CLN3 disease course occurs, reflecting the disease phenotype arising from the presence of the 1kb deletion at the first allele. The extent to which the CLN3 protein is truncated or its function abolished on the second allele does not appear important, since classic disease presentation occurred both in a case where the second allele was the most severely truncating known (Kwon et al., 2005), and in another where only the C-terminal 15 residues of CLN3 were lost (Munroe et al., 1997). Certain missense mutations in combination with the 1kb deletion also give rise to a classic juvenile phenotype, highlighting single residues of the CLN3 protein that are probably critical for function, thus abolishing all or most function from the second allele. Examples are the missense mutations p.Val330Phe, p.Gln352His, and p.Arg334Cys, all affecting highly conserved residues (Figure 8.1). p.Gln352His also destroys a splice donor site, so a defect in splicing may be the underlying defect (Leman et al., 2005).

However, several missense mutations give rise to an atypical disease course. p.Leu101Pro, p.Leu170Pro, p.Glu295Lys, and p.Arg334His, in combination with the 1kb deletion mutation, all result in a protracted disease course (Munroe et al., 1997, Wisniewski et al., 1998a, Lauronen et al., 1999). p.Arg334His can also be associated with a classic disease course, indicating some variability (Munroe et al., 1997). In contrast, the p.Arg334Cys mutation, which affects the same residue, has so far always been associated with a CLN3 disease, classic juvenile phenotype (Munroe et al., 1997, Lauronen et al., 1999). In some cases (e.g. p.Gln295Lys), disease features other than blindness may be very mild or delayed in their onset, even to the extent that cognitive and motor functions remain unaffected for several decades (Järvelä et al., 1997, Wisniewski et al., 1998a, Åberg et al 2009). In these missense mutations CLN3 function is not completely abolished, and indeed, work in yeast suggests that the function that remains is additional to that retained by the 1kb deletion (Haines et al., 2009). Thus, more CLN3 function remains in these patients than in those homozygous for the 1kb deletion.

A small number of CLN3 disease, juvenile patients are homozygous for mutations other than the 1kb deletion. There are six characterized mutations, all frameshift or nonsense, and they should cause major disruption to the protein structure, the most severe being a homozygous approximately 6kb deletion (Taschner et al., 1995). All (if, as likely, the 5′ boundary of the 6kb deletion is downstream of exon 6) of these patients are predicted to produce a transcript that either includes CLN3 residues encoded by the first six exons or, as a result of alternative splicing, residues encoded by exons 7–15. Yeast modelling data suggests that these should exhibit a function, like the 1kb mutant protein, that affects lysosome size (Haines et al., 2009). Most of these mutations are associated with a CLN3 disease, classic juvenile course (Munroe et al., 1997). Two siblings homozygous for a C-terminal deletion (S. Mole, unpublished data) have a slightly more severe disease course than classic juvenile CLN3 disease and have enlarged lysosomes, as does one young patient who is a compound heterozygote for c.1056+3A>C and p. Asp416Gly, a mutation that does not completely abolish CLN3 function (Haines et al., 2009, S. Mole, unpublished data).

At present, mutation analysis of *CLN3* tends to be carried out in children presenting with visual failure, those who are found to have vacuolated lymphocytes, and those with a neurodegenerative disease presentation. There is a strong possibility that mutations in *CLN3* also cause more severe or milder disease. It has been postulated that other mutations in *CLN3* may not always result in the recognized hallmarks of CLN3 disease, classic juvenile including fingerprint profiles of the storage material visible using electron microscopy, vacuolated lymphocytes, and visual failure. There is also a possibility that CLN3 may itself modify disease caused by mutations in other genes, because healthy carriers of the now presumed 1kb deletion have subclinical eye changes (Gottlob et al., 1988) that must reflect cellular changes from decreased CLN3 function.

The small patient numbers and the variability in clinical phenotype that exists even amongst patients with the same mutations place limits on the *CLN3* genotype–phenotype interpretations. However, cell biology studies in mammalian cells and yeasts help in understanding the cellular mechanisms that underlie the observed CLN3 disease, juvenile genotype–phenotype correlations. Overexpressed CLN3 (or yeast Btn1) truncated protein equivalent to that caused by the 1kb deletion does not appear to traffic out of the ER (Järvelä et al., 1999, Haines et al., 2009). In contrast, the missense mutations p.Leu101Pro, p.Leu170Pro, p.Glu295Lys, p.Val330Phe, and p.Arg334His do not abolish trafficking of the mutant CLN3 protein to the endosome-lysosome system, nor, in the case of p.Glu295Lys to presynaptic vesicles in neurons (Järvelä et al., 1999, Haskell et al., 2000).

The hypothesis that the 1kb deletion does not completely abolish CLN3 function stems from work in both mammalian cells and yeast (Kitzmüller et al., 2008). Two *CLN3* RNA transcripts were present in cells from a CLN3 disease, classic juvenile patient homozygous for the 1kb deletion, both predicted to encode the first 153 amino acids of CLN3, with one also containing residues 264–438. Using RNA interference to specifically deplete these transcripts in cells from a patient resulted in a significant increase in the size of the lysosomes in these cells suggesting that one or both of these mutant CLN3 transcripts was biologically active. Supporting this conclusion, constructs expressed in mammalian cells or in *S. pombe* that mimic the common 1kb deletion mutation of CLN3 are biologically active and cause a decrease in the size of lysosomes or vacuoles, the opposite effect to that of depleting *CLN3* transcripts or deleting the *S. pombe CLN3* orthologue *btn1*. The proposal that residual CLN3 function may be associated with a classic juvenile CLN3 disease course remains to be reconciled with the prediction that aberrant mRNA transcripts produced in patients with premature termination codons are removed during RNA surveillance by nonsense mediated decay (Amrani et al., 2006).

Genotype–morphotype correlation

The storage material in cells from CLN3 disease patients has the ultrastructural appearance of fingerprint profiles, sometimes together with curvilinear and rectilinear profiles (Elleder et al., 1999). CLN3 disease, protracted juvenile does not appear to differ significantly from CLN3 disease, classic juvenile, with respect to autopsy findings of the brain (Goebel et al., 1976), and to the ultrastructure of the storage material which is of a fingerprint type in cerebral neurons (Goebel et al., 1976) (Figure 8.17) and within lymphocytic vacuoles (Wisniewski et al., 1998b). Some rare cases have an unusual ultrastructural phenotype. Two siblings heterozygous for the 1kb deletion and the p.Glu295Lys mutation had a very slow disease progression and storage with granular deposits in addition to fingerprint and curvilinear profiles in skin and rectum (Wisniewski et al., 1998a). The same atypical mixture of storage

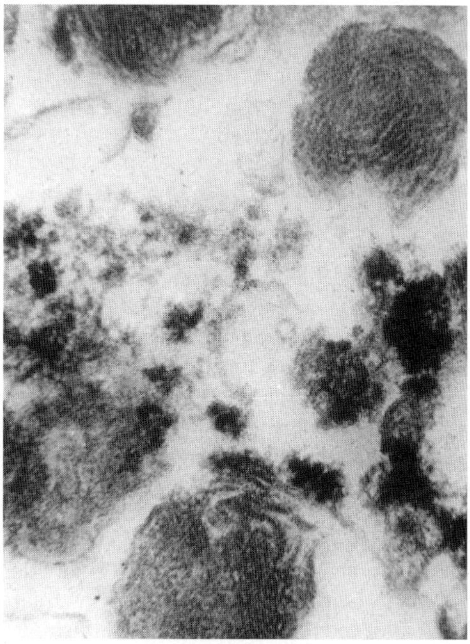

Figure 8.17 CLN3 disease, protracted juvenile: fingerprint profiles in a postmortem cerebral neuron, ×49, 500.

material was seen in a patient homozygous for the 1kb deletion, who had a variant disease course, although with the usual vacuolated lymphocytes (Åberg et al., 1998). Cells from three patients, none of whom carry the 1kb deletion, have strikingly enlarged lysosomes visible under light microscopy (S. Mole, unpublished data).

DIAGNOSIS

The clinical diagnosis of CLN3 disease, juvenile should be straightforward and simple, provided the physician considers this possibility. A history of gradual visual loss in an otherwise healthy young school-child is very suggestive of CLN3 disease, juvenile. Exclusion of refractive errors suggests retinal disease. The experienced ophthalmologist will be alerted by the fundoscopic findings alone at this stage, but electroretinography may be necessary to confirm the retinopathy and will usually show the potentials to be almost or totally extinguished.

A regular blood smear should be checked by light microscopy for the presence of several large clear vacuoles in the cytoplasm of a significant proportion (>10%) of lymphocytes (Figure 8.9). Approximately 50% of samples showing vacuolated lymphocytes were subsequently found to be due to CLN3 disease in a national referral laboratory (Anderson et al., 2005). A separate blood sample is used for the preparation of lymphocytes for electron microscopy in doubtful cases, and a sample is used for the preparation of DNA.

The combination of typical ophthalmological findings and vacuolated lymphocytes in the peripheral blood is strongly supportive of the diagnosis. A molecular genetic analysis should be requested and will show the typical 1kb deletion in *CLN3* in the majority of cases (see 'Molecular genetics' section). When the deletion is not found or is present only in one allele, sequencing of the whole gene is necessary. If this is not easily available, electron microscopy of white blood cells or other tissues is helpful. In diagnostically difficult cases a skin biopsy is taken. The tissue is divided, one part being used for electron microscopy and the other one for establishing a fibroblast culture. Presymptomatic diagnosis can be made on the basis of the ultrastructural appearances of a white blood cell pellet (buffy coat preparation).

Differential diagnosis

The history of a patient with classic juvenile CLN3 disease is so unique that few other conditions have to be considered in the differential. Late-manifesting forms of CLN1 disease (palmitoyl protein thiosterase 1 deficiency), CLN2 disease (tripeptidyl peptidase 1 deficiency), and CLN10 disease (cathepsin D deficiency) can present in a similar way and are diagnosed by testing for the respective enzyme deficiencies. In any young patient diagnosed as having 'retinitis pigmentosa', investigation should not stop at the ophthalmological level, and an extra-ocular condition should be ruled out. In the presence of an isolated retinopathy in a young child, gyrate atrophy of the retina with hyperornithinaemia should be excluded by the measurement of urine and plasma amino acids, and Refsum disease excluded by measuring phytanic acid in blood. If learning difficulties or other neurological symptoms are present, peroxisomal, mitochondrial, and other lysosomal disorders together with retinopathy-associated genetic syndromes must be considered. Additional diagnostic considerations can be found in Chapter 3.

Prenatal and carrier diagnostics

In most families it will be now possible to test for the presence of the 1kb deletion or other defined mutation in an at-risk pregnancy or suspected carrier. Otherwise, care should be taken since fetal disease-specific inclusions in CLN3 disease, classic juvenile seem to differ in ultrastructure from their postnatal counterparts (see 'Extracerebral storage' section).

CLINICAL MANAGEMENT

At present there is no specific disease-modifying treatment for CLN3 disease, juvenile. Many therapies have been tried on theoretical grounds. However, to date there is no evidence of long-term benefit for any. Clinical management, therefore, must be palliative.

Palliative care not only utilizes medical and physical approaches, but integrates the psychological and spiritual aspects of patient care also. The World Health Organization has developed a definition of palliative care for children who are suffering of a life-limiting illness in which a holistic approach of patient care is described (see Chapter 5). These principles apply fully to the clinical management of CLN3 disease, juvenile. In this section therefore, attention will be paid not only to medical treatment, but also to psychological aspects, daily activities, and family support.

Diagnosis

The time of uncertainty before a definite diagnosis can be given is a nerve-racking period for parents and family. Once the diagnosis has been made, the parents and carers should be appropriately informed about the nature of the disease. It is important for parents to gain an understanding of the nature of the condition and the shortened life expectancy. Written information and contact details of family support groups should be provided. Family expectations for the future will be adjusted. Epilepsy should be discussed early so that family and carers are prepared in advance of the first seizure. The educational goals at home and at school can be adjusted as the disease progresses with guidance from the multidisciplinary team. If there are other children in the family, the disease will have a major impact on their lives too. Younger siblings may also develop the disease and parents may need some guidance regarding testing and informing their other children about the condition.

Much can be done using traditional and complementary treatment strategies to manage symptoms and maintain and promote skills in order to optimize quality of life. Doctors have an important role in this process, but other professionals (for example, school staff, community nurses, and social workers) who are familiar with CLN3 disease, juvenile, are perhaps of greater importance in the long term.

Education

Children with CLN3 disease, juvenile and other neurodegenerative diseases benefit from a specialized educational programme. A different approach is needed for those with progressive disease compared with those children with congenital intellectual disabilities. Teachers must be well informed about the special needs and the cognitive and psychological problems of this group. Children and youngsters usually enjoy school. It enhances their self-esteem. There is considerable and well-documented experience in the field of education in CLN3 disease, juvenile (Proceedings of 'First International Conference on Batten Disease and Education' held in Örebro, Sweden, 2006).

Seizures

The predominant seizure type is generalized tonic–clonic, but any type of seizure may occur, from subtle partial to myoclonic status. Epilepsy in CLN3 disease, juvenile is generally regarded as a progressive myoclonic epilepsy syndrome, even if there is no obvious myoclonic component. Treatment depends on the severity of the epilepsy. In the beginning seizures may be infrequent and not very intrusive. Anti-epileptic drugs may not be necessary initially. When the seizure frequency increases, sodium valproate and lamotrigine, individually or in combination, are currently the drugs of choice. Practice varies throughout Europe and North America regarding which drug is used at first. More recently topiramate and levetiracetam have been shown to be effective. Levetiracetam also appears to improve the parkinsonian tremor seen in some young people. The use of these newer agents and their possible side effects should be evaluated further. Benzodiazepines like clobazam and clonazepam are useful in combination therapy, but they may cause problems because of bronchial hypersecretion (especially clonazepam). It is generally agreed that carbamazepine, gabapentin, and phenytoin may worsen myoclonic seizures in CLN3 disease, juvenile.

Monotherapy may be sufficient for some years, but as the disease progresses, epilepsy usually becomes difficult to control. A balance between reasonable seizure control and medication side effects must be struck. The ultimate goal must always be to improve quality of life. Clusters of seizures can be managed with rectal or oro-buccal benzodiazepines. Rectal paraldehyde is also usually effective. A short course of oral clobazam or diazepam may be used to terminate a period of frequent seizures.

Emotional and mental health

Emotional, behavioural, and psychotic problems are common at all stages of CLN3 disease, juvenile. In childhood, emotional and behavioural problems may be evident early in the disease course, and later on psychotic symptoms may arise. According to a recent study, 74% of young persons (mean age 15.2 years) with CLN3 disease, juvenile show symptoms which are borderline or clinically significant. Symptoms include restlessness, anxiety, panic attacks, aggressiveness, hallucinations, delusions, and, for a minority (10%), symptoms of depression.

A familiar environment with a structured, meaningful daily programme and a quiet, peaceful, undemanding approach have been found to be most helpful for young people with CLN3 disease, juvenile. They are able to feel safe, becoming more self-confident, and their independence skills can be maintained as long as possible. Promoting self-esteem is very important. Activities must be adapted to individual abilities according to the stage of the disease and likes and dislikes. The abilities and mood may show day-to-day variation and this may demand much flexibility and creativity of parents and caretakers. If, despite such measures, anxiety has a negative effect on daily functioning, benzodiazepines such as oxazepam, may be effective.

Extreme restlessness and/or aggressive behaviour, delusions and hallucinations may be managed using newer atypical (less dopamine receptor blockade than the classical antipsychotics) antipsychotic drugs such as risperidone or olanzapine, or older drugs such as sulpiride or pipamperone. Chlorpromazine is also very effected and can be used in small doses or as required. Risperidone is probably most widely used, but positive experience with the other drugs also exists. These drugs must be used with caution, but possible side effects should not deter from using them if necessary. Hallucinations may be extremely frightening and interfere with all daily activities. If depression seems to be the underlying problem, selective serotonin reuptake inhibitors (SSRIs) such as citalopram have been found to be beneficial in young people with CLN3 disease, juvenile.

Often there is an association in time between seizures, hallucinations, sleep disturbance, and feeding problems. Optimizing anti-epileptic medication regimens, incidental treatment with antipsychotics, or temporarily increasing the dose of antipsychotics, giving attention to other potential medical problems (for example, constipation and infection) may all contribute to improvement of the situation.

Myoclonic jerks, which may be severe and particularly disturbing, are difficult to treat. The muscle relaxant drugs baclofen and tizanidine may be effective.

Sleep disturbance

Sleep disturbance is common and is likely to worsen with age and disease progression. In general, a quiet environment and set routines before going to bed are helpful. Drugs like benzodiazepines or chloral hydrate are often (preferably for short duration only) necessary. When paroxysmal epileptic activity disturbs sleep, clonazepam may be effective. The use of melatonin in CLN3 disease, juvenile was not helpful in most of the patients in one Finnish study (Hätönen et al., 1999).

Motor problems

Motor problems become troublesome in the second decade and include: losing balance easily, frequent falls, slightly stooped posture, slow shuffling gait, difficulties in initiating movements, in getting up, problems with stairs and steps, and increasing difficulties with all daily self-care activities. The motor problems are of cerebellar and extrapyramidal origin. Activities of all kinds are important to maintain and promote motor skills: walking, swimming, tandem cycling, horseback riding, etc. These activities should be encouraged from childhood, as they seem to slow the progression of motor disabilities and enhance physical well-being (and self-esteem). Later on the motor activities can be supported by physical therapies.

In an open study in Finland there was a favourable response to levodopa during the first year of treatment, although there was a great variation in response. The experience in practice is variable. Further evaluation is necessary, especially concerning the long-term effects.

In the later stages of the disease, mobility aids, adapted seating and standing frames, wheelchairs, and housing adaptations including wheelchair access and ramps, are necessary to maintain mobility as long as possible.

Communication

Communication is compromised not only by difficulties with articulation, with initiating a phrase or sentence, but also by word finding difficulties and short-term memory problems, etc. For parents, the loss of communication is one of the saddest features of this disease. An experienced speech and language therapist can be very helpful early on, in promoting speech, and may be able to offer alternative ways of communication later. Favourite things and subjects, family traditions, important life events, etc. can be collected and recorded in a paper or electronic life story book. In the later stages, this life-story work will prove invaluable in maintaining meaningful relationships with family, carers, and professionals.

Nutrition

In childhood and adolescence, attention must be paid to a regular and well-balanced diet with sufficient fibre content to avoid constipation. In young adults, chewing and swallowing may become difficult. Attention to seating and posture, food volumes and texture, and especially the rate of food presentation during meals are essential. The advice of a speech and language therapist about these aspects together with the use of adapted cutlery, etc, is mandatory in optimizing feeding strategies. Feeding by a gastrostomy tube may be considered because of increased risk of choking, aspiration, and malnutrition. Adequate hydration and nutrition by tube feeding improve general well-being and ensure reliable drug administration. The placement of a gastrostomy tube should be carefully discussed with the parents, and with the young person, if still able to participate in decision-making.

Family care and support

CLN3 disease, juvenile is characterized by the fact that parents are confronted with the loss of their child not once, but again and again over the years. Parents and siblings have needs that also change over time: coming to terms with the diagnosis, coping with deterioration over the years, understanding the illness, and getting access to appropriate medical, educational, and social help. As CLN3 disease, juvenile is rare, it is vital for parents to be referred to a specialist or a centre with experience of the condition. A key worker, who coordinates care and liaises with all professionals involved, is essential, as usually many professionals are involved. In many countries parent support organizations have been set up (see Chapter 24 for details) for peer support, practical advice, and help. Parents should be given the details of such organizations. For many families they have been of great value.

Bereavement counselling is needed at the time of the diagnosis, but also during the course of the disease. Psychologists, pastors, close friends, and other family members may give vital support in this respect, and may themselves need information and support from professionals and voluntary agencies.

EXPERIMENTAL THERAPY

There is no curative therapy yet available for CLN3 disease, juvenile. However, current strategies are examining immunomodulation, blocking classes of glutamate receptors and targeted eye therapy (Cooper, 2008).

If most juvenile CLN3 disease patients retain partial CLN3 function, then the mutant protein produced by the 1kb deleted allele is capable of staving off early onset of disease. Thus, therapeutic approaches that either enhance this function or mimic the effect of this function in neurons may considerably extend and increase the quality of life of patients. Manipulation of an intrinsic intracellular activity appears to offset the loss of *Cln3* in a mouse, and some CLN3 disease patients who are homozygous for the 1kb deletion have a markedly protracted disease course presumably due to other genetic factors (A. Schulz, unpublished data). Identification of these additional factors may provide tools that can be similarly manipulated in patients to provide protection against the loss of CLN3 function.

REFERENCES

Åberg L, Jarvela I, Rapola J, Autti T, Kirveskari E, Lappi M, Sipila L, & Santavuori P (1998) Atypical juvenile neuronal ceroid lipofuscinosis with granular osmiophilic deposit-like inclusions in the autonomic nerve cells of the gut wall. *Acta Neuropathol*, 95, 306–312.

Åberg L, Liewendahl K, Nikkinen P, Autti T, Rinne JO, & Santavuori P (2000a) Decreased striatal dopamine transporter density in JNCL patients with parkinsonian symptoms. *Neurology*, 54, 1069–1074.

Åberg LE, Bäckman M, Kirveskari E, & Santavuori P (2000b) Epilepsy and antiepileptic drug therapy in juvenile neuronal ceroid lipofuscinosis. *Epilepsia*, 41, 1296–1302.

Åberg LE, Tiitinen A, Autti TH, Kivisaari L, & Santavouri P (2002) Hyperandrogenism in girls with juvenile neuronal ceroid lipofuscinosis. *Eur J Paediatr Neurol*, 6, 199–205.

Adams H, de Blieck EA, Mink JW, Marshall FJ, Kwon J, Dure L, Rothberg PG, Ramirez-Montealegre D, & Pearce DA (2006) Standardized assessment of behavior and adaptive living skills in juvenile neuronal ceroid lipofuscinosis. *Dev Med Child Neurol*, 48, 259–264.

Amrani N, Sachs MS, & Jacobson A (2006) Early nonsense: mRNA decay solves a translational problem. *Nat Rev Mol Cell Biol*, 7, 415–425.

Anderson G, Smith VV, Malone M, & Sebire NJ (2005) Blood film examination for vacuolated lymphocytes in the diagnosis of metabolic disorders; retrospective experience of more than 2,500 cases from a single centre. *J Clin Pathol*, 58, 1305–1310.

Autti T, Raininko R, Santavuori P, Vanhanen SL, Poutanen VP, & Haltia M (1997) MRI of neuronal ceroid lipofuscinosis. II. Postmortem MRI and histopathological study of the brain in 16 cases of neuronal ceroid lipofuscinosis of juvenile or late infantile type. *Neuroradiology*, 39, 371–377.

Autti T, Raininko R, Vanhanen SL, & Santavuori P (1996) MRI of neuronal ceroid lipofuscinosis. I. Cranial MRI of 30 patients with juvenile neuronal ceroid lipofuscinosis. *Neuroradiology*, 38, 476–482.

Bäckman ML, Santavuori PR, Åberg LE, & Aronen ET (2005) Psychiatric symptoms of children and adolescents with juvenile neuronal ceroid lipofuscinosis. *J Intellect Disabil Res*, 49, 25–32.

Baldwin SA, Beal PR, Yao SY, King AE, Cass CE, & Young JD (2004) The equilibrative nucleoside transporter family, SLC29. *Pflugers Arch*, 447, 735–743.

Bensaoula T, Shibuya H, Katz ML, Smith JE, Johnson GS, John SK, & Milam AH (2000) Histopathologic and immunocytochemical analysis of the retina and ocular tissues in Batten disease. *Ophthalmology*, 107, 1746–1753.

Boustany RM (1992) Neurology of the neuronal ceroid-lipofuscinoses: late infantile and juvenile types. *Am J Med Genet*, 42, 533–535.

Braak H & Braak E (1993) Pathoarchitectonic pattern of iso- and allocortical lesions in juvenile and adult neuronal ceroid-lipofuscinosis. *J Inherit Metab Dis*, 16, 259–262.

Braak H & Goebel HH (1978) Loss of pigment-laden stellate cells: a severe alteration of the isocortex in juvenile neuronal ceroid-lipofuscinosis. *Acta Neuropathol*, 42, 53–57.

Braak H & Goebel HH (1979) Pigmentoarchitectonic pathology of the isocortex in juvenile neuronal ceroid-lipofuscinosis: axonal enlargements in layer IIIab and cell loss in layer V. *Acta Neuropathol*, 46, 79–83.

Brockmann K, Pouwels PJ, Christen HJ, Frahm J, & Hanefeld F (1996) Localized proton magnetic resonance spectroscopy of cerebral metabolic disturbances in children with neuronal ceroid lipofuscinosis. *Neuropediatrics*, 27, 242–248.

Brooks AI, Chattopadhyay S, Mitchison HM, Nussbaum RL, & Pearce DA (2003) Functional categorization of gene expression changes in the cerebellum of a Cln3-knockout mouse model for Batten disease. *Mol Genet Metab*, 78, 17–30.

Brück W & Goebel HH (1998) Microglia activation in neuronal ceroid-lipofuscinosis. *Clin Neuropathol*, 5, 276 (poster P29).

Bruun I, Reske-Nielsen E, & Oster S (1991) Juvenile ceroid-lipofuscinosis and calcifications of the CNS. *Acta Neurol Scand*, 83, 1–8.

Cao Y, Espinola JA, Fossale E, Massey AC, Cuervo AM, MacDonald ME, & Cotman SL (2006) Autophagy is disrupted in a knock-in mouse model of juvenile neuronal ceroid lipofuscinosis. *J Biol Chem*, 281, 20483–20493.

Cardona F & Rosati E (1995) Neuronal ceroid-lipofuscinoses in Italy: an epidemiological study. *Am J Med Genet*, 57, 142–143.

Carpenter S, Karpati G, & Andermann F (1972) Specific involvement of muscle, nerve, and skin in late infantile and juvenile amaurotic idiocy. *Neurology*, 22, 170–186.

Carpenter S, Karpati G, Andermann F, Jacob JC, & Andermann E (1977) The ultrastructural characteristics of the abnormal cytosomes in Batten-Kufs' disease. *Brain*, 100, 137–156.

Chan CH, Mitchison HM, & Pearce DA (2008) Transcript and in silico analysis of CLN3 in juvenile neuronal ceroid lipofuscinosis and associated mouse models. *Hum Mol Genet*, 17, 3332–3339.

Chan CH, Ramirez-Montealegre D, & Pearce DA (2009) Altered arginine metabolism in the central nervous system (CNS) of the $Cln3^{-/-}$ mouse model of juvenile Batten disease. *Neuropathol Appl Neurobiol*, 35, 189–207.

Chang JW, Choi H, Kim HJ, Jo DG, Jeon YJ, Noh JY, Park WJ, & Jung YK (2007) Neuronal vulnerability of CLN3 deletion to calcium-induced cytotoxicity is mediated by calsenilin. *Hum Mol Genet*, 16, 317–326.

Chattopadhyay S, Ito M, Cooper JD, Brooks AI, Curran TM, Powers JM, & Pearce DA (2002a) An autoantibody inhibitory to glutamic acid decarboxylase in the neurodegenerative disorder Batten disease. *Hum Mol Genet*, 11, 1421–1431.

Chattopadhyay S, Kriscenski-Perry E, Wenger DA, & Pearce DA (2002b) An autoantibody to GAD65 in sera of patients with juvenile neuronal ceroid lipofuscinoses. *Neurology*, 59, 1816–1817.

Chattopadhyay S & Pearce DA (2000) Neural and extraneural expression of the neuronal ceroid lipofuscinoses genes CLN1, CLN2, and CLN3: functional implications for CLN3. *Mol Genet Metab*, 71, 207–211.

Chattopadhyay S & Pearce DA (2002) Interaction with Btn2p is required for localization of Rsglp: Btn2p-mediated changes in arginine uptake in Saccharomyces cerevisiae. *Eukaryot Cell*, 1, 606–612.

Claussen M, Heim P, Knispel J, Goebel HH, & Kohlschutter A (1992) Incidence of neuronal ceroid-lipofuscinoses in West Germany: variation of a method for studying autosomal recessive disorders. *Am J Med Genet*, 42, 536–538.

Codlin S, Haines RL, Burden JJ, & Mole SE (2008a) Btn1 affects cytokinesis and cell-wall deposition by independent mechanisms, one of which is linked to dysregulation of vacuole pH. *J Cell Sci*, 121, 2860–2870.

Codlin S, Haines RL, & Mole SE (2008b) btn1 affects endocytosis, polarization of sterol-rich membrane domains and polarized growth in Schizosaccharomyces pombe. *Traffic*, 9, 936–950.

Codlin S & Mole SE (2009) S. pombe btn1, the orthologue of the Batten disease gene CLN3, is required for vacuole protein sorting of Cpy1p and Golgi exit of Vps10p. *J Cell Sci*, 122, 1163–1173.

Cooper JD (2008) Moving towards therapies for juvenile Batten disease? *Exp Neurol*, 211, 329–331.

Cooper JD, Russell C, & Mitchison HM (2006) Progress towards understanding disease mechanisms in small vertebrate models of neuronal ceroid lipofuscinosis. *Biochim Biophys Acta*, 1762, 873–889.

Croopnick JB, Choi HC, & Mueller DM (1998) The subcellular location of the yeast Saccharomyces cerevisiae homologue of the protein defective in the juvenile form of Batten disease. *Biochem Biophys Res Commun*, 250, 335–341.

de los Reyes E, Dyken PR, Phillips P, Brodsky M, Bates S, Glasier C, & Mrak RE (2004) Profound infantile neuroretinal dysfunction in a heterozygote for the CLN3 genetic defect. *J Child Neurol*, 19, 42–46.

Eiberg H, Gardiner RM, & Mohr J (1989) Batten disease (Spielmeyer-Sjogren disease) and haptoglobins (HP): indication of linkage and assignment to chr. 16. *Clin Genet*, 36, 217–218.

Eksandh LB, Ponjavic VB, Munroe PB, Eiberg HE, Uvebrant PE, Ehinger BE, Mole SE, & Andreasson S (2000) Full-field ERG in patients with Batten/Spielmeyer-Vogt disease caused by mutations in the CLN3 gene. *Ophthalmic Genet*, 21, 69–77.

Elleder M, Goebel HH, & Koppang N (1989) Lectin histochemical study of lipopigments: results with concanavalin A. *Adv Exp Med Biol*, 266, 243–258.

Elleder M, Lake BD, Gobel HH, Rapola J, Haltia M, & Carpenter S (1999) Definitions of the ultrastructural patterns found in NCL. In Goebel HH, Mole SE, & Lake BD (Eds.) *The Neuronal Ceroid Lipofuscinoses (Batten Disease)*, pp. 5–15. Amsterdam, IOS Press.

Elleder M, Sokolova J, & Hrebicek M (1997) Follow-up study of subunit c of mitochondrial ATP synthase (SCMAS) in Batten disease and in unrelated lysosomal disorders. *Acta Neuropathol*, 93, 379–390.

Elleder M, Voldrich L, Ulehlova L, Dimitt S, & Armstrong D (1988) Light and electron microscopic appearance of the inner ear in juvenile ceroid lipofuscinosis (CL). *Pathol Res Pract*, 183, 301–307.

Elshatory Y, Brooks AI, Chattopadhyay S, Curran TM, Gupta P, Ramalingam V, Hofmann SL, & Pearce DA (2003) Early changes in gene expression in two models of Batten disease. *FEBS Lett*, 538, 207–212.

Ezaki J, Takeda-Ezaki M, Koike M, Ohsawa Y, Taka H, Mineki R, Murayama K, Uchiyama Y, Ueno T, & Kominami E (2003) Characterization of Cln3p, the gene product responsible for juvenile neuronal ceroid lipofuscinosis, as a lysosomal integral membrane glycoprotein. *J Neurochem*, 87, 1296–1308.

Fossale E, Wolf P, Espinola JA, Lubicz-Nawrocka T, Teed AM, Gao H, Rigamonti D, Cattaneo E, MacDonald ME, & Cotman SL (2004) Membrane trafficking and mitochondrial abnormalities precede subunit c deposition in a cerebellar cell model of juvenile neuronal ceroid lipofuscinosis. *BMC Neurosci*, 5, 57.

Gachet Y, Codlin S, Hyams JS, & Mole SE (2005) btn1, the Schizosaccharomyces pombe homologue of the human Batten disease gene CLN3, regulates vacuole homeostasis. *J Cell Sci*, 118, 5525–5536.

Goebel HH, Pilz H, & Gullotta F (1976) The protracted form of juvenile neuronal ceroid-lipofuscinosis. *Acta Neuropathol*, 36, 393–396.

Goebel HH, Zeman W, Patel VK, Pullarkat RK, & Lenard HG (1979) On the ultrastructural diversity and essence of residual bodies in neuronal ceroid-lipofuscinosis. *Mech Ageing Dev*, 10, 53–70.

Golabek AA, Kaczmarski W, Kida E, Kaczmarski A, Michalewski MP, & Wisniewski KE (1999) Expression studies of CLN3 protein (battenin) in fusion with the green fluorescent protein in mammalian cells in vitro. *Mol Genet Metab*, 66, 277–282.

Gottlob I, Leipert KP, Kohlschutter A, & Goebel HH (1988) Electrophysiological findings of neuronal ceroid lipofuscinosis in heterozygotes. *Graefes Arch Clin Exp Ophthalmol*, 226, 516–521.

Gregory CY & Bird AC (1995) Cell loss in retinal dystrophies by apoptosis—death by informed consent! *Br J Ophthalmol*, 79, 186–190.

Haines RL, Codlin S, & Mole SE (2009) The fission yeast model for the lysosomal storage disorder Batten disease predicts disease severity caused by mutations in CLN3. *Dis Model Mech*, 2, 84–92.

Hainsworth DP, Liu GT, Hamm CW, & Katz ML (2009) Funduscopic and angiographic appearance in the neuronal ceroid lipofuscinoses. *Retina*, 29, 657–668.

Hall N, Lake B, Palmer D, Jolly R, & Patrick A (1990) Glycoconjugates in storage cytosomes from ceroid-lipofuscinosis (Batten's disease) and in lipofuscin from old age brain. In Porta AE (Ed.) *Lipofuscin and Ceroid Pigments*, pp. 225–241. New York, Plenum Press.

Haskell RE, Carr CJ, Pearce DA, Bennett MJ, & Davidson BL (2000) Batten disease: evaluation of CLN3 mutations on protein localization and function. *Hum Mol Genet*, 9, 735–744.

Hätönen T, Kirveskari E, Heiskala H, Sainio K, Laakso ML, & Santavuori P (1999) Melatonin ineffective in neuronal ceroid lipofuscinosis patients with fragmented or normal motor activity rhythms recorded by wrist actigraphy. *Mol Genet Metab*, 66, 401–406.

Heikkilä E, Hatonen TH, Telakivi T, Laakso ML, Heiskala H, Salmi T, Alila A, & Santavuori P (1995) Circadian rhythm studies in neuronal ceroid-lipofuscinosis (NCL). *Am J Med Genet*, 57, 229–234.

Herrmann P, Druckrey-Fiskaaen C, Kouznetsova E, Heinitz K, Bigl M, Cotman SL, & Schliebs R (2008) Developmental impairments of select neurotransmitter systems in brains of Cln3(Deltaex7/8) knock-in mice, an animal model of juvenile neuronal ceroid lipofuscinosis. *J Neurosci Res*, 86, 1857–1870.

Hobert JA & Dawson G (2007) A novel role of the Batten disease gene CLN3: association with BMP synthesis. *Biochem Biophys Res Commun*, 358, 111–116.

Hofman I (1990) *The Batten-Spielmeyer-Vogt Disease*. Doorn, Bartiméus Foundation.

Holopainen JM, Saarikoski J, Kinnunen PK, & Jarvela I (2001) Elevated lysosomal pH in neuronal ceroid lipofuscinoses (NCLs). *Eur J Biochem*, 268, 5851–5856.

Janes RW, Munroe PB, Mitchison HM, Gardiner RM, Mole SE, & Wallace BA (1996) A model for Batten disease protein CLN3: functional implications from homology and mutations. *FEBS Lett*, 399, 75–77.

Järvelä I, Autti T, Lamminranta S, Åberg L, Raininko R, & Santavuori P (1997) Clinical and magnetic resonance imaging findings in Batten disease: analysis of the major mutation (1.02-kb deletion). *Ann Neurol*, 42, 799–802.

Järvelä I, Lehtovirta M, Tikkanen R, Kyttala A, & Jalanko A (1999) Defective intracellular transport of CLN3 is the molecular basis of Batten disease (JNCL). *Hum Mol Genet*, 8, 1091–1098.

Järvelä I, Sainio M, Rantamaki T, Olkkonen VM, Carpen O, Peltonen L, & Jalanko A (1998) Biosynthesis and intracellular targeting of the CLN3 protein defective in Batten disease. *Hum Mol Genet*, 7, 85–90.

Järvelä IE, Mitchison HM, O'Rawe AM, Munroe PB, Taschner PE, de Vos N, Lerner TJ, D'Arigo KL, Callen DF, Thompson AD, Knight M, Marrone BL, Mund MO, Meincke L, Breuning MH, Gardiner RM, Doggett NA, Mole SE (1995) YAC and cosmid contigs spanning the Batten disease (CLN3) region at 16p12.1-p11.2. *Genomics*, 29, 478–489.

Kaczmarski W, Wisniewski KE, Golabek A, Kaczmarski A, Kida E, & Michalewski M (1999) Studies of membrane association of CLN3 protein. *Mol Genet Metab*, 66, 261–264.

Kama R, Robinson M, & Gerst JE (2007) Btn2, a Hook1 ortholog and potential Batten disease-related protein, mediates late endosome-Golgi protein sorting in yeast. *Mol Cell Biol*, 27, 605–621.

Kida E, Kaczmarski W, Golabek AA, Kaczmarski A, Michalewski M, & Wisniewski KE (1999) Analysis of intracellular distribution and trafficking of the CLN3 protein in fusion with the green fluorescent protein in vitro. *Mol Genet Metab*, 66, 265–271.

Kim Y, Ramirez-Montealegre D, & Pearce DA (2003) A role in vacuolar arginine transport for yeast Btn1p and for human CLN3, the protein defective in Batten disease. *Proc Natl Acad Sci U S A*, 100, 15458–15462.

Kirveskari E, Partinen M, Salmi T, Sainio K, Telakivi T, Hamalainen M, Larsen A, & Santavuori P (2000) Sleep alterations in juvenile neuronal ceroid-lipofuscinosis. *Pediatr Neurol*, 22, 347–354.

Kitzmüller C, Haines RL, Codlin S, Cutler DF, & Mole SE (2008) A function retained by the common mutant CLN3 protein is responsible for the late onset of juvenile neuronal ceroid lipofuscinosis. *Hum Mol Genet*, 17, 303–312.

Kovács AD & Pearce DA (2008) Attenuation of AMPA receptor activity improves motor skills in a mouse model of juvenile Batten disease. *Exp Neurol*, 209, 288–291.

Kovács AD, Weimer JM, & Pearce DA (2006) Selectively increased sensitivity of cerebellar granule cells to AMPA receptor-mediated excitotoxicity in a mouse model of Batten disease. *Neurobiol Dis*, 22, 575–585.

Kremmidiotis G, Lensink IL, Bilton RL, Woollatt E, Chataway TK, Sutherland GR, & Callen DF (1999) The Batten disease gene product (CLN3p) is a Golgi integral membrane protein. *Hum Mol Genet*, 8, 523–531.

Kwon JM, Rothberg PG, Leman AR, Weimer JM, Mink JW, & Pearce DA (2005) Novel CLN3 mutation predicted to cause complete loss of protein function does not modify the classical JNCL phenotype. *Neurosci Lett*, 387, 111–114.

Kyttälä A, Ihrke G, Vesa J, Schell MJ, & Luzio JP (2004) Two motifs target Batten disease protein CLN3 to lysosomes in transfected nonneuronal and neuronal cells. *Mol Biol Cell*, 15, 1313–1323.

Kyttälä A, Yliannala K, Schu P, Jalanko A, & Luzio JP (2005) AP-1 and AP-3 facilitate lysosomal targeting of Batten disease protein CLN3 via its dileucine motif. *J Biol Chem*, 280, 10277–10283.

Lake BD, Young EP, & Winchester BG (1998) Prenatal diagnosis of lysosomal storage diseases. *Brain Pathol*, 8, 133–149.

Lamminranta S, Åberg LE, Autti T, Moren R, Laine T, Kaukoranta J, & Santavuori P (2001) Neuropsychological test battery in the follow-up of patients with juvenile neuronal ceroid lipofuscinosis. *J Intellect Disabil Res*, 45, 8–17.

Larsen A, Sainio K, Åberg L, & Santavuori P (2001) Electroencephalography in juvenile neuronal ceroid lipofuscinosis: visual and quantitative analysis. *Eur J Paediatr Neurol*, 5 Suppl A, 179–183.

Lauronen L, Heikkila E, Autti T, Sainio K, Huttunen J, Aronen HJ, Korvenoja A, Ilmoniemi RJ, & Santavuori P (1997) Somatosensory evoked magnetic fields from primary sensorimotor cortex in juvenile neuronal ceroid lipofuscinosis. *J Child Neurol*, 12, 355–360.

Lauronen L, Munroe PB, Jarvela I, Autti T, Mitchison HM, O'Rawe AM, Gardiner RM, Mole SE, Puranen J, Hakkinen AM, Kirveskari E, & Santavuori P (1999) Delayed classic and protracted phenotypes of compound heterozygous juvenile neuronal ceroid lipofuscinosis. *Neurology*, 52, 360–365.

Lee TS, Poon SH, & Chang P (2010) Dissimilar neuropsychiatric presentations of two siblings with juvenile neuronal ceroid lipofuscinosis (Batten disease). *J Neuropsychiatry Clin Neurosci*, 22, 123.E14–15.

Leman AR, Pearce DA, & Rothberg PG (2005) Gene symbol: CLN3. Disease: Juvenile neuronal ceroid lipofuscinosis (Batten disease). *Hum Genet*, 116, 544.

Lerner TJ, Boustany RM, MacCormack K, Gleitsman J, Schlumpf K, Breakefield XO, Gusella JF, & Haines JL (1994) Linkage disequilibrium between the juvenile neuronal ceroid lipofuscinosis gene and marker loci on chromosome 16p 12.1. *Am J Hum Genet*, 54, 88–94.

Lim MJ, Alexander N, Benedict JW, Chattopadhyay S, Shemilt SJ, Guerin CJ, Cooper JD, & Pearce DA (2007) IgG entry and deposition are components of the neuroimmune response in Batten disease. *Neurobiol Dis*, 25, 239–251.

Lim MJ, Beake J, Bible E, Curran TM, Ramirez-Montealegre D, Pearce DA, & Cooper JD (2006) Distinct patterns of serum immunoreactivity as evidence for multiple brain-directed autoantibodies in juvenile neuronal ceroid lipofuscinosis. *Neuropathol Appl Neurobiol*, 32, 469–482.

Lou HC & Kristensen K (1973) A clinical and psychological investigation into juvenile amaurotic idiocy in Denmark. *Dev Med Child Neurol*, 15, 313–323.

Luiro K, Kopra O, Blom T, Gentile M, Mitchison HM, Hovatta I, Tornquist K, & Jalanko A (2006) Batten disease (JNCL) is linked to disturbances in mitochondrial, cytoskeletal, and synaptic compartments. *J Neurosci Res*, 84, 1124–1138.

Luiro K, Kopra O, Lehtovirta M, & Jalanko A (2001) CLN3 protein is targeted to neuronal synapses but excluded from synaptic vesicles: new clues to Batten disease. *Hum Mol Genet*, 10, 2123–2131.

Luiro K, Yliannala K, Ahtiainen L, Maunu H, Jarvela I, Kyttala A, & Jalanko A (2004) Interconnections of CLN3, Hook1 and Rab proteins link Batten disease to defects in the endocytic pathway. *Hum Mol Genet*, 13, 3017–3027.

MacLeod PM, Dolman CL, Chang E, Applegarth DA, & Bryant B (1976) The neuronal ceroid lipofuscinoses in British Columbia: a clinical epidemiologic and ultrastructural study. *Birth Defects Orig Artic Ser*, 12, 289–296.

Mao Q, Foster BJ, Xia H, & Davidson BL (2003) Membrane topology of CLN3, the protein underlying Batten disease. *FEBS Lett*, 541, 40–46.

March PA, Wurzelmann S, & Walkley SU (1995) Morphological alterations in neocortical and cerebellar GABAergic neurons in a canine model of juvenile Batten disease. *Am J Med Genet*, 57, 204–212.

Metcalfe DJ, Calvi AA, Seamann MNJ, Mitchison HM, & Cutler DF (2008) Loss of the Batten disease gene CLN3 prevents exit from the TGN of the mannose 6-phosphate receptor. *Traffic*, 11, 1905–1914.

Michalewski MP, Kaczmarski W, Golabek AA, Kida E, Kaczmarski A, & Wisniewski KE (1998) Evidence for phosphorylation of CLN3 protein associated with Batten disease. *Biochem Biophys Res Commun*, 253, 458–462.

Michalewski MP, Kaczmarski W, Golabek AA, Kida E, Kaczmarski A, & Wisniewski KE (1999) Posttranslational modification of CLN3 protein and its possible functional implication. *Mol Genet Metab*, 66, 272–276.

Mitchison HM, Bernard DJ, Greene ND, Cooper JD, Junaid MA, Pullarkat RK, de Vos N, Breuning MH, Owens JW, Mobley WC, Gardiner RM, Lake BD, Taschner PE, & Nussbaum RL (1999) Targeted disruption of the Cln3 gene provides a mouse model for Batten disease. The Batten Mouse Model Consortium [corrected]. *Neurobiol Dis*, 6, 321–334.

Mitchison HM, Lim MJ, & Cooper JD (2004) Selectivity and types of cell death in the neuronal ceroid lipofuscinoses. *Brain Pathol*, 14, 86–96.

Mitchison HM, Munroe PB, O'Rawe AM, Taschner PE, de Vos N, Kremmidiotis G, Lensink I, Munk AC, D'Arigo KL, Anderson JW, Lerner TJ, Moyzis RK, Callen DF, Breuning MH, Doggett NA, Gardiner RM, & Mole SE (1997a) Genomic structure and complete nucleotide sequence of the Batten disease gene, CLN3. *Genomics*, 40, 346–350.

Mitchison HM, O'Rawe AM, Taschner PE, Sandkuijl LA, Santavuori P, de Vos N, Breuning MH, Mole SE, Gardiner RM, & Jarvela IE (1995) Batten disease gene, CLN3: linkage disequilibrium mapping in the Finnish population, and analysis of European haplotypes. *Am J Hum Genet*, 56, 654–662.

Mitchison HM, Taschner PE, Kremmidiotis G, Callen DF, Doggett NA, Lerner TJ, Janes RB, Wallace BA, Munroe PB, O'Rawe AM, Gardiner RM, & Mole SE (1997b) Structure of the CLN3 gene and predicted structure, location and function of CLN3 protein. *Neuropediatrics*, 28, 12–14.

Mitchison HM, Thompson AD, Mulley JC, Kozman HM, Richards RI, Callen DF, Stallings RL, Doggett NA, Attwood J, McKay TR, et al. (1993) Fine genetic mapping of the Batten disease locus (CLN3) by haplotype analysis and demonstration of allelic association with chromosome 16p microsatellite loci. *Genomics*, 16, 455–460.

Mole SE, Zhong NA, Sarpong A, Logan WP, Hofmann S, Yi W, Franken PF, van Diggelen OP, Breuning MH, Moroziewicz D, Ju W, Salonen T, Holmberg V, Jarvela I, & Taschner PE (2001) New mutations in the neuronal ceroid lipofuscinosis genes. *Eur J Paediatr Neurol*, 5 Suppl A, 7–10.

Munroe PB, Mitchison HM, O'Rawe AM, Anderson JW, Boustany RM, Lerner TJ, Taschner PE, de Vos N, Breuning MH, Gardiner RM, & Mole SE (1997) Spectrum of mutations in the Batten disease gene, CLN3. *Am J Hum Genet*, 61, 310–316.

Munroe PB, Rapola J, Mitchison HM, Mustonen A, Mole SE, Gardiner RM, & Jarvela I (1996) Prenatal diagnosis of Batten's disease. *Lancet*, 347, 1014–1015.

Narayan SB, Rakheja D, Pastor JV, Rosenblatt K, Greene SR, Yang J, Wolf BA, & Bennett MJ (2006) Overexpression of CLN3P, the Batten disease protein, inhibits PANDER-induced apoptosis in neuroblastoma cells: further evidence that CLN3P has anti-apoptotic properties. *Mol Genet Metab*, 88, 178–183.

Narayan SB, Tan L, & Bennett MJ (2008) Intermediate levels of neuronal palmitoyl-protein Delta-9 desaturase in heterozygotes for murine Batten disease. *Mol Genet Metab*, 93, 89–91.

Nugent T, Mole SE, & Jones D (2008) The transmembrane topology of Batten disease protein CLN3 determined by consensus computational prediction constrained by experimental data. *FEBS Letters*, 582, 1019–1024.

Osório NS, Sampaio-Marques B, Chan CH, Oliveira P, Pearce DA, Sousa N, & Rodrigues F (2009) Neurodevelopmental delay in the Cln3Deltaex7/8 mouse model for Batten disease. *Genes Brain Behav*, 8, 337–345.

Østergaard JR, Egeblad H, & Molgaard H (2005) *The evolution of cardiac involvement in juvenile neuronal ceroid lipofuscinoses. NCL-2005*: The 10th International Congress on Neuronal Ceroid Lipofuscinoses, p.28.

Padilla-Lopez S & Pearce DA (2006) Saccharomyces cerevisiae lacking Btn1p modulate vacuolar ATPase activity to regulate pH imbalance in the vacuole. *J Biol Chem*, 281, 10273–10280.

Pane MA, Puranam KL, & Boustany RM (1999) Expression of cln3 in human NT2 neuronal precursor cells and neonatal rat brain. *Pediatr Res*, 46, 367–374.

Pearce DA, Carr CJ, Das B, & Sherman F (1999a) Phenotypic reversal of the btn1 defects in yeast by chloroquine: a yeast model for Batten disease. *Proc Natl Acad Sci U S A*, 96, 11341–11345.

Pearce DA, Ferea T, Nosel SA, Das B, & Sherman F (1999b) Action of BTN1, the yeast orthologue of the gene mutated in Batten disease. *Nat Genet*, 22, 55–58.

Pearce DA, McCall K, Mooney RA, Chattopadhyay S, & Curran TM (2003) Altered amino acid levels in sera of a mouse model for juvenile neuronal ceroid lipofuscinoses. *Clin Chim Acta*, 332, 145–148.

Pearce DA, Nosel SA, & Sherman F (1999c) Studies of pH regulation by Btn1p, the yeast homolog of human Cln3p. *Mol Genet Metab*, 66, 320–323.

Pearce DA & Sherman F (1998) A yeast model for the study of Batten disease. *Proc Natl Acad Sci U S A*, 95, 6915–6918.

Pears MR, Cooper JD, Mitchison HM, Mortishire-Smith RJ, Pearce DA, & Griffin JL (2005) High resolution 1H NMR-based metabolomics indicates a neurotransmitter cycling deficit in cerebral tissue from a mouse model of Batten disease. *J Biol Chem*, 280, 42508–42514.

Persaud-Sawin DA & Boustany RM (2005) Cell death pathways in juvenile Batten disease. *Apoptosis*, 10, 973–985.

Persaud-Sawin DA, McNamara JO, 2nd, Rylova S, Vandongen A, & Boustany RM (2004) A galactosylceramide binding domain is involved in trafficking of CLN3 from Golgi to rafts via recycling endosomes. *Pediatr Res*, 56, 449–463.

Pisoni RL, Flickinger KS, Thoene JG, & Christensen HN (1987a) Characterization of carrier-mediated transport systems for small neutral amino acids in human fibroblast lysosomes. *J Biol Chem*, 262, 6010–6017.

Pisoni RL, Thoene JG, Lemons RM, & Christensen HN (1987b) Important differences in cationic amino acid transport by lysosomal system c and system y+ of the human fibroblast. *J Biol Chem*, 262, 15011–15018.

Pontikis CC, Cella CV, Parihar N, Lim MJ, Chakrabarti S, Mitchison HM, Mobley WC, Rezaie P, Pearce DA, & Cooper JD (2004) Late onset neurodegeneration in the $Cln3^{-/-}$ mouse model of juvenile neuronal ceroid lipofuscinosis is preceded by low level glial activation. *Brain Res*, 1023, 231–242.

Pontikis CC, Cotman SL, MacDonald ME, & Cooper JD (2005) Thalamocortical neuron loss and localized astrocytosis in the Cln3Deltaex7/8 knock-in mouse model of Batten disease. *Neurobiol Dis*, 20, 823–836.

Portera-Cailliau C, Sung CH, Nathans J, & Adler R (1994) Apoptotic photoreceptor cell death in mouse models of retinitis pigmentosa. *Proc Natl Acad Sci U S A*, 91, 974–978.

Pullarkat RK & Morris GN (1997) Farnesylation of Batten disease CLN3 protein. *Neuropediatrics*, 28, 42–44.

Puranam KL, Guo WX, Qian WH, Nikbakht K, & Boustany RM (1999) CLN3 defines a novel antiapoptotic pathway operative in neurodegeneration and mediated by ceramide. *Mol Genet Metab*, 66, 294–308.

Raitta K & Santavuori P (1981) *Ophthalmological Findings and Main Clinical Characteristics in Childhood Types of Neuronal Ceroid Lipofuscinoses*. Amsterdam, Elsevier North Holland Biomedical Press.

Rakheja D, Narayan SB, Pastor JV, & Bennett MJ (2004) CLN3P, the Batten disease protein, localizes to membrane lipid rafts (detergent-resistant membranes). *Biochem Biophys Res Commun*, 317, 988–991.

Ramirez-Montealegre D & Pearce DA (2005) Defective lysosomal arginine transport in juvenile Batten disease. *Hum Mol Genet*, 14, 3759–3773.

Richardson SC, Winistorfer SC, Poupon V, Luzio JP, & Piper RC (2004) Mammalian late vacuole protein sorting orthologues participate in early endosomal fusion and interact with the cytoskeleton. *Mol Biol Cell*, 15, 1197–1210.

Rinne JO, Ruottinen HM, Nagren K, Åberg LE, & Santavuori P (2002) Positron emission tomography shows reduced striatal dopamine D1 but not D2 receptors in juvenile neuronal ceroid lipofuscinosis. *Neuropediatrics*, 33, 138–141.

Rowan SA & Lake BD (1995) Tissue and cellular distribution of subunit c of ATP synthase in Batten disease (neuronal ceroid-lipofuscinosis). *Am J Med Genet*, 57, 172–176.

Rusyn E, Mousallem T, Persaud-Sawin DA, Miller S, & Boustany RM (2008) CLN3p impacts galactosylceramide transport, raft morphology, and lipid content. *Pediatr Res*, 63, 625–631.

Sarpong A, Schottmann G, Ruther K, Stoltenburg G, Kohlschutter A, Hubner C, & Schuelke M (2009) Protracted course of juvenile ceroid lipofuscinosis associated with a novel CLN3 mutation (p.Y199X). *Clin Genet*, 76, 38–45.

Song JW, Misgeld T, Kang H, Knecht S, Lu J, Cao Y, Cotman SL, Bishop DL, & Lichtman JW (2008) Lysosomal activity associated with developmental axon pruning. *J Neurosci*, 28, 8993–9001.

Spalton DJ, Taylor DS, & Sanders MD (1980) Juvenile Batten's disease: an ophthalmological assessment of 26 patients. *Br J Ophthalmol*, 64, 726–732.

Stein CS, Yancey PH, Martins I, Sigmund RD, Stokes JB, & Davidson BL (2010) Osmoregulation of ceroid neuronal lipofuscinosis type 3 (CLN3) in the renal medulla. *Am J Physiol Cell Physiol*, 298, C1388–C1400.

Storch S, Pohl S, & Braulke T (2004) A dileucine motif and a cluster of acidic amino acids in the second cytoplasmic domain of the Batten disease-related CLN3 protein are required for efficient lysosomal targeting. *J Biol Chem*, 279, 53625–53634.

Storch S, Pohl S, Quitsch A, Falley K, & Braulke T (2007) C-terminal prenylation of the CLN3 membrane glycoprotein is required for efficient endosomal sorting to lysosomes. *Traffic*, 8, 431–444.

Taschner PE, de Vos N, Thompson AD, Callen DF, Doggett N, Mole SE, Dooley TP, Barth PG, & Breuning MH (1995) Chromosome 16 microdeletion in a patient with juvenile neuronal ceroid lipofuscinosis (Batten disease). *Am J Hum Genet*, 56, 663–668.

Telakivi T, Partinen M, & Salmi T (1985) Sleep disturbance in patients with juvenile neuronal ceroid lipofuscinosis: a new application of the SCSB-method. *J Ment Defic Res*, **29** (Pt 1), 29–35.

The International Batten Disease Consortium (1995) Isolation of a novel gene underlying Batten disease, CLN3. *Cell*, 82, 949–957.

Tuxworth RI, Vivancos V, O'Hare MB, & Tear G (2009) Interactions between the juvenile Batten disease gene, CLN3, and the Notch and JNK signalling pathways. *Hum Mol Genet*, 18, 667–678.

Tyynelä J, Cooper JD, Khan MN, Shemilts SJ, & Haltia M (2004) Hippocampal pathology in the human neuronal ceroid-lipofuscinoses: distinct patterns of storage deposition, neurodegeneration and glial activation. *Brain Pathol*, 14, 349–357.

Tyynelä J, Suopanki J, Baumann M, & Haltia M (1997) Sphingolipid activator proteins (SAPs) in neuronal ceroid lipofuscinoses (NCL). *Neuropediatrics*, 28, 49–52.

Uusi-Rauva K, Luiro K, Tanhuanpaa K, Kopra O, Martin-Vasallo P, Kyttala A, & Jalanko A (2008) Novel interactions of CLN3 protein link Batten disease to dysregulation of fodrin-Na+, K+ ATPase complex. *Exp Cell Res*, 314, 2895–2905.

Uvebrant P & Hagberg B (1997) Neuronal ceroid lipofuscinoses in Scandinavia. Epidemiology and clinical pictures. *Neuropediatrics*, 28, 6–8.

Vitiello SP, Benedict JW, Padilla-Lopez S, & Pearce DA (2010) Interaction between Sdo1p and Btn1p in the

Saccharomyces cerevisiae model for Batten disease. *Hum Mol Genet*, 19, 931–942.
Walenta JH, Didier AJ, Liu X, & Kramer H (2001) The Golgi-associated hook3 protein is a member of a novel family of microtubule-binding proteins. *J Cell Biol*, 152, 923–934.
Walkley SU (1998) Cellular pathology of lysosomal storage disorders. *Brain Pathol*, 8, 175–193.
Walkley SU, March PA, Schroeder CE, Wurzelmann S, & Jolly RD (1995) Pathogenesis of brain dysfunction in Batten disease. *Am J Med Genet*, 57, 196–203.
Weimer JM, Benedict JW, Elshatory YM, Short DW, Ramirez-Montealegre D, Ryan DA, Alexander NA, Federoff HJ, Cooper JD, & Pearce DA (2007) Alterations in striatal dopamine catabolism precede loss of substantia nigra neurons in a mouse model of juvenile neuronal ceroid lipofuscinosis. *Brain Res*, 1162, 98–112.
Weimer JM, Benedict JW, Getty AL, Pontikis CC, Lim MJ, Cooper JD, & Pearce DA (2009) Cerebellar defects in a mouse model of juvenile neuronal ceroid lipofuscinosis. *Brain Res*, 1266, 93–107.
Weimer JM, Chattopadhyay S, Custer AW, & Pearce DA (2005) Elevation of Hook1 in a disease model of Batten disease does not affect a novel interaction between Ankyrin G and Hook1. *Biochem Biophys Res Commun*, 330, 1176–1181.
Weimer JM, Custer AW, Benedict JW, Alexander NA, Kingsley E, Federoff HJ, Cooper JD, & Pearce DA (2006) Visual deficits in a mouse model of Batten disease are the result of optic nerve degeneration and loss of dorsal lateral geniculate thalamic neurons. *Neurobiol Dis*, 22, 284–293.
Wisniewski KE, Gordon-Krajcer W, & Kida E (1993) Abnormal processing of carboxy-terminal fragment of beta precursor protein (beta PP) in neuronal ceroid-lipofuscinosis (NCL) cases. *J Inherit Metab Dis*, 16, 312–316.
Wisniewski KE, Kida E, Gordon-Majszak W, & Saitoh T (1990a) Altered amyloid beta-protein precursor processing in brains of patients with neuronal ceroid lipofuscinosis. *Neurosci Lett*, 120, 94–96.
Wisniewski KE, Kida E, Patxot OF, & Connell F (1992) Variability in the clinical and pathological findings in the neuronal ceroid lipofuscinoses: review of data and observations. *Am J Med Genet*, 42, 525–532.
Wisniewski KE & Maslinska D (1990) Lectin histochemistry in brains with juvenile form of neuronal ceroid-lipofuscinosis (Batten disease). *Acta Neuropathol*, 80, 274–279.
Wisniewski KE, Maslinska D, Kitaguchi T, Kim KS, Goebel HH, & Haltia M (1990b) Topographic heterogeneity of amyloid B-protein epitopes in brains with various forms of neuronal ceroid lipofuscinoses suggesting defective processing of amyloid precursor protein. *Acta Neuropathol*, 80, 26–34.
Wisniewski KE, Zhong N, Kaczmarski W, Kaczmarski A, Kida E, Brown WT, Schwarz KO, Lazzarini AM, Rubin AJ, Stenroos ES, Johnson WG, & Wisniewski TM (1998a) Compound heterozygous genotype is associated with protracted juvenile neuronal ceroid lipofuscinosis. *Ann Neurol*, 43, 106–110.
Wisniewski KE, Zhong N, Kaczmarski W, Kaczmarski A, Sklower-Brooks S, & Brown WT (1998b) Studies of atypical JNCL suggest overlapping with other NCL forms. *Pediatr Neurol*, 18, 36–40.
Zhong N, Wisniewski KE, Hartikainen J, Ju W, Moroziewicz DN, McLendon L, Sklower Brooks SS, & Brown WT (1998) Two common mutations in the CLN2 gene underlie late infantile neuronal ceroid lipofuscinosis. *Clin Genet*, 54, 234–238.

Chapter 9

CLN5

L. Åberg, T. Autti, J.D. Cooper, M. Elleder, M. Haltia, A. Jalanko, C. Kitzmüller, O. Kopra, S.E. Mole, A. Nuutila, L. Peltonen, M.-L. Punkari, J. Rapola, and J. Tyynelä

INTRODUCTION

A variant of late infantile NCL was first recognized as a distinct genetic and clinical entity in Finland, and the gene, *CLN5*, identified in 1998. Subsequently, other cases of CLN5 disease, late infantile variant, were described outside Finland, as well as other late infantile variants that were caused by mutations in different genes.

MOLECULAR GENETICS

Isolation of the *CLN5* gene

Using genome-wide scanning, the *CLN5* gene was assigned to 13q21–q32 by linkage analysis in 16 Finnish families with common ancestors (Savukoski et al., 1994, Varilo et al., 1996). Assuming one founder mutation in Finland, all the affected chromosomes were expected to share the same haplotype in the vicinity of the disease locus. The *CLN5* locus was restricted by haplotype analyses of disease alleles and linkage disequilibrium. The initial 3cM region identified by linkage analyses was restricted to less than 1cM, and three markers flanking a 300kb region revealed a 100% allelic association with the disease, confirming that the *CLN5* gene was located in this chromosomal region.

A PAC contig was assembled over the critical 300kb region, and the order and orientation of the clones were systematically analysed. The size of the clones and the distances between them, as well as clone overlaps, were determined by visual mapping using the Fibre-FISH technique (Heiskanen et al., 1996, Klockars et al., 1996).

Traditional strategies were used for the identification of transcripts encoded by the critical DNA region: multiple cDNA libraries were screened using the PACs, and CpG islands associated with the 5′ ends of genes were cloned, giving an estimation of the number of genes in this DNA region. As part of the Human Genome Project the PAC contig was also completely sequenced. Analyses of transcribed sequences resulted in the identification of six genes from the critical chromosomal region, including three novel cDNAs with no homologies in the public databases. One of these was found to be the *CLN5* gene based on mutations identified in late infantile variant patients (Savukoski et al., 1998).

The *CLN5* gene consists of four exons and encodes several potential methionine start sites in exon 1 (Figure 9.1). No other genes encode proteins similar to CLN5 in the human genome.

Mutations in *CLN5*

Twenty-seven different mutations in *CLN5* are now identified in late infantile variant patients of Finnish and non-Finnish origin (Savukoski et al., 1998, Holmberg et al., 2000, Pineda-Trujillo et al., 2005, Bessa et al., 2006, Cismondi et al., 2008, Lebrun et al., 2009, Sleat et al., 2009, Xin et al., 2010; and others unpublished, but recorded in the NCL mutation database at http://www.ucl.ac.uk/ncl) (Figure 9.1 and see Chapter 20). These consist of ten missense mutations, 11 small deletions or insertions causing frameshifts, one large deletion, and five nonsense mutations.

The most common mutation has so far been found exclusively in families from Finland. This Finnish major mutation (*CLN5* 'Fin major') was identified in 94% of Finnish disease chromosomes. It is a 2bp deletion in exon 4 (c.1175delAT) resulting in the change p. Tyr392X in the corresponding polypeptide. This is predicted to result in a truncated polypeptide of 391 amino acids compared to the expected 407 amino acids. The second most common mutation was first identified in a single family with two affected children carrying the *CLN5* 'Fin minor' haplotype in both alleles. A G>A transversion in exon 1 (c.225G>A) causes the substitution p.Trp75X, resulting in a predicted protein of only 74 amino acids. This has also been found in a family from Sweden that, like Finnish families, is compound heterozygote for the p.Trp75X and a C insertion at amino acid position 223 (c.669insC) causing a frameshift and a premature stop codon predicted at position 253.

All mutations except 'Fin major' have been identified in families from many different countries that include Finland, UK, Afghanistan, Argentina, Canada, China, Colombia, the Czech Republic, Egypt, Italy, the Netherlands, Portugal, Pakistan, Sweden, USA, or with Asian, Hispanic, and Arabian (Qatar and Yemen) origin (Holmberg

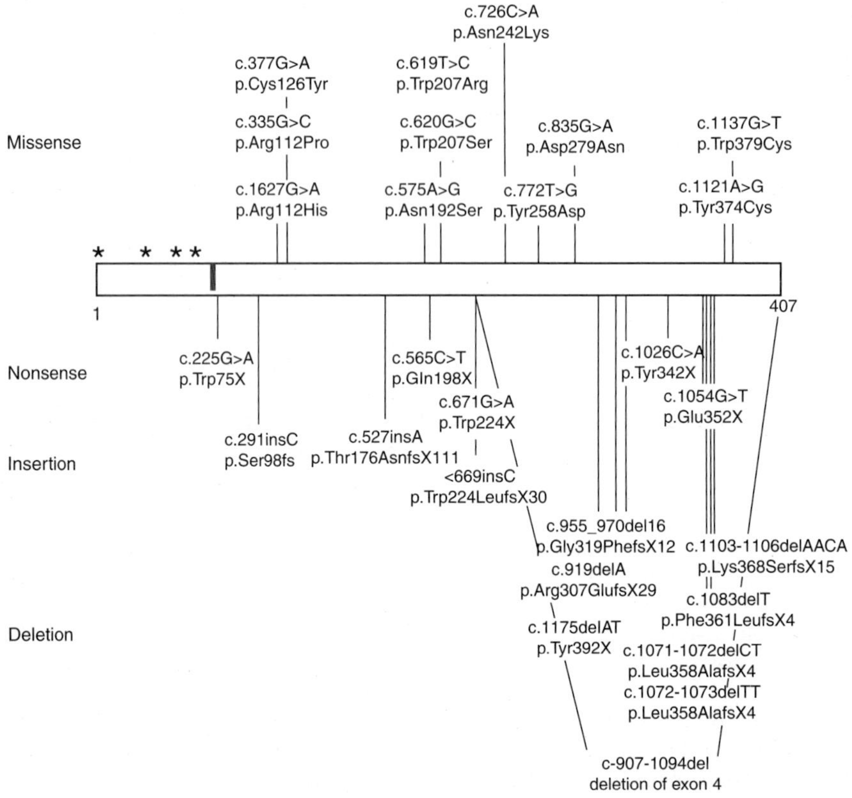

Figure 9.1 A schematic presentation of the CLN5 protein and the identified mutations. * represents several potential methionine start sites in exon 1 of the human protein, of which only the third is conserved.

et al., 2000, Pineda-Trujillo et al., 2005, Bessa et al., 2006, Cannelli et al., 2007, Cismondi et al., 2008, Kohan et al., 2008, Kousi et al., 2009, Lebrun et al., 2009, Sleat et al., 2009, Xin et al., 2010; and unpublished). In many cases, these mutations have so far been described in one or very few families. There may be further founding effects where mutations are confined to families clearly originating from the same country. For example, one mutation (c.919delA, p.Arg307GlufsX29) was reported in a family living in the USA that originated from Egypt, and has also been detected in a family still living in Egypt.

The carrier frequency of the *CLN5* 'Fin major' mutation varies within Finland. Local carrier frequency in the western coastline communities is 1:24, whereas carrier frequency in the rest of Finland is less than 1:100. The carrier frequency is even lower outside Finland. The extremely high carrier frequency in a limited subpopulation of Finland supports the young age of the Finnish *CLN5* mutation, as had been suggested by the still observable regional clustering of cases, genealogical data, and haplotype analyses (Varilo et al., 1996).

Nine polymorphisms have been reported (Savukoski et al., 1998, Xin et al., 2010), also recorded at http://www.ucl.ac.uk/ncl, two of which change amino acids. Two polymorphisms are common and are found in families of varied ethnic origin: One in exon 4 (c.1103A>G; p.Lys368Arg) has a carrier frequency of nearly 20% in the Finnish population and 10% in the USA population, and one in exon 1 (c.4C>T; p.Arg2Cys) has a carrier frequency of 10% in the USA population. One further change (c.335G>C; p.Arg112Pro) may also be a polymorphism as it was found on the same disease allele as that carrying c.835G>A (p.Asp279Asn) (Bessa et al., 2006).

Notably, variation c.4C>T has been found in cases of CLN6 disease and a CLN7 disease. The CLN7 disease patient was homozygous for the relatively common CLN7 mutation c.881C>A (p.Thr294Lys) (M. Elleder, personal communication), yet had juvenile onset and vacuolated lymphocytes, raising the possibility that this change in CLN5 modified the CLN7 disease slightly in some way.

CELL BIOLOGY

Tissue expression of *CLN5*

Hybridization analyses of human *CLN5* have revealed the expression of three transcripts of 2.0kb, 3.0kb, and 4.5kb in all tissues. The appearance of multiple transcripts suggests alternative splicing of the *CLN5* mRNA (Savukoski et al., 1998). Alternative splicing is also a feature of the mouse *Cln5* gene, which is expressed as two transcripts of 2.3kb and 2.9kb in all tissues, and additional mRNAs have been detected in mouse skeletal muscle and in lung (Holmberg et al., 2004). Alternatively spliced mRNAs can also be detected in the EST (expressed sequence tag) sequence database (http://www.ncbi.nih.gov), but their possible translation into different CLN5 protein isoforms has not been experimentally analysed.

In the mouse brain, *Cln5* mRNA shows low expression levels in embryonic day 13 and postnatal day 7, but expression is much more abundant at postnatal day 30, suggesting developmental regulation. The spatial and temporal expression analysis of *Cln5* mRNA has revealed ubiquitous expression in the brain by embryonic day 15. The most abundant expression in the embryonic mouse brain localizes to developing cerebral cortex, cerebellum, and in the ganglionic eminence. In the adult brain, the most intense signal can be detected in the Purkinje cell layer of the cerebellum, in the cerebral cortex, as well as in the hippocampal principal cell layers (Holmberg et al., 2004). Data from embryonic human brain during the period from 37–84 days of gestation also reveal increasing expression during brain development. In the developing cerebral cortex, *CLN5* mRNA expression localizes in the neuroblasts migrating toward the intermediate and cortical plate zones. Similar to mouse expression data, human *CLN5* mRNA expresses also in the thalamus and the developing cerebellum, where the expression is detectable mainly in the future Purkinje cells. In summary, the expression pattern of *CLN5* is very similar to the NCL gene *CLN1/PPT1* (Heinonen et al., 2000).

The distribution of mouse CLN5 protein has further been analysed by immunohistochemistry in developing postnatal mouse brain from P7–P60. In line with its mRNA expression, the CLN5 protein is observed in the cerebral cortex, cerebellum, as well as in the hippocampal formation. The most intense immunoreactivity is detected in cerebellar Purkinje cells, diverse cortical neurons, and hippocampal pyramidal cells, although some glial staining can also be seen. Interestingly, in the hippocampus, the most intense *Cln5* immunopositivity is detected in CA3 pyramidal cells, whereas the labelling in CA1 region shows weaker immunostaining (Holmberg et al., 2004). The distribution of CLN5 protein in developing human brain has been studied mainly in the cortical regions and the distribution pattern is in line with the mRNA expression. At embryonic day 37, some CLN5 immunostaining is seen in the ventricular zone and in some peripheral cells. Later, at day 76 after fertilization, CLN5 immunoreactivity is localized to cells leaving the ventricular zone and migrating peripherally toward the cortical region (Heinonen et al., 2000).

The expression patterns of *Cln5/CLN5* in the mouse and human brain provide a striking parallel to pathological findings from CLN5 disease, late infantile variant patients where a selective neuronal loss has been observed especially in the cerebellum and also in the cerebral cortex and thalamic regions (Autti et al., 1992, Vanhanen et al., 1995a, Vanhanen et al., 1995b) and reviewed in (Haltia, 2003). Recent RNA analyses showed upregulation of *Ppt1* mRNA in 4-month-old $Cln5^{-/-}$ mice, suggestive of a compensatory response, but not the other way round (Lyly et al., 2009).

Protein structure and modifications

The human *CLN5* gene is thought to encode a 407-amino acid polypeptide with a predicted molecular weight of 46kD. The CLN5 protein was initially described as a transmembrane protein (Savukoski et al., 1998), or existing in either soluble or transmembrane forms (Vesa et al., 2002). It was finally revealed to be a soluble lysosomal glycoprotein (Holmberg et al., 2004, Schmiedt et al., 2010) that undergoes cleavage prior to transport to the lysosome.

The 5′ region of the *CLN5* mRNA contains four in-frame initiation methionines (Figure 9.1), with only the third conserved in the Devon cattle and dog CLN5 proteins (see Chapter 19), and these and other species (e.g. mouse, chicken, zebrafish) having only one. CLN5 is not homologous to any known protein but the sequence contains two hydrophobic sequences, predicted to be transmembrane helices by several protein prediction programs (Savukoski et al., 1998). *In vitro* translation analysis of the *CLN5* cDNA demonstrated the production of four polypeptides with apparent molecular weights from 39–47kD (Isosomppi et al., 2002, Vesa et al., 2002). It has been a challenge to derive antibodies capable of detecting endogenous CLN5.

Based on the amino acid sequence, CLN5 has eight potential N-glycosylation sites and expression of the human *CLN5* cDNA in BHK-21 and COS-1 cells revealed a 60–75kD glycosylated polypeptide (Isosomppi et al., 2002, Vesa et al., 2002). EndoH treatment of the CLN5 polypeptide resulted in a 40kD or 47kD polypeptide and PNGase F treatment resulted in a polypeptide with apparent molecular weight of 38kD or 45kD. These observations suggest that the CLN5 protein possesses both high-mannoses-type as well as complex-type sugars (Isosomppi et al., 2002, Vesa et al., 2002). Other potential modification sites of CLN5 include phosphorylation and myristoylation, but these have not been experimentally analysed. Overexpression studies utilizing *CLN5* cDNA constructs mutated at the individual initiator methionines, have further shown that the longest CLN5 polypeptide of 47kD, translated from the first methionine, represents a membrane-bound form of CLN5 (Vesa et al., 2002).

The mouse *Cln5* gene encodes a predicted polypeptide of 341 amino acids with a predicted N-terminal signal sequence. The mouse CLN5 sequence is highly homologous to the human protein from amino acid 102. The same region is further conserved in three other species, including pig, catfish, and frog. For species other than human, an N-terminal hydrophobic stretch is observed at the region corresponding to amino acids 75–91 of the human polypeptide. Experimental analyses have demonstrated the soluble nature of the mouse CLN5 protein (Holmberg et al., 2004). Additionally, it has been shown that deletion of the mouse *Cln5* gene causes an identical tissue pathology to that observed in Finnish patients with CLN5 disease, late infantile variant, suggesting that the soluble form of CLN5 represents the functional entity relevant to the disease phenotype (Kopra et al., 2004).

Intracellular localization and possible function

Overexpressed CLN5 protein was originally shown to localize to lysosomes in studies in BHK-21, HeLa, and COS-1 cells (Isosomppi et al., 2002, Vesa et al., 2002, Holmberg et al., 2004). The endogenous mouse CLN5 protein has been visualized immunohistochemically in the mouse brain, where it appears in granular structures in neuronal extensions that remain unidentified (Holmberg et al., 2004). Early studies of disease-causing mutations (e.g. p. Asp279Asn) showed no dramatic effect on the intracellular localization of CLN5 protein (Vesa et al., 2002), although the polypeptide containing the 'Fin major' mutation (p.Tyr392X) is retained in the Golgi complex in BHK-21 cells (Isosomppi et al., 2002), whereas in COS-1 cells it is detected also in lysosomes (Vesa et al., 2002). This suggests that some CLN5 disease mutations do not cause severe misfolding of the protein and instead, may directly compromise the function of CLN5. However, more recent studies of previously uncharacterized CLN5 mutant proteins found that these disease mutations disturb its lysosomal trafficking, in some cases causing retention in the endoplasmic reticulum (Lebrun et al., 2009, Schmiedt et al., 2010). Since the level of lysosomal targeting of mutant proteins does not correlate with disease onset, it may be that CLN5 also functions elsewhere in the cell. CLN5 protein was identified in the human brain mannose 6-phosphoproteome by two-dimensional gel electrophoresis (Sleat et al., 2005), strongly indicating that it is mannose 6-phosphorylated and transported to the lysosome using this system. There is also evidence that soluble CLN5 protein can undergo mannose 6-phosphate receptor-independent trafficking to the lysosomes (Schmiedt et al., 2010).

CLN5 interaction partners have been investigated using *in vitro* binding pull-down and co-immunoprecipitation analyses (Vesa et al., 2002, Lyly et al., 2009) and, unexpectedly, a large number of interactions with other NCL proteins have been described. CLN5 was first reported to interact with both CLN2/TPP1 and CLN3 polypeptides (Vesa et al., 2002). All mutant forms of CLN5 tested retained their ability to interact with CLN3, suggesting that the interaction domain mediating this interaction is located N-terminally from CLN5 amino acid 224. In contrast, all disease mutations abolished the CLN5–CLN2 interaction, suggesting that the CLN2/TPP1 interaction is mediated by the C-terminal end of CLN5. More recently, CLN5 was also found to interact with CLN1/PPT1, CLN6, and CLN8 (Lyly et al., 2009), and the interactions with CLN2/TPP1 and CLN3 were confirmed. It is possible that these proteins participate in a common pathway in neuronal cell metabolism, since mutations in many of these genes cause NCL with a similar age of onset, and altered TPP1 enzyme levels have been reported in cells from CLN5 patients (Sleat et al., 1998). Interestingly, overexpression of CLN1/PPT1 rescues the lysosomal trafficking defect of CLN5 'Fin major' mutant protein (Lyly et al., 2009). CLN5 is also reported to interact with subunits of F_1-ATP synthase (Lyly et al., 2009), as does CLN1/PPT1 (Lyly et al., 2008).

CLINICAL DATA

Clinical data for CLN5 disease, late infantile variant in Finnish families, caused by the 'Fin major' mutation, is presented first, followed by comments for other mutations where notable.

Epidemiology

CLN5 disease, late infantile variant was originally thought to be confined to Finland, where it has a prevalence of 2.6 per million inhabitants (Uvebrant and Hagberg, 1997). However, it is also found elsewhere, albeit rarely, in Europe (UK, the Czech Republic, Italy, The Netherlands, Portugal, Sweden), in North (USA, Canada) and South America (Argentina, Colombia) and in many other countries including Afghanistan, China, Egypt, Pakistan, or with Asian, Hispanic, and Arabian (Qatar and Yemen) origin (Holmberg et al., 2000, Pineda-Trujillo et al., 2005, Bessa et al., 2006, Cannelli et al., 2007, Cismondi et al., 2008, Kohan et al., 2008, Kousi et al., 2009, Lebrun et al., 2009, Sleat et al., 2009, Xin et al., 2010; and unpublished). In many cases, the non-Finnish mutations have so far been described in one or very few families.

Even within Finland, the disease is found mostly in the area of southern Ostrobothnia, where the prevalence is around 1:5,000 within the local child population 15 years or younger.

Age of onset and first symptoms

The early years are usually normal and the leading sign is most often slowing-down of psychomotor development, usually noticed between the ages of 5–7 years (Santavuori et al., 1991, Xin et al., 2010). However, in the juvenile onset Colombian patients, the disease presented with visual failure, loss of strength, and tremor in the lower extremities at the later age of 9 years (Pineda-Trujillo et al., 2005). One case from Argentina had very early onset at 4 months—this child may have had other problems (Cismondi et al., 2008). Several patients with late infantile variants presented with behavioural problems (Cannelli et al., 2007, R. Williams, unpublished data; R. Badii unpublished data). Two presented at 17 years old, so were classed as adult disease, one with cognitive regression followed 3 years later with visual failure, and the other with motor difficulties closely followed by onset of seizures and visual failure (Xin et al., 2010).

Progression of symptoms

Besides cognitive decline, clumsiness and visual failure are characteristic features at an early stage of the disease. Between the ages of 9–11 years, there is often a rapid progression of symptoms. From the age of 12 years onwards, the children need help with all activities of daily living. The disease leads to premature death, usually between the ages of 12–23 years. For the two adult onset patients, there was a delay of 6–8 years between the first and subsequent major symptoms.

Ophthalmological findings

Mild visual impairment is observed in most patients at the first examination. Functional blindness becomes obvious a few years later. Ophthalmologic examination at an early stage reveals macular dystrophy, which may be cystic. By the age of 7–9 years, optic atrophy is present. In addition, the macula becomes sharply outlined, differing from the appearance of the macula in CLN3 disease, juvenile onset (Santavuori et al., 1991). Giant visual evoked potentials (VEPs) are usually seen between the ages of 8–9.5 years, whereas the electroretinogram (ERG) is already abnormal at an early stage and is abolished by the age of 8–9.5 years.

Epilepsy syndrome

Children experience the first epileptic seizure at a mean age of 9 years (Santavuori et al., 1991). Seizures are usually generalized, but may be partial. In addition, myoclonus is observed from the age of 6–13 years onwards which interferes considerably with daily activities. Optical illusions, reported by many of the children, may be seizures, though they are difficult to differentiate from symptoms related to declining vision.

In the electroencephalogram (EEG), posterior spikes to low-frequency photic stimulation are found between 7–13 years of age (Holmberg et al., 2000). Giant somatosensory evoked potentials (SEPs), often observed in patients with myoclonus (Berkovic et al., 1991), are a characteristic finding around the age of 7.5–9.5 years (Santavuori et al., 1991).

Dementia

Cognitive decline is an early sign of the disease and progresses rapidly. By the age of 9 years, none of the patients studied had an IQ above 66 (Santavuori et al., 1991).

Motor disturbances and speech

Slight clumsiness appears at the age of 3–6 years, whereas more pronounced motor problems are apparent by the age of 6–8 years. Ataxia is noticed at the age of 7–10 years, and independent walking ability is lost between 9–11 years. Spastic contractures develop later. Speech becomes impaired and an inability to produce speech is noticed by the age of 11 years. However, the understanding of speech is better preserved, and some patients still understand everyday speech at the age of 14–15 years.

Psychiatric and behavioural disturbances

Most patients with CLN5 disease, late infantile variant do not have behavioural problems. However, disturbances of sleep–wake rhythm are common.

Feeding

Feeding difficulties usually appear at the age of 9–13 years. Swallowing difficulties and slow eating can cause the children to lose weight as the disease progresses. The weight decrease is mostly due to inadequate energy supply, with the myoclonus and stiffening perhaps increasing the energy demand further.

Puberty

The pubertal development and the age of menarche are within normal range.

Brain imaging

In all patients imaged, magnetic resonance imaging (MRI) has been abnormal at the time of diagnosis, showing severe cerebellar atrophy (Figure 9.2). In addition, on T_2-weighted images the thalamic signal intensity is low when compared to that of the caudate nuclei, while increased signal intensity is detected in periventricular white matter and in the posterior limbs of the internal capsules. Cerebral atrophy is progressive (Autti et al., 1992).

Clinical biochemistry

No vacuolated lymphocytes are found in CLN5 disease, late infantile variant.

MORPHOLOGY

Macroscopic features

In patients from Finland with CLN5 disease, late infantile variant, the macroscopic abnormalities are limited to the brain which shows

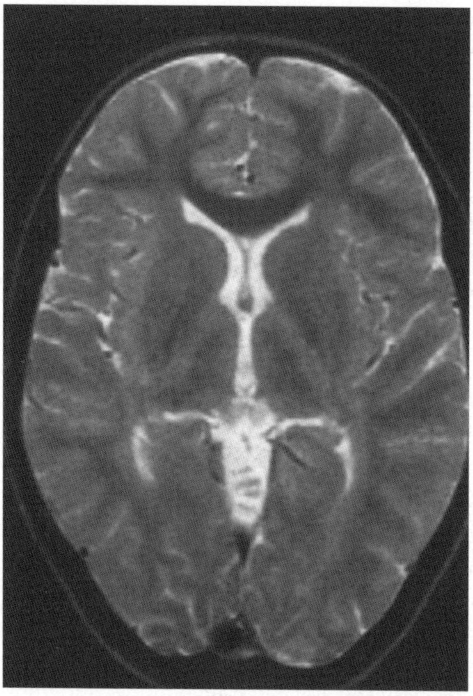

Figure 9.2 CLN5 disease, late infantile variant: MRI of a 7-year-old girl. The T_2-weighted axial images show decreased signal intensity of the thalami. Posterior limbs of the internal capsules show abnormally high signal intensity.

severe generalized cerebral and extreme cerebellar atrophy (Figure 9.3), the total brain weights having varied from 450–660g at autopsy. The cerebral cortex is generally thinner than normal, while the white matter is reduced in amount, and greyish and tough in consistency. The ventricles are diffusely enlarged (Tyynelä et al., 1997). In two siblings of Romany origin, who died at 11 years 8 months and 11 years and 6 months, brain weight was reduced to 590g (50%) and 790g (63%) respectively (M. Elleder, unpublished data). There was brain atrophy with dilatation of the ventricles and the cerebellum was decreased in size.

Histopathology of the central nervous system

A diagnostic brain biopsy specimen, taken in 1971 from the frontal cortex of a 6-year-old boy and therefore typical of early stage disease, showed a well-preserved general cytoarchitecture. All neurons contained moderate intracytoplasmic accumulations of storage granules.

In late stage disease, there is advanced loss of neurons in the cerebral cortex, often in a laminar pattern particularly involving layers III and V. There may even be spongiosis. In addition to the neuronal perikarya, there is storage in axon hillocks resulting in fusiform axonal enlargements (spindles or meganeurites) in the remaining cortical neurons, particularly in the superficial part of layer III (Tyynelä et al., 1997). There is extensive cerebral cortical astrocytosis.

In all patients there is pronounced intraneuronal storage in the hippocampal sectors CA2–4,

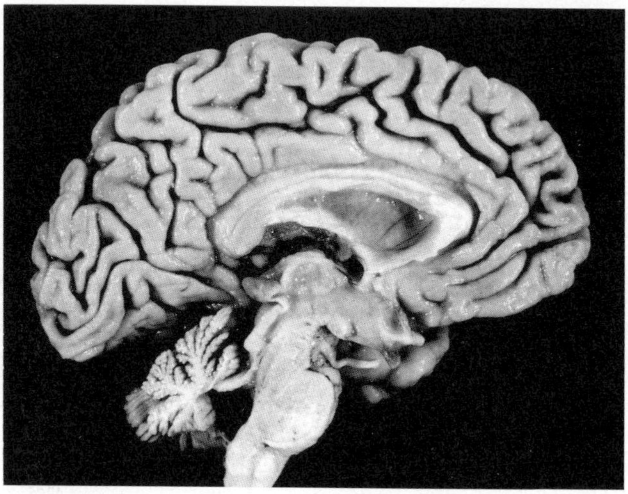

Figure 9.3 CLN5 disease, late infantile variant: the severely atrophic brain of a 14-year-old female patient. Note the particularly striking shrinkage of the cerebellum. Scale in millimetres.

while the CA1 area is relatively unaffected (Tyynelä et al., 1997, Tyynelä et al., 2004).

In the cerebellum, there is advanced atrophy with almost complete destruction of Purkinje cells and of neurons in the granular layer of the cerebellar cortex. The remaining Purkinje cells display variable degrees of autofluorescent storage mainly in the perikarya. The dendrites of these cells display moderate storage with a variable degree of hypertrophy best demonstrated by neurofilament staining. The latter occasionally culminated in cactus-like formations (Figure 9.4). Those neurons remaining in the granular layer show small aggregates of perinuclear storage lysosomes. Neurons in the dentate nucleus display massive storage, but only occasional drop out. An olivary nucleus was not available for analysis.

With the exception of severe loss of neurons in the thalami, subcortical structures generally show only mild-to-moderate neuronal loss, but moderate-to-pronounced intraneuronal ballooning (Tyynelä et al., 1997), particularly in large striatal neurons and in many of the nigral and spinal motor neurons. The latter display occasional cell dropout. However, there are also neurons in these sites that display little storage.

Astrocytosis is present in all the regions mentioned, especially in the cerebellum. Astrocytes display a moderate degree of storage. There is a slight increase in CD68+ microglial cells, which are frequently enlarged by autofluorescent material. Occasionally they form resorptive nodules, presumably around regressively changed neurons.

The cerebral white matter displays, in some cases, moderate-to-severe loss of myelin and gliosis, particularly advanced in the periventricular white matter and in the cerebellar folia.

Postmortem magnetic resonance imaging

Postmortem MRI in CLN5 disease, late infantile variant showed high signal intensity in the periventricular white matter, a finding correlated with the advanced myelin loss and gliosis in that area (Autti et al., 1997).

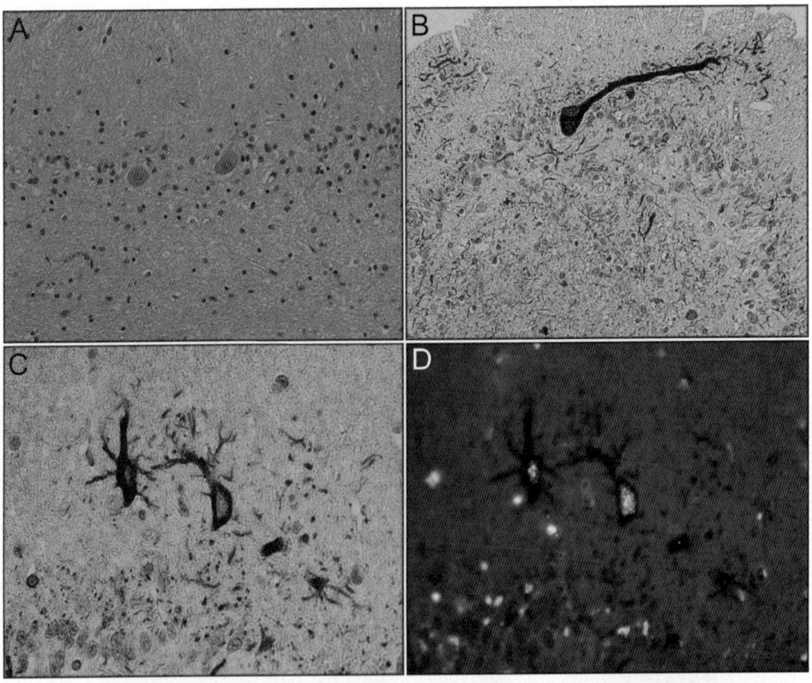

Figure 9.4 CLN5 disease, late infantile variant: cerebellar cortex with massive reduction of the number of Purkinje cells, absence of the granular cell layer, and Bergmann gliosis (HE) (A). Dendrites of the persisting Purkinje cells are strongly stained for neurofilaments (B, C) which clearly depict their shape which is either thickened linear (B) or torpedo like with pronounced arborization. Note that there are numerous autofluorescent lysosomes in the dendrites and in the astrocytes (D) easily demonstrable in immunostained sections (compare C with D). (A, B) ×20; (C, D) ×40.

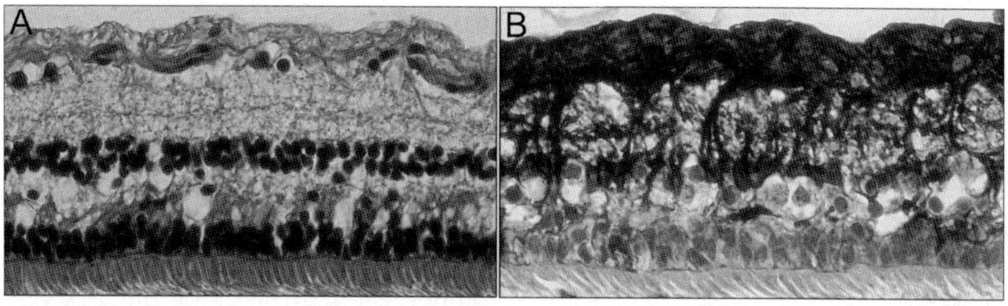

Figure 9.5 CLN5 disease, late infantile variant: retina. Absence of neurons in the ganglion layer. Neurons in both outer and inner nuclear layers are reduced. Note persistence of the photoreceptor layer (A). Pronounced astrogliosis (GFAP) dominates in the ganglion layer (B). (A, B) ×20.

Retinal pathology

In two siblings of Romany origin (M. Elleder, unpublished data), there was an overall reduction in the retinal thickness with a pronounced reduction of neurons in the ganglion layer. Generally, neurons in both outer and inner nuclear layers were reduced in number, but both layers remained separated. Occasionally, the neurons were reduced and both layers fused. Neurofilament staining showed reduced axons in the ganglion layer and irregular staining in the internal plexiform layer. The photoreceptor layer was only slightly altered, and the retinal pigment epithelium layer was minimally altered. Autofluorescent lysosomes were numerous in the remaining neurons of the ganglion layer, but were quite rare in the outer and inner nuclear layer neurons. Dispersed discrete storage lysosomes were interspersed with melanin pigment granules in the retinal pigment epithelium, and were absent in choroidal melanocytes. There was pronounced glial fibrillary acidic protein (GFAP)-positive astrogliosis with most in the ganglion layer, less in the nuclear layers, and least in the outer nuclear layer (Figure 9.5).

Histochemical, immunohistochemical, and biochemical features of the storage material

As with other NCL types, there was a notable increase in the size of the storage lysosomes in CLN5 disease. In paraffin sections the intraneuronal storage granules are autofluorescent, positive with Luxol fast blue, periodic acid–Schiff, and Sudan black B (Figures 9.6 and 9.7). As in CLN2 disease, classic late infantile (Goebel et al., 1996), the storage bodies show strong immunoreactivity for subunit c of the mitochondrial ATP synthase (Figure 9.8), but also for sphingolipid activator proteins A and D (Figure 9.9) (Tyynelä et al., 1997). Quantitative sequence analysis of purified CLN5 disease, late infantile variant brain storage material revealed that subunit c of the mitochondrial ATP synthase is the major component of the cytosomes (Tyynelä et al., 1997). Thus, CLN5 disease, late infantile variant is another form of NCL with subunit c storage.

Subunit c accumulation varies, due to the absence of this component in the fingerprint

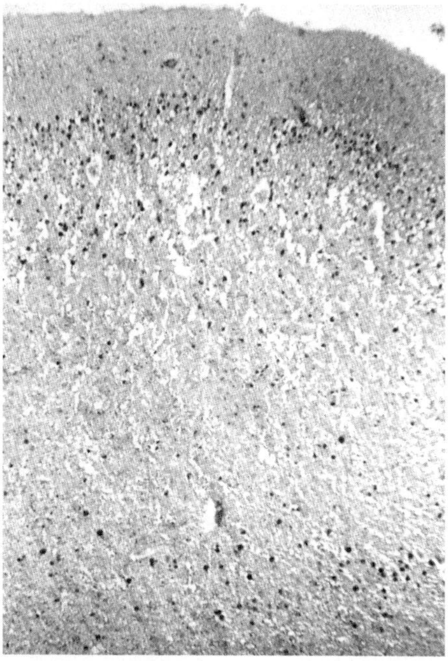

Figure 9.6 CLN5 disease, late infantile variant: pronounced cortical neuronal loss, particularly involving layers III–V, with spongy change. The remaining neurons show moderate-to-severe storage (black). Paraffin section, Sudan black B, ×35.

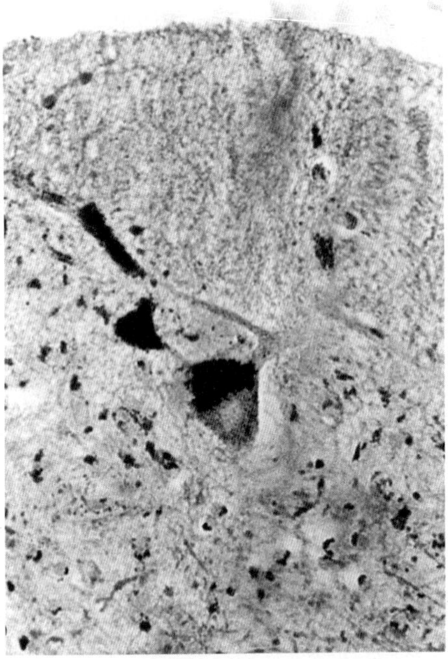

Figure 9.7 CLN5 disease, late infantile variant: storage granules in the dilated dendrites of a cerebellar Purkinje cell. Note complete loss of granule cells. Paraffin section, Sudan black B, ×200.

inclusions (see Chapter 4), and partly due to the so-called secondary transformation of the stored material, as in CLN2 disease, classical late infantile (see Chapter 7). Most of the storage lysosomes gave a strong immunohistochemical (immunoperoxidase) signal for cathepsin D, which blocked autofluorescence in sections mounted in proper mounting medium. Frequently, and especially for the larger storage lysosomes, the signal for cathepsin D was low or absent and the autofluorescence was easily detectable.

Most storage, as in other NCL types, was in the cerebral neuronal perikarya, in the cortical areas and also in the axon hillocks. Storage was generalized throughout the CNS. Much less autofluorescent storage was seen in astrocytes. Storage was discrete in the ependyma and in the plexus choroideus epithelium. It was barely detectable in the oligodendroglia. Microglial phagocytes contained mostly phagocytosed storage material. The main sequal of storage was neuronal degeneration.

Extracerebral storage

Extracerebral storage is generalized, of various intensities, manifesting autofluorescence, increased acid phosphatase activity, and increased cathepsin D immunohistochemical signal. It is especially pronounced in cardiomyocytes, peripheral neurons, skin eccrine glands, skeletal muscle, and in parietal cells of the gastric mucosa, and is less in hepatocytes, smooth muscle cells, kidney tubules, adrenal cortex, adipocytes, thyrocytes and pancreas. Subunit c is detectable only in lysosomal storage of higher intensity. Its absence, e.g. in hepatocytes, is not due to presence of fingerprint type inclusions. There are the beginning signs of hypertrophy of

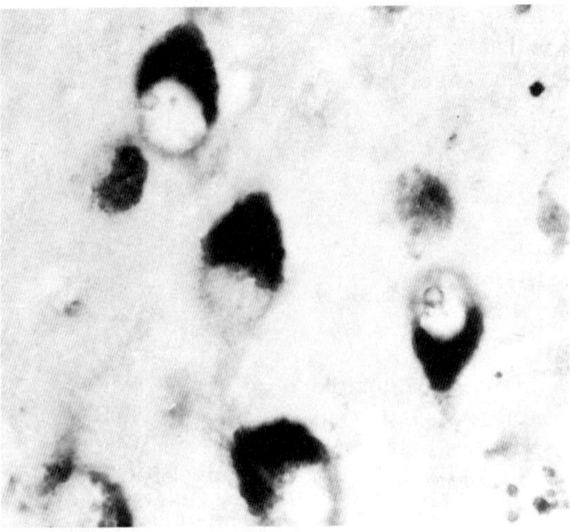

Figure 9.8 CLN5 disease, late infantile variant: cortical nerve cells show moderate amounts of storage granules immunoreactive for mitochondrial ATP synthase subunit c. Six-year-old male patient. Paraffin section, immunoperoxidase, ×500.

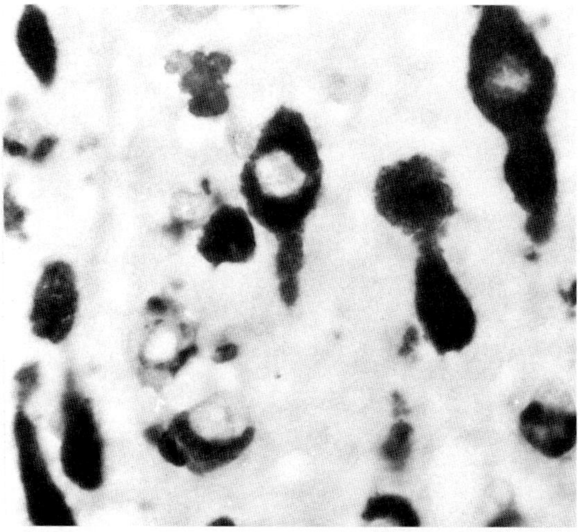

Figure 9.9 CLN5 disease, late infantile variant: cortical nerve cells show numerous axonal spindles filled with storage bodies immunoreactive for sphingolipid activator proteins A and D. Fourteen-year-old female patient. Paraffin section, immunoperoxidase, ×500.

cardiomyocytes. The distribution and immunohistochemical staining pattern of the storage material is similar to that in CLN6 disease.

Ultrastructure

As in all types of NCL, characteristic cytoplasmic inclusions (Figure 9.10) encircled by the lysosomal membrane are present in many different cell types (Santavuori et al., 1982). Their ultrastructure includes fingerprint (FP), and curvilinear (CL) profiles as in CLN2 disease, classic late infantile and CLN3 disease, classic juvenile. In addition, many of the inclusion bodies show a variety of features in which the FP or CL seem to be modified and dissolved to nondescript lamellar structures. These features correspond to the rectilinear (RL) complex (Figures 9.11–9.14).

Autonomic ganglion cells of the plexus of the vermiform appendix and rectum show well-preserved bodies with pure FP. They are indistinguishable from those seen in CLN3 disease,

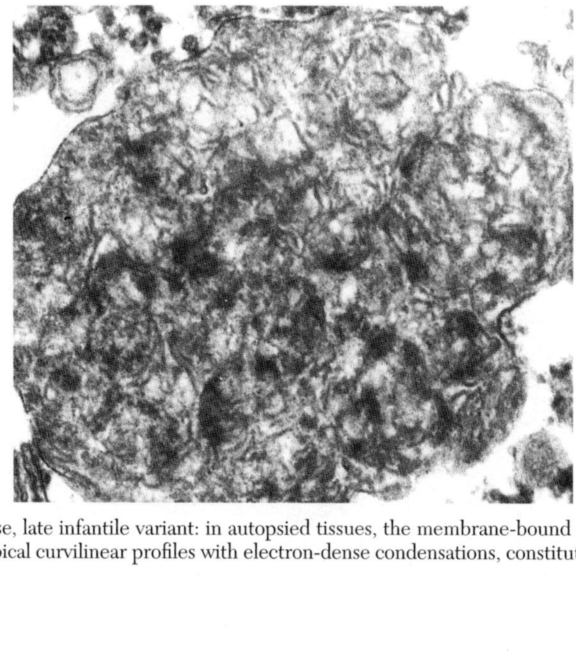

Figure 9.10 CLN5 disease, late infantile variant: in autopsied tissues, the membrane-bound storage cytosomes are composed of rectilinear or atypical curvilinear profiles with electron-dense condensations, constituting the rectilinear complex, ×20,000.

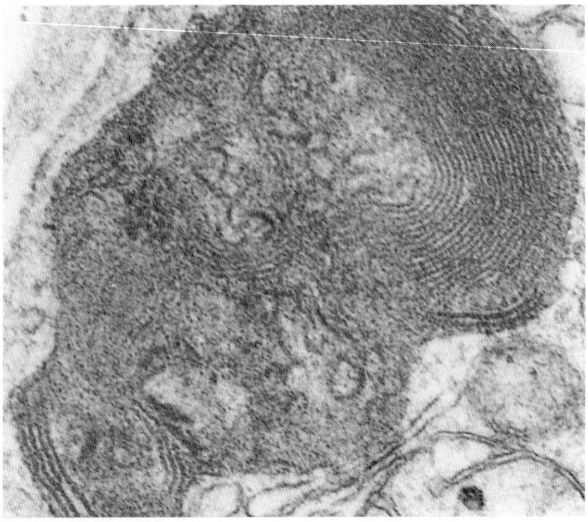

Figure 9.11 CLN5 disease, late infantile variant: cytoplasmic inclusions in an autonomic ganglion cell showing internal structure of FP, but straightening of the lamellae and dissolving to granular and circular structures in the middle part of the inclusion, ×22,000.

classic juvenile and other late infantile/early juvenile variants, with the possible exception that they are not within cytoplasmic vacuoles as found in many CLN3 disease, classic juvenile patients.

Extraneural cells (endothelium, pericytes, smooth muscle, Schwann cells) of skin and rectal mucosa show inclusions that are predominantly either classic CL-bodies or those of the RL complex. Blood lymphocytes contain inclusions with FP mixed with amorphic electron-dense globules (Figure 9.15) (Rapola and Lake, 2000). This observation corrects the findings presented in the original clinical and pathological report of the disease (Santavuori et al., 1982).

Essentially, there were no recognizable differences between the ultrastructure of CLN5 disease and that in CLN6, CLN7, and CLN8 diseases late infantile variants, or CLN3 disease, juvenile.

Cytosomes ultrastructurally compatible with NCL were found in the endothelial and pericytic cells of chorionic villi at the 14th gestational week (Rapola et al., 1999). The cytosomes were similar to those reported in a fetus with CLN3 disease, classic juvenile (Munroe et al., 1996).

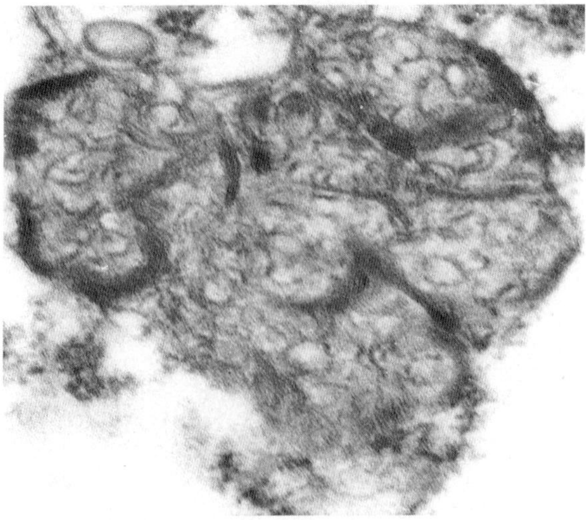

Figure 9.12 CLN5 disease, late infantile variant: cytoplasmic inclusion in a dermal sweat gland with the characteristic appearance of mixed FP and CL profiles, ×20,000.

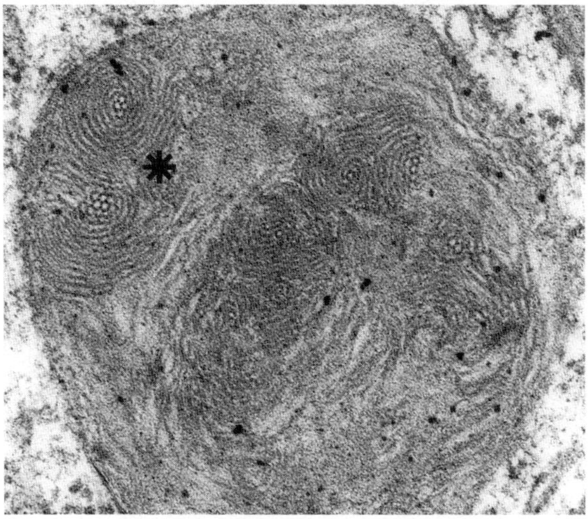

Figure 9.13 CLN5 disease, late infantile variant: cytoplasmic inclusion in an autonomic ganglion cell showing typical hexagonal lattice structure of FP (asterisk) and unwinding of the remaining part to a membranous lamellar body, ×24,000.

DISEASE MECHANISM

CLN5 is generally considered to be a soluble lysosomal glycoprotein, although it may also function elsewhere in the cell (Holmberg et al., 2004, Schmiedt et al., 2010). It has been suggested that the formation of complexes with other NCL proteins, such as CLN2/TPP1 (Vesa et al., 2002), and more recently with CLN1/PPT1, CLN3, CLN6, and CLN8 (Lyly et al., 2009), are functionally significant. Some mutations may cause CLN5 to be retained in the endoplasmic reticulum or Golgi apparatus, so that mutant protein does not reach the lysosome (Isosomppi et al., 2002, Lebrun et al., 2009, Schmiedt et al., 2010). Although there remains no defined role for CLN5, in general the consequences of its mutation are a relatively late infantile onset and slowly progressing neurodegenerative disorder, as well as later onset forms. Pathologically, human CLN5 deficiency displays a pronounced atrophy of the cerebellum and more generalized effects upon the cortical mantle (Savukoski et al., 1998, Haltia, 2003) and selective effects upon hippocampal neuron survival (Tyynelä et al., 2004). *Cln5* deficient

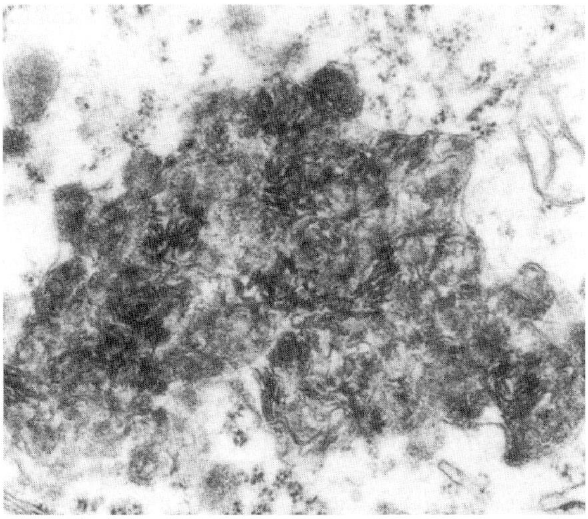

Figure 9.14 CLN5 disease, late infantile variant: a neuronal inclusion of the cerebral cortex showing structures compatible with the rectilinear complex. Biopsy specimen, ×14,000.

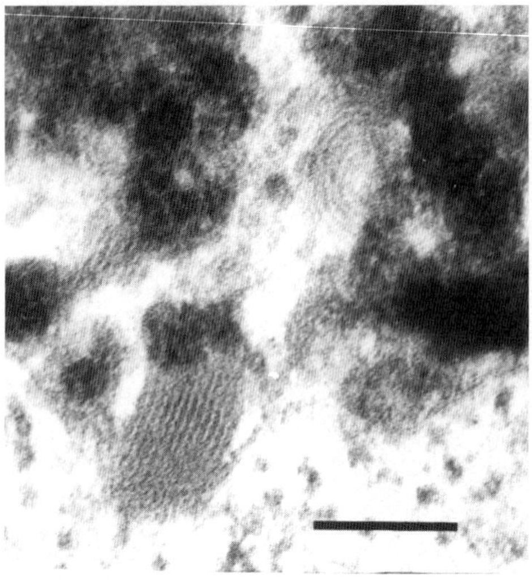

Figure 9.15 Finnish vLINCL: cytoplasmic inclusion in a blood lymphocyte with FP and amorphic electron-dense globules (bar 100nm).

mice also display a relatively slowly progressing neurological phenotype that includes the typical pathological features of murine NCL including selective effects on neuronal survival and localized glial activation (Kopra et al., 2004; von Schantz et al., 2009). However, compared with other forms of NCL, *Cln5* deficient mice are unique so far in displaying a significant loss of cortical neuron populations before effects on thalamic relay neurons become evident (von Schantz et al., 2009). Although gene expression profiling has implied that the same cellular pathways are affected in both *Ppt1* and *Cln5*-deficient mice (von Schantz et al., 2008), it is apparent that the consequences of mutations in *Cln5* are radically different in the thalamocortical system. The mechanisms that underlie this distinctive feature of CLN5 disease pathogenesis are currently unexplained, but these findings highlight that studying the relative staging of pathogenesis of different forms of NCL can be particularly informative.

CORRELATIONS

Genotype–phenotype correlation

Most mutations found in *CLN5* cause a late infantile variant NCL with very little variation in clinical phenotype. Patients carrying some combination of the Finnish major, Finnish minor, Dutch, or Swedish mutations (p. Tyr392X, p.Tyr75X, p.Asp279Asn, and c.669_670insC or p.Trp224LeufsX30, respectively) present the usual disease progression, although the consequences of these mutations on the protein level are predicted to be very different (Holmberg et al., 2000). A patient from Portugal, who was found to be compound heterozygous for the Dutch mutation and two novel mutations on the same disease allele (p. Gln189X and p.Arg112Pro), also shows a classic CLN5 disease, late infantile variant disease phenotype (Bessa et al., 2006).

However, mutations also cause disease with an onset in the juvenile age range; p.Arg112His was found in three siblings from a Colombian family, the first occurrence of a mutation of *CLN5* outside Europe. In these children, disease started at 9 years with visual failure rather than mental retardation as the presenting symptom and the disease progressed rapidly (Pineda-Trujillo et al., 2005). The fact that the missense mutation in these patients occurs in an amino acid that is also mutated in the Portuguese patient would suggest that the more conservative change of Arg to His in position 112 disrupts the function of CLN5 to a lesser degree than the change of Arg to Pro. One Spanish patient with onset at 7 years carried mutation c.1103–1106delAACA (Kohan et al., 2008). Two patients from Italy with an age of onset at 5 and 7 years, respectively, carried p.Tyr258Asp. Behavioural disturbances and mental deterioration were the dominant disease manifestations at onset (Cannelli et al., 2007).

Very recently, the same *CLN5* mutation, c.1121A>G or p.Tyr374Cys, was found in two patients with adult onset (both at 17 years, carrying mutations c.[377G>A]+[1121A>G]; c.[1121A>G]+[907-1094del188] respectively) (Xin et al., 2010). Using a separate sample, one of these patients had previously been found to carry a change (c.1883C>G, p.Thr628Arg) in the *CLCN6* gene on one disease chromosome (Poët et al., 2006) that had been postulated to modify the disease phenotype. In contrast, a child with infantile (4 months) onset carried mutation c.291_292insC (p.Ser98LeufsX13) (Cismondi et al., 2008).

Thus, mutations in *CLN5* should be considered as a possible cause in NCL with a wide range of onset.

Genotype–morphotype correlation

The usual phenotype of CLN5 disease, late infantile variant is characterized by storage material similar to that found in other late infantile variants and consists of FP profiles and CL bodies. Although the sample size of individuals with a disease progression that differs from that in the classic CLN5 disease, late infantile variant form is very small, there seems to be a distinction in the appearance of the storage material. Cells from the Colombian patients harbouring the p.Arg112His mutations were reported to contain only FP profiles, occasionally associated with lipid droplets, with no CL or RL profiles being found (Pineda-Trujillo et al., 2005). Three CLN5 disease, juvenile onset cases had only FP and CL (Xin et al., 2010). The storage material of the Italian patients carrying the p.Val258Asp mutation on the other hand was polymorphic and consisted of FP profiles, granular deposits, and variants of RL profiles (Cannelli et al., 2007), a pattern that was also seen in one of the adult onset patients reported by (Xin et al., 2010). The other had granular osmiophilic deposits and FP in different tissue types.

DIAGNOSIS

Diagnosis and differential diagnosis

At presentation, symptoms including learning disability, motor clumsiness, and visual failure, suggest the possibility of a neurodegenerative disease. The probability of NCL is further supported by ophthalmological, neurophysiological, and neuroradiological examinations. Early cerebellar and thalamic involvement on brain imaging, typical EEG abnormalities, together with the lack of vacuolated lymphocytes and supporting ophthalmological findings are highly suggestive of a late infantile variant. The diagnosis is confirmed by *CLN5* mutation testing.

Biochemical features and enzyme tests

None are applicable.

Gene mutation

Many disease-causing mutations have now been identified in patients with CLN5 disease (see above, and Chapter 20). The most common of these mutations, the 'Finnish major' mutation, c.1175delAT (p.Lys368Arg), together with another mutation, c. 225G>A (p.Trp75X), is now screened routinely in suspected Finnish patients (http://www.hus.fi/HUSLAB). Other mutations have been described in only a few patients of diverse ethnic origin, necessitating sequencing of the whole *CLN5* gene in non-Finnish cases.

Ultrastructure

The storage material, observed in tissues of patients with CLN5 disease, late infantile variant, consists of RL, atypical CL and FP profiles (Tyynelä et al., 1997). However, cases of later onset may be more heterogenous and also contain granular material.

Other family members, prenatal diagnosis, carrier diagnosis

Prenatal diagnosis can be carried out in fetuses at risk, by genetic screening of a chorionic villus sample. Electron microscopic examination may not reveal inclusion bodies in chorionic villus samples early in pregnancy (Rapola et al., 1999). In one case, cytosomes ultrastructurally compatible with NCL were found in the endothelial and pericytic cells of chorionic villi of an affected fetus at the 14th gestational week (Rapola et al., 1999). In Finland, where CLN5 disease, late infantile variant is more prevalent, carrier diagnosis is available after genetic counselling.

CLINICAL MANAGEMENT

Drug therapy

For epileptic seizures and myoclonus, the first choice of antiepileptic drug is valproate. If side effects develop, an alternative drug can be tried. Either lamotrigine or levetiracetam can be used as an alternative to valproate. However, if sufficient seizure control cannot be achieved with monotherapy, combination therapy is recommended: valproate–lamotrigine, valproate–levetiracetam, and lamotrigine–levetiracetam combinations have been used. Despite medication, epilepsy may become intractable with age. The addition of a third antiepileptic drug may be needed: usually clonazepam. Side effects of clonazepam, including hypersecretion, hypersalivation, and sedation, may be troublesome however. In prolonged seizures, phenobarbitone and benzodiazepines have been used. For myoclonic jerks, dystonia, and prevention of contractures, baclofen and tizanidine are useful

Feeding

Due to swallowing difficulties, slow eating, and weight loss, most patients eventually receive a gastrostomy. This helps to ensure adequate energy and fluid intake, as well as providing a route for reliable drug administration. In addition, the risk of aspiration may be reduced. Good nutritional state enhances general well-being and decreases the risk of decubitus.

Rehabilitation

In school, special classes and personal assistance are needed for children with CLN5 disease, late infantile variant. After school, most youngsters attend special day-care centres for the mentally disabled. Individual physiotherapy is important to support the ability to move around independently as long as possible. Later on, prevention of spastic contractures becomes important.

EXPERIMENTAL THERAPY

There is currently no curative therapy available for children and teenagers with mutations in *CLN5*. However, the identification that at least a portion of CLN5 is trafficked via the mannose 6-phosphate pathway (Sleat et al., 2005), means that therapeutic approaches that depend upon cross-correction, including gene therapy and stem cell transplants, are likely to be tested. Indeed, the availability of both mouse (Kopra et al., 2004) and large animal (Frugier et al., 2008) models of *Cln5/CLN5* deficiency means that the practical issues of scaling up therapeutic delivery can be directly addressed.

REFERENCES

Autti T, Raininko R, Launes J, Nuutila A, & Santavuori P (1992) Jansky-Bielschowsky variant disease: CT, MRI, and SPECT findings. *Pediatr Neurol*, 8, 121–126.

Autti T, Raininko R, Santavuori P, Vanhanen SL, Poutanen VP, & Haltia M (1997) MRI of neuronal ceroid lipofuscinosis. II. Postmortem MRI and histopathological study of the brain in 16 cases of neuronal ceroid lipofuscinosis of juvenile or late infantile type. *Neuroradiology*, 39, 371–377.

Berkovic SF, So NK, & Andermann F (1991) Progressive myoclonus epilepsies: clinical and neurophysiological diagnosis. *J Clin Neurophysiol*, 8, 261–274.

Bessa C, Teixeira CA, Mangas M, Dias A, Sa Miranda MC, Guimaraes A, Ferreira JC, Canas N, Cabral P, & Ribeiro MG (2006) Two novel CLN5 mutations in a Portuguese patient with vLINCL: insights into molecular mechanisms of CLN5 deficiency. *Mol Genet Metab*, 89, 245–253.

Cannelli N, Nardocci N, Cassandrini D, Morbin M, Aiello C, Bugiani M, Criscuolo L, Zara F, Striano P, Granata T, Bertini E, Simonati A, & Santorelli FM (2007) Revelation of a novel CLN5 mutation in early juvenile neuronal ceroid lipofuscinosis. *Neuropediatrics*, 38, 46–49.

Cismondi IA, Cannelli N, Aiello C, Santorelli FM, Kohan R, Ramírez AMO, & Halac IN (2008) Novel human pathological mutations: Gene symbol: CLN5: Neuronal Ceroid Lipofuscinosis, Finnish Variant. *Hum Genet*, 123, 537–555.

Frugier T, Mitchell NL, Tammen I, Houweling PJ, Arthur DG, Kay GW, van Diggelen OP, Jolly RD, & Palmer DN (2008) A new large animal model of CLN5 neuronal ceroid lipofuscinosis in Borderdale sheep is caused by a nucleotide substitution at a consensus splice site (c.571+1G>>>A) leading to excision of exon 3. *Neurobiol Dis*, 29, 306–315.

Goebel HH, Gerhard L, Kominami E, & Haltia M (1996) Neuronal ceroid-lipofuscinosis—late-infantile or Jansky-Bielschowsky type—revisited. *Brain Pathol*, 6, 225–228.

Haltia M (2003) The neuronal ceroid-lipofuscinoses. *J Neuropathol Exp Neurol*, 62, 1–13.

Heinonen O, Salonen T, Jalanko A, Peltonen L, & Copp A (2000) CLN-1 and CLN-5, genes for infantile and variant late infantile neuronal ceroid lipofuscinoses, are expressed in the embryonic human brain. *J Comp Neurol*, 426, 406–412.

Heiskanen M, Kallioniemi O, & Palotie A (1996) Fiber-FISH: experiences and a refined protocol. *Genet Anal*, 12, 179–184.

Holmberg V, Jalanko A, Isosomppi J, Fabritius AL, Peltonen L, & Kopra O (2004) The mouse ortholog of the neuronal ceroid lipofuscinosis CLN5 gene encodes a soluble lysosomal glycoprotein expressed in the developing brain. *Neurobiol Dis*, 16, 29–40.

Holmberg V, Lauronen L, Autti T, Santavuori P, Savukoski M, Uvebrant P, Hofman I, Peltonen L, & Jarvela I (2000) Phenotype-genotype correlation in eight patients with Finnish variant late infantile NCL (CLN5). *Neurology*, 55, 579–581.

Isosomppi J, Vesa J, Jalanko A, & Peltonen L (2002) Lysosomal localization of the neuronal ceroid lipofuscinosis CLN5 protein. *Hum Mol Genet*, 11, 885–891.

Klockars T, Savukoski M, Isosomppi J, Laan M, Jarvela I, Petrukhin K, Palotie A, & Peltonen L (1996) Efficient construction of a physical map by fiber-FISH of the CLN5 region: refined assignment and long-range contig covering the critical region on 13q22. *Genomics*, 35, 71–78.

Kohan R, Cannelli N, Aiello C, Santorelli FM, Cismondi AI, Milà M, Ramírez AMO, & Halac IN (2008) Novel human pathological mutations: Gene symbol: CLN5: Neuronal Ceroid Lipofuscinosis, Finnish Variant. *Hum Genet*, 123, 537–555 (552).

Kopra O, Vesa J, von Schantz C, Manninen T, Minye H, Fabritius AL, Rapola J, van Diggelen OP, Saarela J, Jalanko A, & Peltonen L (2004) A mouse model for Finnish variant late infantile neuronal ceroid lipofuscinosis, CLN5, reveals neuropathology associated with early aging. *Hum Mol Genet*, 13, 2893–2906.

Kousi M, Siintola E, Dvorakova L, Vlaskova H, Turnbull J, Topcu M, Yuksel D, Gokben S, Minassian BA, Elleder M, Mole SE, & Lehesjoki AE (2009) Mutations in CLN7/MFSD8 are a common cause of variant late-infantile neuronal ceroid lipofuscinosis. *Brain*, 132, 810–819.

Lebrun AH, Storch S, Ruschendorf F, Schmiedt ML, Kyttala A, Mole SE, Kitzmuller C, Saar K, Mewasingh LD, Boda V, Kohlschutter A, Ullrich K, Braulke T, & Schulz A (2009) Retention of lysosomal protein CLN5 in the endoplasmic reticulum causes neuronal ceroid lipofuscinosis in Asian sibship. *Hum Mutat*, 30, E651–661.

Lyly A, Marjavaara SK, Kyttala A, Uusi-Rauva K, Luiro K, Kopra O, Martinez LO, Tanhuanpaa K, Kalkkinen N, Suomalainen A, Jauhiainen M, & Jalanko A (2008) Deficiency of the INCL protein Ppt1 results in changes in ectopic F1-ATP synthase and altered cholesterol metabolism. *Hum Mol Genet*, 17, 1406–1417.

Lyly A, von Schantz C, Heine C, Schmiedt ML, Sipila T, Jalanko A, & Kyttala A (2009) Novel interactions of CLN5 support molecular networking between neuronal ceroid lipofuscinosis proteins. *BMC Cell Biol*, 10, 83.

Munroe PB, Rapola J, Mitchison HM, Mustonen A, Mole SE, Gardiner RM, & Jarvela I (1996) Prenatal diagnosis of Batten's disease. *Lancet*, 347, 1014–1015.

Pineda-Trujillo N, Cornejo W, Carrizosa J, Wheeler RB, Munera S, Valencia A, Agudelo-Arango J, Cogollo A, Anderson G, Bedoya G, Mole SE, & Ruiz-Linares A (2005) A CLN5 mutation causing an atypical neuronal ceroid lipofuscinosis of juvenile onset. *Neurology*, 64, 740–742.

Rapola J, Lahdetie J, Isosomppi J, Helminen P, Penttinen M, & Jarvela I (1999) Prenatal diagnosis of variant late infantile neuronal ceroid lipofuscinosis (vLINCL[Finnish]; CLN5). *Prenat Diagn*, 19, 685–688.

Rapola J & Lake BD (2000) Lymphocyte inclusions in Finnish-variant late infantile neuronal ceroid lipofuscinosis (CLN5). *Neuropediatrics*, 31, 33–34.

Santavuori P, Rapola J, Nuutila A, Raininko R, Lappi M, Launes J, Herva R, & Sainio K (1991) The spectrum of Jansky-Bielschowsky disease. *Neuropediatrics*, 22, 92–96.

Santavuori P, Rapola J, Sainio K, & Raitta C (1982) A variant of Jansky-Bielschowsky disease. *Neuropediatrics*, 13, 135–141.

Savukoski M, Kestila M, Williams R, Jarvela I, Sharp J, Harris J, Santavuori P, Gardiner M, & Peltonen L (1994) Defined chromosomal assignment of CLN5 demonstrates that at least four genetic loci are involved in the pathogenesis of human ceroid lipofuscinoses. *Am J Hum Genet*, 55, 695–701.

Savukoski M, Klockars T, Holmberg V, Santavuori P, Lander ES, & Peltonen L (1998) CLN5, a novel gene encoding a putative transmembrane protein mutated in Finnish variant late infantile neuronal ceroid lipofuscinosis. *Nat Genet*, 19, 286–288.

Schmiedt ML, Bessa C, Heine C, Ribeiro MG, Jalanko A, & Kyttala A (2010) The neuronal ceroid lipofuscinosis protein CLN5: new insights into cellular maturation, transport, and consequences of mutations. *Hum Mutat*, 31, 356–365.

Sleat DE, Ding L, Wang S, Zhao C, Wang Y, Xin W, Zheng H, Moore DF, Sims KB, & Lobel P (2009) Mass spectrometry-based protein profiling to determine the cause of lysosomal storage diseases of unknown etiology. *Mol Cell Proteomics*, 8, 1708–1718.

Sleat DE, Lackland H, Wang Y, Sohar I, Xiao G, Li H, & Lobel P (2005) The human brain mannose 6-phosphate glycoproteome: a complex mixture composed of multiple isoforms of many soluble lysosomal proteins. *Proteomics*, 5, 1520–1532.

Sleat DE, Sohar I, Pullarkat PS, Lobel P, & Pullarkat RK (1998) Specific alterations in levels of mannose 6-phosphorylated glycoproteins in different neuronal ceroid lipofuscinoses. *Biochem J*, 334 (Pt 3), 547–551.

Tyynelä J, Cooper JD, Khan MN, Shemilts SJ, & Haltia M (2004) Hippocampal pathology in the human neuronal ceroid-lipofuscinoses: distinct patterns of storage deposition, neurodegeneration and glial activation. *Brain Pathol*, 14, 349–357.

Tyynelä J, Suopanki J, Santavuori P, Baumann M, & Haltia M (1997) Variant late infantile neuronal ceroid-lipofuscinosis: pathology and biochemistry. *J Neuropathol Exp Neurol*, 56, 369–375.

Uvebrant P & Hagberg B (1997) Neuronal ceroid lipofuscinoses in Scandinavia. Epidemiology and clinical pictures. *Neuropediatrics*, 28, 6–8.

Vanhanen SL, Raininko R, Autti T, & Santavuori P (1995a) MRI evaluation of the brain in infantile neuronal ceroid-lipofuscinosis. Part 2: MRI findings in 21 patients. *J Child Neurol*, 10, 444–450.

Vanhanen SL, Raininko R, Santavuori P, Autti T, & Haltia M (1995b) MRI evaluation of the brain in infantile neuronal ceroid-lipofuscinosis. Part 1: Postmortem MRI with histopathologic correlation. *J Child Neurol*, 10, 438–443.

Varilo T, Savukoski M, Norio R, Santavuori P, Peltonen L, & Jarvela I (1996) The age of human mutation: genealogical and linkage disequilibrium analysis of the CLN5 mutation in the Finnish population. *Am J Hum Genet*, 58, 506–512.

Vesa J, Chin MH, Oelgeschlager K, Isosomppi J, DellAngelica EC, Jalanko A, & Peltonen L (2002) Neuronal ceroid lipofuscinoses are connected at molecular level: interaction of CLN5 protein with CLN2 and CLN3. *Mol Biol Cell*, 13, 2410–2420.

von Schantz C, Kielar C, Hansen SN, Pontikis CC, Alexander NA, Kopra O, Jalanko A, & Cooper JD (2009) Progressive thalamocortical neuron loss in Cln5 deficient mice: Distinct effects in Finnish variant late infantile NCL. *Neurobiol Dis*, 34, 308–319.

von Schantz C, Saharinen J, Kopra O, Cooper JD, Gentile M, Hovatta I, Peltonen L, & Jalanko A (2008) Brain gene expression profiles of Cln1 and Cln5 deficient mice unravels common molecular pathways underlying neuronal degeneration in NCL diseases. *BMC Genomics*, 9, 146.

Xin W, Mullen TE, Kiely R, Min J, Feng X, Cao Y, O'Malley L, Shen Y, Chu-Shore C, Mole SE, Goebel HH, & Sims K (2010) CLN5 mutations are frequent in juvenile and late-onset non-Finnish patients with NCL. *Neurology*, 74, 565–571.

Chapter 10

CLN6

J. Alroy, T. Braulke, I.A. Cismondi, J.D. Cooper, D. Creegan, M. Elleder, C. Kitzmüller, R. Kohan, A. Kohlschütter, S.E Mole, I. Noher de Halac, R. Pfannl, A. Quitsch, and A. Schulz

INTRODUCTION

Mutations in *CLN6* cause one of the earliest variant NCLs recognized (Lake and Cavanagh, 1978), originally termed early juvenile NCL, and are now known to underlie one of the many types of late infantile variant NCLs. Patients are of diverse ethnic origin. The function of CLN6 is unknown.

MOLECULAR GENETICS

Gene identification

The gene for a late infantile variant form of NCL, *CLN6*, was mapped to chromosome 15q21–23 by homozygosity mapping in two consanguineous families of Indian origin (Sharp et al., 1997). Refined genetic mapping in an extended group of 31 variant families led to the *CLN6* critical region being narrowed to less than 1cM between markers *D15S988* and *D15S1000* (Sharp et al., 1999, Sharp et al., 2001). A BAC contig of cloned genomic DNA was constructed across this critical region (Sharp et al., 2001) and new polymorphic markers derived that were used to further refine the critical region to a distance which was encompassed by seven BACs. At the same time, a common haplotype was identified in a subset of CLN6 disease families from Costa Rica that was estimated to span approximately 1.6Mb (Gao et al., 2002). Genes and transcripts were identified using homology searches and gene prediction programs, and included known and novel genes. The *CLN6* gene was finally identified independently by two groups, by sequencing DNA from patients to identify mutations in these genes (Gao et al., 2002, Wheeler et al., 2002). The gene mutated in the *nclf* mouse model was identified at the same time (Gao et al., 2002, Wheeler et al., 2002).

Gene structure

CLN6 comprises seven exons which span a genomic region of approximately 22kb. The open reading frame is 936 nucleotides, which encodes a 311-amino acid protein with seven predicted transmembrane domains (Gao et al., 2002, Wheeler et al., 2002). There is 90% identity between the human and mouse sequences.

Transcripts of nearly 2.4kb and 3.7kb are present in all human tissues tested (Gao et al., 2002, Wheeler et al., 2002). Additional ones of 1.1kb and 5.9kb may be present in skeletal muscle (Wheeler et al., 2002).

Mutation spectrum

Forty-one mutations have been reported to cause CLN6 disease (Gao et al., 2002, Wheeler et al., 2002, Sharp et al., 2003, Teixeira et al., 2003, Siintola et al., 2005, Cismondi et al., 2008, Al-Muhaizea et al., 2009, Cannelli et al., 2009, Kousi et al., 2009; and others recorded in the NCL mutation database at http://www.ucl.ac.uk/ncl). These consist of 19 missense mutations, 14 small insertion and/or deletions predicted to cause frameshifts, or in one case affect splicing, one intragenic deletion that removes two exons, three mutations that affect splice sites, and four nonsense mutation.

One mutation (c.316insC), an insertion of a single cytosine in a run of six cytosine residues, is identical to that in *nclf*, the naturally occurring mouse model for CLN6 disease.

No major founder effect for CLN6 disease is observed, with many mutations in *CLN6* unique to only one family. Patients from the same country may share the same mutation (Sharp et al., 2003). The most common mutation is c.395–396delCT, which is found mainly in families from India, but also in those from Italy and Saudi Arabia. The second most common mutation is c.794–796delCCT, which is found in families from Sudan, Czech Republic, Italy, Turkey, Saudi Arabia. Diagnostic tests that detect specific mutations in *CLN6* may be worthwhile for certain populations (e.g. Costa Rica, Pakistan, Portugal, India).

mRNA studies in cultured skin fibroblasts from patients confirmed that the c.395–396delCT mutation resulted in a shorter transcript lacking exons 5–7. When compared to age-matched controls, levels of *CLN6* mRNA were particularly reduced in a patient heterozygous for c.[395–396delCT]+[715–718delTTCG],p.[Ser132CysfsX18]+[Phe329ProfsX29]) (Cannelli et al., 2009). The rate of synthesis and the stability of three other mutant CLN6 proteins were reduced in a mutation-dependent manner (c.368G>A, c.460-462delATC, c.316insC, predicted to affect transmembrane domain 3 (p.Gly123Asp), cytoplasmic loop 2 (p.Ile154del) or result in a truncated membrane protein (p.Arg106ProfsX26), respectively) (Kurze et al., 2010). None of these three mutations prevented dimerization of the CLN6 polypeptides.

One polymorphism in *CLN6* has been reported.

Related genes

There are no related genes to *CLN6*. *CLN6* is confined to vertebrates, and mutations in the equivalent gene in mouse and sheep cause NCL in these animals (see Chapters 17 and 18).

CELL BIOLOGY

Protein structure

The *CLN6* gene encodes a highly conserved polytopic membrane protein of 311 amino acids (Gao et al., 2002, Wheeler et al., 2002). CLN6 contains an N-terminal cytoplasmic domain, seven putative transmembrane domains, and a luminal C-terminus (Heine et al., 2007) (Figure 10.1A). The 27kDa CLN6 exhibits no asparagine-linked glycosylation sites and can form homodimers upon overexpression (Heine et al., 2004, Heine et al., 2007) (Figure 10.1B).

Localization

CLN6 is localized in the endoplasmic reticulum (ER) (Heine et al., 2004, Mole et al., 2004). In neuronal cells, the protein is additionally found along neural extensions in subdomains of a tubular ER network (Heine et al., 2007) (Figure 10.2). Mutational analysis has shown that CLN6 contains two ER retention signals, one comprises the N-terminal 49 amino acids and a second dominant motif consists of the distal pair of transmembrane domains (Heine et al., 2007).

Two studies suggest that the proteosomal and lysosomal degradative pathways are sufficient to prevent the accumulation/aggregation of mutant CLN6 polypeptides in the ER (Oresic et al., 2009, Kurze et al., 2010). In one study, mutations (p.Gly123Asp and p.Met241Thr) caused rapid proteasome-mediated degradation of the CLN6 mutant proteins (Oresic et al., 2009), and in a second study, the particularly rapid degradation of the mutant protein arising from c.316insC (p.Arg106ProfsX26), which is an identical mutation to that in the murine *Cln6* gene in the *nclf* mouse model, was strongly inhibited by proteasomal and partially by lysosomal protease inhibitors.

Possible function

CLN6 represents a conserved protein among vertebrates bearing no known functional or sequence homologies with other proteins. Its function is currently unknown, and it is also unclear how mutations in the ER protein CLN6 lead to lysosomal dysfunction. This is, however, not without precedent because the deficiency in the activity of formylglycine-generating enzyme that is essential for a specific post-translational modification of lysosomal sulfatases results in a severe lysosomal storage disorder (Dierks et al., 2005). In CLN6 defective cells the activities of several lysosomal hydrolases and the sorting and proteolytic cleavage of the newly synthesized lysosomal proteinase cathepsin D is normal (Sleat et al., 1998, Heine et al., 2004). This indicates that neither trafficking nor processing of lysosomal hydrolases tested was affected by mutant CLN6. However, it was shown that the lysosomal degradation of an endocytosed protein was reduced suggesting an impaired lysosomal function which is in agreement with findings on increased lysosomal pH in fibroblasts in CLN6 disease patients (Holopainen et al., 2001). To provide clues about the function of the CLN6 protein, experiments were

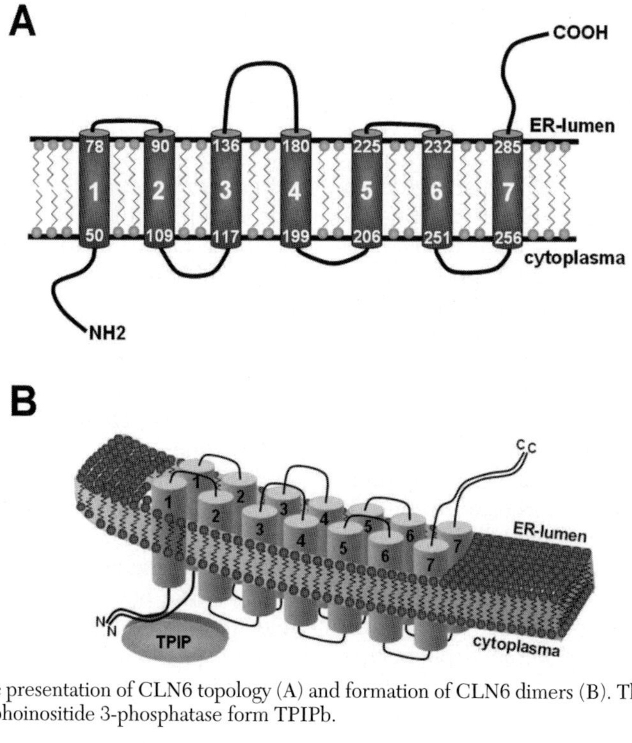

Figure 10.1 Schematic presentation of CLN6 topology (A) and formation of CLN6 dimers (B). The N-terminus of CLN6 interacts with the phosphoinositide 3-phosphatase form TPIPb.

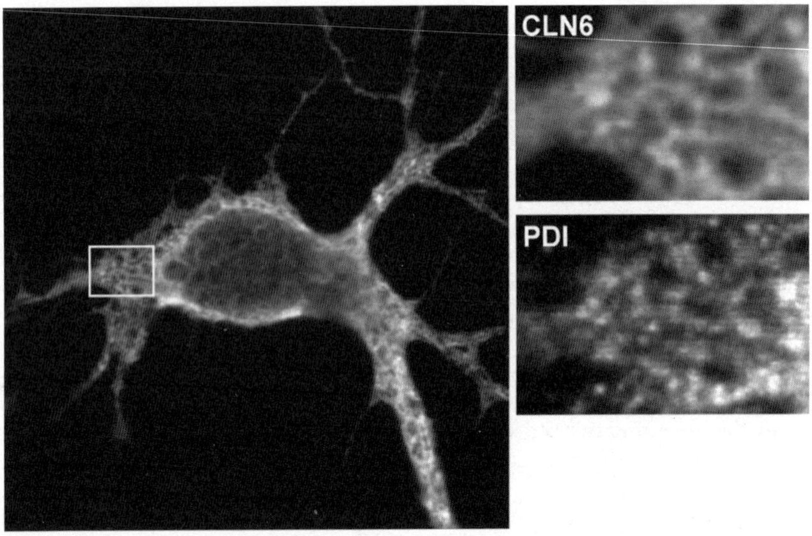

Figure 10.2 Localization of human CLN6 overexpressed in mouse hippocampal primary neurons. Neurons were double immunostained for CLN6 and the ER marker protein disulfide isomerase, PDI. The squares at the right represent a magnified view of the indicated region of the neuronal extension marked by the white rectangle (left) which were stained either for CLN6 or PDI. Note the tubular distribution of CLN6 which differs partially from punctate immunostaining of PDI.

carried out to identify proteins interacting with CLN6. Using the N-terminal 49-amino acid cytoplasmic domain of CLN6 as affinity matrix, the β form of the TPTE and PTEN homologous inositol lipid phosphatase (TPIP) was purified from HEK293 cells (A. Quitsch, personal communication) (Figure 10.1B). TPIP catalyses the conversion of phosphatidylinositol 3,4,5 trisphosphate (PtdIns3,4,5P_3) to PtdIns4,5P_2, an important component of transport vesicles that binds directly to the endocytic adaptor protein AP-2 (Honing et al., 2005). Alterations in the concentration and distribution of phosphoinositides in CLN6 defective cells may result in impaired trafficking of proteins along specific routes.

CLN6, along with other NCL proteins, has been reported to interact with CLN5 (Lyly et al., 2009). CLN6 also interacts with collapsin response mediator protein-2 (CRMP-2), and the CRMP-2 protein level is reduced in the *nclf* mouse brain, particularly in the thalamus (Benedict et al., 2009). This may cause alterations in neurite maturation since the maturation of *nclf* hippocampal neurons was reduced.

There are natural animal models (*nclf* mouse, the New Zealand South Hampshire sheep (OCLN6) and the Merino sheep) carrying defects in the orthologous *CLN6* genes. The course of their neurodegenerative phenotype resembles human CLN6 disease. Therefore, these animals provide a valuable resource for understanding the role of CLN6 for normal brain physiology (Jolly et al., 1989, Bronson et al., 1998, Gao et al., 2002, Wheeler et al., 2002, Tammen et al., 2006). Indeed, with a larger more complex brain than mice, the sheep brain is better suited for modelling human disease (Tammen et al., 2006). This complexity has revealed more pronounced phenotypes in CLN6 deficient sheep, with connectivity being the major determinant of which neuron populations are lost (Oswald et al., 2008). This neuron loss is preceded by an early prominent activation of astrocytes and microglia in presymptomatic sheep, and is most pronounced in the occipital and somatosensory cortex (Oswald et al., 2005). Activated microglia serve as indicators of local neuronal damage predicting subsequent degeneration of neurons and might be linked to the upregulated expression of the radical scavenger manganese-dependent superoxide dismutase (Heine et al., 2003). In addition to fundamental discoveries about the nature of stored material (Palmer et al., 1986a, Palmer et al., 1986b), these sheep have also recently yielded valuable biochemical data about alterations in glutamate:glutamine cycling (Pears et al., 2007) and the amino acid composition and presence of neuropeptides within the cerebrospinal fluid (Kay et al., 2009).

Another approach to gain insight into the function of CLN6 and pathophysiological mechanisms underlying the disease, is the analysis of transcript profiles. Twelve genes have been reported to be upregulated in fibroblasts cell lines from CLN6 disease patients. These are involved in cholesterol homeostasis, extracellular matrix remodelling, and immuno/inflammatory response (Teixeira et al., 2006). Microarray studies of brain cortex from presymptomatic *nclf* mice revealed reduced expression levels of genes encoding GABA receptor subunits, components of intracellular vesicular transport machinery, and proteins involved in RNA metabolism (A. Quitsch, personal communication).

Lipid profiles were examined in different areas of brains from the *nclf* mouse models for CLN6 disease. This mouse, like *Ctsd*$^{-/-}$ mice, exhibited increased levels of GM2 and GM3 gangliosides (Jabs et al., 2008). However, other changes in the *Ctsd*$^{-/-}$ mice were not shared by the *nclf* mice.

CLINICAL DATA

CLN6 disease, late infantile is, from a clinical standpoint, a rare variant of late infantile NCL. Clinical features of CLN6 disease are similar to those observed in CLN2 disease, classic late infantile with a slight tendency to manifest later and with a somewhat more prolonged course. The onset of first symptoms in children affected by CLN6 disease can range from late infantile to early juvenile or juvenile age (18 months to 8 years) (Mole et al., 2005). While the age of onset and the rate of progression of symptoms in children affected by CLN6 disease may vary to some extent, the order in which symptoms develop is consistent in most cases. First symptoms comprise seizures and motor difficulties. As in CLN2 disease, classic late infantile seizures may be partial, generalized tonic–clonic, secondarily generalized, or sometimes absent.

Motor deterioration can present with ataxia, spasticity, and myoclonus. Early signs might initially be interpreted as developmental delay, but soon developmental regression becomes obvious. After a short period of 1–2 years, seizures and motor deterioration are followed by visual failure, loss of speech, and cognitive decline. During the later stages of the disease, children lose independent mobility and the ability to swallow. Many receive nutritional support using a nasogastric or gastrostomy tube.

Children affected by CLN6 disease have been identified in ethnic groups from several different countries including Argentina, Costa Rica, Greece, Italy, India, Morocco, North America, Pakistan, Portugal, Sudan, Turkey, and Venezuela. Particular *CLN6* mutations may predominate in certain ethnic groups and may influence age of onset and progress of the disease in these populations. Clinical data on patients with late infantile variant NCL have been published, but relatively few patients described have proven mutations in the *CLN6* gene (summarized in Table 10.1). Some earlier descriptions of patients with apparent CLN6 disease should be treated with caution as more recent data have shown that mutations in the *CLN5*, *CLN7*, or *CLN8* genes may cause a very similar disease phenotype, and these early patients have not all been characterized at a genetic level.

Children affected by CLN6 disease from Costa Rica, Portugal, Pakistan, the Czech Republic and Italy were compared (Sharp et al., 2003) (Table 10.1). Patients from Costa Rica generally carried the most frequent mutation, p.Glu72X, and their course of disease was rather uniform. Onset of first symptoms occurred between the ages of 3–5 years. Rapid progression of the disease led to visual failure, loss of ambulation, and frequent seizures by the age of 6–8 years. Death occurred between the ages of 14–17 years, which is later than in patients from other ethnic backgrounds. In five Portuguese cases described, the age at onset of symptoms ranged from 2.5–4.5 years, followed by onset of seizures at 3–5 years, visual failure at 4–6 years, and becoming bedridden by the age 6–8 years. The genetic background of these patients was similar, and they were all homozygous for the amino acid deletion p.Ile154del. These data show that some but not all differences in the clinical course of CLN6 disease can be associated with ethnic origin and the particular disease-causing mutation(s) within that population.

Neurophysiology

Few studies have described the neurophysiological findings in children affected by CLN6 disease in detail.

Table 10.1 Clinical course of CLN6 patients

Country of origin	Whole group	Costa Rica*	N. Portugal*	Pakistan*	Czech Republic, Italy*	Turkey#	Turkey#	New-foundland°
Number of families	25	7	3	3	5	1	1	5
Number of affected	33	7	5	5	6	2	1	7
Age at onset ofdisease	1.6-4.9 (27)	3-4.5 (6)	2.5-4.5 (4)	1.6-4 (4)	2-4.2 (4)	2.5 (2)		3.0-4.9 (7)
Age at onset of seizures	2.5-7.2 (25)	3-6 (5)	3.7-5 (3)	3-4 (4)	3-4.5 (3)	2.5 (2)	4 (1)	3.0-7.2 (7)
Age at visual failure	3-6 (17)	3-6 (6)	4.5-5.9 (2)	4 (1)	>4 (1)			4.0-6.0 (7)
Age at loss of ambulation	2-8 (15)	6-8 (6)	4.2-6.5 (4)	6 (2)	2-5.6 (3)			
Age at death	9-16.8 (17)	14.5-16.8 (4)	10.5-11.7 (4)	9 (2)				8.0-14.9 (7)
Mutation		p.Glu72X	p.Ile154del	c.316dupC	Not known	p.Tyr221X	c.542+ 5G>T	p.Val91Glu*fs*X42

Table modified (Sharp et al., 2003). Clinical symptoms of 33 CLN6 disease patients arranged as a whole group or as subsets according to country of origin and genetic data. Ages are given as ranges in years (number of cases for which data are available).
* data according to (Sharp et al., 2003).
# data according to (Siintola et al., 2005).
° data according to (Moore et al., 2008).

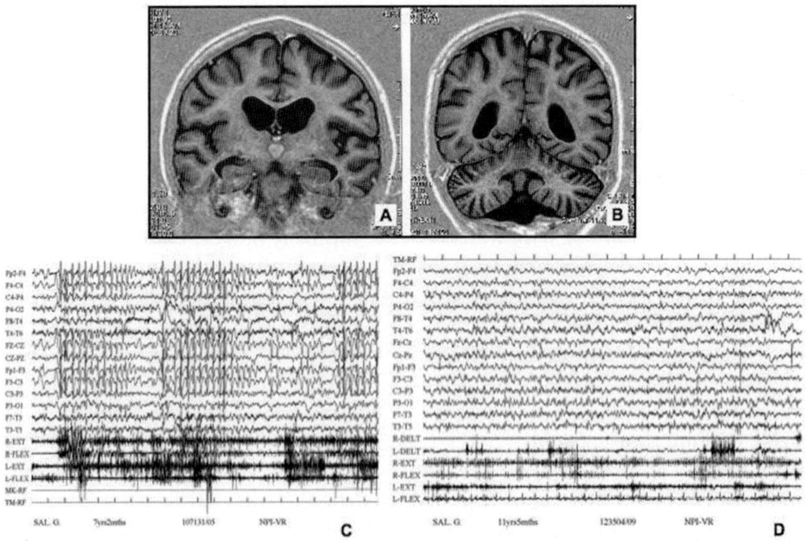

Figure 10.3 CLN6 disease, late infantile: in T_2-IR MRI coronal sections (A and B), of a child age 8 years, there is diffuse cortical atrophy involving both the cerebral and cerebellar hemispheres. The corpus callosum is thinned and the ventricular system is diffusely enlarged. EEG findings in the same child at age 8 and 12. At 8 years (C) there are subcontinuous bursts of slow spike–wave complexes of great amplitude often giving origin to an atypical absence, and diffuse deterioration of background activity with a predominance of delta-theta components. At 12 years (D) there are subcontinuous spikes and theta waves of small amplitude (involving the centroparietal regions, mainly of the right hemisphere) related to rhythmic myoclonias, generating a myoclonic status predominating on the right side. Figure provided by Professor Dalla Bernardina, Verona, Italy.

ELECTROENCEPHALOGRAM

As in CLN2 disease, classic late infantile, children affected by CLN6 disease can have an electro-encephalogram (EEG) showing high-amplitude discharges posteriorly in response to intermittent photic stimulation (Peña et al., 2001). The EEG of a child heterozygous for c.519delT and c.896C>T mutations, with a clinical onset at age 5, demonstrates changes as the disease progresses over a 4-year period (Figure 10.3). The EEG of a child from Argentina, at the age of 4 years, showed preserved background activity during wakefulness and sleep, with occasional 5–6 second bursts of high voltage slow waves and evidence of bilateral multifocal temporal onset and rapid generalization (I. Noher de Halac, personal communication). One patient with verified CLN6 disease from the Czech Republic had profoundly abnormal background activity with generalized spike-and-wave episodes (discharges), and no focal abnormality detected (M. Elleder, unpublished data).

ELECTRORETINOGRAM

There are relatively few reports of electroretinogram (ERG) results in children with CLN6 disease. They all state that during later stages of the disease the ERG becomes extinguished (Sharp et al., 2003). The child from Argentina, at aged 4, had mildly delayed visual evoked potentials and an apparently normal ERG.

Neuroradiology

Magnetic resonance imaging (MRI) in children affected by CLN6 disease shows progressive cerebral and cerebellar atrophy (Pena et al., 2001, Cannelli et al., 2009) (Figure 10.3), in this example 3 years after clinical onset. Hyperintense signals on T_2-weighted MRI scans have been seen in the periventricular white matter and hypointense signals in the thalami and putamina in a Costa Rican child affected by CLN6 disease (Peña et al., 2001). MRI in a presymptomatic child at around 3 years showed mild cerebellar atrophy (Cannelli et al., 2009). In a patient from Argentina (mutations p.Arg103Trp and p.Phe185LeufsX17) MRI was normal at 4 years, but by 6 years there were signs of cerebral and diffuse cerebellar atrophy, with no basal ganglia abnormalities.

MORPHOLOGY

Macroscopy

Gross findings from two children with CLN6 disease are described. The first is of a child (mutations c.[485T>G]+[794–796delCCT], p.[Leu162Arg]+[Ser265del]) who died at 7 years (M. Elleder, unpublished data). At postmortem, there was atrophy of the brain, with reduction (70%) of the brain weight to 883g (compared to 1263g of control weight). Macroscopically, there was moderate brain atrophy with dilatation of the ventricles, but no visible alteration of the cerebellum. In the cortex there was laminar degeneration variably expressed in the fifth cortical layer. The second brain belongs to a child (mutations c.[357–358insATC]+[890delC], p.[Ile119–Phe120insIle]+[Pro297LeufsX53], W. Xin and K.B. Sims, unpublished data) who died at the age of 13. At postmortem there was marked global brain atrophy with a weight of 455g (mean weight for age 1400g) and moderate cerebellar atrophy (Figure 10.4). Coronal sections of cerebrum showed thinning of the cortex and changes resembling cortical laminar necrosis and moderate ventricular dilatation (Figure 10.4). The white matter showed a firm, rubbery consistency.

Microscopy

In the 7-year-old child there was an increased number of lysosomes, which were distended with autofluorescent storage material (M. Elleder, unpublished data). Most storage, as in other NCL types, was in the brain neuronal perikarya, in the cortical areas and also in their axon hillocks. Storage was generalized throughout the cerebrum, cerebellum, brain stem, and spinal cord. Much less storage intensity was seen in astrocytes. Storage was discrete in the ependyma and the choroid plexus epithelium. It was barely detectable in the oligodendroglia. Microglial phagocytes contained mostly phagocytosed storage material. There was little extracerebral storage.

There was a notable increase in the size of the storage lysosomes in neurons. Subunit c

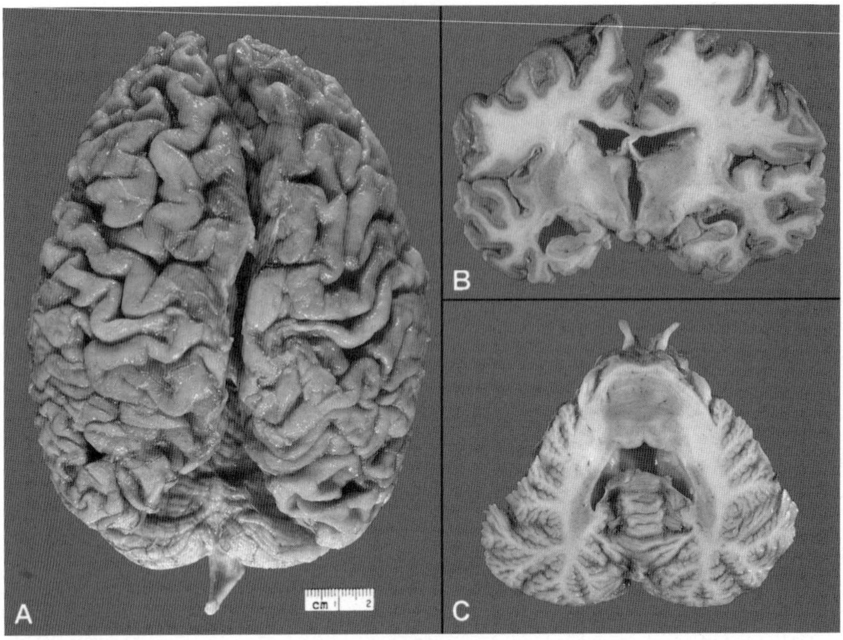

Figure 10.4 CLN6 disease, late infantile: 13-year-old patient. (A) Dorsal view showing moderate cortical atrophy with slender gyri and prominent sulci. (B) Coronal section at the level of the thalami highlighting cortical atrophy and ventricular dilatation. (C) Section of cerebellum and pons showing cerebellar cortical atrophy and fourth ventricular dilatation.

accumulation was not uniform, due to the absence of this component in the fingerprint inclusions, and partly due to the so-called secondary transformation of the stored material, unlike that in CLN2, classical late infantile disease (see Chapter 7). There was strong staining for concanavalin A positive lipid bound mannose, suggesting the presence of the oligosaccharyl diphosphodolichol (Elleder, 1989) in the storage neurons in CLN6, variant late infantile disease. Most of the storage lysosomes gave strong immunohistochemical (immunoperoxidase) signal for cathepsin D, which blocked autofluorescence in sections mounted in proper mounting medium. Frequently, and especially for the larger storage lysosomes, the signal for cathepsin D was low or absent and the autofluorescence was easily detectable.

In this 7-year-old child, neuronal loss was most apparent in the cerebral cortex (M. Elleder, unpublished data). In the entorhinal cortex the neuronal storage was accompanied by moderate neuronal degeneration. However, there was little degeneration in the hippocampus consequent to storage, in contrast to that in CLN7, variant late infantile disease. The basal ganglia and thalamus displayed neuronal storage, and most was present in large striatal neurons.

The cerebellar cortex displayed storage in all cell types (Figure 10.5) but without significant neuronal loss of either Purkinje cells or neurons of the granule layer. This was duplicated in a second case aged 12.5 years, suggesting that in some children with CLN6 disease, variant late infantile the cerebellar cortex is not significantly affected. However, in contrast, in a 13-year-old child described below, the cerebellar cortex is markedly abnormal. In the 7-year-old child, Purkinje cells displayed focal drop out. Storage was in the perikarya, and much less in dendrites, which were slightly hypertrophic, with occasional irregular focal distension. Staining for neurofilaments was increased (Figure 10.5). Clear-cut Bergmann gliosis was not apparent in the 7-year-old child, but was marked in the 13-year-old (see below). Astrocytes displayed moderate perinuclear storage. Microglial macrophages (CD68+), some of them enlarged, were present in low amounts. The dentate nucleus was gliotic (Figure 10.6) and had prominent neuronal storage with dispersed drop out of many neurons—these displayed a continuum of changes ranging from mild hypertrophy of the soma, frequently surrounded by an elaborate fine network of neuronal processes representing nerve preterminals (since there was

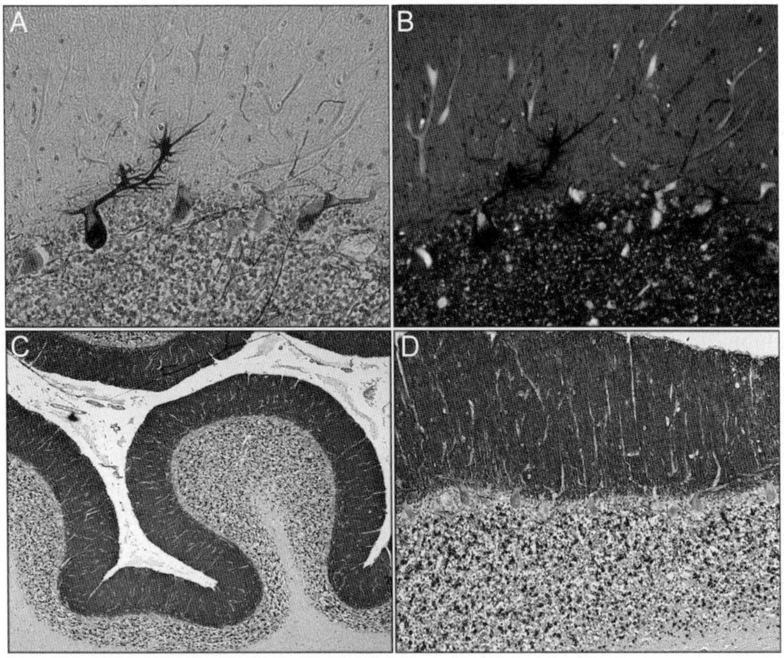

Figure 10.5 CLN6 disease, late infantile: cerebellar cortex with persisting Purkinje cells and neurons of the granular cell layer. Purkinje cells display accentuation of their dendrites by neurofi lament staining (A) and autofluorescence storage is demonstrated in the same immunostained section (B). Synaptophysin staining (C, D) shows absence of any substantial reduction of synapses in both molecular and granular cell layers. Note perfect preservation of the synaptic glomeruli in the granule cell layer. (A, B) Å~ 20; (C) Å~ 4; (D) Å~ 10.

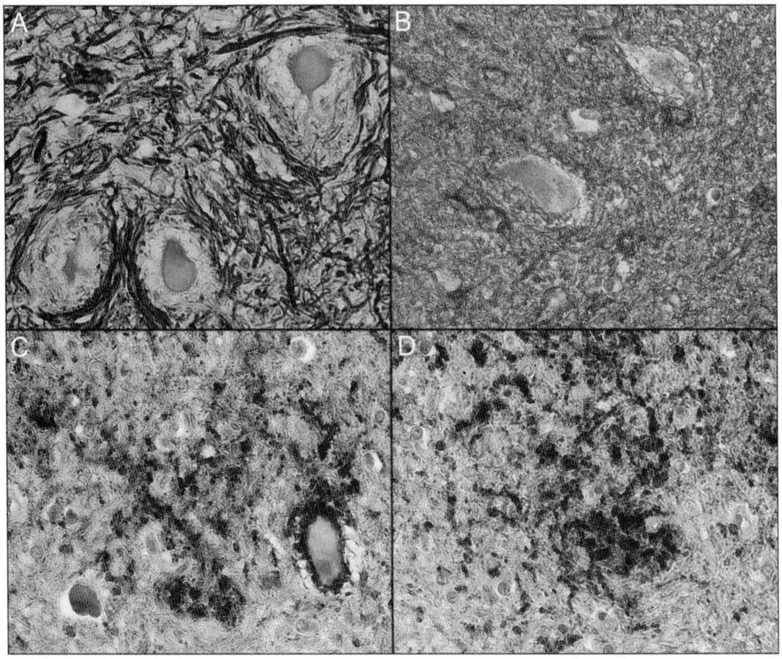

Figure 10.6 CLN6 disease, late infantile: dentate nucleus with storage and various degree of neuronal degeneration. The neurons are surrounded by a delicate network of nerve cell processes stained for neurofilaments (A), synaptophysin (C, D), and astrocytic processes stained for GFAP (B). (A–D) ×40.

strong staining for synaptophysin), to shrinkage and gradual disappearance. This resembles so-called grumose degeneration (Arai, 1989, Cruz-Sanchez et al., 1992), also found in CLN7 disease, variant late infantile. Occasionally there were neuronophagic micronodules composed of CD68+ microglial phagocytes. Similar, but less intensive changes were present in the olivary nucleus. Neuronal storage in the thalamus and the basal ganglia was prominent, most present in the large striatal neurons. Neuronal storage was seen in the bulk of neurons in the medulla oblongata, brainstem region, and in the spinal cord. There was partial drop out of spinal alpha motor neurons. Some of the neurons in the spinal medulla intermediolateral nucleus and in the substantia nigra displayed moderate storage frequently with prominent Nissl substance.

Another pathological feature in the 7-year-old child was astrocytosis, at sites with prominent storage and storage sequelae. Storage in astrocytes did not seem to interfere with their activation. The increase in microglial phagocytes (CD68+) suggests their activation. These frequently contained autofluorescent storage material, the bulk of which may have been scavenged as it was frequently seen in neuronophagic nodules.

In this 7-year-old case, there was discrete extracerebral storage visible by lysosomal accumulation of autofluorescent material, with variable immunohistochemically detectable subunit c. There was also a strong signal for cathepsin D. The list of tissues studied encompassed the peripheral nervous system, heart, liver, skeletal muscle, smooth muscle of the gut and of the vascular wall, adrenal cortex, thyroid, pancreas, skin eccrine glands, gastric mucosa (especially parietal cells), and adipocytes. The degree of extracerebral storage was much lower than that in cases of variant late infantile CLN5 and CLN7 diseases studied in parallel. Despite the low degree of storage in cardiomyocytes, there were initial signs of hypertrophy. Electron microscopy revealed, besides storage, a notable increase of mitochondria with seperation of myofibrils.

The neuropathology in a second child aged 12.5 years, with inferred *CLN6* mutations (from parents, c.[506T>C]+[310C>T]) was practically identical to the 7-year-old case, since the cerebellar cortex displayed only occasional dropout of Purkinje cells, i.e. the numbers of the neuronal cerebellar cortical populations were normal) (M. Elleder, unpublished data).

The findings in the 13-year-old child included a severe loss of neurons in the cerebral cortex, most apparent in the mid-layers, accompanied by reactive gliosis and neuropil loss, highlighted by staining for glial fibrillary acidic protein (GFAP) (Figures 10.7 and 10.8). Remaining neurons in the deep layers (layer 5) showed expanded cytoplasm containing granular and vacuolar material, highlighted by periodic acid–Schiff (PAS) reaction and Luxol fast blue stain (Figures 10.7 and 10.8). These granules were weakly positive for Ziehl–Neelsen acid fast stain. Others have reported positive staining with oil red O and Sudan black (Haltia, 2003, Beaudoin et al., 2004). Cortical neuron morphology ranged from large cells with abundant stored material and intact nuclei, to cells with pyknotic nuclei with chromatin condensation, karyorrhexis and spillage of cytoplasmic contents to the extracellular space, providing evidence of progressive neuronal death, i.e. apoptosis (Figure 10.8). Stored material was seen in all areas examined, including motor and sensory neurons in thalami, basal ganglia, midbrain, pons, and spinal cord. In contrast with the 7-year-old patient (see above), sections of the cerebellum showed marked devastation of the internal granular cell layer and loss of Purkinje cells as well as marked Bergmann gliosis. Remaining Purkinje cells show enlarged cytoplasm with stored autofluorescent material (Figure 10.8). There was striking variation in degeneration of white matter tracts. Extensive degeneration was observed in the corticospinal tract, in contrast with great preservation in proprioceptive, pain, and temperature tracts, cranial nerve III as well as the medial longitudinal fasciculus (MLF) and cross pontine fibres (Figure 10.7) (J. Alroy and R. Pfannl, unpublished data).

Disparity between these two well-studied cases could be due to differences in the extent of neurodegeneration that occurred during the disease, since one died at age 7 and the other at age 13, or to differences in the severity of the underlying mutations that affected disease progression.

ULTRASTRUCTURE

In CLN6 disease, late infantile variant the ultrastructure of the brain storage content is mixed and highly pleomorphic, i.e. rectilinear (short, long), fingerprint profiles and curvilinear-like deposits. Amorphous structures are present occasionally, resembling lipid-like hemidense droplets. Electron microscopic examination of cerebellar cortex from the 13-year-old child shows Purkinje cells with enlarged cytoplasm containing numerous membrane-bound secondary lysosomes packed with rectilinear bodies (Figure 10.9). Similar storage material is found in lymphocytes, endothelial cells, and pericytes (Figure 10.10). In the eccrine sweat gland epithelium of another child, a mixture of fingerprint, curvilinear, and dense bodies is present (Cannelli et al., 2009), usually within lysosomal structures but occasionally free in the cytoplasm. There is also evidence of vacuoles that are either empty or contain osmiophilic inclusions, e.g. in the cytoplasm of smooth muscle cells (Cannelli et al., 2009). The ultrastructure of CLN6 disease can be distinguished from that of CLN1 or CLN2 disease, but not from CLN3, CLN5, CLN7, or CLN8 disease.

A blood smear does not reveal any significant signs of lysosomal storage at the optical microscopy level. In one case, about 1% of lymphocytes displayed vacuolation, but not to the same extent as CLN3 disease, juvenile (M. Elleder, unpublished data). In other cases, lymphocytes in blood films were not observed to be vacuolated, and some contained storage material visible by electron microscopic examination (Cannelli et al., 2009).

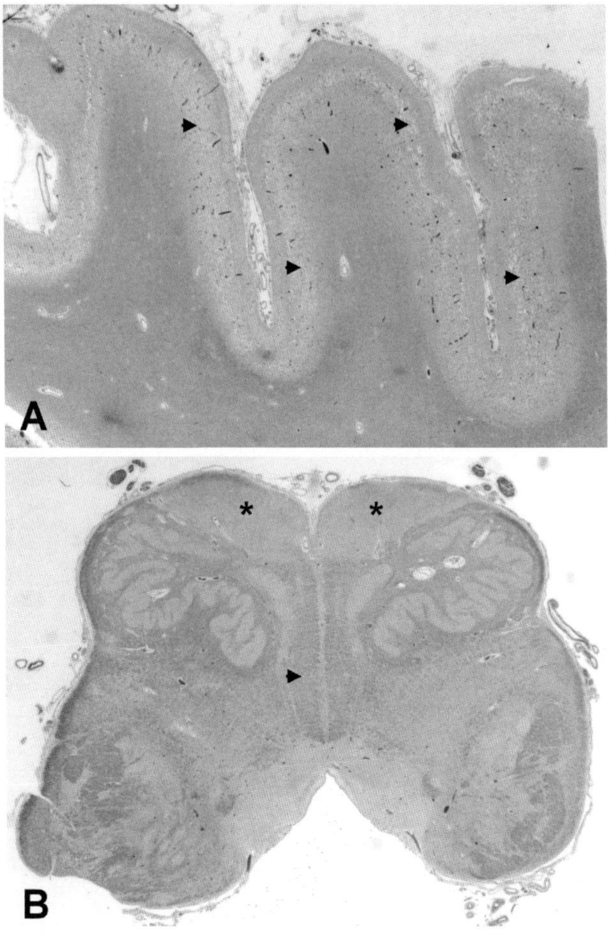

Figure 10.7 CLN6 disease, late infantile: 13-year-old patient. (A) Low-power view of cerebral cortex showing degeneration of primarily mid-layers of the cortex (arrowheads). (B) Cross-section of medulla at the level of inferior olivary nuclei showing marked degeneration of the corticospinal tracts (asterisk) and preservation of sensory tracts including proprioceptive tract (arrow head). Luxol fast blue–hematoxylin–eosin stain.

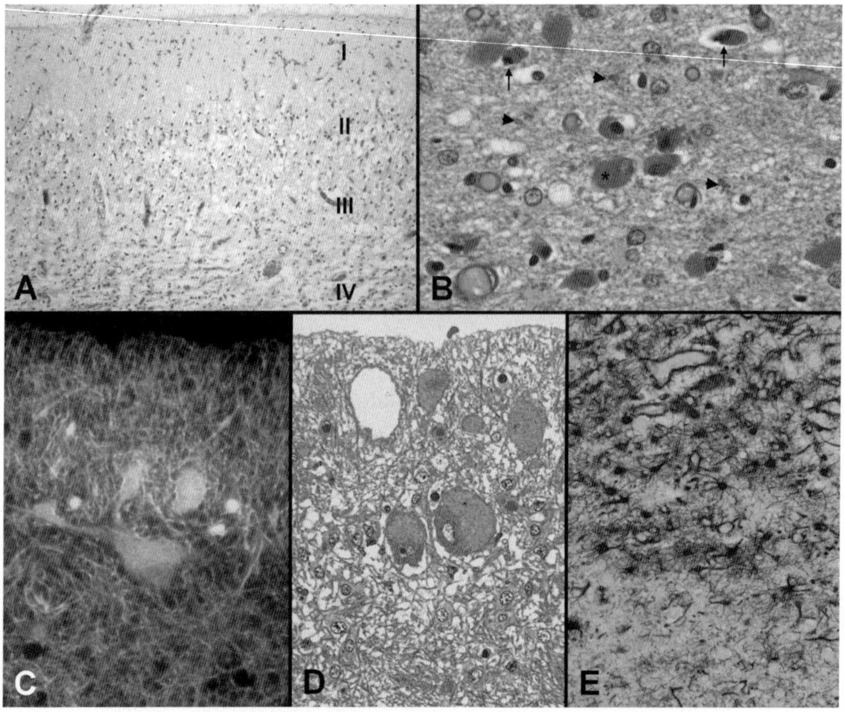

Figure 10.8 CLN6 disease, late infantile: 13-year-old patient. (A) Cerebral cortex demonstrating neuronal loss, particularly in mid-layers (III–IV) and blue-stained neuronal storage material (Luxol fast blue–hematoxylin–eosin). (B) Medium power photomicrograph of cerebral cortex highlighting PAS-positive granular cytoplasmic material (asterisk). Note pyknotic nuclei (arrow) and extracellular granular debris of storage material in neuropil (arrowhead). (C) High magnification of cerebellar cortex with autofluorescence of stored material. (D) Close-up view of epon-embedded cerebellar cortex highlighting finely vacuolated and granular cytoplasmic material in Purkinje cells (toluidine blue). (E) Reactive gliosis in cerebral cortex (GFAP).

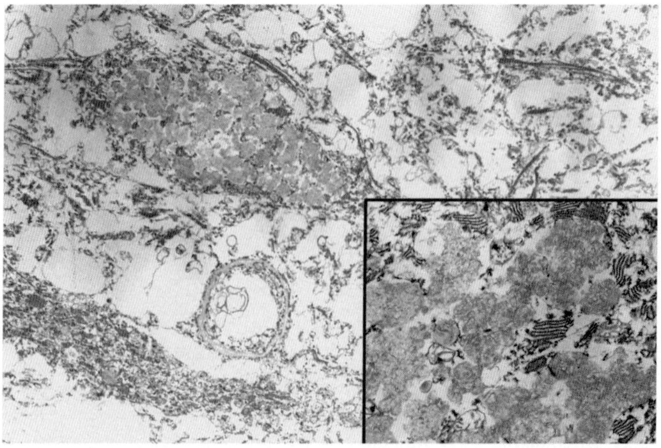

Figure 10.9 CLN6 disease, late infantile: 13-year-old patient. Low magnification electron micrograph of two cerebellar neurons illustrating numerous secondary lysosomes. Inset: close-up view of the lysosomes packed with rectilinear storage material.

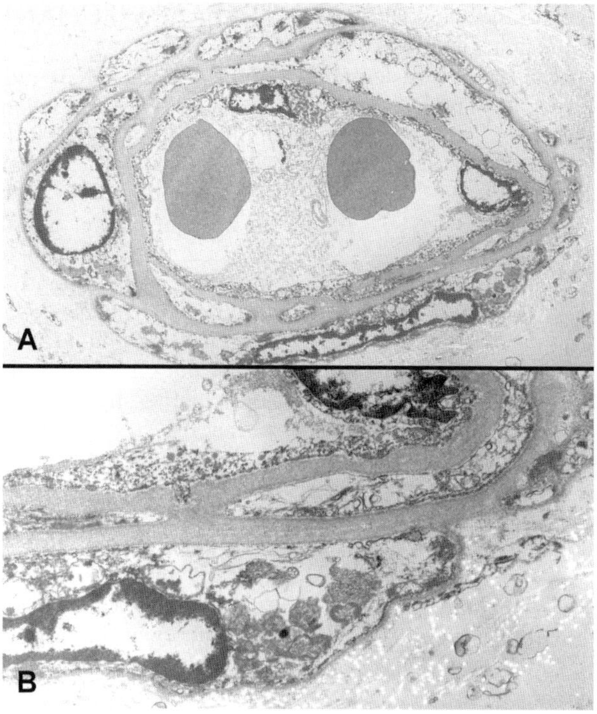

Figure 10.10 CLN6 disease, late infantile: 13-year-old patient. (A) Cerebellar arteriole at low power illustrating erythrocytes, endothelial cells and pericytes. (B) High magnification revealing the presence of secondary lysosomes filled with rectilinear material in pericytes.

RETINAL PATHOLOGY

In one patient with defined mutations there was neuronal depopulation in all retinal layers (Figure 10.11) (M. Elleder, unpublished data). The inner, and especially the outer, nuclear layers were greatly reduced and often fused into one irregular line. The photoreceptor layer was almost absent. The retinal pigment epithelial layer was reasonably preserved and only occasionally rarefied, with melanin-bearing CD68+ macrophages present in the vicinity, as well as deeper in the retina. There was little lysosomal storage, and what was present was most apparent in the remaining neurons of the ganglion layer—in other neurons it was discrete and barely detectable. Discrete autofluorescent lysosomes were seen in the retinal pigment epithelium, but

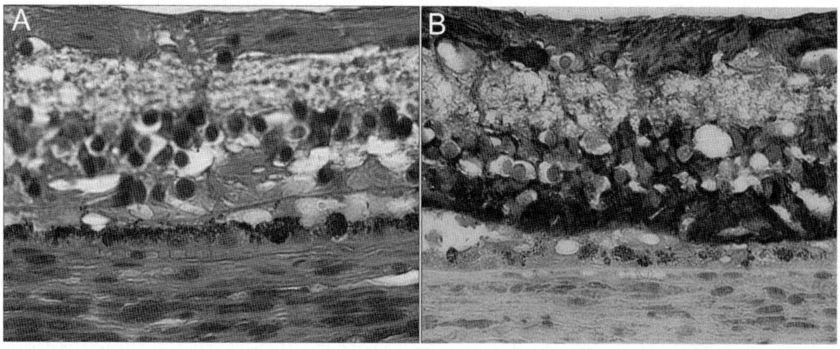

Figure 10.11 CLN6 disease, late infantile: section of the retina showing absence of neurons in the ganglion layer, pronounced depopulation of neurons in both outer and inner nuclear layers, sometimes fusing into a single disorganized line (A). There is strong staining for GFAP in both outer and inner retinal layers (B). Note absence of the photoreceptor layer and various degree of reduction of melanin in the retinal pigment cell epithelium. (A, B) ×20.

were absent in choroidal melanocytes. The ganglion layer and also the remaining neurons of the fused inner and outer nuclear layers were densely gliotic and GFAP-positive. Gliosis replaced even the missing photoreceptor layer. Neurofilaments were absent from the ganglion layer and strongly reduced in the optic nerve.

CONCLUDING REMARKS

The pathology of storage lysosomes in CLN6 disease, late infantile variant in terms of ultrastructure and immunohistochemistry, is indistinguishable from that of variant late infantile CLN5 and CLN7 diseases, and the general pattern of storage distribution is very similar. As in other NCL types, there is a differential sensitivity of neuronal populations with the highest effects in CLN6 disease being in the retinal neurons generally and in certain populations of cerebral cortical neurons. The cause of the sensitivity is unclear. It is worth mentioning that in CLN6 disease, late infantile variant there is remarkably less sensitivity, in comparison to variant late infantile CLN5 and CLN7 diseases, of cerebellar cortical neurons to storage. There even seems to be neurite hypertrophy in some neuronal population, which may be transient. Studies of further cases are needed, however, particularly those with prolonged disease course to determine if the cerebellar cortex remains spared.

Differential diagnosis

The morphological appearance and ultrastructure of the brain and visceral organs of patients with CLN6 disease, variant late infantile are essentially indistinguishable from those of CLN3, juvenile disease. The most helpful investigation is the examination of peripheral lymphocytes, which in CLN3 disease will always have a proportion displaying vacuolation. At the ultrastructural level, patients with CLN6 disease will have lymphocytes with condensed fingerprint profiles, but no vacuolation. These positive lymphocytes may not be plentiful, therefore, at least 100 cells should be examined.

The tendency to condensation should not be interpreted as transition to NCLs containing granular storage material. It is highly recommended that ultrastructural examination of multiple cell types is performed in order to make an accurate NCL diagnosis.

DISEASE MECHANISM

The key challenge in understanding the pathogenesis of CLN6 deficiency lies in linking how mutations in this ER protein (Mole et al., 2004), result in a lysosomal storage disorder. However, defects in CLN6 do appear to have an influence upon lysosomal function (Heine et al., 2004), although how these effects are mediated remains poorly understood. Elevated levels of manganese dependent superoxide dismutase (MnSOD) are observed in both human and ovine CLN6 deficiency, suggesting a role for oxidative stress and/or inflammatory cytokines in disease progression (Heine et al., 2003) and these findings have been replicated in *Cln6*^{nclf} mice (J. Cooper et al., unpublished observations). Characterization of CLN6 deficient South Hampshire sheep has proved particularly informative, revealing the early and remarkably localized activation of astrocytes and microglia that accurately predict the sites of subsequent neuron loss (Oswald et al., 2005). These reactive changes are already evident prenatally, demonstrating that effects upon the CNS start far earlier than was previously suspected (Kay et al., 2006). Consistent with other forms of human and murine NCL, South Hampshire sheep also display a complex pattern of progressive loss of interneurons (Oswald et al., 2008), revealing that cellular location and connectivity rather than phenotypic identity are the major determinants of neuron loss. The phenotype of *Cln6*^{nclf} mice broadly resembles that of South Hampshire sheep (Bronson et al., 1998), displaying many of the characteristic features of murine NCL including localized reactive changes, loss of thalamic relay neurons, and synaptic pathology early in disease progression (Kielar et al., 2009, Cooper et al., unpublished observations), but these phenotypes are markedly less pronounced than in CLN6 deficient sheep.

CORRELATIONS

Genotype–phenotype correlation

Most mutations in *CLN6* are associated with a broadly similar clinical course with an age of onset slightly later than for CLN2 disease, classic late infantile. However, two patients from one study (Cannelli et al., 2009) had onset at 2 years, with delayed language skills. There is some evidence that minor differences in the disease course can be correlated with the country of origin of the family and the disease-causing mutation (Sharp et al., 2003), and there is intrafamilial variation (Cannelli et al., 2009). It can therefore be speculated that the genetic background of patients has a modifying effect on the disease course. One patient, who carries p.Tyr221Ser on one allele and an as yet undefined mutation on the second allele, has been associated with a markedly protracted disease course (Sharp et al., 2003), with delayed onset of visual failure. Recently, a patient from Italy homozygous for p.Tyr221Cys had no visual failure by age 17 (Cannelli et al., 2009). This suggests that mutations that affect other regions of the CLN6 protein besides Tyr221 lead to visual impairment. In these patients, onset of epilepsy also seems to be delayed.

Genotype–morphotype correlation

There are no reports of differences in the appearance of the accumulating lipopigment in patients with different mutations in *CLN6*. However, within the group of NCL late infantile variants the distribution and ultrastructure of storage material in CLN6 disease is very similar to that seen in CLN5 disease and CLN7 disease. There have been some claims that accumulations of subunit c of mitochondrial ATP synthase are absent from hepatic, adrenal, and endocrine pancreatic cells in variant late infantile cases (Elleder et al., 1997), which is in contrast to CLN2 disease. Blood lymphocytes show no vacuolations but contain compact fingerprint-containing lipopigments as seen in CLN5 disease and CLN7 disease.

DIAGNOSIS

The diagnosis of CLN6 disease should be considered in any patient with a clinical picture of late infantile or early juvenile onset NCL with normal PPT1 and TPP1 enzyme activities and no lymphocyte vacuoles.

A diagnosis of CLN6 disease is based on clinicopathological findings and DNA studies. Before commencing genetic testing, electron microscopic examination of a skin or rectal biopsy or isolated blood lymphocytes should be performed to confirm the diagnosis of NCL. The ultrastructure of lipopigments in CLN6 disease comprises fingerprint and curvilinear profiles as well as rectilinear complexes.

The NCL Mutation Database (http://www.ucl.ac.uk/ncl) currently lists all mutations that have been described in the *CLN6* gene. Several recurrent mutations have been described in particular ethnic groups. The remaining mutations described have been family specific, and therefore in many populations the only option may be to screen the entire *CLN6* gene where possible in order to make a genetic diagnosis.

Differential diagnosis

Other NCL variants with late infantile or early juvenile age of onset should be considered in the differential diagnosis for CLN6 disease. CLN1 disease, CLN2 disease, and CLN10 disease can be excluded easily by enzyme analysis of PPT1, TPP1, and CTSD. Lymphocyte vacuoles are a hallmark of juvenile CLN3 disease and are not found significantly in CLN6 disease. Variant late infantile NCLs due to mutations in the *CLN5*, *CLN7*, or *CLN8* genes were originally thought to be confined to specific populations, but are now known to be more widespread and should be considered. Diagnosis of these variants is based on clinicopathological findings and DNA studies. Identification of the specific type of late infantile NCL is of great importance in order to provide genetic counselling for the affected families. Other progressive brain diseases to be considered are mentioned in Chapter 7.

CLINICAL MANAGEMENT

To date, there is no cure for patients with CLN6 disease. As in patients affected with all types of NCL, specialized palliative treatment and care can help to reduce suffering and to improve quality of life.

Anticonvulsants such as valproic acid, lamotrigine, and clobazam are recommended whereas phenytoin and vigabatrin should be avoided. Levetiracetam, piracetam, and zonisamide may be helpful for treatment of myoclonus. Spasticity should be controlled with baclofen in sufficient dosage.

As in classic CLN2 disease, late infantile, physiotherapists and occupational therapists should be involved in addition to paediatricians and paediatric neurologists in order to provide optional management.

EXPERIMENTAL THERAPY

As the function of the CLN6 protein remains unknown, no experimental therapy studies have yet been initiated. In addition, bone marrow transplantation has not been attempted.

REFERENCES

Al-Muhaizea MA, Al-Hassnan ZN, & Chedrawi A (2009) Variant late infantile neuronal ceroid lipofuscinosis (CLN6 gene) in Saudi Arabia. *Pediatr Neurol*, 41, 74–76.

Arai N (1989) 'Grumose degeneration' of the dentate nucleus. A light and electron microscopic study in progressive ranuclear palsy and dentatorubropallidoluysial atrophy. *J Neurol Sci*, 90, 131–145.

Beaudoin D, Hagenzieker J, & Jack R (2004) Neuronal ceroid lipofuscinosis: what are the roles of electron microscopy, DNA, and enzyme analysis in diagnosis. *J Histotechnol*, 27, 237–243.

Benedict JW, Getty AL, Wishart TM, Gillingwater TH, & Pearce DA (2009) Protein product of CLN6 gene responsible for variant late-onset infantile neuronal ceroid lipofuscinosis interacts with CRMP-2. *J Neurosci Res*, 87, 2157–2166.

Bronson RT, Donahue LR, Johnson KR, Tanner A, Lane PW, & Faust JR (1998) Neuronal ceroid lipofuscinosis (nclf), a new disorder of the mouse linked to chromosome 9. *Am J Med Genet*, 77, 289–297.

Cannelli N, Garavaglia B, Simonati A, Aiello C, Barzaghi C, Pezzini F, Cilio MR, Biancheri R, Morbin M, Dalla Bernardina B, Granata T, Tessa A, Invernizzi F, Pessagno A, Boldrini R, Zibordi F, Grazian L, Claps D, Carrozzo R, Mole SE, Nardocci N, & Santorelli FM (2009) Variant late infantile ceroid lipofuscinoses associated with novel mutations in CLN6. *Biochem Biophys Res Commun*, 379, 892–897.

Cismondi IA, Kohan R, Ghio A, Ramirez AM, & Halac IN (2008) Novel human pathological mutations: Gene symbol: CLN6. Disease: Neuronal ceroid lipofuscinosis, late Infantile. *Hum Genet*, 124, 324.

Cruz-Sanchez FF, Rossi ML, Cardozo A, Picardo A, & Tolosa E (1992) Immunohistological study of grumose degeneration of the dentate nucleus in progressive supranuclear palsy. *J Neurol Sci*, 110, 228–231.

Dierks T, Dickmanns A, Preusser-Kunze A, Schmidt B, Mariappan M, von Figura K, Ficner R, & Rudolph MG (2005) Molecular basis for multiple sulfatase deficiency and mechanism for formylglycine generation of the human formylglycine-generating enzyme. *Cell*, 121, 541–552.

Elleder M (1989) Lectin histochemical study of lipopigments with special regard to neuronal ceroid-lipofuscinosis. Results with concanavalin A. *Histochemistry*, 93, 197–205.

Elleder M, Sokolova J, & Hrebicek M (1997) Follow-up study of subunit c of mitochondrial ATP synthase (SCMAS) in Batten disease and in unrelated lysosomal disorders. *Acta Neuropathol*, 93, 379–390.

Gao H, Boustany RM, Espinola JA, Cotman SL, Srinidhi L, Antonellis KA, Gillis T, Qin X, Liu S, Donahue LR, Bronson RT, Faust JR, Stout D, Haines JL, Lerner TJ, & MacDonald ME (2002) Mutations in a novel CLN6-encoded transmembrane protein cause variant neuronal ceroid lipofuscinosis in man and mouse. *Am J Hum Genet*, 70, 324–335.

Haltia M (2003) The neuronal ceroid-lipofuscinoses. *J Neuropathol Exp Neurol*, 62, 1–13.

Heine C, Koch B, Storch S, Kohlschutter A, Palmer DN, & Braulke T (2004) Defective endoplasmic reticulum-resident membrane protein CLN6 affects lysosomal degradation of endocytosed arylsulfatase A. *J Biol Chem*, 279, 22347–22352.

Heine C, Quitsch A, Storch S, Martin Y, Lonka L, Lehesjoki AE, Mole SE, & Braulke T (2007) Topology and endoplasmic reticulum retention signals of the lysosomal storage disease-related membrane protein CLN6. *Mol Membr Biol*, 24, 74–87.

Heine C, Tyynelä J, Cooper JD, Palmer DN, Elleder M, Kohlschutter A, & Braulke T (2003) Enhanced expression of manganese-dependent superoxide dismutase in human and sheep CLN6 tissues. *Biochem J*, 376, 369–376.

Holopainen JM, Saarikoski J, Kinnunen PK, & Jarvela I (2001) Elevated lysosomal pH in neuronal ceroid lipofuscinoses (NCLs). *Eur J Biochem*, 268, 5851–5856.

Honing S, Ricotta D, Krauss M, Spate K, Spolaore B, Motley A, Robinson M, Robinson C, Haucke V, & Owen DJ (2005) Phosphatidylinositol-(4,5)-bisphosphate regulates sorting signal recognition by the clathrin-associated adaptor complex AP2. *Mol Cell*, 18, 519–531.

Jabs S, Quitsch A, Kakela R, Koch B, Tyynelä J, Brade H, Glatzel M, Walkley S, Saftig P, Vanier MT, & Braulke T (2008) Accumulation of bis(monoacylglycero)phosphate and gangliosides in mouse models of neuronal ceroid lipofuscinosis. *J Neurochem*, 106, 1415–1425.

Jolly RD, Shimada A, Dopfmer I, Slack PM, Birtles MJ, & Palmer DN (1989) Ceroid-lipofuscinosis (Batten's disease): pathogenesis and sequential neuropathological changes in the ovine model. *Neuropathol Appl Neurobiol*, 15, 371–383.

Kay GW, Palmer DN, Rezaie P, & Cooper JD (2006) Activation of non-neuronal cells within the prenatal developing brain of sheep with neuronal ceroid lipofuscinosis. *Brain Pathol*, 16, 110–116.

Kay GW, Verbeek MM, Furlong JM, Willemsen MA, & Palmer DN (2009) Neuropeptide changes and neuroactive amino acids in CSF from humans and sheep with neuronal ceroid lipofuscinoses (NCLs, Batten disease). *Neurochem Int*, 55, 783–788.

Kielar C, Wishart TM, Palmer A, Dihanich S, Wong AM, Macauley SL, Chan CH, Sands MS, Pearce DA, Cooper

JD, & Gillingwater TH (2009) Molecular correlates of axonal and synaptic pathology in mouse models of Batten disease. *Hum Mol Genet*, 18, 4066–4080.

Kousi M, Siintola E, Dvorakova L, Vlaskova H, Turnbull J, Topcu M, Yuksel D, Gokben S, Minassian BA, Elleder M, Mole SE, & Lehesjoki AE (2009) Mutations in CLN7/MFSD8 are a common cause of variant late-infantile neuronal ceroid lipofuscinosis. *Brain*, 132, 810–819.

Kurze AK, Galliciotti G, Heine C, Mole SE, Quitsch A, & Braulke T (2010) Pathogenic mutations cause rapid degradation of lysosomal storage disease-related membrane protein CLN6. *Hum Mutat*, 31, E1163–1174.

Lake BD & Cavanagh NP (1978) Early-juvenile Batten's disease—a recognisable sub-group distinct from other forms of Batten's disease. *Analysis of 5 patients. J Neurol Sci*, 36, 265–271.

Lyly A, von Schantz C, Heine C, Schmiedt ML, Sipila T, Jalanko A, & Kyttala A (2009) Novel interactions of CLN5 support molecular networking between neuronal ceroid lipofuscinosis proteins. *BMC Cell Biol*, 10, 83.

Mole SE, Michaux G, Codlin S, Wheeler RB, Sharp JD, & Cutler DF (2004) CLN6, which is associated with a lysosomal storage disease, is an endoplasmic reticulum protein. *Exp Cell Res*, 298, 399–406.

Mole SE, Williams RE, & Goebel HH (2005) Correlations between genotype, ultrastructural morphology and clinical phenotype in the neuronal ceroid lipofuscinoses. *Neurogenetics*, 6, 107–126.

Oresic K, Mueller B, & Tortorella D (2009) Cln6 mutants associated with neuronal ceroid lipofuscinosis are degraded in a proteasome-dependent manner. *Biosci Rep*, 29, 173–181.

Oswald MJ, Palmer DN, Kay GW, Barwell KJ, & Cooper JD (2008) Location and connectivity determine GABAergic interneuron survival in the brains of South Hampshire sheep with CLN6 neuronal ceroid lipofuscinosis. *Neurobiol Dis*, 32, 50–65.

Oswald MJ, Palmer DN, Kay GW, Shemilt SJ, Rezaie P, & Cooper JD (2005) Glial activation spreads from specific cerebral foci and precedes neurodegeneration in presymptomatic ovine neuronal ceroid lipofuscinosis (CLN6). *Neurobiol Dis*, 20, 49–63.

Palmer DN, Barns G, Husbands DR, & Jolly RD (1986a) Ceroid lipofuscinosis in sheep. II. The major component of the lipopigment in liver, kidney, pancreas, and brain is low molecular weight protein. *J Biol Chem*, 261, 1773–1777.

Palmer DN, Husbands DR, Winter PJ, Blunt JW, & Jolly RD (1986b) Ceroid lipofuscinosis in sheep. I. Bis(monoacylglycero)phosphate, dolichol, ubiquinone, phospholipids, fatty acids, and fluorescence in liver lipopigment lipids. *J Biol Chem*, 261, 1766–1772.

Pears MR, Salek RM, Palmer DN, Kay GW, Mortishire-Smith RJ, & Griffin JL (2007) Metabolomic investigation of CLN6 neuronal ceroid lipofuscinosis in affected South Hampshire sheep. *J Neurosci Res*, 85, 3494–3504.

Peña JA, Cardozo JJ, Montiel CM, Molina OM, & Boustany R (2001) Serial MRI findings in the Costa Rican variant of neuronal ceroid-lipofuscinosis. *Pediatr Neurol*, 25, 78–80.

Sharp JD, Wheeler RB, Lake BD, Fox M, Gardiner RM, & Williams RE (1999) Genetic and physical mapping of the CLN6 gene on chromosome 15q21-23. *Mol Genet Metab*, 66, 329–331.

Sharp JD, Wheeler RB, Lake BD, Savukoski M, Jarvela IE, Peltonen L, Gardiner RM, & Williams RE (1997) Loci for classical and a variant late infantile neuronal ceroid lipofuscinosis map to chromosomes 11p15 and 15q21-23. *Hum Mol Genet*, 6, 591–595.

Sharp JD, Wheeler RB, Parker KA, Gardiner RM, Williams RE, & Mole SE (2003) Spectrum of CLN6 mutations in variant late infantile neuronal ceroid lipofuscinosis. *Hum Mutat*, 22, 35–42.

Sharp JD, Wheeler RB, Schultz RA, Joslin JM, Mole SE, Williams RE, & Gardiner RM (2001) Analysis of candidate genes in the CLN6 critical region using in silico cloning. *Eur J Paediatr Neurol*, 5 Suppl A, 29–31.

Siintola E, Topcu M, Kohlschutter A, Salonen T, Joensuu T, Anttonen AK, & Lehesjoki AE (2005) Two novel CLN6 mutations in variant late-infantile neuronal ceroid lipofuscinosis patients of Turkish origin. *Clin Genet*, 68, 167–173.

Sleat DE, Sohar I, Pullarkat PS, Lobel P, & Pullarkat RK (1998) Specific alterations in levels of mannose 6-phosphorylated glycoproteins in different neuronal ceroid lipofuscinoses. *Biochem J*, 334 (Pt 3), 547–551.

Tammen I, Houweling PJ, Frugier T, Mitchell NL, Kay GW, Cavanagh JA, Cook RW, Raadsma HW, & Palmer DN (2006) A missense mutation (c.184C>T) in ovine CLN6 causes neuronal ceroid lipofuscinosis in Merino sheep whereas affected South Hampshire sheep have reduced levels of CLN6 mRNA. *Biochim Biophys Acta*, 1762, 898–905.

Teixeira C, Guimaraes A, Bessa C, Ferreira MJ, Lopes L, Pinto E, Pinto R, Boustany RM, Sa Miranda MC, & Ribeiro MG (2003) Clinicopathological and molecular characterization of neuronal ceroid lipofuscinosis in the Portuguese population. *J Neurol*, 250, 661–667.

Teixeira CA, Lin S, Mangas M, Quinta R, Bessa CJ, Ferreira C, Sa Miranda MC, Boustany RM, & Ribeiro MG (2006) Gene expression profiling in vLINCL CLN6-deficient fibroblasts: Insights into pathobiology. *Biochim Biophys Acta*, 1762, 637–646.

Wheeler RB, Sharp JD, Schultz RA, Joslin JM, Williams RE, & Mole SE (2002) The gene mutated in variant late-infantile neuronal ceroid lipofuscinosis (CLN6) and in nclf mutant mice encodes a novel predicted transmembrane protein. *Am J Hum Genet*, 70, 537–542.

Chapter 11

CLN7

M. Elleder, M. Kousi, A.-E. Lehesjoki, S.E. Mole, E. Siintola, and M. Topçu

INTRODUCTION

Mutations in *MFSD8* (*CLN7*) underlie one of the many types of variant late infantile NCL, and patients are of diverse ethnic origins. The function of MFSD8 can be predicted as a transporter, from its similarity with other proteins, but what it transports is not yet known.

MOLECULAR GENETICS

Gene identification

The *CLN7* locus on chromosome 4q28.1–q28.2 was identified following a genome-wide single nucleotide polymorphism (SNP) scan and homozygosity mapping in ten families of mainly Turkish origin. The underlying gene, *MFSD8*, was identified by demonstrating six homozygous mutations in one of the positional candidate genes (Siintola et al., 2007).

Gene structure

MFSD8 (GenBank accession number NM_152778) spans 48.24kb of genomic DNA (NCBI AceView, http://www.ncbi.nlm.nih.gov/IEB/Research/Acembly/). The gene consists of 13 exons (Figure 11.1), of which exons 2–13 contain a 1557bp open reading frame encoding a 518-amino acid polypeptide.

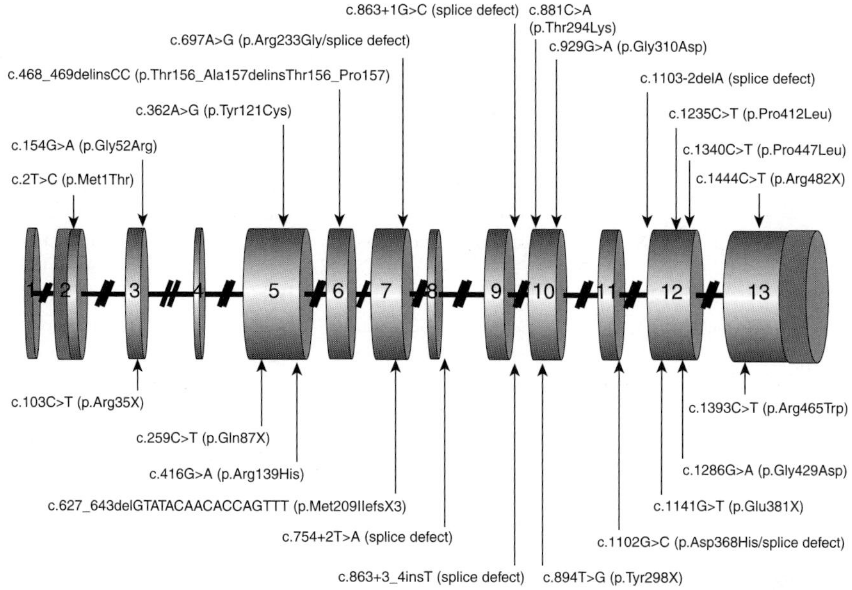

Figure 11.1 *CLN7* gene schema. Genomic structure of *MFSD8* and relative positions of the late infantile variant associated mutations. *MFSD8* consists of 13 exons (cylinders 1–13). The exons are shown to scale. The introns are shown as lines and are not to scale. The coding regions are shown in light grey and the untranslated regions in dark grey. The positions of the disease-associated mutations are indicated by arrows.

Mutation spectrum

There are currently a total of 22 mutations known in *CLN7*. These include 12 missense, four nonsense, four small insertions or deletions, and two that probably affect splice sites (Table 11.1 and Figure 11.1) (Siintola et al., 2007, Aiello et al., 2009, Aldahmesh et al., 2009, Kousi et al., 2009, Stogmann et al., 2009). Originally identified in a group of mainly Turkish late infantile variant NCL patients, *MFSD8* mutations have since been identified in phenotypically similar patients of various ethnic origins (Table 11.1). Two synonymous coding polymorphisms have been reported.

Related genes

The *MFSD8* encoded protein belongs to the major facilitator superfamily (MFS) of proteins. These are single-polypeptide transporter proteins that carry various small solutes (Pao et al., 1998). The substrate specificity (sugars, drugs, inorganic and organic cations, and various metabolites, etc.) varies between MFS phylogenetic subfamilies (Pao et al., 1998).

CELL BIOLOGY

Protein function and structure

MFSD8 codes for a 518-amino acid and approximately 58kD protein that is predicted to be a polytopic integral membrane protein with 12 membrane-spanning domains (Siintola et al., 2007) (Figure 11.2). Both N- and C-termini are in the cytoplasm, and there are two N-glycosylation sites at N371 and N376 (Steenhuis et al., 2010). MFSD8 contains a MFS domain (MFS_1). Based on this, MFSD8 may function as a transporter. Its substrate specificity, however, is currently not known.

Gene expression

MFSD8 is ubiquitously expressed with the main transcript of approximately 5kb, as shown on human multiple tissue Northern blot (Siintola et al., 2007). In some tissues, transcripts of approximately 1–3kb and/or of approximately 6kb are also detected. *MFSD8* has a complex splicing pattern with several alternatively spliced variants (Siintola et al., 2007). It is not known whether the alternatively spliced mRNA variants produce stable and/or

Table 11.1 *CLN7/MFSD8* mutations

Nucleotide change	Amino acid change/ Predicted consequence	Phenotype	Country of origin	References
c.2T>C	p.Met1Thr	Late infantile variant	Italy	Aiello et al., 2009
c.103C>T	p.Arg35X	Late infantile variant	Turkey Italy	Kousi et al., 2009 Aiello et al., 2009
c.154G>A	p.Gly52Arg	Late infantile variant	Italy	Aiello et al., 2009
c.259C>T	p.Gln87X	Late infantile variant	N. Europe	P. Ray pers comm
c.362A>G	p.Tyr121Cys	Late infantile variant but with no visual failure	Egypt	Stogmann et al., 2009
c.416G>A	p.Arg139His	Late infantile variant	India	Kousi et al., 2009
c.468_469delinsCC	p.Ala157Pro	Juvenile, protracted course into adulthood	Netherlands	Kousi et al., 2009
c.627_643del GTATACAACA CCAGTTT	p.Met209IlefsX3	Late infantile variant	Italy (Sardinia)	Aiello et al., 2009, Kousi et al., 2009
c.697A>G	p.Arg233Gly (or altered splicing)	Late infantile variant	Turkey	Siintola et al., 2007
c.754+2T>A	Altered splicing	Late infantile variant	Turkey Croatia Czech Republic	Siintola et al., 2007 Kousi et al., 2009 Kousi et al., 2009
c.863+1G>C	Altered splicing	Late infantile variant	Turkey	Kousi et al., 2009
c.863+3_4insT	Altered splicing	Late infantile variant	Italy	Aiello et al., 2009
c.881C>A	p.Thr294Lys	Late infantile variant	Turkey Roma from former Czechoslovakia Czech Republic Italy	Kousi et al., 2009 Kousi et al., 2009 Aiello et al., 2009
c.894T>G	p.Tyr298X	Late infantile variant	India	Siintola et al., 2007
c.929G>A	p.Gly310Asp	Late infantile variant	Turkey Italy	Siintola et al., 2007 Aiello et al., 2009
c.1102G>C	p.Asp368His (or altered splicing)	Late infantile variant	Turkey	Siintola et al., 2007
c.1103-2delA	Altered splicing	Late infantile variant	Czech Republic	Kousi et al., 2009
c.1141G>T	p.Glu381X	Late infantile variant	France	Aiello et al., 2009
c.1235C>T	p.Pro412Leu	Late infantile variant	Saudi Arabia	Aldahmesh et al., 2009
c.1286G>A	p.Gly429Asp	Late infantile variant	Turkey	Siintola et al., 2007
c.1340C>T	p.Pro447Leu	Late infantile variant	Italy	Aiello et al., 2009
c.1393C>T	p.Arg465Trp	Late infantile variant	Albania/Greece	Kousi et al., 2009
c.1444C>T	p.Arg482X	Late infantile variant	France	Aiello et al., 2009

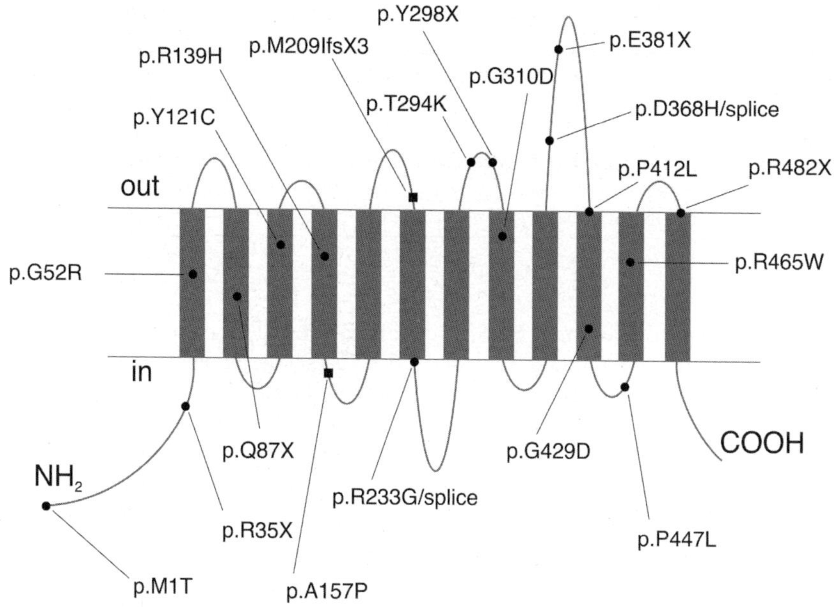

Figure 11.2 MFSD8 protein structure. The predicted topology of the MFSD8 protein with 12 transmembrane domains. The sites of the late infantile variant associated exon mutations are shown. 'Out' refers to the lumen of the lysosome and 'in' to the cytoplasm.

functional transcripts or if they represent a posttranscriptional regulatory mechanism of *MFSD8* expression.

Protein localization

In transiently transfected COS-1 and HeLa cells, HA-tagged MFSD8 protein localizes to the lysosomal compartment (Siintola et al., 2007). Lysosomal localization of MFSD8 requires a major consensus acidic dileucine-based motif in the N-terminus, two minor tandem tyrosine-based signals in the C-terminus, and additional, presumably unconventional sorting signals (Storch et al. 2010, Sharifi et al., 2010). MFSD8 follows the direct trafficking route of the endocytic pathway en route to the lysosomes, justified by recognition of the major dileucine-motif by AP1 adaptor coat protein complexes (Sharifi et al., 2010). Of the missense mutations tested to date (Table 11.1), none affect the subcellular localization of the MFSD8 protein (Siintola et al., 2007, Kousi et al., 2009).

Tissue distribution/expression

In Northern blot analysis, *MFSD8* was detected with very low expression levels in all tissues analyzed (Siintola et al., 2007). The ubiquitous expression is also supported by expressed sequence tags (ESTs) originating from various tissues. The expression of *CLN7/MFSD8*, along with other lysosomal genes, was altered in mice fed a high iron diet (Johnstone and Milward, 2010), perhaps reflecting the build-up of lipofuscin that can occur with iron overload or iron disorders.

CLINICAL DATA

Turkish variant late infantile NCL was first considered to be a distinct clinical and genetic entity (Wheeler et al. 1999). However, recent molecular genetic analyses have shown that several genes (at least *CLN8, CLN6,* and *CLN7/MFSD8*) underlie this late infantile variant phenotype (Ranta et al. 2004, Siintola et al., 2005, Siintola et al., 2007). Originally identified

Table 11.2 **Clinical features of CLN7 disease, late infantile variant**

Onset (years)	Late infantile (1.5–6)
Early symptoms	Seizures, developmental regression
Later symptoms	Myoclonus, epileptic seizures, motor, mental, visual, and speech impairment, ataxia, sleep and personality disorders, stereotypic hand movements
Disease course	Rapidly progressive, premature death

in a group of mainly Turkish patients, *MFSD8* mutations have since been identified in late infantile variant patients of various ethnic origins including France, Italy, Egypt, India, the Netherlands, Croatia, Slovakia, the Czech Republic, Saudi Arabia, Albania/Greece (Siintola et al., 2007, Aiello et al., 2009, Aldahmesh et al., 2009, Kousi et al., 2009, Stogmann et al., 2009; unpublished data) (Table 11.1). The prevalence of *MFSD8*-associated NCL disease is unknown.

The onset of symptoms in all but one patient with *MFSD8* mutations varies from 1.5–6 years (Topçu et al., 2004, Siintola et al., 2007, Aiello et al., 2009, Aldahmesh et al., 2009, Kousi et al., 2009, Stogmann et al., 2009) (Table 11.2). The presenting symptoms are most commonly seizures and developmental regression (Topçu et al., 2004, Siintola et al., 2007, Kousi et al., 2009, Stogmann et al., 2009). However, in three cases it was failing vision (Aiello et al., 2009, Aldahmesh et al., 2009), and in three cases it was motor regression (Aiello et al., 2009).

The progress of the disease is rapid and various symptoms develop in the majority of patients early in the disease course. These include motor and cognitive regression, speech impairment, seizures, visual failure, ataxia, and myoclonus (Kousi et al., 2009). However, one family had no visual failure (Stogmann et al., 2009). Sleep and personality disorders, as well as stereotypic hand movements, usually develop. Some of the patients have parkinsonian-like features including a face without expression, increase in salivation, and extrapyramidal system involvement. Swallowing problems are prominent in the vegetative state. There is early loss of ambulation and patients die prematurely. Despite similar disease progression in all patients carrying *MFSD8* mutations, some intra- and interfamilial variation has been described. In one family with five affected siblings, two died at 13 years of age, while the other three remain alive at ages 8, 10, and 15 respectively (Stogmann et al., 2009). In another family the eldest sibling is still alive at 18 years (Aldahmesh et al., 2009). Also one patient (homozygous for the c.468–469delinsCC mutation that leads to an in-frame substitution of a single amino acid) showed a later onset (at 11 years) and a much more protracted disease course even into adulthood (Kousi et al., 2009).

MORPHOLOGY

Macroscopy

In subjects later confirmed genetically as CLN7 disease, gross examination at postmortem reveals atrophy of the brain, with weights ranging from 590–883g (age range 5–12 years) (Elleder et al., 1997a). The normal brain weights for these ages are from 1237–1351g. The degree of atrophy was approximately proportional to the duration of the symptoms, with the greatest weight loss in this study found in the 12-year-old (590g), and minimal in one patient with the shortest clinical course of 2 years (Elleder et al., 1997a). More recently, the reduction at postmortem was calculated for three children homozygous for c.881C>A as 33% in a 7-year-old, 44% at 8 years, and 40% at 12 years; and in two children homozygous for c.754+2T>A as 54% at 9 years, and 57% at 18 years.

Macroscopy was dominated by atrophy of both cerebrum and cerebellum. Frequently there was spontaneous detachment of the cortex from the adjacent white matter even in fixed brains, reflecting laminar degeneration in the lower cortical layers. The increase in brain atrophy was paralleled by distension of the ventricular system, which was most prominent in the case dying at aged 12. The white matter appeared normal on slicing and there was no evidence of demyelination. Visceral organs appeared normal.

Microscopy

STORAGE MATERIAL FEATURES

Storage lysosomes are distended by autofluorescent material. Frequently these are enlarged, their size varying from 0.5–5μm. Generally, they contain high amounts of mitochondrial ATP synthase subunit c (SCMAS), identified immunohistochemically. The intensity of the signal varies, as in other NCL types, since the fingerprint profiles, which represent part of the stored material, are unreactive for subunit c (see Chapter 4). However, correlation of autofluorescence with subunit c staining and electron microscopy (EM) suggests that the lysosomal accumulation of subunit c is low. By this it differs from CLN2 disease in which immunodetectable SCMAS is present even when there is little storage (see Chapter 7). The signal for cathepsin D is generally strong but variable, and correlation with autofluorescence shows that a population of storage autofluorescent lysosomes may be free of detectable cathepsin D. This raises the question about the nature and derivation of these storage compartments. The practical implication is that the most sensitive detection of the storage process in routine paraffin sections is autofluorescence. Secondary transformation of storage material is present but not as much as in CLN2 disease (Chapter 7). Sizable neuronal spheroid inclusions composed of the transformed material are not seen.

The lysosomal storage is generalized, but mostly expressed in neurons (in the perikarya and axon hillocks), much less in astrocytes (perikarya), and discrete in oligodendroglia, ependyma, and in the choroid plexus epithelium. Glial macrophages mostly contain scavenged storage material; however, primary storage cannot be excluded. Astrocytes and glial phagocytes are activated. Oligodendroglia are inert and myelination does not display any demonstrable primary alteration. Cell degeneration is confined to neurons

Neuronal storage is ubiquitous and generalized, affecting all brain and spinal cord neurons. The storage material is finely granular with varying degrees of clumping, and stains with Sudan black, periodic acid–Schiff (PAS) and Luxol fast blue, and is brightly autofluorescent. The neurons also immunostain strongly for SCMAS. Less positive immunostaining is observed in the astrocytes and vascular smooth muscle and endothelial cells, but the ependyma is generally negative.

Neuronal storage is most pronounced in layers II–VI, layer I being minimally affected. Laminar degeneration is confined mostly to cortical layer V, but in some regions other layers were affected as well. Areas devoid of storage neurons are replaced by hypertrophic astrocytes and contain various amounts of phagocytes, either individual or aggregated into resorptive nodules (most probably due to active neuronophagy) and loaded with scavenged autofluorescent debris. This pattern was seen in all cases but is further aggravated by age 12. In older cases, the cortex becomes progressively thinned, astrogliosed, and infiltrated with individual microglial phagocytes containing autofluorescent debris. There is also partial spongiform transformation and some storage neurons persist. There can also be pronounced neovascularization of the cortex.

Neuronal storage is pronounced in the basal ganglia and thalamus, and most intense in striatal neurons. There are no overt regressive changes except for diffuse astrogliosis and focal neuronophagic granulomas. The number of dispersed small CD68+ microglial cells is generally high. In older cases the dominant finding in the striatum is a spongy state combined with oedema, and pronounced vascularization. Storage neurons are present and viable, astrocytes are enlarged with decreased staining for glial fibrillary acidic protein (GFAP). There are no signs of glial phagocyte activation.

The hippocampus was studied in three cases (aged 7, 8, and 9). There is discrete uniform neuronal storage in the dentate gyrus with only focal discrete reduction of their number. Neurons in all CA sectors are distended by storage. Moderate neuronal drop out is ubiquitous but occurs most expressed in the CA2 sector (Figure 11.3).

Various intensities of storage occur in the brainstem and spinal cord that is confined to part of the neuronal soma. Neuronal ballooning also occurs. Individual neurons in the nigral nucleus and in the spinal cord are almost or completely free of storage, and some of them are remarkably enlarged, with prominent Nissl substance. In the nigral nucleus there are occasional neuromelanin pigmented neurons that do not express features compatible with storage. There are also enlarged neurons free of discernible pigmentation in standard histological

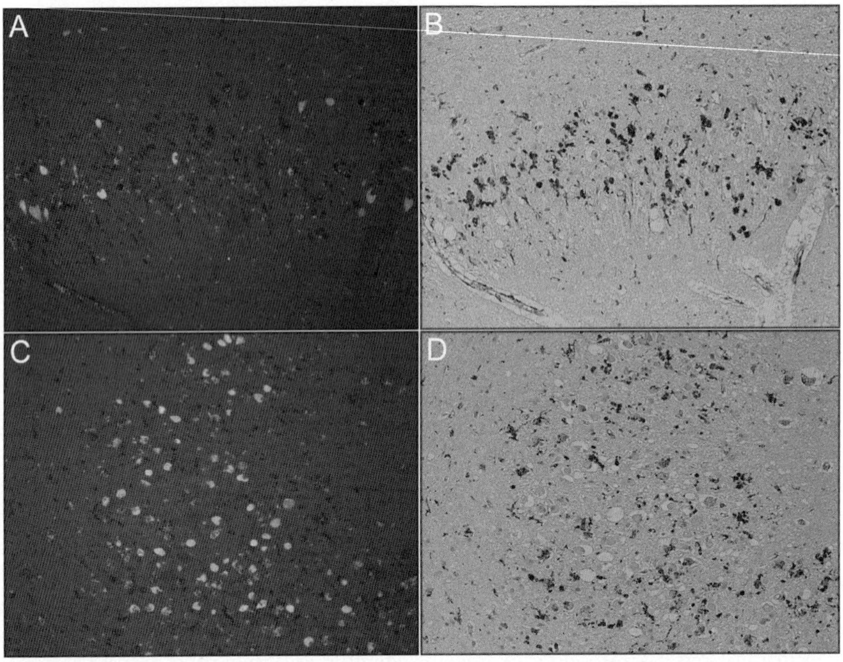

Figure 11.3 CLN7 disease: hippocampus (age 7). Paraffin sections immunostained for CD68 (PGM1) antigen that detects macrophages and simultaneously examined for autofluorescence in neurons (compare adjacent panels). (A, B) CA2 sector showing a number of enlarged scavenging macrophages and reduced population of neurons loaded with autofluorescent lysosomes. (C, D) Sector CA3. The number of storage neurons is only partially reduced. Macrophages are more dispersed and are small. (A–D) ×10.

staining but positive in the Masson reaction (which is negative in storage neurons in NCL generally). This raises the question of the relationship between lysosomal storage and neuromelanin deposition in CLN7 disease, and perhaps other NCL types as well.

CENTRAL NERVOUS SYSTEM PATHOLOGY

Neuronal loss is most marked in layer V of the cerebral cortex, with the occipital cortex being most affected. The progressive reduction of the cortical neurons is proportional to disease length.

In the cerebellum, the cortex is markedly affected, with almost complete loss of the granular layer, regardless of age. In contrast, Purkinje cells are progressively lost in proportion to disease length, and by 12 years only isolated Purkinje cells persist (Figure 11.4) which display storage in the perikarya, with less in the dendrites. Some of these cells are markedly hypertrophic. Their dendrite system is often enlarged, with variable degrees of storage and hypertrophy. The dendrite hypertrophy frequently culminates in focal torpedo-like or spheroid-like expansions with excessive ramification (Figure 11.4). There is always intensive astrogliosis, frequently with several layers of Bergmann astroglia. Remaining Purkinje cells are often encircled by a collar of GFAP-positive astrocyte processes. There is variable admixture of individual dispersed CD68+ microglia frequently in the form of resorptive nodules. These were most obvious in the patient who died at age 9 years, where the cerebellar cortex was dispersedly infiltrated with resorptive nodules.

The dentate nucleus, which displays storage, is always affected by neuronal loss and consequent shrinkage. This correlates with illness length, although in less prolonged cases many dentate neurons are surrounded by fine neuronal processes that stain for synaptophysin, indicating that they are preterminal nerve endings. This may correspond to 'grumose degeneration' (Arai, 1989, Cruz-Sanchez et al., 1992). The neuronal processes are intermingled with astrocytic processes (Figure 11.5). Severe astrogliosis is a feature, together with dispersed individual CD68+ glia that in some cases exert

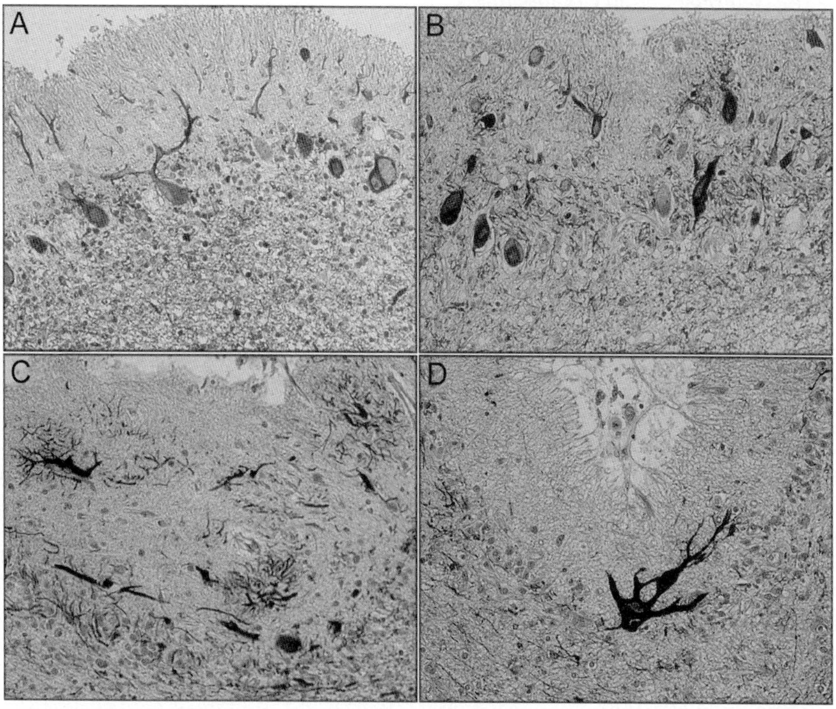

Figure 11.4 CLN7 disease: cerebellar cortex with progressive depopulation of both Purkinje cells and the granule cell layer neurons with disease progression; (A) 7 years, (B) 8 years, (C) 9 years, (D) 18 years. Staining for neurofilaments depicts modification of the Purkinje cell dendrites. Note pronounced hypertrophy of the remaining Purkinje cell in (D). (A–D) ×20.

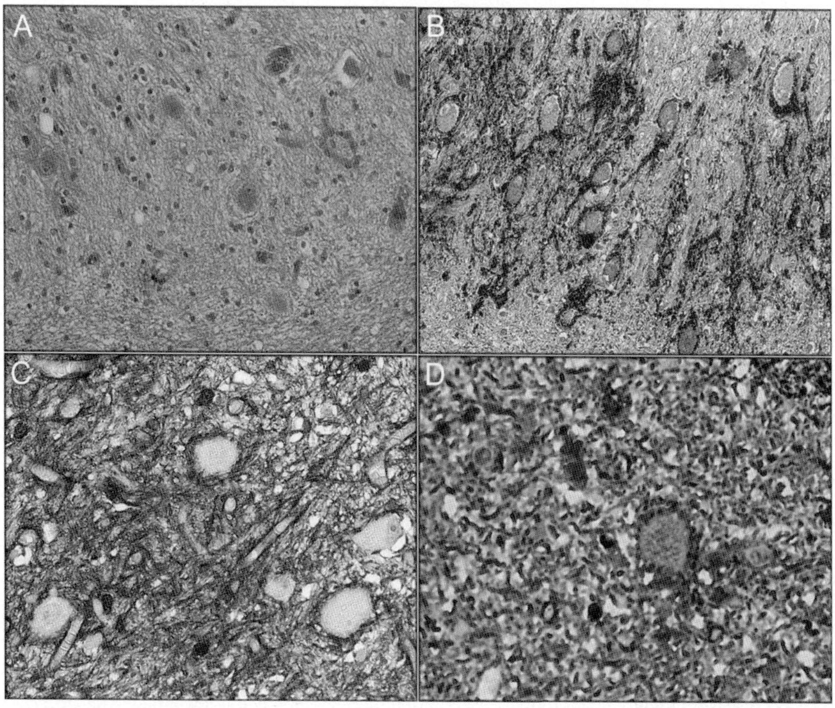

Figure 11.5 CLN7 disease: dentate nucleus with neuronal storage and progressive degeneration (aged 7). Neurons are surrounded by a delicate network of fibres (A), stained for synaptophysin (B), GFAP (C), and neurofilaments (D). (A–D) ×40.

prominent neuronophagy. Similar changes are seen in the inferior olivary nuclei. The progressive reduction of the olivary neurons is proportional to the course length. The neuropathology of six further patients has recently been reported (Sharifi et al., 2010).

The myelin was well preserved in all cases. Generally the white matter contained many small microglial CD68+ cells.

RETINAL PATHOLOGY

There is a progressive reduction of retinal neurons in proportion to disease length (Figure 11.6). In two patients homozygous for the mutation c.881C>A there was a marked reduction of neurons in the ganglion layer and in both internal and external nuclear layers which were rarefied, disorganized, and almost completely fused. There was a focal spongy appearance in the internal plexiform layer. The photoreceptor layer was practically missing (Figure 11.6). The retinal pigment epithelium was rich in melanin in one case, but seriously depleted of it in the older case (Figure 11.6). The content of melanin granules was inversely proportional to the autofluorescent storage granules in the retinal pigment epithelium. Signs of retinitis pigmentosa were minimal. Only discrete individual melanin granules and scarce melanophages were observed in the external part of the retina. Autofluorescent storage lysosomes were present in the remaining cells of the ganglion layer, and a few discrete storage lysosomes were seen in the remnants of the nuclear layers. There was severe astrogliosis that was GFAP positive in the ganglion layer and in the fused and reduced nuclear layers (Figure 11.6).

EXTRACEREBRAL STORAGE

Extracerebral storage is of low intensity and manifested by an increased amount of autofluorescent lysosomes with a strong signal for cathepsin D. The degree of immunodetectable amount of ATP synthase subunit c ranged from absence to strong signal. It was often strong in the heart and skeletal muscle. The liver displayed significant ATP synthase subunit c storage only in the oldest case studied, who was homozygous for the mutation c.881C>A. In other younger cases, lysosomal storage in hepatocytes was seen by EM, or by its autofluorescence and an increased signal for cathepsin D. There were no signs of organ damage with the exception of the heart. Cardiomyocytes displayed a definite tendency to evolution of a mild hypertrophic cardiomyopathy proportional to the length of the clinical course. In the age range 7–9 years there were initial changes that were well recognizable histologically. In a patient homozygous for c.754+2T>A that died aged 18 years, there was a moderate disarray of cardiac trabecules (Figure 11.7). Cardiology reports were not available.

Visceral storage, identified by autofluorescence, sudanophilia, acid phosphatase positivity, and EM is generalized and similar in distribution to CLN2 disease. SCMAS is found using immunohistochemistry to be accumulated in muscle cells (smooth, skeletal, and cardiac), exocrine pancreas, eccrine sweat glands, and renal tubules. In contrast with CLN2 disease,

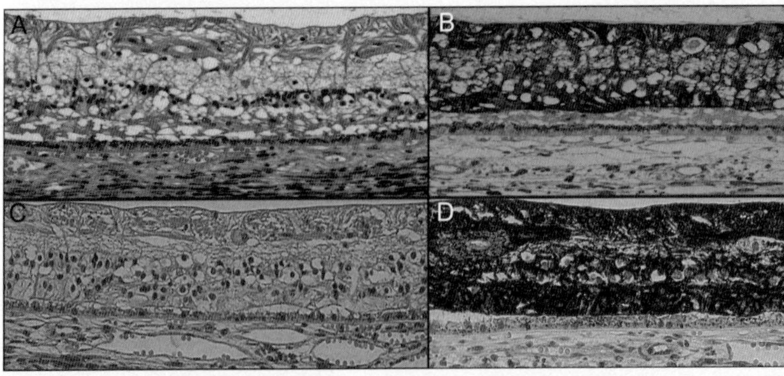

Figure 11.6 CLN7 disease: age-dependant retinal degeneration (upper panels age 7, lower panels age 9). (A, C) (HE staining): neuronal population is more reduced at age 9. (B, D) (GFAP staining): astrogliosis is extensive throughout the whole retina. Note reduction of melanin in the retinal pigment epithelium (C, D). (A–D) ×20.

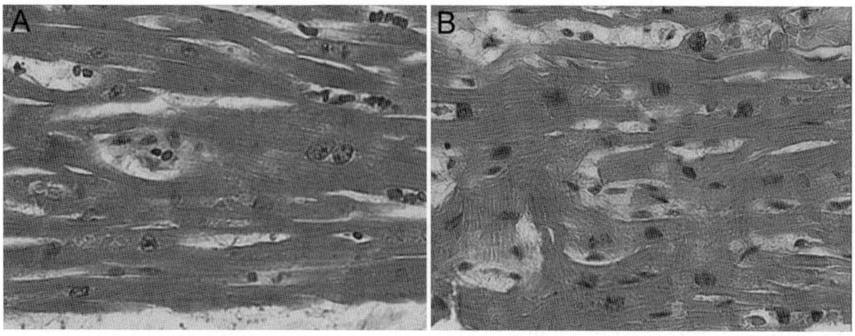

Figure 11.7 CLN7 disease: myocardium showing hypertrophy of cardiomyocytes and partial disarray of heart trabecules. HE staining A (age 12), B (age 18), ×40.

where liver, adrenals, and endocrine pancreas are strongly immunostained for SCMAS, there is no SCMAS staining in CLN7 disease (or CLN3 disease) in these sites despite evidence of lysosomal storage. Absence of SCMAS storage in these sites has been confirmed by polyacrylamide gel electrophoresis (SDS PAGE) studies on extracted tissues (Elleder et al., 1997b). In rectal biopsies, within the smooth muscle of the muscularis mucosae and muscularis propria small strongly acid phosphatase cells are present among the muscle cells. These 'histiocytes' are found also in CLN3 disease, but are absent in CLN2 disease. Intestinal neurons are variably SCMAS-positive and may be negative in spite of other evidence of storage.

Lymphocytes in blood films are not vacuolated, in contrast with CLN3 disease.

ULTRASTRUCTURE

On EM examination there are fingerprint profiles and/or curvilinear bodies (Topçu et al., 2004, Siintola et al., 2007, Kousi et al., 2009) or a complex of fingerprint profiles and rectilinear inclusions, occasionally associated with curvilinear bodies (Kousi et al., 2009) (Figure 11.8).

The ultrastructure of the cerebral neuronal storage material is a mixture of rectilinear complex and fingerprint profiles. There may be a significant tendency to condensation with consequent loss of the distinct membranous pattern. The transformation of storage material into perikaryonal spheroids (Elleder and Tyynelä, 1998) is less marked than in CLN2 disease or CLN1 disease. The ultrastructure of the visceral storage material is very similar to that found in CLN3

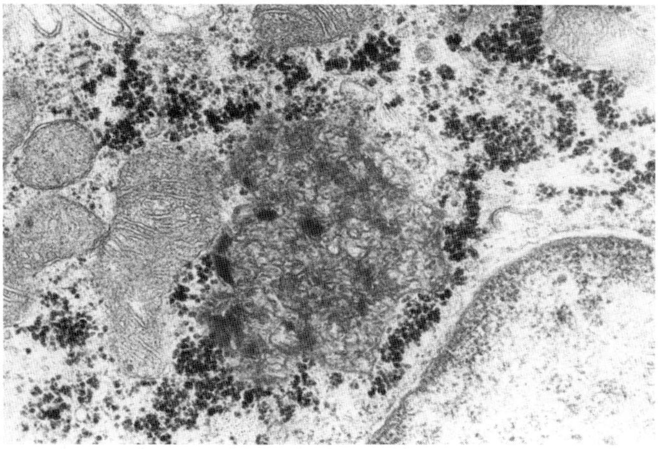

Figure 11.8 CLN7 disease: skin biopsy, epithelial cell. A mixture of irregular curvilinear or rectilinear profiles and fingerprint profiles.

disease and CLN5 disease. In the eccrine sweat gland epithelium there is a mixture of fingerprint, curvilinear, and rectilinear complex profiles with an admixture of curved stacks of membranes, the proportion of each varying from cell to cell. There is, in general, less evidence of vacuolar change than is seen in CLN3 disease. Smooth muscle cells and endothelial cells (from skin and rectal biopsies) contain curvilinear, fingerprint, and rectilinear complex profiles. Intestinal neuron inclusions are of pure fingerprint profiles with no evidence of curvilinear or rectilinear complex bodies. As in the sweat gland epithelium the vacuolar component often seen in CLN3 disease is generally absent. Skeletal muscle inclusions are of the rectilinear complex type. Lymphocytes (in the order of 2–10%) contain electron dense, condensed storage material in which it may be difficult to demonstrate the laminae except for some fingerprint profiles. Often these membrane-bound storage inclusions contain a small, adherent lipid droplet.

Typical NCL ultrastructural material was not found in two families with CLN7 disease (Aldahmesh et al., 2009, Stogmann et al., 2009), although these studies were incomplete since limited tissues were examined (see Chapter 4).

Differential diagnosis

The morphological appearance and ultrastructure of the brain and visceral organs of patients with CLN7 disease can be similar to those of CLN3 disease and CLN6 disease. The subtle lack of vacuolar changes in sweat gland epithelium and intestinal neurons may help to differentiate the two conditions, but the most helpful investigation is the examination of peripheral lymphocytes, which in CLN3 disease will always have a proportion displaying vacuoles. At the ultrastructural level patients with CLN7 disease will have lymphocytes with condensed fingerprint profiles with no vacuolation. These positive lymphocytes may not be plentiful, therefore at least 100 cells should be examined.

The tendency to condensation should not be interpreted as transition to NCLs containing granular storage material. It is highly recommended that ultrastructural examination of multiple cell types is performed in order to make an accurate NCL diagnosis.

DISEASE MECHANISM

There are no data to explain the disease mechanism. A mouse model does not yet exist.

CORRELATIONS

No obvious genotype–phenotype correlation has been detected in late infantile variant patients with *MFSD8* mutations (Siintola et al., 2007, Kousi et al., 2009). However, a patient homozygous for c.468–469delinsCC mutation changing an alanine to a proline at p.157 presented with visual failure at age 11 and had a remarkably delayed and protracted disease course, such that he was employed up to age 25. Other symptoms did not appear until the third decade (onset of motor impairment at 24 years, seizures at 25), and many were delayed into the fourth decade (mental regression at 30, speech problems at 36, chairbound at 39) (Kousi et al., 2009). The patient is currently 44 years old.

Five siblings carrying p.Tyr121Cys did not develop visual failure (Stogmann et al., 2009). Another patient with juvenile onset and vacuolated lymphocytes, at least at the time of sample taking, was homozygous for *CLN7* mutation c.881C>A (p.Thr294Lys) (M. Elleder, personal communication). This patient also carried a common *CLN5* variation c.4T>C, raising the possibility that this change modified the CLN7 disease in some way.

DIAGNOSIS

The diagnosis of CLN7 disease is based on the typical clinical findings combined with neurophysiological and neuroradiological investigations, ultrastructural analysis of the storage material, and molecular genetic analysis of the *CLN7/MFSD8* gene (Tables 11.1–3).

Neurophysiology

Characteristic electroencephalogram (EEG) findings include diffuse background slowing with occipital spikes more prominent during sleep.

Table 11.3 **Laboratory findings of CLN7 disease, late infantile variant**

Neurophysiology	EEG	Diffuse background slowing with occipital spikes more prominent during sleep
	ERG	No response
	VEP	Initially delay in P1 latency followed by absent response in advanced disease
Neuroimaging		Cerebellar and cerebral atrophy, increased intensity in the cerebellum and periventricular white matter in T2-weighted and FLAIR sequences, brain stem atrophy, hypointensity of the thalami, thin corpus callosum
Electron microscopy	Lymphocytes	FP
	Rectal biopsy	CL or FP/CL
	Muscle biopsy	FP/CL
	Skin biopsy	FP or FP/RL complex occasionally with CL
Molecular genetics	MFSD8 gene	Nonsense, missense, splice-site affecting, deletion/insertion, deletion insertion mutations (mainly homozygous)

CL, curvilinear; FP, fingerprint; RL rectilinear.

Sleep studies may show bioelectric status during sleep. EEG abnormalities and seizures are less prominent compared with those seen in CLN8 disease, late infantile variant. At the onset of the disease visual evoked potentials (VEPs) show delay in P1 latency and electroretinogram shows no response. As the disease progresses VEPs show no response.

Neuroimaging

The brain magnetic resonance imaging findings are abnormal from the early stages of the disease. Varying degrees of progressive cerebellar and/or cerebral atrophy have been reported for several patients (Topçu et al., 2004, Siintola et al., 2007, Kousi et al., 2009). Other findings include brainstem atrophy, thinning of the corpus callosum, increased signal intensity in the periventricular white matter, and hypointensity of the thalami.

ELECTRON MICROSCOPY OF PERIPHERAL TISSUE

In patients with suspected CLN7 disease, an ultrastructural examination of the storage material in peripheral tissues should be performed. In CLN7 disease patients the storage material has shown a fingerprint appearance in lymphocytes (Topçu et al., 2004) or curvilinear bodies and/or fingerprint profiles in rectal and/or muscle biopsy samples (Siintola et al., 2007, Kousi et al., 2009). In skin biopsy samples EM findings have revealed fingerprint profiles (Siintola et al., 2007) or a complex of fingerprint profiles and rectilinear inclusions occasionally associated with curvilinear bodies (Kousi et al., 2009).

MOLECULAR GENETIC TESTING OF *MFSD8*

In patients consistent with a variant late infantile phenotype, genetic testing for *CLN7/MFSD8*, as well as for *CLN5*, *CLN6*, and *CLN8*, should be considered. Additionally, in differential diagnosis of any NCL with juvenile onset, patients that remain negative for *CLN3* mutations should be screened for *CLN7/MFSD8* defects. Mutations in *MFSD8* have been found in patients of various ethnic origins. Screening for *MFSD8* mutations is performed by sequencing the exons and exon–intron boundaries from patient genomic DNA.

In families with proven mutations, prenatal diagnosis can be offered in subsequent pregnancies. This has already been used successfully to show that a fetus was not affected (M. Elleder, personal communication).

CLINICAL MANAGEMENT

Treatment is mainly supportive and symptomatic. Antiepileptic medication is necessary to control seizures, which may respond to phenobarbital and valproic acid. Although response to levetiracetam is more prominent in CLN8 disease, some occasional patients with *CLN7/MFSD8* mutations may respond to levetiracetam as well. Intravenous immunoglobulin treatment (1g/kg total dose, 2-day infusion, monthly for a year) was effective in terms of decreasing seizure frequency and slowing clinical deterioration in three patients (unpublished data).

In addition to seizures, behavioural and sleep problems are frequent. Patients with behavioural problems, agitation, and hyperactivity may be referred to a child psychiatrist. Sleep problems may respond to melatonin. Progressive motor impairment may require physical treatment to prevent contractions, for spasticity treatment oral baclofen may be considered. Other daily problems to be managed include drooling, feeding impairment, and progressive visual loss.

EXPERIMENTAL THERAPY

No experimental therapeutic trials for CLN7 disease have been reported so far. The use of antioxidants (vitamin E at high dosage) and intravenous immunoglobulin have been tested but their values in the majority of CLN7 disease patients remain unproven.

REFERENCES

Aiello C, Terracciano A, Simonati A, Discepoli G, Cannelli N, Claps D, Crow YJ, Bianchi M, Kitzmuller C, Longo D, Tavoni A, Franzoni E, Tessa A, Veneselli E, Boldrini R, Filocamo M, Williams RE, Bertini ES, Biancheri R, Carrozzo R, Mole SE, & Santorelli FM (2009) Mutations in MFSD8/CLN7 are a frequent cause of variant-late infantile neuronal ceroid lipofuscinosis. *Hum Mutat*, 30, E530–540.

Aldahmesh MA, Al-Hassnan ZN, Aldosari M, & Alkuraya FS (2009) Neuronal ceroid lipofuscinosis caused by MFSD8 mutations: a common theme emerging. *Neurogenetics*, 10, 307–311.

Arai N (1989) 'Grumose degeneration' of the dentate nucleus. A light and electron microscopic study in ranuclear palsy and dentatorubropallidoluysial atrophy palsy and dentatorubropallidoluysial atrophy. *J Neurol Sci*, 90, 131–145.

Cruz-Sanchez FF, Rossi ML, Cardozo A, Picardo A, & Tolosa E (1992) Immunohistological study of grumose degeneration of the dentate nucleus in progressive supranuclear palsy. *J Neurol Sci*, 110, 228–231.

Elleder M, Franc J, Kraus J, Nevsimalova S, Sixtova K, & Zeman J (1997a) Neuronal ceroid lipofuscinosis in the Czech Republic: analysis of 57 cases. Report of the 'Prague NCL group'. *Eur J Paediatr Neurol*, 1, 109–114.

Elleder M, Sokolova J, & Hrebicek M (1997b) Follow-up study of subunit c of mitochondrial ATP synthase (SCMAS) in Batten disease and in unrelated lysosomal disorders. *Acta Neuropathol*, 93, 379–390.

Elleder M & Tyynelä J (1998) Incidence of neuronal perikaryal spheroids in neuronal ceroid lipofuscinoses (Batten disease). *Clin Neuropathol*, 17, 184–189.

Johnstone D & Milward EA (2010) Genome-wide microarray analysis of brain gene expression in mice on a short-term high iron diet. *Neurochem Int*, 56, 856–863.

Kousi M, Siintola E, Dvorakova L, Vlaskova H, Turnbull J, Topcu M, Yuksel D, Gokben S, Minassian BA, Elleder M, Mole SE, & Lehesjoki AE (2009) Mutations in CLN7/MFSD8 are a common cause of variant late-infantile neuronal ceroid lipofuscinosis. *Brain*, 132, 810–819.

Pao SS, Paulsen IT, & Saier MH, Jr. (1998) Major facilitator superfamily. *Microbiol Mol Biol Rev*, 62, 1–34.

Sharifi A, Kousi M, Sagné C, Bellenchi GC, Morel L, Darmon M, Hulková H, Ruivo R, Debacker C, El Mestikawy S, Elleder M, Lehesjoki AE, Jalanko A, Gasnier B, Kyttälä A (2010) Expression and lysosomal targeting of CLN7, a major facilitator superfamily transporter associated with variant late-infantile neuronal ceroid lipofuscinosis. *Hum Mol Genet*, 19, 4497–4514.

Siintola E, Topcu M, Aula N, Lohi H, Minassian BA, Paterson AD, Liu XQ, Wilson C, Lahtinen U, Anttonen AK, & Lehesjoki AE (2007) The novel neuronal ceroid lipofuscinosis gene MFSD8 encodes a putative lysosomal transporter. *Am J Hum Genet*, 81, 136–146.

Siintola E, Topcu M, Kohlschutter A, Salonen T, Joensuu T, Anttonen AK, & Lehesjoki AE (2005) Two novel CLN6 mutations in variant late-infantile neuronal ceroid lipofuscinosis patients of Turkish origin. *Clin Genet*, 68, 167–173.

Steenhuis P, Herder S, Gelis S, Braulke T, & Storch S (2010) Lysosomal targeting of the CLN7 membrane glycoprotein and transport via the plasma membrane require a dileucine motif. *Traffic*, 11, 987–1000.

Stogmann E, El Tawil S, Wagenstaller J, Gaber A, Edris S, Abdelhady A, Assem-Hilger E, Leutmezer F, Bonelli S, Baumgartner C, Zimprich F, Strom TM, & Zimprich A (2009) A novel mutation in the MFSD8 gene in late infantile neuronal ceroid lipofuscinosis. *Neurogenetics*, 10, 73–77.

Topçu M, Tan H, Yalnizoglu D, Usubütün A, Saatci I, Aynaci M, Anlar B, Topaloglu H, Turanli G, Kose G, & Aysun S (2004) Evaluation of 36 patients from Turkey with neuronal ceroid lipofuscinosis: clinical, neurophysiological, neuroradiological and histopathologic studies. *Turk J Pediatr*, 46, 1–10.

Chapter 12

CLN8

C. Aiello, N. Cannelli, J.D. Cooper, M. Haltia, R. Herva, U. Lahtinen, A.-E. Lehesjoki, S.E. Mole, F. M. Santorelli, E. Siintola, and A. Simonati

INTRODUCTION

Mutations in the *CLN8* gene are responsible for at least two very different clinical entities. The first to be described was northern epilepsy (NE), also known as progressive epilepsy with mental retardation (EPMR) (Hirvasniemi et al., 1994, Hirvasniemi et al., 1995), which is an autosomal recessive childhood epilepsy syndrome seen most often in Finland. Unexpectedly, neuropathological studies established its inclusion as one of the NCLs (Haltia et al., 1999, Herva et al., 2000) and *CLN8* was identified as the causative gene. EPMR can be considered a mutation-specific disease phenotype. Subsequently patients from Turkey with a late infantile variant NCL were identified who also had mutations within the same gene, and many *CLN8* mutations have now been found in patients from different ethnic backgrounds. Further investigation of *CLN8* may provide valuable genetic and therapeutic information. CLN8 disease should be considered in the differential diagnosis of young children

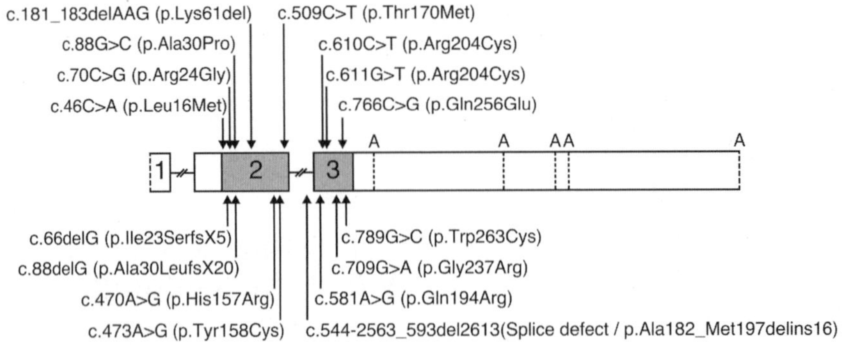

Figure 12.1 *CLN8* gene schema. Genomic structure of *CLN8* and positions of the disease-associated mutations. *CLN8* is transcribed from three exons (boxes 1–3). The coding regions are shown in grey and the untranslated regions in white. The positions of the disease-associated mutations are indicated by arrows. Suggested polyadenylation sites are indicated with 'A'. The intragenic genomic deletion depicted in italics is likely to lead to mRNA instability (Reinhardt et al., 2010) or possibly a truncated protein.

presenting with an otherwise unexplained epileptic encephalopathy.

MOLECULAR GENETICS

Gene identification

The gene underlying EPMR was localized by linkage analysis to chromosome 8p23 in a large Finnish pedigree (OMIM 610003) (Tahvanainen et al., 1994). Later, the human *CLN8* gene was identified by positional cloning (Ranta et al., 1996, Ranta et al., 1999). The murine *Cln8* gene localized to the same genomic region as the gene underlying a naturally occurring NCL mouse model, the motor neuron degeneration (*mnd*) mouse, and a homozygous insertion (c.267–268insC) was identified in *Cln8* in these *mnd* mice (Ranta et al., 1999).

Gene structure

CLN8 (GenBank accession number NM_018941) consists of three exons, the first of which is not translated (Ranta et al., 1999) (Figure 12.1). The gene spans 30.80kb of genomic DNA (NCBI AceView, http://www.ncbi.nlm.nih.gov/IEB/Research/Acembly/). In human multiple tissue Northern blot, transcripts of 1.4kb, 3.4kb, and 7.5kb are present in all tissue samples, corresponding most likely to the different poly(A) sites (Ranta et al., 1999). The open reading frame of 861bp encodes a 286-amino acid polypeptide (Ranta et al., 1999).

Mutation spectrum

To date, 16 mutations have been identified in the *CLN8* gene (NCL Mutation Database, http://www.ucl.ac.uk/ncl/mutation; Table 12.1, Figure 12.1). These include 12 missense mutations, three small deletions that in two cases are predicted to lead to a frameshift and truncated proteins, and one large deletion that probably causes mRNA instability since no mutant transcripts were detected in the patient (Reinhardt et al., 2010), or alternatively, could lead to a frameshift and a predicted truncated protein. Surprisingly, no nonsense mutations have been described. Two variations occur together on the same disease allele (c.[46C>A; 509C>T]; p.[Leu16Met; Thr170Met]). The most common *CLN8* mutation, c.70C>G (p.Arg24Gly), occurs in homozygous form in all but one Finnish EPMR patients (Ranta et al., 1999). In this patient, c.70C>G occurs in compound heterozygous form with another missense mutation (c.709G>A, p.Gly237Arg) (Siintola et al., 2006). *CLN8* mutations have also been detected in patients originating from countries around the Mediterranean (Turkey, Italy, Israel), and Germany and Pakistan causing the more severe CLN8 disease, late infantile variant (OMIM 600143) (Ranta et al., 2004, Cannelli et al., 2006, Zelnik et al., 2007, Kousi et al., 2009, Vantaggiato et al., 2009,

Table 12.1 **CLN8 mutations (modified from the NCL Mutation Database, http://www.ucl.ac.uk/ncl/mutation)**

Nucleotide change	Amino acid change/Predicted consequence	Phenotype	Country of origin	References
c.[46C>A/509C>T]	p.[Leu16Met/ Thr170Met]	Late infantile variant	Turkey	Ranta et al., 2004
c.66delG	p.Ile23SeffsX5	Late infantile variant	Italy	Cannelli et al., 2006
c.70C>G	p.Arg24Gly	EPMR	Finland	Ranta et al., 1999
c.88delG	p.Ala30Leufs×20	Late infantile variant	Turkey	Ranta et al., 2004
c.88G>C	p.Ala30Pro	Late infantile variant	Italy	Cannelli et al., 2006
c.181–183delAAG	p.Lys61del	Late infantile variant	Italy	Vantaggiato et al., 2009
c.470A>G	p.His157Arg	Late infantile variant	Turkey	Kousi et al., 2009
c.473A>G	p.Tyr158Cys	Late infantile variant	Italy Pakistan	Cannelli et al., 2006 A.-E. Lehesjoki pers. comm.
c.544–2563 _593del2613	2613bp deletion (mRNA instability/splice defect/p.Ala182_ Met197 delinsLys-SerLysMetGlnIle-HisIleHisProAla-LeuHisArgValArg)	Late infantile variant, rapid progression	Turkey	Reinhardt et al., 2010
c.581A>G	p.Gln194Arg	Late infantile variant	Italy	Cannelli et al., 2006
c.610C>T	p.Arg204Cys	Late infantile variant	Turkey	Ranta et al., 2004
c.611G>T	p.Arg204Leu	Late infantile variant	Germany	Reinhardt et al., 2010
c.709G>A	p.Gly237Arg	EPMR	Finland	Siintola et al., 2006
c.766C>G	p.Gln256Glu	Late infantile variant	Israel	Zelnik et al., 2007
c.789G>C	p.Trp263Cys	Late infantile variant	Turkey	Ranta et al., 2004

Reinhardt et al., 2010). One missense mutation (p.Arg204Cys) is known to affect an amino acid that is absolutely conserved across the TLC (TRAM–Lag1p–CLN8) superfamily of proteins to which CLN8 belongs (Ranta, 2004, Winter and Ponting, 2002).

Two polymorphisms have also been described (Ranta, 1999).

Related genes

CLN8 is conserved across vertebrates, but not in invertebrates (Siintola et al., 2006). Sequence similarity searches have shown that CLN8 belongs to a large eukaryotic protein family of TLC-domain homologues (SMART accession number SM00724) that share modest identity at the amino acid level, but have a conserved domain structure with at least five transmembrane α-helixes and few highly or absolutely conserved amino acid residues (Winter and Ponting, 2002). They are postulated to function in lipid metabolism, transport, or sensing. Members of this family have been shown to facilitate early events of protein secretion, e.g. translocation of nascent polypeptide chains into the endoplasmic reticulum (ER) and export of glycosylphosphatidylinositol-anchored proteins out of the ER. A number of TLC proteins function as ceramide synthases with specificity for fatty acids of varying lengths (Mizutani et al., 2005).

CELL BIOLOGY

Protein structure, localization, and function

The *CLN8* gene encodes a novel 33kDa polytopic non-glycosylated membrane protein that is a resident of the ER and the ER–Golgi intermediate compartment (ERGIC) (Lonka et al., 2000). This localization is conserved whether CLN8 is expressed in non-neuronal or neuronal cells (Lonka et al., 2004). The precise topology of CLN8 has not been determined, but at least five transmembrane domains are predicted (Figure 12.2). The C-terminus of the protein is probably located in the cytoplasm as it carries a functional dilysine-based ER-retention signal. Inactivation of this signal disrupts the recycling of CLN8 back to the ER and results in an accumulation in the Golgi complex. However, known patient mutations do not alter the localization of CLN8 (Lonka et al., 2000, Lonka et al., 2004, Vantaggiato et al., 2009).

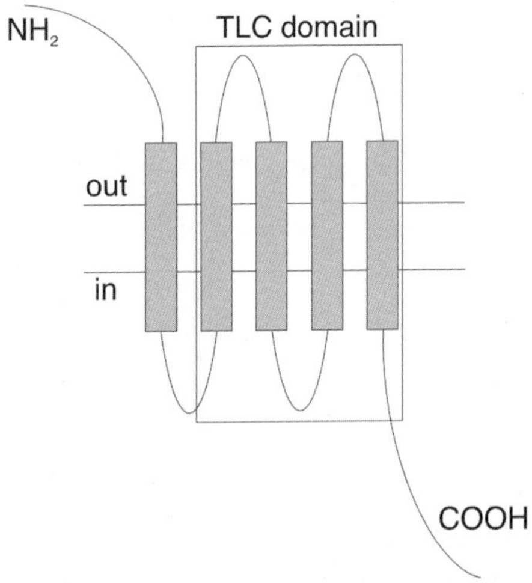

Figure 12.2 CLN8 protein structure. Schematic view of the predicted topology of CLN8. The topology of CLN8 is not known in detail. Because of long hydrophobic regions in the protein, each prediction program predicts it to contain different number of transmembrane domains, varying from four to seven. The prediction with five transmembrane domains is shown here, based on the HMMTOP (http://www.enzim.hu/hmmtop/) prediction program. The approximate site of the predicted TLC domain is indicated with a box. 'In' refers to cytoplasm and 'out' to the lumen of the endoplasmic reticulum.

The molecular function of CLN8 is unknown at present, but lipidomic analysis suggests that sphingolipid metabolism is disturbed in CLN8-deficient cells (Hermansson et al., 2005). A novel NCL phenotype that may be termed CLN9 disease (see Chapter 14) is characterized by decreased sphingolipid levels that can be partially reversed by introducing either TLC-domain ceramide synthases, or, interestingly, *CLN8* into the cells (Schulz et al., 2006). Although catalytic activity has not been demonstrated for CLN8, these two lines of evidence suggest that it might act as a regulatory factor in sphingolipid synthesis.

Recent work using ectopically expressed CLN8 in neuronal cells, validated through a gene silencing approach, suggests that CLN8 plays a role in cell proliferation during neuronal differentiation and in protection against cell death (Vantaggiato et al., 2009), but not in cell migration. The precise biochemical function of CLN8 remains to be identified.

Gene expression and tissue distribution

The *CLN8* mRNA is expressed ubiquitously at low levels in embryonic and adult mouse tissues (Lonka et al., 2005) and in adult human tissues (Ranta et al., 1999). In prenatal mouse embryos *Cln8* is most prominently expressed in the developing gastrointestinal tract, dorsal root ganglia, and brain. In postnatal mouse brain, highest expression is found in the cortex and hippocampus. Expression of *Cln8* in the developing and mature brain combined with regional differences in the expression suggests roles for Cln8 in maturation, differentiation, and supporting the survival of specific neuronal populations. So far, lack of antibodies recognizing endogenous CLN8 has hampered any attempts to examine tissue distribution by immunohistochemical methods.

Table 12.2 **Clinical features of CLN8 disease**

	Late infantile variant	EPMR
Onset (years)	Late infantile (2–7) (early developmental delay)	Early juvenile (5–10)
Early symptoms	Myoclonus (→myoclonic seizures) Unsteady gait Visual failure	Epilepsy (generalized tonic–clonic seizures) (cognitive decline)
Later symptoms	School-age Rapid cognitive decline Behavioural abnormalities Central/peripheral visual impairment epilepsy Neurological symptoms (spasticity, dystonia, tremors, etc.)	Adulthood Mental deterioration Behavioural abnormalities Motor impairment (late) (Speech loss) (Seizures)
Disease course	Rapidly progressive	Slowly progressive

CLINICAL DATA

Introduction

Mutations in *CLN8* cause childhood onset NCL that has remarkable phenotypic differences according to the underlying mutation. It was first described in Finland and termed NE or EPMR. The disease was characterized by an early juvenile onset and slowly progressive course, with epilepsy and cognitive deterioration (Hirvasniemi et al., 1994), and found to be associated with one homozygous missense mutation in the *CLN8* gene (Ranta et al., 1999). Later, many mutations in *CLN8* were detected in patients from different ethnic backgrounds (Table 12.1) and affected with a more severe late infantile variant NCL phenotype with early onset myoclonus and visual failure, partially overlapping with CLN2 disease, classic late infantile, other late infantile variants, and juvenile onset NCLs (Ranta et al., 2004, Cannelli et al., 2006, Zelnik et al., 2007, Kousi et al., 2009, Vantaggiato et al., 2009, Reinhardt et al., 2010). Therefore two distinct *CLN8*-associated phenotypes, EPMR and late infantile variant, have been characterized using clinical, neurophysiological, neuroradiological, and molecular criteria (Tables 12.2 and 12.3). The more

Table 12.3 **Laboratory findings in CLN8 disease**

		Late infantile variant	EPMR
Neurophysiology	EEG	Slowed background activity Decreased amplitude Focal and generalized abnormalities No photic response	Slowed background activity Multifocal paroxysms No photic response
	ERG	Decreased amplitude → extinction	Not reported
	VEP	High amplitude → decreased → extinction	Abnormal in some patients
Neuroimaging		Cerebral and cerebellar atrophy, enlarged ventricles, white matter involvement (early onset and progressive course)	Cerebellar atrophy (late)
Electron microscopy	(Skin biopsy, buffy coat)	Heterogeneous cytosomes: finger prints, curvilinear-like profiles, loose or granular matrix	Not reported
Molecular genetics	*CLN8* gene	Missense, frameshift mutations (both as homozygous and heterozygous)	c.70C>G homozygous mutation (p.Arg24Gly) in all except one patient

severe phenotype is probably due to complete loss of CLN8 function and EPMR can be considered a mutation-specific phenotype.

CLN8 disease, late infantile variant

Children with CLN8 disease, late infantile variant show a more severe clinical phenotype than EPMR patients (Topçu et al., 2004, Cannelli et al., 2006, Zelnik et al., 2007, Kousi et al., 2009, Vantaggiato et al., 2009, Reinhardt et al., 2010). All children have developmental delay, with delay of independent walking (17–18 months) and speech (2–3 years). The onset of symptoms is between the ages of 2–7 years; myoclonic seizures and an unsteady gait are commonly the initial symptoms, other seizures follow soon after. At this stage the differential diagnosis is of an epileptic encephalopathy. Cognitive decline, and both cortical and retinal visual impairment usually occur; behavioural abnormalities are also frequent. Rapid disease progression with loss of cognitive skills is observed over 2 years from the time of diagnosis. By the age of 8–10 years severe deterioration of neurological and cognitive skills is apparent together with medication-resistant epilepsy. Spasticity, dystonia, tremors, and other extrapyramidal signs are also commonly observed. In the second decade of life children are unable to walk or stand without support. Seizures may evolve over the course of the disease: myoclonic seizures are seen early; focal and generalized seizures occur at all stages of the disease; atypical absences are also seen. Seizures are very difficult to control with medication. The life-expectancy of children affected by CLN8 disease, late infantile variant is not yet known. The eldest patients known are now in their second decade, and their general health remains good. One patient died at 10 years from cardiac failure (Vantaggiato et al., 2009).

CLN8 disease, progressive epilepsy with mental retardation/northern epilepsy

The main clinical features are epilepsy, slowly progressive mental decline, and, later, motor impairment with severe speech loss. Developmental milestones are normal until disease onset (Hirvasniemi et al., 1994, Hirvasniemi et al., 1995).

Symptoms usually start between the ages of 5–10 years, often with generalized, tonic–clonic seizures. At the same time some mental decline occurs, which can be misdiagnosed as a secondary effect of the epilepsy. Seizure frequency increases until puberty. Cognitive deterioration is more rapid during puberty. Behavioural disturbances can occur at this time, for example, irritability, restlessness, inactivity, and these features may continue into adulthood. The most frequent seizure type throughout the disease is generalized tonic–clonic. Less common are complex partial seizures. Myoclonic seizures may occur but they are never prominent. Epilepsy is partially responsive to treatment. The number of seizures decreases spontaneously after puberty, even with no change in treatment, and by the second to third decade they become relatively sporadic. On the other hand, cognitive decline continues and in some cases loss of speech has been reported. Motor function is also impaired, with cerebellar signs. In a number of cases, visual acuity is reduced (without evidence of retinal degeneration). The disease has a chronic course and survival to the sixth or seventh decade has been reported. CLN8 disease, EPMR is very unusual amongst the NCLs of childhood onset in this respect.

The disease course has been subdivided into three stages, according to the characteristics of the clinical evolution: the early progression of the disease (stage 1, from onset to puberty), the slowed clinical evolution (stage 2, up to young adulthood), and the stage of permanent disability, which is reached during the fourth decade (stage 3) (Hirvasniemi et al., 1995).

MORPHOLOGY

Macroscopy

Autopsy data are so far only available on three CLN8 disease, EPMR patients who had died at 23 (accidental death), 38, and 61 years of age. Their respective fresh brain weights were 1530g, 1024g, and 1300g. Apart from oedema in the first and generalized gyral atrophy in the second patient, the external appearances as well as the cut surfaces of the brains were unremarkable. General autopsy findings did not include any specific macroscopic abnormalities related to their neurological disease (Herva et al., 2000).

Histology

The most striking histological abnormality in the autopsied CLN8 disease, EPMR patients was the presence of cytoplasmic storage material particularly within nerve cells but also, to a lesser extent, in many other cell types throughout the body, including the heart muscle cells, Kupffer cells of the liver, epithelium of the distal and collecting tubules of the kidney, adrenal medulla, and follicular epithelium of the thyroid gland. Although storage cytosomes could be seen in virtually all neurons, their amount varied greatly between different neuronal populations, resulting in a characteristic and unusually distinct distribution pattern (Herva et al., 2000). The most prominent storage occurred in the hippocampus, particularly in the CA2–4 sectors, while Sommer's sector (CA1) and the neurons of the fascia dentata were relatively spared. In the CA2 area the storage phenomenon was coupled with slight neuronal loss, astrocytosis, and an occasional figure of neuronophagy (Tyynelä et al., 2004). The presubiculum also showed prominent storage. In the isocortex the deep part of lamina III showed pronounced perikaryal ballooning of the large pyramidal cells, while conspicuous axonal enlargements (spindles or meganeurites filled with storage cytosomes) were a frequent feature in the less ballooned nerve cells of the more superficial parts of this layer. Slight to moderate storage without evident neuronal loss occurred in the basal ganglia and thalamus. In the cerebellar cortex the numerically well-preserved granule cells contained some finely granular storage material, while the Purkinje cells were intact, with few exceptions, and the dentate, pontine, and inferior olivary neurons showed moderate storage. The pigmented brainstem neurons were largely intact but most cranial nerve nuclei and spinal anterior and posterior horn cells showed slight to moderate accumulation of storage granules. The storage granules were Luxol fast blue- and periodic acid–Schiff (PAS)-positive, sudanophilic (Figure 12.3), and autofluorescent in ultraviolet light (Figure 12.4). With the exception of a few areas such as the hippocampal CA2 region, neuronal loss as well as astrocytic and microglial reactions were very modest (Herva et al., 2000).

No vacuolated lymphocytes have been observed or reported in peripheral blood smears of CLN8 disease, EPMR patients (Herva et al., 2000) or CLN8 disease, late infantile variant (Topçu et al., 2004, Cannelli et al., 2006, Zelnik et al., 2007, Kousi et al., 2009, Vantaggiato et al., 2009, Reinhardt et al., 2010).

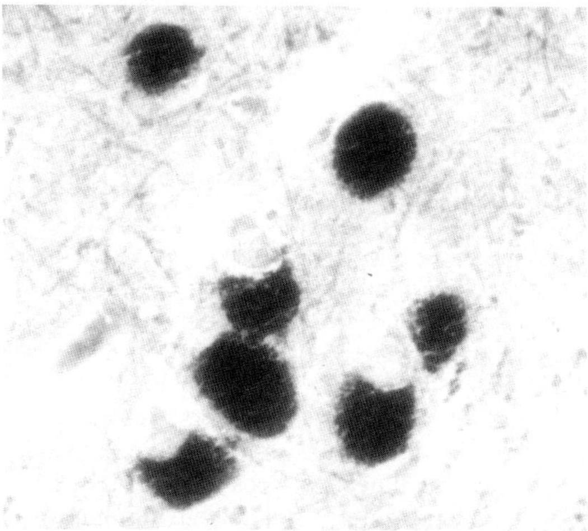

Figure 12.3 CLN8 disease, EPMR: neurons show moderate amounts of intracytoplasmic sudanophilic storage granules (black). Paraffin section of the pontine nuclei, Sudan black B stain, ×500.

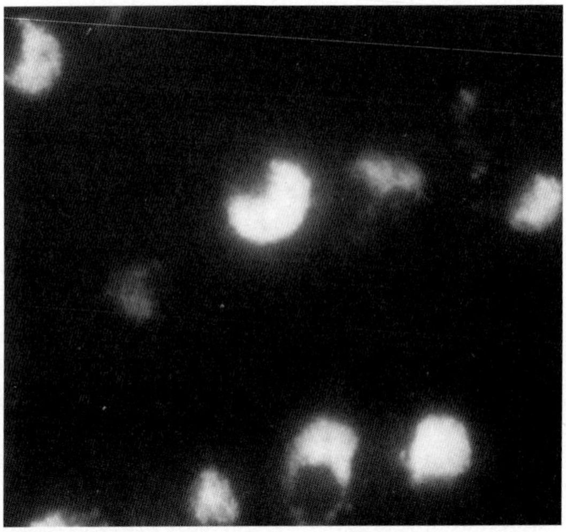

Figure 12.4 CLN8 disease, EPMR: the intraneuronal storage material displays bright autofluorescence in ultraviolet light. Unstained paraffin section of the pontine nuclei, ×500.

Immunocytochemistry

Immunocytochemical staining of EPMR brain tissue revealed accumulation of both subunit c of mitochondrial ATP synthase and sphingolipid activator proteins (SAPs) in the neurons. The storage material in other tissues was also strongly stained for subunit c. This is in line with biochemical data indicating that EPMR is a subunit-c-storing form of NCL. Strikingly, the intraneuronal storage deposits were also strongly positive for β-amyloid protein. In contrast, no extracellular β-amyloid protein deposits or immunoreactivity for hyperphosphorylated tau protein were seen (Herva et al., 2000).

Ultrastructure

Isolated blood lymphocytes obtained from six Turkish late infantile patients with four different *CLN8* mutations contained storage cytosomes with condensed fingerprint profiles (Figure 12.5) while a mixture of curvilinear profiles and fingerprint patterns was reported in two skin biopsies (Ranta et al., 2004, Topçu et al., 2004). Three Italian late infantile variant patients with four further mutations in the *CLN8* gene showed mixed osmiophilic inclusions, including curvilinear or curvilinear-like bodies, fingerprint profiles and, more rarely, GROD-like deposits in skin (eccrine sweat gland cells, fibrocytes, Schwann cells) and muscle biopsies or blood lymphocytes (Cannelli et al., 2006) (Figure 12.6). A 10-year-old male Israeli-Arab patient with yet another *CLN8* mutation showed abundant fingerprint profiles but only rare curvilinear or rectilinear structures or granular deposits in the epithelial cells of eccrine sweat glands (Zelnik et al., 2007). One Italian patient had curvilinear, or curvilinear and fingerprint profiles, but no GRODs, in eccrine sweat glands in a skin biopsy (Vantaggiato et al., 2009).

In two autopsied EPMR patients the intraneuronal electron-dense storage cytosomes were of irregular shape and surrounded by a unit membrane. They contained loosely packed structures, resembling curvilinear profiles (Figure 12.7). Limited electron-dense areas with a granular ultrastructure were also seen (Herva et al., 2000).

DISEASE MECHANISM

In common with other forms of NCL, the normal function of the *CLN8* gene product is not known and like CLN6, it is unclear how mutations in this ER resident protein lead to the accumulation of storage material within the lysosome. The sequence homology of CLN8 to the family of TLC-domain proteins suggests a possible role in lipid synthesis or transport, but this remains unproven. Depending upon the precise mutation that is present, human *CLN8* deficiency results in either a late infantile variant presentation or the milder and more protracted

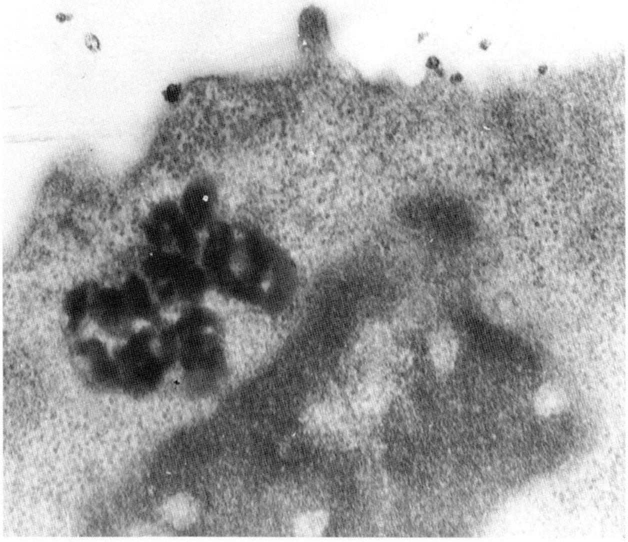

Figure 12.5 CLN8 disease, late infantile variant: cytoplasmic inclusion with fingerprint and electron-dense granular material in a lymphocyte (original magnification ×16,000). Courtesy of Dr Alp Usubütün, Hacettepe University School of Medicine, Ankara, Turkey.

disease, EPMR. Neuropathologically, EPMR displays a less pronounced neurodegenerative presentation than the late infantile onset NCLs (Herva et al., 2000), with selective accumulation of storage material, neuron loss, and glial activation within the hippocampal formation, cortex, and cerebellum (Herva et al., 2000, Tyynelä et al., 2004).

The truncation mutation present in the *Cln8^{mnd}* mouse is predicted to completely abolish its function and therefore more closely mimics late infantile onset CLN8 deficiency rather than EPMR (Ranta et al., 1999). Similar to *Cln6^{nclf}*, these *Cln8^{mnd}* mice display pathological features typical of murine NCL with selective effects on neuron survival, localized glial

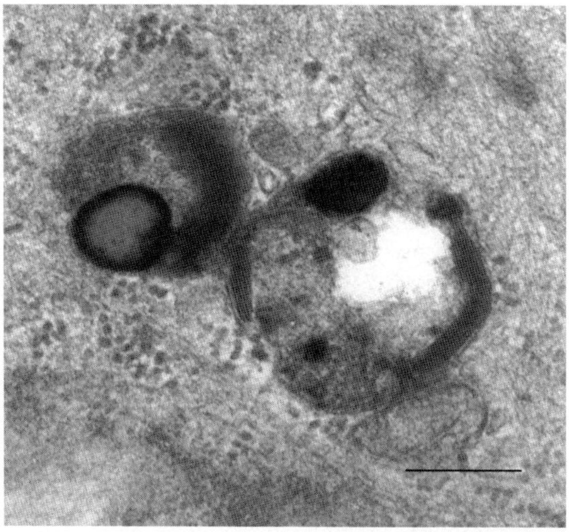

Figure 12.6 CLN8 disease, late infantile variant: ultrastructural findings in skin biopsy from a 12-year-old child carrying the homozygous mutation c.88G>C (electron micrograph: thin section, uranyl acetate and lead citrate stain). Fibrocytic process: two adjacent cytosomes containing fingerprint profiles, ceroid and an osmiophilic body in a loose matrix (bar = 1.5μm). Courtesy of Professor Alessandro Simonati, University of Verona School of Medicine, Verona, Italy.

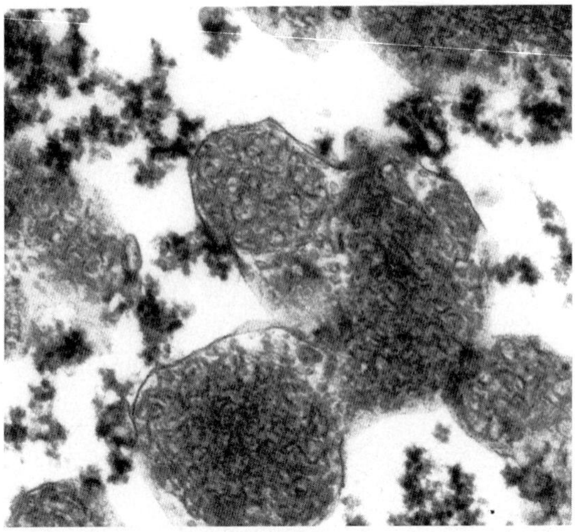

Figure 12.7 CLN8 disease, EPMR: the intraneuronal storage cytosomes are surrounded by a unit membrane and contain electron-dense structures, resembling curvilinear profiles. Transmission electron micrograph, ×25,000.

activation, and synaptic pathology that precedes neuron loss (Fujita et al., 1998, Cooper et al., 1999, Mennini et al., 2004; J. Cooper et al. unpublished observations). These effects are pronounced within the spinal cord (Fujita et al., 1998, Mennini et al., 2004), but also include different subpopulations of cortical and hippocampal neurons and pronounced effects within the thalamocortical system (Cooper et al., 1999; J. Cooper et al. unpublished observations). A variety of disease mechanisms have been proposed in *Cln8*^{mnd} mice including the expression of pro-inflammatory cytokines, oxidative stress and excitotoxicity (Fujita et al., 1998, Griffin et al., 2002, Guarneri et al., 2004, Mennini et al., 2004).

CORRELATIONS

Known mutations in *CLN8* are associated with two distinct phenotypes. The missense mutation common in Finnish patients, p.Arg24Gly (Ranta et al., 1999), results in a protracted form of NCL, EPMR. The other mutations, identified in patients of wide ethnic origin (Ranta et al., 2004, Cannelli et al., 2006, Zelnik et al., 2007, Kousi et al., 2009, Vantaggiato et al., 2009, Reinardt et al 2010) (Table 12.1), when not heterozygous with p.Arg24Gly, are associated with a more severe, late infantile variant phenotype with rapid progression and premature death. The majority of these mutations are missense mutations within the TLC domain, one of which (p.Arg204Cys) affects an amino acid absolutely conserved within the TLC protein family (Winter and Ponting, 2002, Ranta et al., 2004). Several of the mutations may dramatically affect the protein structure and/or expression, since they create frameshifts leading to premature stop codons and possibly degradation of the gene product at the mRNA or protein level. One mutation, which is an intragenic genomic deletion, has been reported to cause a more rapidly progressing CLN8 disease (Reinhardt et al., 2010). No mutant transcripts were detected in the patient, suggesting that this mutation leads to mRNA instability. In theory, the genomic deletion could also lead to the expression of small amounts of a truncated protein (p.Ala182AspfsX49). Since no nonsense mutations have been described, it is difficult at this stage to confidently predict the severity of disease arising from complete absence of CLN8 function.

Systematic morphological analyses on the storage material from tissue material in patients with a number of different mutations have not been performed, so no conclusive correlations between genotype and the morphological phenotype can be made.

DIAGNOSIS

An integrated approach is necessary for the diagnosis of CLN8 disease. It includes neurophysiological investigation, neuroradiological studies, ultrastructural analysis of peripheral tissues (either lymphocyte pellet or skin biopsy), and molecular genetic analysis of *CLN8* (Williams et al., 2006).

Neurophysiology

CLN8 DISEASE, LATE INFANTILE VARIANT

At the onset of symptoms, the electroencephalogram (EEG) shows focal and generalized abnormalities (slow waves, spike–waves complexes, diffuse spikes); polyspike waves synchronous to myoclonic jerks are also present. Progressive slowing of the EEG background activity and decreased amplitude are observed later. Deterioration of sleep organization is also observed, with loss of physiological sleep stages and normal sleep phenomena (Striano et al., 2007). Progressive signal attenuation (with later possible extinction) is observed in the electroretinogram (ERG). High amplitude visual evoked potentials are recorded during the early stages of the disease, followed by progressive attenuation of the evoked responses. The pattern of evolution of the neurophysiological findings shares some similarities with those observed in CLN2 disease, classic late infantile. These findings are consistent with storage accumulation within cortical neurons and retinal ganglion cells, and progressive death of these cell populations.

CLN8 DISEASE, EPMR

During the first stage (stage of progression) of EPMR, a progressive slowing of the background EEG activity is recorded. Moreover, multifocal paroxysms become evident, both as slow wave and spikes and polyspikes. During the second stage, alpha activity reappears and slow (delta) rhythm is reduced as are the epileptiform discharges. This EEG pattern persists unchanged for many years. Sleep organization is not altered (Hirvasniemi et al., 1994). ERG is unaffected; high amplitude visual evoked potentials are not recorded. The neurophysiological findings in EPMR are therefore not like those of the other childhood onset NCLs, nor are the patterns of evolution of both EEG and evoked potentials consistent with that usually seen in other storage diseases.

Brainstem auditory evoked responses (BAERs) are normal in both variants.

Neuroimaging

Late cerebellar and cerebral atrophy has been reported in CLN8 disease, EPMR patients (Hirvasniemi and Karumo, 1994), whereas in CLN8 disease, late infantile variant brain magnetic resonance imaging (MRI) studies have shown evolution of the neurodegeneration from early in the disease course (Figure 12.8). Progressive cerebral and cerebellar atrophy occurs, associated with thinning of the corpus callosum and enlargement of the lateral ventricles, leading to severe brain atrophy. White matter hyperintensity (of the posterior limb of the internal capsule) is also reported. Magnetic resonance spectroscopy is consistent with both grey and white matter involvement (Striano et al., 2007).

Electron microscopy of peripheral tissue

Lymphocyte pellets and skin biopsy samples are suitable for ultrastructural examination.

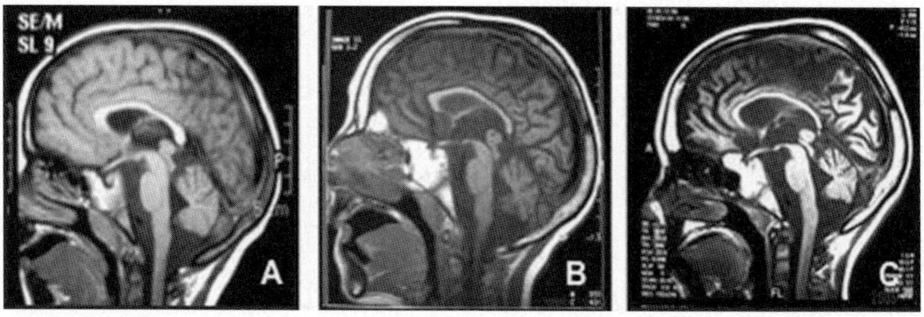

Figure 12.8 CLN8 disease, late infantile variant: MRI scan of a child with CLN8 disease, late infantile carrying heterozygous mutations c.581A>G and c.66delG. Sagittal scans were taken at disease onset (age 4 years, A), age 6 years (B), and age 11 years (C). There is a progressive atrophy of the telencephalic and cerebellar cortices as well as of the corpus callosum along the disease course.

A heterogeneous ultrastructural pattern of the cytosomes is characteristic of CLN8 disease, with fingerprint and curvilinear-like profiles embedded in either a loose or a granular matrix, as well as, in some cases, osmiophilic bodies (Herva et al., 2000, Cannelli et al., 2006, Zelnik et al., 2007, Vantaggiato et al., 2009). These features are not specific for any NCL subtype, but the mixed pattern of the inclusions may suggest appropriate genetic testing. No vacuolations are present in circulating lymphocytes.

Molecular genetic testing

While a single homozygous missense mutation has been reported to account for the majority of CLN8 disease, EPMR patients in Finland (Ranta et al., 1999, Siintola et al., 2006), a variety of mutations account for the late infantile variant phenotype in patients from other populations. Thus, *CLN8* testing should be considered in the genetic screening of late infantile variant NCL alongside *CLN5*, *CLN6*, and *MFSD8/CLN7* mutation analysis. Moreover, CLN8 disease should be included in the differential diagnosis of a late infantile onset epileptic encephalopathy.

CLINICAL MANAGEMENT

There is no specific pharmacological treatment for either of the two diseases associated with mutations in *CLN8*. Anti-epileptic drugs are necessary to control seizures. Amongst CLN8 disease, late infantile variant patients, the response to anti-epileptic drugs is poor. In the early stages of the disease valproate and clonazepam may be beneficial. Myoclonic seizures can be worsened with the use of certain medications, such as lamotrigine (Striano et al., 2007). In CLN8 disease, EPMR patients the seizures may be transiently controlled by valproate and phenobarbitone, and best results may be obtained with clonazepam (Hirvasniemi et al., 1994).

Most medical management strategies should be directed towards maintaining and improving the quality of life of the patients throughout the disease course. In CLN8 disease, EPMR, mental retardation and behavioural disturbances are the predominant problems for caregivers. Adults affected by CLN8 disease, EPMR are cared for in residential settings for adults with learning disabilities, where they may participate in a variety of activities, tailored to the individual needs. Some patients may require pharmacological treatment for behaviour. However since neuroleptics tend to increase seizure susceptibility, decisions regarding medication should be considered carefully.

During the early stages of CLN8 disease, late infantile variant, cognitive decline and behavioural problems (and seizures) represent the major issues to be managed at both home and school. Within a short time major physical difficulties become evident, and support must be provided for the progressive functional impairment. Walking difficulties may require the use of orthotics and physiotherapy to prevent contractures. Drooling and feeding difficulties, due to impaired swallowing, may necessitate gastrostomy placement. Progressive visual loss and sleep disturbances are also frequent problems, which patients and their families have to manage daily.

EXPERIMENTAL THERAPY

No experimental therapeutic trials have been developed for CLN8 disease so far. The use of antioxidants (vitamin E at high dosage) has been tested in some cases but its value remains unproven. The *Cln8*^{mnd} mouse model was treated with the trophic factor IGF-1 (Cooper et al., 1999), but this displayed very limited effects and has not been taken further.

REFERENCES

Cannelli N, Cassandrini D, Bertini E, Striano P, Fusco L, Gaggero R, Specchio N, Biancheri R, Vigevano F, Bruno C, Simonati A, Zara F, & Santorelli FM (2006) Novel mutations in CLN8 in Italian variant late infantile neuronal ceroid lipofuscinosis: Another genetic hit in the Mediterranean. *Neurogenetics*, 7, 111–117.

Cooper JD, Messer A, Feng AK, Chua-Couzens J, & Mobley WC (1999) Apparent loss and hypertrophy of interneurons in a mouse model of neuronal ceroid lipofuscinosis: evidence for partial response to insulin-like growth factor-1 treatment. *J Neurosci*, 19, 2556–2567.

Fujita K, Yamauchi M, Matsui T, Titani K, Takahashi H, Kato T, Isomura G, Ando M, & Nagata Y (1998) Increase of glial fibrillary acidic protein fragments in the spinal cord of motor neuron degeneration mutant mouse. *Brain Res*, 785, 31–40.

Griffin JL, Muller D, Woograsingh R, Jowatt V, Hindmarsh A, Nicholson JK, & Martin JE (2002) Vitamin E deficiency and metabolic deficits in neuronal ceroid lipofuscinosis described by bioinformatics. *Physiol Genomics*, 11, 195–203.

Guarneri R, Russo D, Cascio C, D'Agostino S, Galizzi G, Bigini P, Mennini T, & Guarneri P (2004) Retinal oxidation, apoptosis and age- and sex-differences in the mnd mutant mouse, a model of neuronal ceroid lipofuscinosis. *Brain Res*, 1014, 209–220.

Haltia M, Tyynelä J, Hirvasniemi A, Herva R, Ranta US, & Lehesjoki AE (1999) CLN8 - Northern epilepsy. In Goebel HH, Mole SE, & Lake BD (Eds.) *The Neuronal Ceroid Lipofuscinoses (Batten Disease)*, pp. 117–124. Amsterdam, IOS Press.

Hermansson M, Kakela R, Berghall M, Lehesjoki AE, Somerharju P, & Lahtinen U (2005) Mass spectrometric analysis reveals changes in phospholipid, neutral sphingolipid and sulfatide molecular species in progressive epilepsy with mental retardation, EPMR, brain: a case study. *J Neurochem*, 95, 609–617.

Herva R, Tyynelä J, Hirvasniemi A, Syrjakallio-Ylitalo M, & Haltia M (2000) Northern epilepsy: a novel form of neuronal ceroid-lipofuscinosis. *Brain Pathol*, 10, 215–222.

Hirvasniemi A, Herrala P, & Leisti J (1995) Northern epilepsy syndrome: clinical course and the effect of medication on seizures. *Epilepsia*, 36, 792–797.

Hirvasniemi A & Karumo J (1994) Neuroradiological findings in the northern epilepsy syndrome. *Acta Neurol Scand*, 90, 388–393.

Hirvasniemi A, Lang H, Lehesjoki AE, & Leisti J (1994) Northern epilepsy syndrome: an inherited childhood onset epilepsy with associated mental deterioration. *J Med Genet*, 31, 177–182.

Kousi M, Siintola E, Dvorakova L, Vlaskova H, Turnbull J, Topçu M, Yuksel D, Gokben S, Minassian BA, Elleder M, Mole SE, & Lehesjoki AE (2009) Mutations in CLN7/MFSD8 are a common cause of variant late-infantile neuronal ceroid lipofuscinosis. *Brain*, 132, 810–819.

Lonka L, Aalto A, Kopra O, Kuronen M, Kokaia Z, Saarma M, & Lehesjoki AE (2005) The neuronal ceroid lipofuscinosis Cln8 gene expression is developmentally regulated in mouse brain and up-regulated in the hippocampal kindling model of epilepsy. *BMC Neurosci*, 6, 27.

Lonka L, Kyttala A, Ranta S, Jalanko A, & Lehesjoki AE (2000) The neuronal ceroid lipofuscinosis CLN8 membrane protein is a resident of the endoplasmic reticulum. *Hum Mol Genet*, 9, 1691–1697.

Lonka L, Salonen T, Siintola E, Kopra O, Lehesjoki AE, & Jalanko A (2004) Localization of wild-type and mutant neuronal ceroid lipofuscinosis CLN8 proteins in non-neuronal and neuronal cells. *J Neurosci Res*, 76, 862–871.

Mennini T, Bigini P, Cagnotto A, Carvelli L, Di Nunno P, Fumagalli E, Tortarolo M, Buurman WA, Ghezzi P, & Bendotti C (2004) Glial activation and TNFR-I upregulation precedes motor dysfunction in the spinal cord of mnd mice. *Cytokine*, 25, 127–135.

Mizutani Y, Kihara A, & Igarashi Y (2005) Mammalian Lass6 and its related family members regulate synthesis of specific ceramides. *Biochem J*, 390, 263–271.

Ranta S, Lehesjoki AE, Hirvasniemi A, Weissenbach J, Ross B, Leal SM, de la Chapelle A, & Gilliam TC (1996) Genetic and physical mapping of the progressive epilepsy with mental retardation (EPMR) locus on chromosome 8p. *Genome Res*, 6, 351–360.

Ranta S, Topçu M, Tegelberg S, Tan H, Ustübütün A, Saatci I, Dufke A, Enders H, Pohl K, Alembik Y, Mitchell WA, Mole SE, & Lehesjoki AE (2004) Variant late infantile neuronal ceroid lipofuscinosis in a subset of Turkish patients is allelic to Northern epilepsy. *Hum Mutat*, 23, 300–305.

Ranta S, Zhang Y, Ross B, Lonka L, Takkunen E, Messer A, Sharp J, Wheeler R, Kusumi K, Mole S, Liu W, Soares MB, Bonaldo MF, Hirvasniemi A, de la Chapelle A, Gilliam TC, & Lehesjoki AE (1999) The neuronal ceroid lipofuscinoses in human EPMR and mnd mutant mice are associated with mutations in CLN8. *Nat Genet*, 23, 233–236.

Reinhardt K, Grapp M, Schlachter K, Bruck W, Gartner J, & Steinfeld R (2010) Novel CLN8 mutations confirm the clinical and ethnic diversity of late infantile neuronal ceroid lipofuscinosis. *Clin Genet*, 77, 79–85.

Schulz A, Mousallem T, Venkataramani M, Persaud-Sawin DA, Zucker A, Luberto C, Bielawska A, Bielawski J, Holthuis JC, Jazwinski SM, Kozhaya L, Dbaibo GS, & Boustany RM (2006) The CLN9 protein, a regulator of dihydroceramide synthase. *J Biol Chem*, 281, 2784–2794.

Siintola E, Lehesjoki AE, & Mole SE (2006) Molecular genetics of the NCLs—status and perspectives. *Biochim Biophys Acta*, 1762, 857–864.

Steenhuis P, Herder S, Gelis S, Braulke T, & Storch S (2010) Lysosomal targeting of the CLN7 membrane glycoprotein and transport via the plasma membrane require a dileucine motif. Traffi c, 11, 987–1000.

Striano P, Specchio N, Biancheri R, Cannelli N, Simonati A, Cassandrini D, Rossi A, Bruno C, Fusco L, Gaggero R, Vigevano F, Bertini E, Zara F, Santorelli FM, & Striano S (2007) Clinical and electrophysiological features of epilepsy in Italian patients with CLN8 mutations. *Epilepsy Behav*, 10, 187–191.

Tahvanainen E, Ranta S, Hirvasniemi A, Karila E, Leisti J, Sistonen P, Weissenbach J, Lehesjoki AE, & de la Chapelle A (1994) The gene for a recessively inherited human childhood progressive epilepsy with mental retardation maps to the distal short arm of chromosome 8. *Proc Natl Acad Sci U S A*, 91, 7267–7270.

Topçu M, Tan H, Yalnizoglu D, Usubutun A, Saatci I, Aynaci M, Anlar B, Topaloglu H, Turanli G, Kose G, & Aysun S (2004) Evaluation of 36 patients from Turkey with neuronal ceroid lipofuscinosis: clinical, neurophysiological, neuroradiological and histopathologic studies. *Turk J Pediatr*, 46, 1–10.

Tyynelä J, Cooper JD, Khan MN, Shemilts SJ, & Haltia M (2004) Hippocampal pathology in the human neuronal ceroid-lipofuscinoses: distinct patterns of storage deposition, neurodegeneration and glial activation. *Brain Pathol*, 14, 349–357.

Vantaggiato C, Redaelli F, Falcone S, Perrotta C, Tonelli A, Bondioni S, Morbin M, Riva D, Saletti V, Bonaglia MC, Giorda R, Bresolin N, Clementi E, & Bassi MT (2009) A novel CLN8 mutation in late-infantile-onset neuronal

ceroid lipofuscinosis (LINCL) reveals aspects of CLN8 neurobiological function. *Hum Mutat*, 30, 1104–1116.
Williams RE, Åberg L, Autti T, Goebel HH, Kohlschutter A, & Lonnqvist T (2006) Diagnosis of the neuronal ceroid lipofuscinoses: an update. *Biochim Biophys Acta*, 1762, 865–872.
Winter E & Ponting CP (2002) TRAM, LAG1 and CLN8: members of a novel family of lipid-sensing domains? *Trends Biochem Sci*, 27, 381–383.
Zelnik N, Mahajna M, Iancu TC, Sharony R, & Zeigler M (2007) A novel mutation of the CLN8 gene: is there a Mediterranean phenotype? *Pediatr Neurol*, 36, 411–413.

Chapter 13

CLN10

J.D. Cooper, S. Partanen, E. Siintola, R. Steinfeld, P. Strömme, and J. Tyynelä

INTRODUCTION

Congenital NCL was first reported in the 1940s, and since then a handful of cases have been described in the literature. The first molecular explanation for congenital NCL was given in 2006 when a mutation in the gene encoding cathepsin D was identified in one patient, also proving the recessive inheritance of the disease. Simultaneously, a patient with a later childhood onset cathepsin D deficiency was described, and now cases with onset as late as adulthood are known. Thus, complete lack of cathepsin D and its enzymatic activity causes the congenital form of NCL, whereas a partial inactivation of the enzyme leads to a later-onset form of NCL. Cathepsin D deficiency should therefore be considered as a diagnosis in convulsing newborns with microcephaly, as well as in patients with later-onset forms of NCL characterized by visual impairment, ataxia, and cognitive decline.

MOLECULAR GENETICS

Gene identification

As the cathepsin D gene (*CTSD*) had previously been identified as a causative gene for naturally occurring NCL in sheep and American bulldogs (Tyynelä et al., 2000, Awano et al., 2006), it was also considered as a candidate gene for human NCL. Disease-causing mutations in human *CTSD*, at chromosome 11p15.5, were

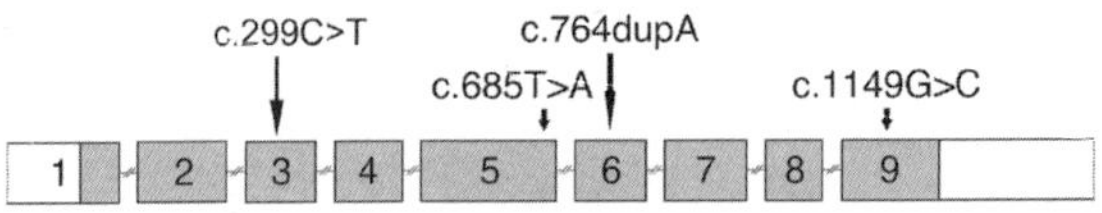

Figure 13.1 Schematic presentation of the human *CTSD* genomic structure. The gene is composed of 9 exons (shown as grey boxes). Locations of the disease-associated mutations are indicated by arrows. Nucleotide changes associated with diseases are indicated by arrows: c.299C>T, c.685T>A, c.764dupA, and c.1149G>C.

identified in two separate NCL phenotypes (OMIM 610127) (Siintola et al., 2006, Steinfeld et al., 2006).

Gene structure

CTSD (GenBank accession number M11233) consists of nine exons (Figure 13.1). The gene spans 29.77 kb of genomic DNA (NCBI AceView, http://www.ncbi.nlm.nih.gov/IEB/Research/Acembly/). The open reading frame of 1239 bp encodes a 412 amino acid polypeptide.

Mutation spectrum

To date, four mutations in three patients have been identified in *CTSD* (Figure 13.2). Two mutations have been reported in patients with congenital NCL. A homozygous duplication (c.764dupA) in exon 6 was present in a patient of Pakistani origin (Siintola et al., 2006). The duplication creates a premature stop codon (p. Tyr255X), predicting a truncation of the protein by 158 amino acids. Transient expression of this c.764dupA *CTSD* in BHK cells showed complete lack of enzyme activity. CTSD immunostaining was absent in samples from the patient's brain (Siintola et al., 2006) suggesting that either the mutant polypeptide is degraded or that none is produced due to degradation at the mRNA level. c.299C>T was found in exon 3 of *CTSD* in a patient of Caucasian origin (Fritchie et al., 2009). This mutation causes a transition of a conserved Ser-residue (p.Ser100Phe) adjacent to the catalytic site of the enzyme activity, and is therefore likely to directly affect the enzyme. The mutant protein appeared stable and normally processed but little cathepsin D activity was detected in the fibroblasts from the patient (Fritchie et al., 2009).

Compound heterozygosity for two *CTSD* missense mutations ([g.6517T>A]+[g.10267G>C] or [p.Phe229Ile]+[p.Trp383Cys]), resulting in CTSD deficiency, caused a late infantile onset NCL-like neurodegenerative disease in a German patient. The mutation p.Phe229Ile affects a highly conserved amino acid residue, but nevertheless is associated with significant residual enzymatic activity. The other mutation, p.Trp383Cys, may cause major conformational changes, resulting in disturbed post-translational processing, mistargeting, and complete loss of enzymatic activity of CTSD (Steinfeld et al., 2006).

It is expected that more mutations will be described, as patients with congenital and

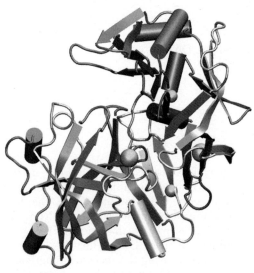

Figure 13.2 Crystal structure of the human CTSD protein visualized by the VMD program (Humphrey et al., 1996). The N-terminal domain is shown in dark and the C-terminal domain in light. Amino acids associated with disease-causing mutations are marked with spheres, the large sphere indicating the location of the alteration leading to congenital NCL. Courtesy of Dr Liisa Laakkonen, Division of Biochemistry, Department of Biological and Environmental Sciences, University of Helsinki, Finland.

atypical presentation of NCL are investigated for possible cathepsin D deficiency.

Related genes

Cysteine cathepsins have also been associated with neurodegeneration in mice: cathepsin F-deficient mice develop a late onset NCL disease (Tang et al., 2006), while a double deficiency of cathepsin B and L results in an early onset NCL-like phenotype, brain atrophy, and early death in mice (Felbor et al., 2002). It has been suggested that cathepsins B and D act together in regulating cell survival and death (Isahara et al., 1999, Jäättelä et al., 2004).

CELL BIOLOGY

Enzyme structure, localization, and function

CTSD (EC 3.4.23.5) is a lysosomal enzyme belonging to the pepsin family of aspartic proteases (Press et al., 1960). It has a bilobed structure with a deep active-site cleft in between the two lobes. Each of the lobes has a key aspartic acid residue, which together form the active site of the enzyme (Metcalf and Fusek, 1993, Rawlings and Barrett, 1995). CTSD is synthesized as an inactive preproprotein, with an N-terminal signal sequence mediating its transport across the endoplasmic reticulum (ER) membrane (Hasilik and Neufeld, 1980a, Rawlings and Barrett, 1995). In the ER it receives two high-mannose oligosaccharide chains, which become phosphorylated in the *trans*-Golgi network and target the enzyme to the lysosome via the mannose-6-phosphate receptor trafficking route (Hasilik and Neufeld, 1980b). Depending on the cell type, alternative targeting of CTSD to the lysosome also exists (Dittmer et al., 1999) which utilizes the receptor sortilin (Canuel et al., 2009, Zeng et al., 2009). The low lysosomal pH facilitates the proteolytic cleavage of the propeptide, creating an active single-chain form of CTSD, which is further processed into a two-chain mature enzyme composed of the 30kDa heavy chain and the 14kDa light chain (Hasilik and Neufeld, 1980a). This propeptide may be significantly active if secreted (Vetvicka, 2009).

CTSD plays an important role in lysosomal protein turnover, antigen processing, and disease (Saftig et al., 1995). CTSD has an acidic pH optimum varying from 3.5–5.0, and its enzymatic activity is selectively inhibited by pepstatin A (Aoyagi et al., 1972). CTSD is also likely to participate in limited proteolysis by activating tissue and cell specific substrates, such as peptide hormones, insulin-like growth factor II, rhodopsin, and myelin basic protein (Benuck et al., 1978, Diment et al., 1989, Claussen et al., 1997). Apart from its enzymatic activity, CTSD has a complex role outside the lysosome in regulating cell proliferation and apoptosis, particularly in cancer (Fusek and Vetvicka, 1994, Glondu et al., 2001, Kågedal et al., 2001, Glondu et al., 2002, Benes et al., 2008). Some of its effects may be exerted by its secreted zymogen, procathepsin D (Vetvicka, 2009). It has also been suggested that CTSD may be a key factor in a lysosome-mediated programmed cell death pathway (Jäättelä et al., 2004), contributing towards protection against Parkinson's disease (Qiao et al., 2008), and may slightly increase the risk of Alzheimer's disease (Schuur et al., 2009).

Gene expression and tissue distribution of CTSD

CTSD is expressed in most tissues but the amount varies between different cell types. It is particularly abundant in all types of macrophages, which harbour many lysosomes (Whitaker and Rhodes, 1983). Within the central nervous system, CTSD is strongly expressed in neurons and microglial cells, less in oligodendrocytes, and hardly at all in astrocytes (Whitaker and Rhodes, 1983). CTSD expression is developmentally regulated. During development of the rat nervous system, its highest expression coincides with the most active period of myelination, around postnatal day 15 (Snyder and Whitaker, 1983, Suopanki et al., 2000). Activity and localization of CTSD also changes during aging and in certain pathological conditions, e.g. in Alzheimer's disease (Nakanishi et al., 1994, Cataldo et al., 1995, Nakanishi et al., 1997).

CLINICAL DATA

Incidence

The congenital form of human NCL was first described during the 1940s (Norman and Wood, 1941), and altogether ten cases have been reported in the literature (Brown et al., 1954, Sandbank, 1968, Humphreys et al., 1985, Garborg et al., 1987, Barohn et al., 1992, Siintola et al., 2006). Although the disease is rare, it is likely to be underdiagnosed, as affected fetuses may be aborted or stillborn.

Age of onset and symptoms

CLN10 disease, congenital NCL begins *in utero*. Affected fetuses may show signs of intrauterine growth retardation with a silent pattern on cardiotopography (CTG), and a proportionally small biparietal diameter. Seizures may also occur during fetal life. In one case the mother observed decreased normal fetal movements, together with abnormal fetal movements, which on an ultrasound examination at 36 weeks' gestation were thought to represent seizure activity (Siintola et al., 2006). At birth, affected infants present with intractable seizures, spasticity, and central apnoea with cyanosis. Survival is limited to only a few days, seldom to weeks.

CLN10 disease, late infantile variant

Partial inactivation of CTSD is associated with a more protracted neurodegenerative disease in humans (Steinfeld et al., 2006). A human patient described in the literature who is compound heterozygous for the missense mutations p.Phe229Ile and p.Trp383Cys had subtle signs of visual disturbance such as night blindness at the age of 4 years. At early school-age she suffered from ataxia and partial blindness. Fundoscopy revealed retinitis pigmentosa. In the course of the disease she developed progressive cognitive decline, loss of speech, retinal atrophy, and loss of motor skills. From her mid-teens she has been wheelchair-bound and severely mentally retarded (Steinfeld et al., 2006).

Brain imaging

Cerebral computed tomography (CT) examination of the newborns diagnosed with CLN10 disease, congenital NCL shows generalized cerebral and cerebellar brain atrophy, with enlarged lateral ventricles, increased amounts of cerebrospinal fluid (CSF) over the cerebral hemispheres, widening of the subarachnoid spaces, and a small cerebellum (Strömme et al. unpublished data). Brain magnetic resonance imaging (MRI) of a CLN10 disease, congenital NCL patient with c.299C>T mutation confirmed had microcephaly with sloping forehead and very small frontal lobes. Diffuse abundance of the extra-axial CSF spaces and minimal hydrocephalus was also noted (Fritchie et al., 2009). Cranial MRI of the patient with CLN10 disease, late infantile variant also showed features characteristic of a neurodegenerative disease with extensive cerebral and cerebellar atrophy (Steinfeld et al., 2006).

Biochemical features

CTSD enzyme activity in cells and tissues can be assayed, and CTSD deficiencies are associated with an abnormally low enzymatic activity and abnormal enzyme kinetics (Siintola et al., 2006, Steinfeld et al., 2006, Fritchie et al., 2009). Multiple lysosomal enzyme activities are also elevated in CTSD deficiencies. The neuronal storage material is positive for sphingolipid activator proteins (see below). *Ctsd*$^{-/-}$ mice have increased levels of GM2 and GM3 gangliosides, and staining for these is found preferentially in neurons and glial cells (Jabs et al., 2008). There is also a 20-fold elevation of the unusual lysophospholipid bis (monoacylglycero) phosphate in the brain, accompanied by sporadic accumulation of unesterified cholesterol. The impaired processing of the sphingolipid activator protein precursor may provide the mechanistic link to the storage of lipids in *Ctsd*$^{-/-}$ mice brains.

MORPHOLOGY

Electron microscopy

The autofluorescent storage material, typical of NCL diseases, is widely spread within the central nervous system of CLN10 disease, congenital NCL patients. In addition to brain tissue, only the thymus has been reported to contain ceroid lipofuscin in one of the patients (Brown et al., 1954). The ultrastructure of the storage deposits in the remaining neurons as well as in activated glial cells shows granular ultrastructure (Figure 13.3) (Humphreys et al., 1985, Garborg et al., 1987, Barohn et al., 1992, Fritchie et al., 2009). The skin biopsy specimen also revealed granular storage material in non-myelinated Schwann cells of the patient with CTSD deficiency and late-onset disease (Steinfeld et al., 2006), and granular material was found in the late onset patients (R. Steinfeld, unpublished data).

Autopsy findings, histopathology, and immunohistopathology

All patients with CLN10 disease, congenital NCL have been noted to be microcephalic and brain weight in examined cases has ranged from 65–200g (Barohn et al., 1992, Siintola et al., 2006, Fritchie et al., 2009). Other features include obliteration of the fontanelles, overriding sutures, a receding forehead, broad bridge of the nose, and low set and external malformation of the ears, particularly microtia. Ophthalmological findings have not been reported. In one consanguineous family with three affected infants, two out of four otherwise healthy siblings had reduced hearing, necessitating a hearing aid in one (Siintola

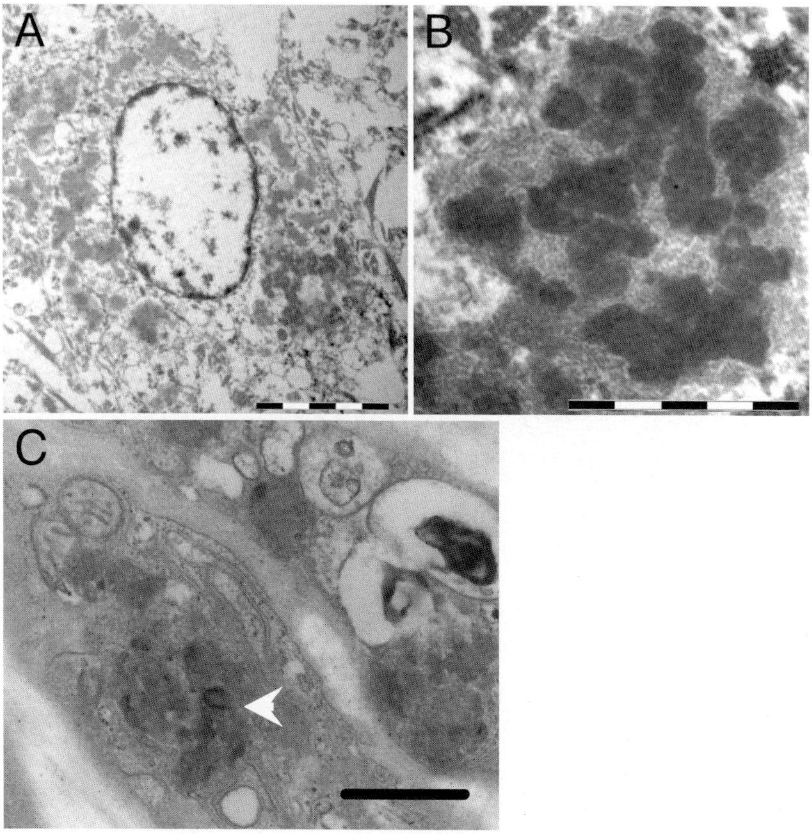

Figure 13.3 Electron microscopic ultrastructure of storage deposits in CLN10 disease, congenital NCL. (A) A general view of a cortical neuron filled with electron dense storage deposits, scale bar 5μm. (B) High magnification revealing the granular ultrastructure of the neuronal storage material, scale bar 1μm. Courtesy of Dr Magnus Röger and Prof. Jan Maehlen Ullevål University Hospital, Oslo, Norway.

et al., 2006). Malformations, apart from a claw hand and adducted thumbs, have not been observed outside the head and neck.

All patients show nearly identical neuropathological changes at autopsy with extremely pronounced cerebral and cerebellar atrophy and extensive loss of neurons and myelin. The cerebral cortex contains a large number of activated astrocytes and microglia (Figure 13.4). Within the cerebellum, the number of Purkinje cells and granule cells is severely reduced. The white matter also shows dramatic pathological changes

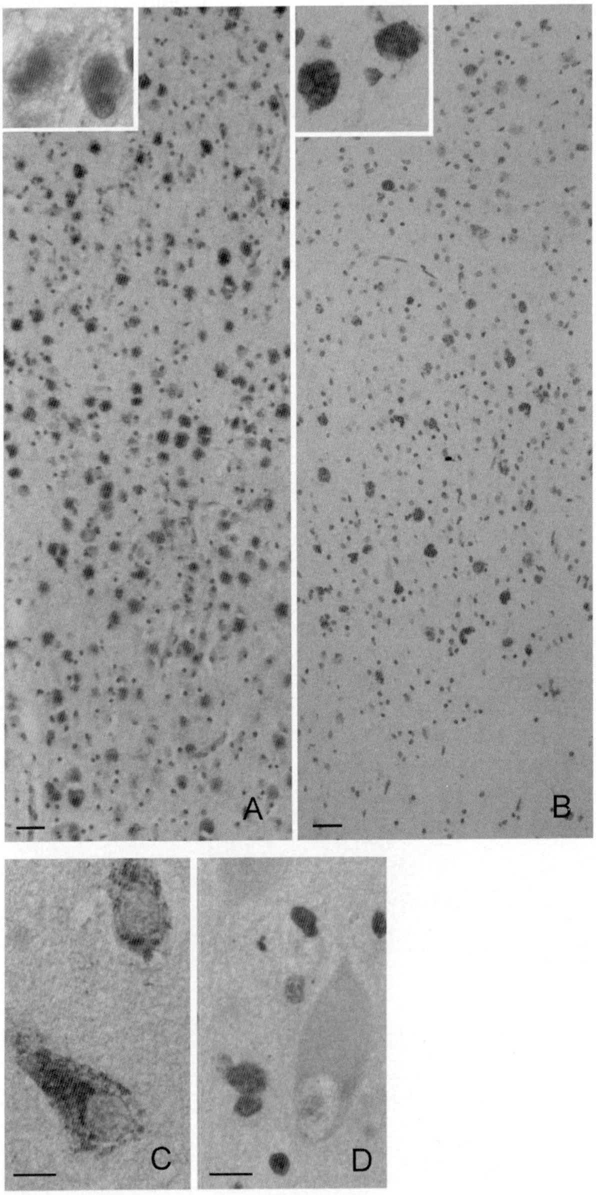

Figure 13.4 Immunohistological stainings of paraffin-embedded brain tissue samples. (A) Extreme activation of astrocytes and (B) microglial cells is evident in the cerebral cortex of patients with congenital NCL, as revealed by staining the tissue with antibodies against (A) glial fibrillary acidic protein and (B) CD68. (C) CTSD staining is punctate in normal human neurons, while (D) no staining is observed in neurons of patients with congenital NCL. Scale bar 25μm in (A) and (B); 5μm in (C) and (D).

with loss of myelin and pronounced astrocytic activation (Sandbank, 1968, Humphreys et al., 1985, Garborg et al., 1987, Siintola et al., 2006, Fritchie et al., 2009). Outside of the central nervous system, the thymus contains abundant amounts of autofluorescent storage material (Brown et al., 1954).

Immunohistological studies showed lack of CTSD in three patients with congenital NCL (Figure 13.4) (Siintola et al., 2006) and lack of enzyme activity in one (Fritchie et al., 2009). However, it is likely that patients with residual CTSD staining will be discovered in the future. The storage material can be stained with antibodies against sphingolipid activator proteins, but not with antibodies against mitochondrial ATP synthase subunit c (Siintola et al., 2006).

DISEASE MECHANISM

At present it is unknown how the deficiency of a lysosomal protease, CTSD, results in a selective death of neurons within the central nervous system. There is certainly an increasing recognition of the complex role played by CTSD (Benes et al., 2008). The metabolic pathways that are involved are likely to be highly conserved among species, since CTSD deficiency also leads to neurodegeneration and accumulation of storage material in the fly model *Drosophila* (Myllykangas et al., 2005). In mice, humans, and sheep with CTSD deficiency, the whole brain including the cerebrum and cerebellum, as well as the white and grey matter, are severely affected. Both neuronal loss and glial activation are observed in all these species (Humphreys et al., 1985, Garborg et al., 1987, Barohn et al., 1992, Koike et al., 2000, Tyynelä et al., 2000, Siintola et al., 2006, Haapanen et al., 2007, Partanen et al., 2008, Fritchie et al., 2009). However, the different areas of the brain show different degrees of pathological change: in *Ctsd* deficient mice, the somatosensory thalamocortical system is more severely affected than the neighbouring brain areas, suggesting that these pathways may be a primary target of the disease (Partanen et al., 2008). Of the molecular mechanisms, oxidative stress is likely to play a role in the pathogenesis. In particular, nitric oxide has been implicated as a factor in neuronal death in *Ctsd* knockout mice (Nakanishi et al., 2001, Koike et al., 2003). Recent compelling evidence also indicates autophagy (Koike et al., 2005) and synaptic alterations (Partanen et al., 2008, Mutka et al., 2010) as key mediators of neuronal death in *Ctsd* knockout mice. Indeed, reorganization of the presynaptic compartment occurs before synaptic elimination and the subsequent neuron loss, which again occurs first within the thalamus and only subsequently in the cortex (Partanen et al., 2008). These synaptic changes are accompanied by demyelination and altered cholesterol trafficking (Mutka et al., 2010), further emphasizing the early involvement of the axon and synapse in CTSD deficiency. Unexpectedly, CTSD deficiency in mice, sheep, and human cases was also recently shown to result in misprocessing of alpha-synuclein, a protein that is associated with the development of Parkinson's disease (Cullen et al., 2009).

Deficiency of certain neuronal chloride channels, including *Clcn6* and *Clcn7*, has been suggested to produce an NCL-like phenotype in mice (Kasper et al., 2005, Poët et al., 2006; Pressey et al., 2010). Indeed, the rapidly progressing phenotypes of *Ctsd* knockout mice, *Clcn7* knockout mice, and grey lethal mice (*gl*) mice, which bear a mutation in *Ostm1*, the β-subunit critical for *Clcn7* function, are remarkably similar (Pressey et al., 2010, and A. Haapanen et al. unpublished observations). CLCN7 deficiency causes osteopetrosis in human, the malignant form of which is associated with severe involvement of the central nervous system (Kornak et al., 2001). *CLCN6* has been associated with two cases of late onset NCL and it remains a candidate gene for mild forms of human NCL (Poët et al., 2006). However, more detailed characterization of *Clcn6* knockout mice reveals that these mice do not display many of the features typical of murine NCL (Pressey at al., 2010).

CORRELATIONS

Four mutations have been described in human patients. Mutation p.Tyr255X is predicted to result in truncation of CTSD by 158 amino acids and causes complete lack of enzyme activity. Mutation p.Ser100Phe affects a conserved amino acid residue adjacent to the active site of CTSD and results in the production of inactive but stable enzyme, resembling the findings in lambs with congenital NCL. Mutation p. Phe229Ile affects a highly conserved amino acid residue, but nevertheless is associated with significant residual enzymatic activity. p.Trp383Cys may cause major conformational changes resulting in disturbed post-translational processing, mistargeting since it is associated with complete loss of enzymatic activity of CTSD (Steinfeld et al., 2006).

It appears that the complete inactivation or lack of CTSD results in prenatal onset, congenital NCL in humans (Siintola et al., 2006, Fritchie et al., 2009), while less pathogenic mutations with preservation of residual enzyme activity lead to a milder phenotype, with a later onset, of the disease (Steinfeld et al., 2006). This suggestion is supported by observations in other species: complete inactivation of CTSD leads to a congenital form of the disease in lambs and to an early onset disease in mice, while partial inactivation of CTSD leads to a later onset form of the disease in American Bulldogs (Saftig et al., 1995, Tyynelä et al., 2000, Awano et al., 2006) (see Chapters 17 and 18). The CTSD-deficient sheep are severely affected at birth. They tremble and are unable to stand, and die within a few days (Tyynelä et al., 2000). *Ctsd* deficient mice, however, appear normal at birth, but soon develop blindness and epilepsy, and die at the age of 26 days (Saftig et al., 1995, Koike et al., 2000). Of the multiple existing mouse models of NCL diseases, *Ctsd* knockout mice exhibit the earliest onset and most severe phenotype. In contrast, American Bulldogs carrying the homozygous missense mutation p.Met199Ile have 36% residual CTSD activity left and start to develop progressive ataxia and exaggerated movements relatively late, between 0.9–3.5 years. The life expectancy of these dogs is reduced to 30–50% when compared with non-affected dogs (Awano et al., 2006).

It is likely that a wider disease phenotype will come to be recognized in the future as atypical NCL patients are investigated for CTSD deficiency and *CTSD* mutations. New mutations will be added to the mutation database at http:/www.ucl.ac.uk/ncl.CatD.

Granular ultrastructure is typical for the storage material found in CLN10 disease in humans, sheep, and fly (Humphreys et al., 1985, Garborg et al., 1987, Barohn et al., 1992, Tyynelä et al., 2000, Myllykangas et al., 2005, Steinfeld et al., 2006, Fritchie et al., 2009). However, the mouse storage material possesses either granular or fingerprint ultrastructure (Koike et al., 2000).

DIAGNOSIS

The clinical diagnosis of CLN10 disease, congenital NCL should be suspected when an infant presents with intractable seizures and microcephaly. In some cases epilepsy begins during fetal life and the seizure activity can be confirmed by antenatal real-time ultrasound examination. Other features may include low-set ears or malformations of the external ears. Survival is usually limited to only a few days.

The early symptoms associated with the reported later onset form of CTSD deficiency somewhat resemble those of the CLN3 disease, classic juvenile, since both NCL types initially present with visual disturbances. However, ataxia was an early symptom in the patient with CTSD deficiency, whereas motor deficits commonly develop later in CLN3 disease, classic juvenile patients. Therefore, patients with early visual impairment suspected to suffer from a form of NCL, should undergo enzymatic testing for CTSD deficiency. The presence of granular storage material in the Schwann cells of the skin is also indicative of CTSD deficiency, provided CLN1/PPT1 deficiency has been excluded. Subsequently, the correct diagnosis should be confirmed by molecular analysis of the *CTSD* gene.

CLINICAL MANAGEMENT AND EXPERIMENTAL THERAPY

At present, only symptomatic treatment is available for CLN10 disease. Prenatal treatment of congenital NCL would require the appropriate substances or vectors to reach the fetal brain through the placenta early in pregnancy. In patients with later onset CTSD deficiency, treatment serves to ameliorate the motor and behavioural complications as well as feeding difficulties. Experimental strategies to treat CLN10 disease might arise from gene therapy, stem cell therapy, and/or enzyme replacement therapy. Work in model organisms may identify new targets suitable for therapeutic intervention, such as genetic modifiers for cathepsin D deficiency in *Drosophila* models (Kuronen et al., 2009).

REFERENCES

Aoyagi T, Morishima H, Nishizawa R, Kunimoto S, & Takeuchi T (1972) Biological activity of pepstatins, pepstanone A and partial peptides on pepsin, cathepsin D and renin. *J Antibiot* (Tokyo), 25, 689–694.

Awano T, Katz ML, O'Brien DP, Taylor JF, Evans J, Khan S, Sohar I, Lobel P, & Johnson GS (2006) A mutation in the cathepsin D gene (CTSD) in American Bulldogs with neuronal ceroid lipofuscinosis. *Mol Genet Metab*, 87, 341–348.

Barohn RJ, Dowd DC, & Kagan-Hallet KS (1992) Congenital ceroid-lipofuscinosis. *Pediatr Neurol*, 8, 54–59.

Benes P, Vetvicka V, & Fusek M (2008) Cathepsin D—many functions of one aspartic protease. *Crit Rev Oncol Hematol*, 68, 12–28.

Benuck M, Grynbaum A, & Marks N (1978) Breakdown of somatostatin and substance P by cathepsin D purified from calf brain by affinity chromatography. *Brain Res*, 143, 181–185.

Brown NJ, Corner BD, & Dodgson MC (1954) A second case in the same family of congenital familial cerebral lipoidosis resembling amaurotic family idiocy. *Arch Dis Child*, 29, 48–54.

Canuel M, Libin Y, & Morales CR (2009) The interactomics of sortilin: an ancient lysosomal receptor evolving new functions. *Histol Histopathol*, 24, 481–492.

Cataldo AM, Barnett JL, Berman SA, Li J, Quarless S, Bursztajn S, Lippa C, & Nixon RA (1995) Gene expression and cellular content of cathepsin D in Alzheimer's disease brain: evidence for early up-regulation of the endosomal-lysosomal system. *Neuron*, 14, 671–680.

Claussen M, Kubler B, Wendland M, Neifer K, Schmidt B, Zapf J, & Braulke T (1997) Proteolysis of insulin-like growth factors (IGF) and IGF binding proteins by cathepsin D. *Endocrinology*, 138, 3797–3803.

Cullen V, Lindfors M, Ng J, Paetau A, Swinton E, Kolodziej P, Boston H, Saftig P, Woulfe J, Feany MB, Myllykangas L, Schlossmacher MG, & Tyynelä J (2009) Cathepsin D expression level affects alpha-synuclein processing, aggregation, and toxicity in vivo. *Mol Brain*, 2, 5.

Diment S, Martin KJ, & Stahl PD (1989) Cleavage of parathyroid hormone in macrophage endosomes illustrates a novel pathway for intracellular processing of proteins. *J Biol Chem*, 264, 13403–13406.

Dittmer F, Ulbrich EJ, Hafner A, Schmahl W, Meister T, Pohlmann R, & von Figura K (1999) Alternative mechanisms for trafficking of lysosomal enzymes in mannose 6-phosphate receptor-deficient mice are cell type-specific. *J Cell Sci*, 112 (Pt 10), 1591–1597.

Felbor U, Kessler B, Mothes W, Goebel HH, Ploegh HL, Bronson RT, & Olsen BR (2002) Neuronal loss and brain atrophy in mice lacking cathepsins B and L. *Proc Natl Acad Sci U S A*, 99, 7883–7888.

Fritchie K, Siintola E, Armao D, Lehesjoki AE, Marino T, Powell C, Tennison M, Booker JM, Koch S, Partanen S, Suzuki K, Tyynelä J, & Thorne LB (2009) Novel mutation and the first prenatal screening of cathepsin D deficiency (CLN10). *Acta Neuropathol*, 117, 201–208.

Fusek M & Vetvicka V (1994) Mitogenic function of human procathepsin D: the role of the propeptide. *Biochem J*, 303 (Pt 3), 775–780.

Garborg I, Torvik A, Hals J, Tangsrud SE, & Lindemann R (1987) Congenital neuronal ceroid lipofuscinosis. *A case report. Acta Pathol Microbiol Immunol Scand A*, 95, 119–125.

Glondu M, Coopman P, Laurent-Matha V, Garcia M, Rochefort H, & Liaudet-Coopman E (2001) A mutated cathepsin-D devoid of its catalytic activity stimulates the growth of cancer cells. *Oncogene*, 20, 6920–6929.

Glondu M, Liaudet-Coopman E, Derocq D, Platet N, Rochefort H, & Garcia M (2002) Down-regulation of cathepsin-D expression by antisense gene transfer inhibits tumor growth and experimental lung metastasis of human breast cancer cells. *Oncogene*, 21, 5127–5134.

Haapanen A, Ramadan UA, Autti T, Joensuu R, & Tyynelä J (2007) In vivo MRI reveals the dynamics of pathological changes in the brains of cathepsin D-deficient mice and correlates changes in manganese-enhanced MRI with microglial activation. *Magn Reson Imaging*, 25, 1024–1031.

Hasilik A & Neufeld EF (1980a) Biosynthesis of lysosomal enzymes in fibroblasts. Synthesis as precursors of higher molecular weight. *J Biol Chem*, 255, 4937–4945.

Hasilik A & Neufeld EF (1980b) Biosynthesis of lysosomal enzymes in fibroblasts. Phosphorylation of mannose residues. *J Biol Chem*, 255, 4946–4950.

Humphrey W, Dalke A, & Schulten K (1996) VMD: visual molecular dynamics. *J Mol Graph*, 14, 33–38, 27–28.

Humphreys S, Lake BD, & Scholtz CL (1985) Congenital amaurotic idiocy—a pathological, histochemical, biochemical and ultrastructural study. *Neuropathol Appl Neurobiol*, 11, 475–484.

Isahara K, Ohsawa Y, Kanamori S, Shibata M, Waguri S, Sato N, Gotow T, Watanabe T, Momoi T, Urase K, Kominami E, & Uchiyama Y (1999) Regulation of a novel pathway for cell death by lysosomal aspartic and cysteine proteinases. *Neuroscience*, 91, 233–249.

Jäättelä M, Cande C, & Kroemer G (2004) Lysosomes and mitochondria in the commitment to apoptosis: a potential role for cathepsin D and AIF. *Cell Death Differ*, 11, 135–136.

Jabs S, Quitsch A, Kakela R, Koch B, Tyynelä J, Brade H, Glatzel M, Walkley S, Saftig P, Vanier MT, & Braulke T (2008) Accumulation of bis(monoacylglycero)phosphate and gangliosides in mouse models of neuronal ceroid lipofuscinosis. *J Neurochem*, 106, 1415–1425.

Kågedal K, Johansson U, & Ollinger K (2001) The lysosomal protease cathepsin D mediates apoptosis induced by oxidative stress. *FASEB J*, 15, 1592–1594.

Kasper D, Planells-Cases R, Fuhrmann JC, Scheel O, Zeitz O, Ruether K, Schmitt A, Poet M, Steinfeld R, Schweizer M, Kornak U, & Jentsch TJ (2005) Loss of the chloride channel ClC-7 leads to lysosomal storage disease and neurodegeneration. *EMBO J*, 24, 1079–1091.

Koike M, Nakanishi H, Saftig P, Ezaki J, Isahara K, Ohsawa Y, Schulz-Schaeffer W, Watanabe T, Waguri S, Kametaka S, Shibata M, Yamamoto K, Kominami E, Peters C, von Figura K, & Uchiyama Y (2000) Cathepsin D deficiency induces lysosomal storage with ceroid lipofuscin in mouse CNS neurons. *J Neurosci*, 20, 6898–6906.

Koike M, Shibata M, Ohsawa Y, Nakanishi H, Koga T, Kametaka S, Waguri S, Momoi T, Kominami E, Peters C, Figura K, Saftig P, & Uchiyama Y (2003) Involvement of two different cell death pathways in retinal atrophy of cathepsin D-deficient mice. *Mol Cell Neurosci*, 22, 146–161.

Koike M, Shibata M, Waguri S, Yoshimura K, Tanida I, Kominami E, Gotow T, Peters C, von Figura K, Mizushima N, Saftig P, & Uchiyama Y (2005) Participation of autophagy in storage of lysosomes in neurons from mouse models of neuronal ceroid-lipofuscinoses (Batten disease). *Am J Pathol*, 167, 1713–1728.

Kornak U, Kasper D, Bosl MR, Kaiser E, Schweizer M, Schulz A, Friedrich W, Delling G, & Jentsch TJ (2001) Loss of the ClC-7 chloride channel leads to osteopetrosis in mice and man. *Cell*, 104, 205–215.

Kuronen M, Talvitie M, Lehesjoki AE, & Myllykangas L (2009) Genetic modifiers of degeneration in the cathepsin D deficient Drosophila model for neuronal ceroid lipofuscinosis. *Neurobiol Dis*, 36, 488–493.

Metcalf P & Fusek M (1993) Two crystal structures for cathepsin D: the lysosomal targeting signal and active site. *EMBO J*, 12, 1293–1302.

Mutka AL, Haapanen A, Kakela R, Lindfors M, Wright AK, Inkinen T, Hermansson M, Rokka A, Corthals G, Jauhiainen M, Gillingwater TH, Ikonen E, & Tyynelä J (2010) Murine cathepsin D deficiency is associated with dysmyelination/myelin disruption and accumulation of cholesteryl esters in the brain. *J Neurochem*, 112, 193–203.

Myllykangas L, Tyynelä J, Page-McCaw A, Rubin GM, Haltia MJ, & Feany MB (2005) Cathepsin D-deficient Drosophila recapitulate the key features of neuronal ceroid lipofuscinoses. *Neurobiol Dis*, 19, 194–199.

Nakanishi H, Amano T, Sastradipura DF, Yoshimine Y, Tsukuba T, Tanabe K, Hirotsu I, Ohono T, & Yamamoto K (1997) Increased expression of cathepsins E and D in neurons of the aged rat brain and their colocalization with lipofuscin and carboxy-terminal fragments of Alzheimer amyloid precursor protein. *J Neurochem*, 68, 739–749.

Nakanishi H, Tominaga K, Amano T, Hirotsu I, Inoue T, & Yamamoto K (1994) Age-related changes in activities and localizations of cathepsins D, E, B, and L in the rat brain tissues. *Exp Neurol*, 126, 119–128.

Nakanishi H, Zhang J, Koike M, Nishioku T, Okamoto Y, Kominami E, von Figura K, Peters C, Yamamoto K, Saftig P, & Uchiyama Y (2001) Involvement of nitric oxide released from microglia-macrophages in pathological changes of cathepsin D-deficient mice. *J Neurosci*, 21, 7526–7533.

Norman RM & Wood N (1941) Congenital form of amaurotic family idiocy. *J Neurol Psych*, 4, 175–190.

Partanen S, Haapanen A, Kielar C, Pontikis C, Alexander N, Inkinen T, Saftig P, Gillingwater TH, Cooper JD, & Tyynelä J (2008) Synaptic changes in the thalamocortical system of cathepsin D-deficient mice: a model of human congenital neuronal ceroid-lipofuscinosis. *J Neuropathol Exp Neurol*, 67, 16–29.

Poët M, Kornak U, Schweizer M, Zdebik AA, Scheel O, Hoelter S, Wurst W, Schmitt A, Fuhrmann JC, Planells-Cases R, Mole SE, Hubner CA, & Jentsch TJ (2006) Lysosomal storage disease upon disruption of the neuronal chloride transport protein ClC-6. *Proc Natl Acad Sci U S A*, 103, 13854–13859.

Press EM, Porter RR, & Cebra J (1960) The isolation and properties of a proteolytic enzyme, cathepsin D, from bovine spleen. *Biochem J*, 74, 501–514.

Pressey SNR, O'Donnell KJ, Stauber T, Fuhrmann JC, Tyynela J, Jentsch TJ, and Cooper JD (2010). Distinct neuropathological phenotypes after disrupting the chloride transport proteins ClC-6 or ClC-7/Ostm1. *J Neuropath Exp Neurol* (In press).

Qiao L, Hamamichi S, Caldwell KA, Caldwell GA, Yacoubian TA, Wilson S, Xie ZL, Speake LD, Parks R, Crabtree D, Liang Q, Crimmins S, Schneider L, Uchiyama Y, Iwatsubo T, Zhou Y, Peng L, Lu Y, Standaert DG, Walls KC, Shacka JJ, Roth KA, & Zhang J (2008) Lysosomal enzyme cathepsin D protects against alpha-synuclein aggregation and toxicity. *Mol Brain*, 1, 17.

Rawlings ND & Barrett AJ (1995) Families of aspartic peptidases, and those of unknown catalytic mechanism. *Methods Enzymol*, 248, 105–120.

Saftig P, Hetman M, Schmahl W, Weber K, Heine L, Mossmann H, Koster A, Hess B, Evers M, von Figura K, et al. (1995) Mice deficient for the lysosomal proteinase cathepsin D exhibit progressive atrophy of the intestinal mucosa and profound destruction of lymphoid cells. *EMBO J*, 14, 3599–3608.

Sandbank U (1968) Congenital amaurotic idiocy. *Pathol Eur*, 3, 226–229.

Schuur M, Ikram MA, van Swieten JC, Isaacs A, Vergeer-Drop JM, Hofman A, Oostra BA, Breteler MM, & van Duijn CM (2009) Cathepsin D gene and the risk of Alzheimer's disease: A population-based study and meta-analysis. *Neurobiol Aging* doi:10.1016/j.neurobiolaging.2009.10.011.

Siintola E, Partanen S, Strömme P, Haapanen A, Haltia M, Maehlen J, Lehesjoki AE, & Tyynelä J (2006) Cathepsin D deficiency underlies congenital human neuronal ceroid-lipofuscinosis. *Brain*, 129, 1438–1445.

Snyder DS & Whitaker JN (1983) Postnatal changes in cathepsin D in rat neural tissue. *J Neurochem*, 40, 1161–1170.

Steinfeld R, Reinhardt K, Schreiber K, Hillebrand M, Kraetzner R, Bruck W, Saftig P, & Gartner J (2006) Cathepsin D deficiency is associated with a human neurodegenerative disorder. *Am J Hum Genet*, 78, 988–998.

Suopanki J, Partanen S, Ezaki J, Baumann M, Kominami E, & Tyynelä J (2000) Developmental changes in the expression of neuronal ceroid lipofuscinoses-linked proteins. *Mol Genet Metab*, 71, 190–194.

Tang CH, Lee JW, Galvez MG, Robillard L, Mole SE, & Chapman HA (2006) Murine cathepsin F deficiency causes neuronal lipofuscinosis and late-onset neurological disease. *Mol Cell Biol*, 26, 2309–2316.

Tyynelä J, Sohar I, Sleat DE, Gin RM, Donnelly RJ, Baumann M, Haltia M, & Lobel P (2000) A mutation in the ovine cathepsin D gene causes a congenital lysosomal storage disease with profound neurodegeneration. *EMBO J*, 19, 2786–2792.

Vetvicka V (2009) Pleiotropic effects of cathepsin D. *Endocr Metab Immune Disord Drug Targets*, 9, 385–391.

Whitaker JN & Rhodes RH (1983) The distribution of cathepsin D in rat tissues determined by immunocytochemistry. *Am J Anat*, 166, 417–428.

Zeng J, Racicott J, & Morales CR (2009) The inactivation of the sortilin gene leads to a partial disruption of prosaposin trafficking to the lysosomes. *Exp Cell Res*, 315, 3112–3124.

Chapter 14

Genetically Unassigned or Unusual NCLs

R.-M. Boustany, C. Ceuterick-de Groote, H.H. Goebel, J.-J. Martin, S.E. Mole, and A. Schulz

INTRODUCTION

There are several groups of NCL patients that remain undefined genetically or are unusual genetically. One group includes those with symptom onset in adulthood. Historically this group was assigned the gene symbol *CLN4*, as it was assumed that this disease was caused by mutations in a distinct gene. There is a second group with juvenile onset, known as the 'CLN9' type, that do not carry mutations in *CLN3*. A third group comprises children with onset in late infancy that do not carry mutations in the genes already known to cause disease with this age of onset (*CLN2/TPP1*, *CLN5*, *CLN6*, *CLN7/MFSD8*, *CLN8*). Disease in this age range is clearly genetically heterogeneous, and there may be several new genes still to be identified. There are also further small groupings of families who do not appear to map to known human gene loci. Some of these families may carry mutations in genes known to cause NCL-like disease in animals but, to date, few of these genes have been studied in human patients.

Work in mouse models suggests that other genes may contribute to NCL-like disease. These include *CLCN6* and *CLCN7*, which have not been fully tested as candidates causing human NCL disease. Another gene, *SGSH*, usually associated with one of the mucopolysaccharidoses (MPSs), was found to be mutated in one patient initially diagnosed with adult onset NCL. This patient, more correctly, has a diagnosis of MPSIII, adult onset.

ADULT ONSET NCL: 'CLN4'

Introduction

Adult onset NCL (ANCL), also called Kufs disease (Kufs, 1925, Kufs, 1927, Kufs, 1929, Kufs, 1931), is clinically distinct from the other NCLs. The storage of lipopigments in ANCL has been predominantly but not exclusively reported in neurons, in contrast with other forms of NCL in which the storage affects the nervous system, visceral organs, conjunctiva, and skin. ANCL is usually considered to be autosomal recessive, but several families (Dyken and Wisniewski, 1995, Josephson et al., 2001, Nijssen et al., 2002, Burneo et al., 2003, Ivan et al., 2005) show autosomal dominant inheritance. This disease has been referred to as Parry disease. The occurrence of familial as well as sporadic cases has been reported in more recent papers (Sadzot et al., 2000, Reif et al., 2003, Sinha et al., 2004, Robertson et al., 2008, Zini et al., 2008). It is important to stress that, in contrast to some types of NCLs that can overlap with ANCL, there is no pigmentary degeneration of the retina in Kufs disease. The terms 'Kufs disease' and 'ANCL' should be reserved for cases where enzyme deficiencies (CTSD, PPT1, and TPP1) and mild mutations in known NCL genes have been excluded or at least considered.

Clinical data

INCIDENCE

Fewer than 100 cases have been reported since the first description of Kufs disease in 1925. It is a rare condition that is difficult to diagnose (Goebel and Braak, 1989). In 1992, only four (1.3 %) out of 319 NCL cases in the Institute for Basic Research Batten Disease Registry were diagnosed with ANCL (Wisniewski and al., 1992). In fact, more than 50% of the reported cases of Kufs disease are thought not to be correctly diagnosed, and may represent a heterogeneous group of lipidoses (Berkovic et al., 1988). There is an equal sex incidence.

AGE AT ONSET AND FIRST SYMPTOMS

Presenting features are behavioural changes, epileptic seizures, ataxia, cerebellar signs, abnormal movements, extrapyramidal signs, spasticity followed by dementia. Autosomal dominant Kufs disease, appears as a distinct clinicopathological phenotype characterized initially by generalized tonic–clonic seizures and dementia.

The disease usually starts around the age of 30 years but onset during adolescence has been reported (29.7±10.1 years with a range of 11–50 years) (Berkovic et al., 1988). Cases of late adult onset with clinical symptoms at age 60–65 years have also been described (Constantinidis et al., 1992). There remains doubt as to their nosology since the spleens of these patients contained cells ballooned by lipid storage. Curiously, there are a few reports of what has been paradoxically called 'childhood' Kufs disease. For example, a 9-year-old boy was reported who developed hyperkinetic behaviour and temporospatial disorientation at age 5 years (Barthez-Carpentier et al., 1991). He was referred for intellectual deterioration. He had poor coordination. There were no visual disturbances and the electroretinogram was normal. At age 14 years, he was bedridden, had marked spasticity, and intractable seizures. He died at age 15 years. No necropsy was performed. A rectal biopsy showed large amounts of osmiophilic granules packed with fingerprint profiles in the cytoplasm of neurons of Auerbach's plexus. The authors felt that the findings were consistent with Kufs disease. They also included eight patients from the literature who were not accepted by Berkovic and colleagues (Berkovic et al., 1988) because of the onset in childhood and the absence of electron microscopy. The existence of 'childhood' Kufs disease cannot be ruled out but histological evidence is essential to support the diagnosis.

Four examples of adut onset NCL were reported among a total of 19 NCL cases (Nardocci et al., 1995). The age at onset varied from 12–50 years. Sadzot et al. collected 12 cases (including their patients) with onset before 20 years of age: three with type B and nine with type A phenotype (Berkovic et al., 1988, Sadzot et al., 2000) (see following section).

In dominant ANCL, disease onset is between the ages of 24–46 years. In one family, disease onset was usually in the fifth decade but earlier in the youngest generation (Nijssen et al., 2002). Although granular osmiophilic deposits (GRODs) were present in the brain, there was no deficiency of either PPT1 or CTSD enzymes in this family (Nijssen et al., 2003).

To be differentiated from adult onset NCL is NCL disease caused by so-called 'milder' mutations in genes usually associated with earlier onset (e.g. *CLN1/PPT1*, *CLN5*, *CLN10/CTSD*). CLN1 disease, adult has palmitoyl protein thioesterase (PPT1) deficiency and GRODs (skin biopsy). This variant of CLN1 disease was first described in two sisters presenting psychiatric symptoms at 31 and 38 years of age (van Diggelen et al., 2001b) (see Chapter 6), and later in another patient presenting in her late teens (Ramadan et al. 2007). More recently, one case diagnosed with ANCL was found to carry mutations in *CLN5* (Sleat et al., 2009). Another case diagnosed with ANCL was found to carry mutations in *SGSH*, which more usually causes the childhood lysosomal storage disorder mucopolysaccharidosis type IIIA (MPSIIIA) (Sleat et al., 2009). To date, most cases of adult onset NCL have not been excluded from all known NCL disease genes and therefore it is a possibility that most late onset cases are 'milder' mutations of other NCL genes, or even genes that cause other types of lysosomal storage disorders. These cases illustrate the value of an NCL classification and diagnostic system that includes genetic data as well as age at onset.

SIGNS AND SYMPTOMS AND THEIR TEMPORAL APPEARANCE

Various clinical and genetic phenotypes of ANCL may be recognized (Berkovic et al., 1988). Two main forms have been characterized. **Clinical phenotype A** presents with a progressive myoclonic epilepsy syndrome with dementia, ataxia, and late-occurring pyramidal and extrapyramidal features. Vision is normal and no pigmentary retinal degeneration is found, although marked photosensitivity is observed in some patients. After a while, the seizures become intractable and in association with the aforementioned features this should arouse the suspicion of Kufs disease. **Clinical phenotype B** is characterized by behavioural changes and dementia, associated with motor disturbances with cerebellar and/or extrapyramidal signs. Again the vision is normal without pigmentary retinal degeneration. Facial dyskinesias are common. Some examples of type B also have a non-progressive epilepsy syndrome. One Kufs patient showed signs suggesting overlap between phenotypes A and B (Loiseau et al., 1990). In another family (Dom et al., 1979, Martin et al., 1987), epilepsy was present but was neither a prominent nor a progressive feature. Both clinical patterns were described in two siblings of an Irish family (Callagy et al., 2000).

Dominant ANCL combines both phenotypes, and dementia is a prominent feature. The clinical course is dominated by generalized tonic–clonic seizures, myoclonus, and dementia. Abnormal speech, hearing impairment, cerebellar dysfunction, essential hypertension and parkinsonism have also been reported in some families.

TYPES OF SEIZURES

Generalized epilepsy is the rule. Myoclonic seizures may be noted occasionally. Motor seizures and massive myoclonic jerks have been described in an ANCL family with dominant inheritance (Boehme et al., 1971). Though myoclonus was not described in one family (Ferrer et al., 1980), it appeared early in the disease in another family (Nijssen et al., 2002). A tonic–clonic seizure was the initial symptom in a family in which myoclonic seizures developed subsequently (Burneo et al., 2003). A 37-year-old woman developed clusters of tonic–clonic seizures as well as focal seizures thought to be of temporo-occipital origin clinically associated with visual hallucinations, wandering, and agitation (Zini et al., 2008).

OPHTHALMOLOGIC FEATURES

Kufs disease differs from other forms of NCL by the lack of funduscopic abnormalities and absence of blindness. Normal or decreased amplitude electroretinograms (ERGs), pattern ERGs, and visual evoked potentials (VEPs) have been documented in patients with Kufs disease (Vercruyssen et al., 1982, Dawson et al., 1985, Berkovic et al., 1988). In contrast with CLN3 disease, classic juvenile and protracted juvenile there is no retinal pigmentary degeneration in ANCL. Since protracted childhood and adult types of NCLs may show symptom and onset overlap, reports of retinal degeneration in Kufs disease may be due to a confusion between these types of NCLs. However, abnormal storage in the retinal ganglion cells was found in a patient diagnosed with Kufs disease. In this patient the pigment epithelium, the photoreceptors, and the other retinal layers were normal (Martin et al., 1987). In another adult patient with NCL, granular lipopigments were found in various retinal layers (Goebel et al., 1998). This patient was found to have mutations in the *CLN5* gene (Xin et al., 2010), and is now diagnosed as having CLN5 disease, adult.

Donnet and colleagues described a patient with Kufs disease with very large VEPs and normal ERGs (Donnet et al., 1992). Storage in ANCL has been described in extraocular eye muscles (Martin et al., 1987), oculomotor nuclei, and the pons (Constantinidis et al., 1992). These findings may explain the poor upward gaze control described in several patients (Dawson et al., 1985, Donnet et al., 1992, Tominaga et al., 1994). Nystagmus has been reported in several patients with Kufs disease (Leonberg et al., 1982). There are a few reports concerning vertical gaze palsy (Constantinidis et al., 1992, Tominaga et al., 1994) and cerebellar abnormalities of smooth pursuit have been recorded on electro-oculograms but, as already mentioned, some doubts may be cast on the diagnosis of Kufs disease in these patients. More recently, abnormal eye examination has been reported in two siblings with Kufs disease (Callagy et al., 2000). A bilateral macular dystrophy has been described in a problematic case of Kufs disease: a 53-year-old female patient (Pasquinelli et al., 2004). Ophthalmologic examination is considered normal in dominant ANCL (Josephson et al., 2001, Burneo et al., 2003), although moderately decreased visual acuity has been reported (Nijssen et al., 2002, Ivan et al., 2005).

Very protracted NCL disease was described in a consanguineous Japanese family with three affected sons, two of which died in their fifties, who presented with visual failure and mental retardation or motor disability in the first or second decade (Anzai et al., 2006). Fingerprint and curvilinear deposits were described in brain autopsy. No genetic investigations were performed.

DETAILS OF MOTOR ABNORMALITIES

Extrapyramidal signs and facial dyskinesias may be noted. Dysmetria, dysdiadochokinesia, and impaired coordination of fine movements may also be detected. Gait ataxia is progressive. Burneo and colleagues mentioned normal cerebellar functions in their family (Burneo et al., 2003) but referred to prominent cerebellar dysfunction in two families presented by Arpa et al. at an annual meeting of the Spanish Neurological Society in 1978. Dysarthria develops and sometimes some degree of expressive dysphasia may occur. Extrapyramidal signs including dyskinesias, hypomimia, dysarthria, dysphagia, and gait disorders also are frequent in dominant ANCL (Josephson et al., 2001, Nijssen et al., 2002). Parkinsonism occurred a few years after disease onset in two families with autosomal dominant inheritance (Nijssen et al., 2002, Burneo et al., 2003).

DETAILS OF THE DEMENTIA

Initially, the diagnosis of depression or paranoid psychosis may be considered (Jakob and Kolkmann, 1973). Behavioural problems may be described. Mental symptoms such as excitement, hallucinations, and delusions or stupor can sometimes be so pronounced that a diagnosis of schizophrenia is made (Tobo et al., 1984). Later, a progressive dementia may be recognized. Though early onset dementia has been considered a prominent feature in autosomal dominant Kufs disease, a differential of other neurodegenerative dementing disorders must be considered. It has been proposed that when seizures and motor disturbances are also present, a diagnosis of Kufs disease might be considered (Josephson et al., 2001). One patient, whose parents originated from the same small village in Italy, presented with rapidly progressive dementia and focal occipital seizures, and developed severe frontotemporal dementia, with fingerprint inclusions found on brain biopsy (Zini et al., 2008).

RATE OF PROGRESSION

The mean length of the illness is 12.5 8.1 years (Berkovic et al., 1988). The course is slowly progressive and leads to death generally due to bronchopneumonia around the age of 40–50 years. Disease course was very short (over 3–4 years) in one patient considered to be affected by Kufs disease (Pasquinelli et al., 2004), while it had an extended duration over several decades in two brothers with an early onset of Kufs disease during adolescence (Sadzot et al., 2000). A 53-year-old man who presented with rapid cognitive decline associated with myoclonic jerks, died 3 years after presentation (Robertson et al., 2008), although he had suffered with adult onset generalized epilepsy that had started two decades earlier. A somewhat prolonged course from onset to death was reported in families with dominant NCL. Death occurred between the ages of 41–59 years.

DIFFERENTIAL DIAGNOSIS

After the critical revision by Berkovic and colleagues (Berkovic et al., 1988) and reviews (Martin, 1991, Martin, 1993), a few other or 'forgotten' examples of ANCL have been reported (Martin and Ceuterick, 1997), which demonstrates the care required before confirming the diagnosis of ANCL or Kufs disease. For example, three cases with autosomal recessive transmission were reported by Trillet et al. (Trillet et al., 1973). The clinical features were compatible with Kufs disease starting during adolescence with a prolonged evolution. The autopsy of one patient showed intraneuronal lipofuscin storage but EM failed to reveal curvilinear, fingerprint, or rectilinear profiles in the inclusions. One adult patient reported by Rumbach and colleagues (Rumbach et al., 1983) did not fit within the classic Kufs disease pattern since the patient showed severely impaired vision with retinitis pigmentosa. Three patients reported by Charles et al. (Charles et al., 1990) seem also to represent questionable examples of Kufs disease. Indeed, brain biopsies of two of the patients showed only large amounts of 'classic' lipofuscin while a normal liver biopsy was the only morphological examination in the third patient. One of the three patients had lesions suggestive of a retinitis pigmentosa, and this again should exclude the diagnosis of Kufs disease. A diagnosis of ANCL with dementia, amyotrophy, and vertical gaze palsy (Tominaga et al., 1994) was doubtful because inclusions with curvilinear profiles were very poorly documented and mini-membranous cytoplasmic bodies were present in the neurons of the locus niger. It may have been an example of juvenile dystonic lipidosis (Niemann–Pick disease type C).

Within the NCLs, a distinction must be made between protracted childhood forms of NCL with onset in adolescence, such as CLN3 disease, juvenile protracted, or CLN1 disease, juvenile, which are accompanied by visual failure and pigmentary retinal degeneration; adult onset CLN1 disease associated with PPT1 deficiency and GRODs (van Diggelen et al., 2001a, Ramadan et al., 2007); adult onset NCL disease caused by mutations in other NCL genes (e.g. CLN5 disease, adult) (Xin et al., 2010); and the autosomal recessive or autosomal dominant Kufs disease. Laboratory features including electron microscopy, appropriate enzymatic assays, and DNA examination should clarify individual cases.

Differential diagnosis of the clinical phenotype A of Kufs disease may include adult forms of storage disorders such as a late form of GM2 gangliosidosis, Gaucher disease, Niemann–Pick disease type C, or juvenile dystonic lipidosis and sialidoses, and more recently mucopolysaccharidosis type IIIA (MPSIIIA) caused by mutations in *SGSH* (Sleat et al., 2009). Extracerebral biopsies will reveal signs of lysosomal storage suggestive of different storage disorders (Ceuterick and Martin, 1998). Enzymatic assays and/or DNA examination should then point towards the true origin of the disorder. Other conditions that may be confused with ANCL include the group of progressive myoclonic epilepsies (PMEs), specifically Unverricht–Lundborg disease, Lafora disease, mitochondrial disease, and Friedreich's ataxia. In the case of mitochondrial cytopathies, a muscle biopsy may support the diagnosis by revealing abnormally structured mitochondria, biochemical abnormalities of respiratory chain enzymes, DNA deletions or point mutations in the mitochondrial or nuclear genome. Dentatorubropallidoluysian atrophy (DRPLA) Friedreich's ataxia and Huntington's chorea can also be excluded using molecular genetic analysis of trinucleotide repeats (Pasquinelli et al., 2004).

The diagnosis of Lafora body disease can be confirmed by axillary skin biopsy and molecular genetic investigation of genes in which pathogenic mutations have been characterized including *EPM2A* and *NHLRC1/EPM2B*. Characteristic periodic acid–Schiff (PAS)-positive inclusions composed of granular filamentous material are indeed observed in peripheral cells of eccrine sweat gland ducts as well as in myoepithelial cells of apocrine sweat glands.

For the clinical phenotype B, there should not be great difficulties in differentiating this condition from Creutzfeldt–Jakob disease which usually has a much more rapid course, myoclonic jerks, periodic sharp wave complexes in the electroencephalogram (EEG) and/or detectable levels of protein 14-3-3 in the cerebrospinal fluid. In about 5–10% of patients, mutations of the prion protein gene on chromosome 20 are also identified. Alzheimer's disease usually begins later than ANCL, except for those familial forms that show mutations in the presenilin genes on chromosomes 1 and 14, or in the amyloid precursor protein gene on chromosome 21. Wilson disease may be excluded on the basis of copper status and genetic analysis. In patients less than 65 years of age with a familial story of frontotemporal dementia, mutations in the tau and progranulin genes located on neighbouring loci on chromosome 17 have been found (Baker et al., 2006, Cruts et al., 2006).

Inheritance

Sporadic cases of Kufs disease have been reported in 16 out of 50 cases of ANCL (Berkovic et al., 1988), and more recently. Autosomal recessive inheritance has been the rule in the majority of the cases. A few examples of autosomal dominant inheritance have been described, and in some instances this type of ANCL is referred to as Parry disease after one of the reported families (Boehme et al., 1971, Ferrer et al., 1980, Leonberg et al., 1982, Dyken and Wisniewski, 1995). Increasing numbers of autosomal dominant ANCL families are being published (Josephson et al., 2001, Nijssen et al., 2002, Burneo et al., 2003).

NEUROPHYSIOLOGY

Neurophysiological investigations may show intense photoparoxysmal responses, an unusual sensitivity to low-frequency photic stimulation, or giant somatosensory evoked potentials (Vercruyssen et al., 1982, Berkovic et al., 1988). These features may be found in other PMEs and are not present in all cases of Kufs disease. Generally, EEG abnormalities are non-specific, and are characterized by features such as slowing of the background rhythms and generalized spike–wave discharges (Vadlamudi et al., 2003). The photopic ERG is usually preserved.

A recent study examined 59 EEGs from six patients of three generations of a family with autopsy proven autosomal dominant adult NCL (Parry disease) (Nijssen et al., 2009). In these patients with epilepsy, myoclonus, dementia, and parkinsonism, EEGs were all severely abnormal, with generalized or bilateral independent periodic epileptiform discharges as the most common pattern. No alpha rhythm was present. No paroxysmal response to photic stimulation was seen. EEG changes over time in the same individuals were modest, despite severe clinical disease progression. Myoclonus did not have a cortical correlate. It was concluded that EEG in autosomal dominant NCL is dominated by generalized periodic epileptiform discharges (GPDs), and that GPDs in adults with myoclonus, parkinsonism, dementia, or epilepsy should raise the possibility of adult NCL, especially with familial occurrence.

NEURORADIOLOGY

Computed tomography (CT) and magnetic resonance imaging findings are unremarkable or non-specific, and may be inconsistent in familial cases. Cortical atrophy is usually found. Some patients show cerebellar atrophy (Callagy et al., 2000, Josephson et al., 2001, Nijssen et al., 2002). Mild, diffuse increased signal intensity in the white matter may be seen on T_2-weighted images (Sadzot et al., 2000, Ivan et al., 2005). Single photon emission CT (SPECT) and positron emission tomography findings are rarely described in ANCL (Nijssen et al., 2002, Reif et al., 2003).

BIOCHEMICAL TESTS

There are no biochemical tests (cerebrospinal fluid (CSF), serum, urine) that are useful for the diagnosis of Kufs disease. Raised CSF protein has been found in one adult NCL case (Sinha et al., 2004).

INVESTIGATIONS OF TWO FAMILIES WITH ANCL

In a family affected by an autosomal recessive form of Kufs disease (Dom et al., 1979, Vercruyssen et al., 1982, Martin et al., 1987), three patients were autopsied (Martin and Ceuterick, 1997), and two of them had submitted, during their life, to skin, peripheral nerve, and skeletal muscle biopsies (Tables 14.1

Table 14.1 **Ultrastructure of extracerebral and brain storage in ANCL**

Tissue		Ultrastructure	References
Skin	Eccrine sweat gland epithelia	FP GRODs LF (large amounts)	Berkovic et al., 1988, Goebel et al., 1997, Martin and Ceuterick, 1997, Gelot et al., 1998, Schreiner et al., 2000, Josephson et al., 2001, Burneo et al., 2003, Nijssen et al., 2003, Reif et al., 2003, Ivan et al., 2005
	Smooth muscle cells	GRODs (*autopsy*) Lipopigments FP-like FP (vascular)	
Muscle	Skeletal muscle fibres	CL + RL	Goebel et al., 1997, Martin and Ceuterick, 1997, Burneo et al., 2003, Nijssen et al., 2003, Reif et al., 2003
	Perimysial capillaries	GRODs (*autopsy*)	
	Heart muscle cells	FP-like FP (*autopsy*) FP, RL (*autopsy*)	
Rectum	Neurons	FP LF (large amounts) FP+GR GRODs, FP LF-like Lipopigments	Barthez-Carpentier et al., 1991, Ruchoux and al., 1996, Gelot et al., 1998, Sadzot et al., 2000, Schreiner et al., 2000, Nijssen et al., 2003, Pasquinelli et al., 2004
	Smooth muscle cells	CL, FP, GR GRODs, FP CP+FP FP	
Liver		FP (*autopsy*) FP, CL	Berkovic et al., 1988, Martin and Ceuterick, 1997
Spleen		CL (*autopsy*)	Goebel et al., 1997
Heart		FP, RL (*autopsy*) CL, cross-hatched, FP (few)	Reske-Nielsen et al., 1981, Sakajiri et al., 1995, Martin and Ceuterick, 1997, Fealey et al., 2009
Brain		GRODs GR GR+CL FP CL Zebra bodies (few)	Boehme et al., 1971, Ferrer et al., 1980, Goebel and Braak, 1989, Charles et al., 1990, O'Neill et al., 1993, Reznik et al., 1995, Martin and Ceuterick, 1997, Elleder and Tyynelä, 1998, Callagy et al., 2000, Sadzot et al., 2000, Josephson et al., 2001, Burneo et al., 2003, Nijssen et al., 2003, Robertson et al., 2008

CL, curvilinear profiles; FP, fingerprint profiles; GR, granular; GRODs, granular osmiophilic deposits; LF, lipofuscin; RL, rectilinear profiles.
Note: extracerebral storage was not found in all patients

and 14.2). The first symptoms appeared between the ages of 30–33 years, and were characterized by epileptic seizures followed by cerebellar signs, myoclonic jerks, and extrapyramidal symptoms. There was no retinitis pigmentosa. Neuropathological examination showed extensive storage of curvilinear bodies in neurons of the central nervous system. There was an obvious diffuse intraneuronal storage affecting the main dendrite, the perikaryon, and the proximal part of the axon. Similar inclusions were found in retinal ganglion cells, in the oculomotor muscles, and in the smooth muscle cells of the ciliary body. The glial cells contained lipofuscin granules and only very seldom fingerprint profiles. Similar inclusions were found in hepatocytes as well as in the myocardium. In the skin, the eccrine sweat glands were filled with clear vacuoles. The vacuoles exhibited very small amounts of curvilinear, rectilinear, and fingerprint profiles, as well as lipid droplets. The muscle biopsies showed large amounts of subsarcolemmal autofluorescent and acid phosphatase-positive granules in comparison with age-matched controls. Electron microscopy confirmed the presence of membrane-bound osmiophilic inclusions containing numerous curvilinear profiles, a few rectilinear profiles, and sometimes a lipid vacuole.

More recently, another family of Dutch origin with the autosomal dominant form of adult NCL, including six affected individuals in three generations, has been reported, with genetic investigations still ongoing (Nijssen et al., 2002, Nijssen et al., 2003). Diagnosis was confirmed by brain biopsy in one patient and autopsies in three others. Disease onset varied from 24 (in the youngest generation) to 46 years of age. Early symptoms consisted of myoclonus affecting the face and arms, epilepsy, moderately impaired visual acuity and hearing loss, cognitive decline, or depression. Parkinsonism occurred a few years after disease onset, with stooped posture, shuffling gait, bradykinesia, and poker-like face. Patients died in the sixth decade (at the age of 51, 56, and 59 years of age). Throughout the brain of these patients, there was abundant storage of autofluorescent PAS-positive lipopigment granules in neurons. Storage material was found in cardiocytes, skeletal muscle, liver, smooth muscle of gut, peripheral nervous system of gut, and in skin eccrine glands (Tables 14.1 and 14.2). Electron microscopy revealed abundant compact GRODs in neurons throughout the central nervous system (CNS). In skeletal muscle, beside subsarcolemmal GRODs, few fingerprints were seen in perimysial capillaries and in eccrine sweat glands in the skin, where many GRODs were seen with lipid droplets. Protein electrophoresis of isolated storage material revealed a major protein band of about 14kDa, recognized in Western blotting by saposin D antiserum (but not subunit c of mitochondrial ATPase antiserum). Activities of PPT1, TPP1, and CTSD were within normal range, ruling out CLN1, CLN2, and CLN10 diseases.

Morphology

NEURONAL STORAGE

The ultrastructure of the neuronal storage material in ANCL has diverse and often mixed patterns (granular, GRODs, curvilinear, rectilinear, and fingerprint profiles) (Figure 14.1), suggesting heterogeneity, and several different forms of ANCL (Mole et al., 2005) (Table 14.1). A granular component is frequently seen (Goebel and Braak, 1989, Charles et al., 1990, Robertson et al., 2008). For many years, this pattern was considered the exclusive type of ultrastructure in an autosomal dominant ANCL family (Boehme et al., 1971, Ferrer et al., 1980), and corresponding to GRODs (Josephson et al., 2001, Burneo et al., 2003, Nijssen et al., 2003). However, it may also appear in affected siblings whose parents are healthy, suggesting an autosomal recessive mode of inheritance (Charles et al., 1990), as well as in sporadic patients (Goebel and Braak, 1989, Charles et al., 1990, Pasquinelli et al., 2004). Also, in

Table 14.2 **Extracerebral tissues in which no storage was found in ANCL**

Tissue	References
Skin (eccrine sweat gland epithelia only)	Loiseau et al., 1990, Barthez-Carpentier et al., 1991, Vital et al., 1991, Goebel et al., 1997, Gelot et al., 1998, Sadzot et al., 2000, Pasquinelli et al., 2004
Conjunctiva	Martin and Ceuterick, 1997, Gelot et al., 1998, Josephson et al., 2001
Skeletal muscle fibres	Berkovic et al., 1988, Vital et al., 1991, Gelot et al., 1998, Sadzot et al., 2000
Heart muscle cells	Pasquinelli et al., 2004
Peripheral nerve	Berkovic et al., 1988, Vital et al., 1991, Martin and Ceuterick, 1997, Gelot et al., 1998, Nijssen et al., 2003
Rectum	Callagy et al., 2000
Liver	Charles et al., 1990
Lymphocytes	Burneo et al., 2003

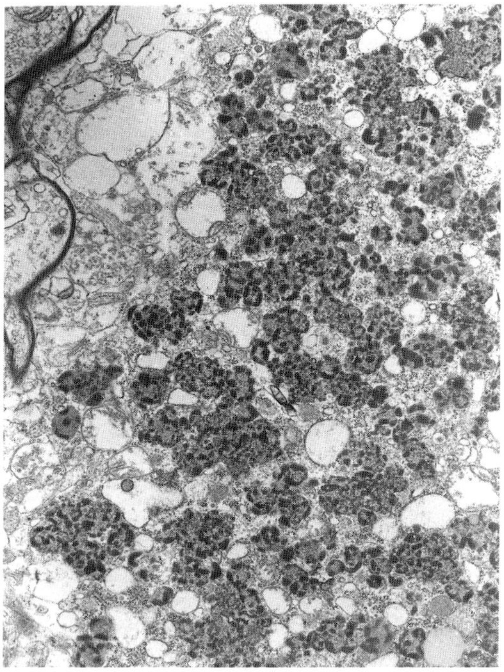

Figure 14.1 Adult NCL: a cortical neuron is loaded with lipopigments, ×8225.

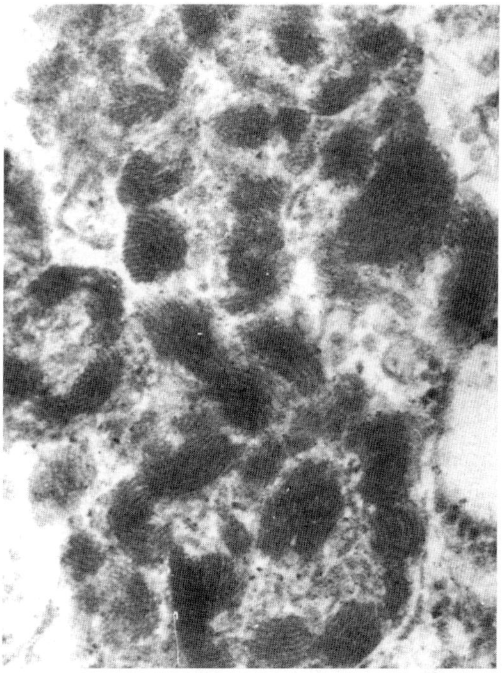

Figure 14.2 Adult NCL: lipopigments in a cortical neuron show fingerprint profiles at higher magnification, ×111, 020.

cerebral neurons of other patients with ANCL, both fingerprint (Figure 14.2) and curvilinear profiles are not infrequently encountered (O'Neill et al., 1993, Reznik et al., 1995, Martin and Ceuterick, 1997, Callagy et al., 2000, Sadzot et al., 2000). Neuronal perikarya containing densely packed curvilinear bodies are also seen in the striatum, the substantia nigra, and the dentate nucleus (Elleder and Tyynelä, 1998). Beside prevailing GRODs (Figure 14.3), a few zebra bodies are found in spinal cord neurons, and numerous fingerprints (Figure 14.4) are noted in sporadic cell neuronal processes (Nijssen et al., 2003). Pallor of the substantia nigra with mild to severe neuronal loss and decreased neuromelanin are noted in few cases of dominant ANCL (Josephson et al., 2001, Burneo et al., 2003, Nijssen et al., 2003). This correlates with parkinsonism in one family (Nijssen et al., 2003).

EXTRACEREBRAL STORAGE

In childhood forms of NCL, extracerebral storage is consistent and ubiquitous. In ANCL this aspect has been incompletely explored and has produced inconsistent results. Extracerebral storage has been sought both by biopsy as well

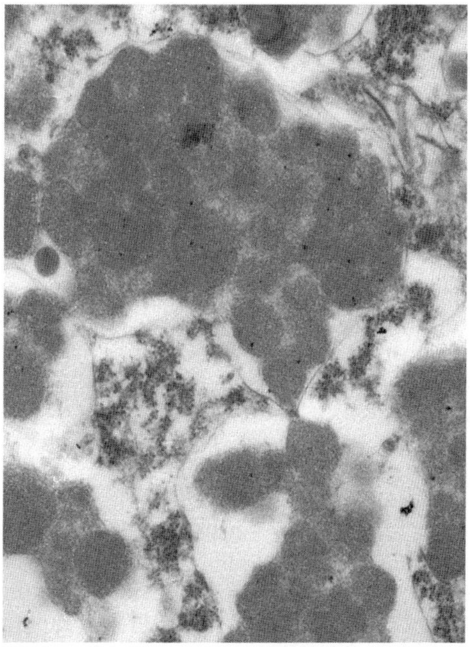

Figure 14.3 Adult NCL (dominant): CNS: neuronal storage in the thalamus with membrane-bound vacuoles containing numerous polyglobular subunits filled with GRODs, ×21, 000.

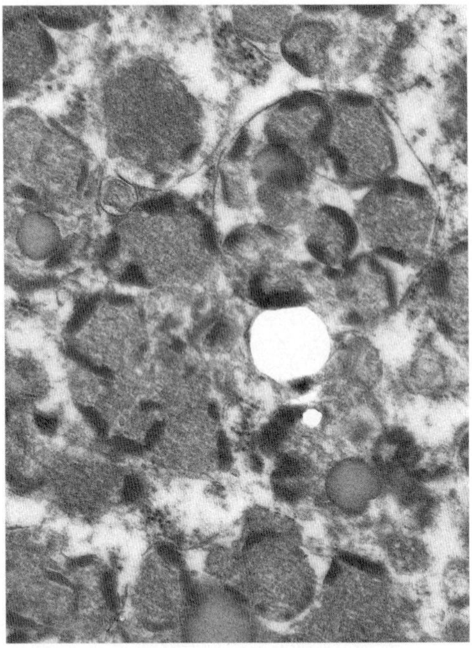

Figure 14.4 Adult NCL (dominant): CNS: cell process in cerebral cortex showing abundant granular inclusions with electron-dense fingerprints, ×65,000.

as at autopsy (Table 14.1). In some patients, fingerprint profiles were observed in eccrine sweat gland epithelial cells (Berkovic et al., 1988, Martin and Ceuterick, 1997), and were also present in dermal vascular smooth muscle cells (Goebel et al., 1997, Reif et al., 2003). The storage is less adequately described or non-specific of NCL in a few papers revealing, respectively, large amounts of 'lipopigments' in sweat glands (Schreiner et al., 2000, Reif et al., 2003) and multilamellated inclusions with fingerprint-like aspects (Ivan et al., 2005). In other ANCL patients, NCL-specific inclusions were not found in skin (Loiseau et al., 1990, Barthez-Carpentier et al., 1991, Vital et al., 1991, Sadzot et al., 2000, Pasquinelli et al., 2004). Curvilinear and rectilinear profiles have been seen in skeletal muscle fibres (Goebel et al., 1997, Martin and Ceuterick, 1997), but others (Berkovic et al., 1988, Vital et al., 1991, Sadzot et al., 2000) could not find NCL-specific inclusions in skeletal muscle. Rectal tissues showed fingerprint profiles within neurons (Barthez-Carpentier et al., 1991) and curvilinear and fingerprint profiles as well as granular material in smooth muscle cells (Ruchoux and al., 1996). Fingerprint profiles were distinct in rectal neurons while intraneuronal granular inclusions with curvilinear profiles were seen in the brain (Sadzot et al., 2000). Thus, the diversity of storage in extracerebral tissues of ANCL still does not allow recognition of a consistent diagnostic pattern. Fingerprint profiles, for instance, were observed in smooth muscle cells of dermal and rectal tissues, but not in dermal eccrine sweat gland epithelial cells nor in rectal neurons in familial ANCL, i.e. occurring in two adult siblings (Gelot et al., 1998). Abnormal accumulation of lipid vacuoles and lipopigments were found in rectal myenteric ganglia but no fingerprints in Kufs disease with early onset dementia (Schreiner et al., 2000).

The ultrastructure of lymphocytes in ANCL has largely been neglected, and NCL-specific inclusions have never been reported. Conjunctiva (Martin and Ceuterick, 1997, Gelot et al., 1998) and peripheral nerve (Berkovic et al., 1988, Vital et al., 1991, Martin and Ceuterick, 1997, Gelot et al., 1998) have always been found to be unaffected, whereas in liver fingerprint or curvilinear profiles were found in some patients (Berkovic et al., 1988) but not in others (Charles et al., 1990). However, postmortem studies on visceral organs revealed fingerprint profiles in liver and heart (Martin and Ceuterick, 1997) and rectilinear profiles in the heart (Martin and Ceuterick, 1997). A 31-year-old woman who presented with biventricular heart failure was found to have CL and cross-hatched deposits, with occasional fingerprints, in vascular smooth muscle cells and focal epithelial cells of myocardial tissue (Fealey et al., 2009). No other tissues were examined. Other cases have been reported with deposits in the heart (Reske-Nielsen et al., 1981, Sakajiri et al., 1995). These heterogeneous ultrastructural findings outside the CNS may require biopsies of several tissues to ascertain ANCL (Tables 14.1 and 14.2). Ultrastructural examination of muscle (Figure 14.5) and skin (eccrine sweat glands; Figure 14.6) biopsies in dominant ANCL, revealed GRODs and lipofuscin (Josephson et al., 2001, Burneo et al., 2003, Nijssen et al., 2003). Few fingerprints were found in smooth muscle cells of perimysial capillaries (Nijssen et al., 2003). Lipofuscin-like inclusions and so-called intraneuronal inclusions were seen in ganglion cells and in nerve cell processes in rectal biopsies (Nijssen et al., 2003). Conjunctival biopsies (Josephson et al., 2001) were non-diagnostic. The histopathological

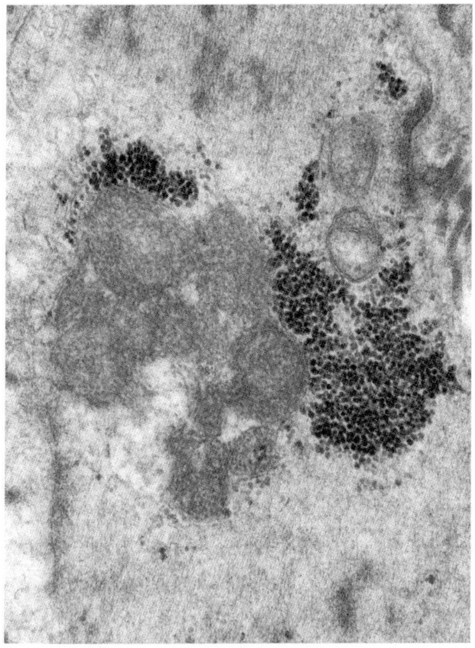

Figure 14.5 Adult NCL (dominant): skeletal muscle: smooth muscle cell of a perimysial capillary with a lipofuscin inclusion composed of GRODs, ×27,600.

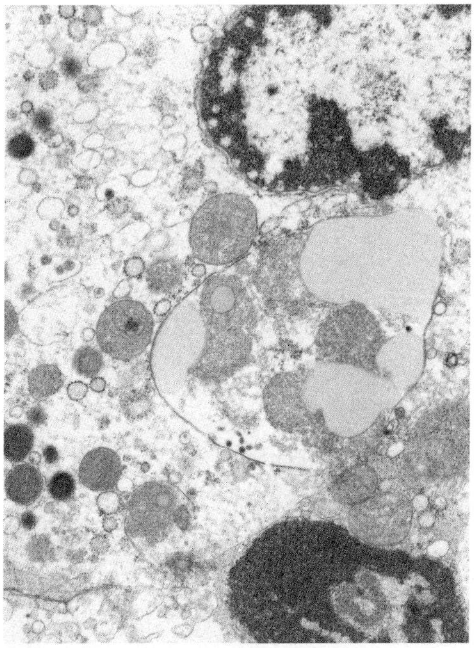

Figure 14.6 Adult NCL (dominant): skin: vacuolar, lipofuscin deposit enclosing GRODs and lipid droplets in an eccrine sweat gland epithelial cell, ×10,700.

reliability in using extraneuronal tissues, and particularly rectal mucosa biopsies, has recently been re-evaluated in Kufs disease (Pasquinelli et al., 2004) which stress the difficulties of this issue.

MACROSCOPY

Atrophy of the brain, usually particularly prominent in the frontal and frontoparietal areas, may vary considerably, leading to reduced brain weights of between 900g (Loiseau et al., 1990) to nearly normal values of 1245g (Goebel and Braak, 1989). Normal brain weight for adult males is 1450g at 21 years, declining to 1370g at 60 years; the female maximum is 1340g at 18 years. The cerebellum may also be atrophic (Goebel and Braak, 1989). In one family (Nijssen et al., 2003) with dominant ANCL, brain weights varied from 896–1144 g. Most dominant ANCL cases showed mild to severe global cerebral and cerebellar atrophy, with markedly depigmented substantia nigra (Josephson et al., 2001, Nijssen et al., 2002, Burneo et al., 2003). Visceral organs are normal.

MICROSCOPY

Loss of nerve cells within the brain is variable. There may be regional differences with rare or moderate neuronal loss despite major intraneuronal storage. In the cerebral cortex it has been described as diffuse (Iseki et al., 1987) or rather selective when applying Braak's pigmento-architectonic technique (Goebel and Braak, 1989). The pigment-laden stellate cells of layers II and III are severely affected, with only mild loss of cells in layer Vb (Martin et al., 1987). Purkinje cells of the cerebellum may also be considerably reduced in number (Iseki et al., 1987). The less obvious loss of neurons in the subcortical grey matter will require precise morphometric studies and include age-matched controls.

Loss of nerve cells may produce secondary demyelination in the white matter (Iseki et al., 1987, Loiseau et al., 1990), and reactive astrocytosis as well as activation of microglial macrophages. This activation has been shown immunohistochemically by a microglial marker (KiM1P) and by demonstrating MHC-II (Brück and Goebel, 1998), whereas antibodies that mark macrophages of acute or chronic inflammatory stages (derived from the circulation rather than from the endogenous CNS microglial population) were not present in ANCL (Brück and Goebel, 1998). This observation suggests that in ANCL the blood–brain barrier in neuron-depleted areas may not be impaired.

Loss of myelinated axons in biopsied sural nerves, possibly as a non-specific feature, has been documented in familial ANCL (Gelot et al., 1998).

Storage occurs within nerve cell bodies (Figure 14.7) and often, as in childhood forms, in the proximal axonal segment, also known as the axon spindle or meganeurite. The staining properties of the storage material in the brain is similar, if not identical, to that in CLN3 disease, juvenile, with strong PAS, Sudan black, and Luxol fast blue staining and bright autofluorescence (Figure 14.8). On rare occasions, distended axon spindles can also be observed in normal ageing, indicating that it may often be difficult to distinguish morphologically between ANCL and normal ageing where lipofuscin may appear increased. Although the emission spectrum of normal lipofuscin is shifted towards the red end, the correct combination of filters is necessary to be able to distinguish this from the autofluorescence of the NCLs (which is more yellow or silvery than orange).

Braak's technique not only identifies loss of neurons but also suggests selective storage, at least at the light microscopic level indicated by changes of neuronal size and shape. In general, the pattern of storage in the neocortex appears to resemble that observed in CLN3 disease, juvenile and protracted juvenile, i.e. within axon spindles in pyramidal cells of layer IIIa and IIIb (Goebel and Braak, 1989, Braak and Braak, 1993), but also with enlargement of neuronal perikarya in pyramidal cells in layer IIIc (Braak and Braak, 1993), in layer V, and even more in layer VI (Martin and Ceuterick, 1997). Although Braak's technique encompasses both salient morphological features in the ANCL type, i.e. loss of neurons and storage, postmortem studies cannot suggest whether degeneration of neurons follows a period of storage within the same types of all individual neurons. Selective involvement is also seen in the allocortex (parahippocampal gyrus and hippocampus). Superficial neurons characteristically arranged in clusters rather than in layers display marked storage, whereas more deeply located neurons of the entorhinal region are scarcely affected. This pattern of involvement closely resembles that seen in

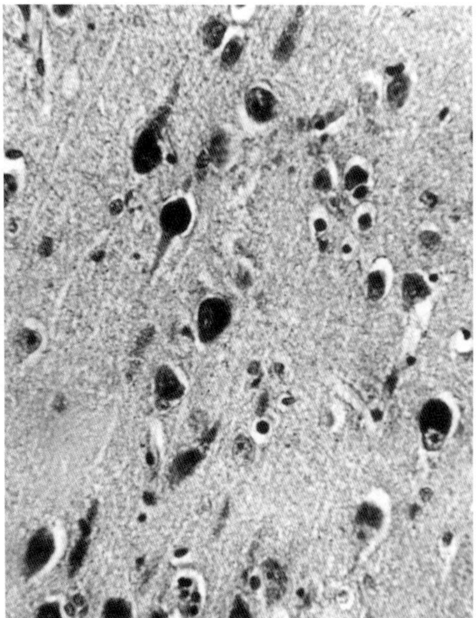

Figure 14.7 Adult NCL: numerous cortical neurons are enlarged by lipopigments, haematoxylin-PAS, ×330.

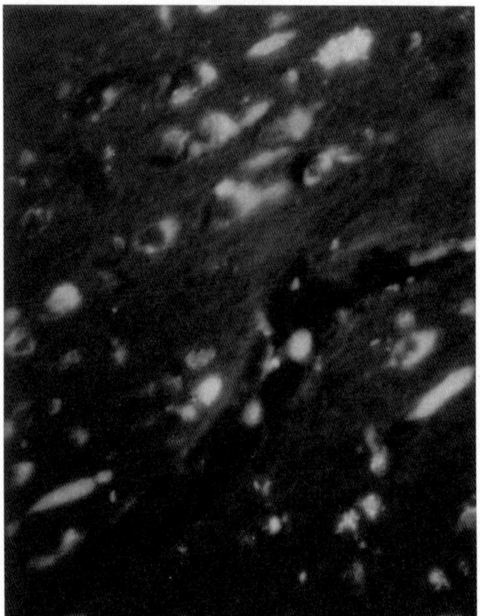

Figure 14.8 Adult NCL: lipopigments in cerebrocortical cells display bright autofluorescence, ×330.

Alzheimer's disease in which neurofibrillary tangles show a similar distribution in the entorhinal allocortex (Braak and Braak, 1993). Further similarities between ANCL and Alzheimer's disease are also seen in the different neuronal populations of the hippocampus. Nerve cells of the fascia dentata are hardly affected, whereas those of the hilar region, the CA-4 projection neurons, can show marked storage, as do the pyramidal cells of the CA-2 and CA-3 regions. Likewise, CA-1 and subicular neurons are less involved.

Subcortically storage is also encountered within nerve cells of the basal ganglia, the thalamus, reticular formation of the brainstem (Reznik et al., 1995, Callagy et al., 2000, Sadzot et al., 2000), and of the spinal anterior horn neurons (Martin and Ceuterick, 1997, Callagy et al., 2000). Similarly a selective storage forming meganeurites, was observed in the amygdaloid nuclei, affecting projection cells of the lateral basal and accessory components whereas the parvocellular granular nucleus and intercalated neurons are not affected (Braak and Braak, 1987).

However, it must be remembered that Braak's technique is one of light microscopy requiring extremely thick sections, i.e. at 100μm and even 800μm. Thus, sub-light-microscopic amounts of storage which cannot be assessed with this technique and the exclusion of those populations of neurons thus found not to be affected, remains to be investigated and confirmed by postmortem electron microscopy, a task not yet systematically performed.

In dominant ANCL, storage was found throughout the CNS in cortical, basal ganglia, thalamus, brainstem, cerebellar, and spinal cord neurons (Josephson et al., 2001, Burneo et al., 2003, Nijssen et al., 2003).

IMMUNOHISTOCHEMISTRY

The storage material contains abnormal amounts of SCMAS (Figure 14.9) (Hall et al., 1991, Elleder et al., 1997) and increased staining for saposins A and D has also been documented (Tyynelä et al., 1997). In a dominant ANCL family (Nijssen et al., 2003), SCMAS were restricted to a subpopulation of neurons, while SAPs appeared uniform throughout the brain. In addition, β-A4 amyloid protein, as well as amyloid precursor protein, epitopes have been found in association with ANCL storage material (Wisniewski et al., 1990a, Wisniewski et al., 1990b). It appears to be a general principle that the amyloid-related proteins accumulate in lipopigments, since they may be seen both in age-related lipofuscin as well as in ANCL-related lipopigments. In this respect, the NCLs seem to be the only group of disorders in which intracellular, i.e. intralysosomal accumulation of amyloid proteins occurs, suggesting an abnormal intralysosomal metabolism rather than an abnormal metabolism of the amyloid proteins. Altered processes and delay in degradation of these compounds have been proposed as causes of non-specific, i.e. not gene-related, accumulation of these proteins within their lysosomal compartment. Precise correlation between the ultrastructure and these immunohistochemical findings has not yet been obtained. However as immunoelectron microscopic studies in CLN2 disease, late infantile and CLN3 disease, juvenile suggested that SCMAS is primarily present in curvilinear profiles and not in fingerprint profiles (Rowan and Lake, 1995), variable immunoreactivity for subunit c of mitochondrial ATP synthase (SCMAS) in ANCL CNS neurons suggests that the ultrastructure would have a curvilinear/fingerprint component while SAP

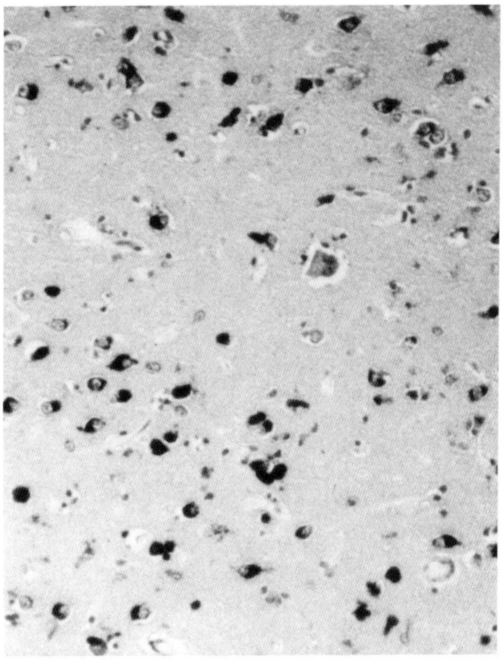

Figure 14.9 Adult NCL: SCMAS in neurons, putamen, ×172.

accumulation would have a GROD pattern. SAP is present in both CLN1 disease and most dominant ANCL in which storage inclusions demonstrate GRODs. Whether such a correlation is also correct for β-A4 amyloid and amyloid precursor protein remains to be established.

While it has not (yet) been possible to re-evaluate the storage in the original tissues studied and described by Kufs (Kufs, 1925), retrospective studies employing modern morphological techniques have led to verification of some earlier descriptions suggestive of ANCL (Goebel and Braak, 1989) and rejecting of others (Martin and Ceuterick, 1997).

RETINAL MORPHOLOGY

One criterion to distinguish ANCL from CLN3 disease, classic juvenile and protracted juvenile is absence of the retinal involvement in ANCL (Berkovic et al., 1988, Martin and Ceuterick, 1997), even in adult patients with early onset during adolescence (Sadzot et al., 2000). Postmortem retinal studies on ANCL are rare but have confirmed preservation of the retinal architecture (Figure 14.10) (Martin et al., 1987, Goebel et al., 1998), and this is corroborated by the demonstration of a lack of microglial activation in the retina (Brück and Goebel, 1998). Although both funduscopic (Charles et al., 1990) and ERG (Rumbach et al., 1983) abnormalities have been reported, there was no morphological confirmation in these cases. The combined appearance of ANCL and retinal degeneration has only once been described clinically and morphologically (Ikeda et al., 1984). In these three unrelated patients, a fortuitous coincidence of ANCL and retinal degeneration of the retinitis pigmentosa (RP)-type, cannot be excluded. The absence of retinal degeneration in childhood cases of NCL has led to the suggestion that they should be classified as ANCL (Barthez-Carpentier et al., 1991, Reznik et al., 1995).

Observations on retinal ultrastructural morphology in ANCL (Ikeda et al., 1984, Martin et al., 1987, Goebel et al., 1998) mention accumulation of storage material in ganglion cells of either granular (Figure 14.11) (Ikeda et al., 1984, Goebel et al., 1998), or curvilinear pattern in conjunction with a granular one (Martin et al., 1987). Storage of the ANCL type was not described in other neuronal cell types of the preserved retina (Martin et al., 1987). However, in another ANCL patient, the perikarya of the

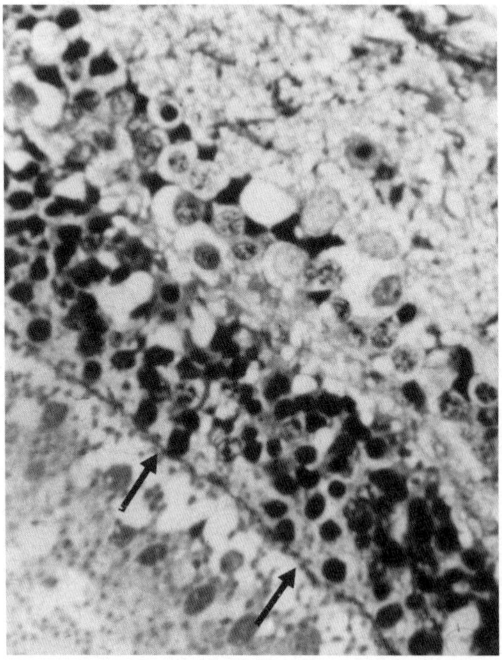

Figure 14.10 Adult NCL: preservation of retina including photoreceptors (arrows), haematoxylin-eosin, ×528.

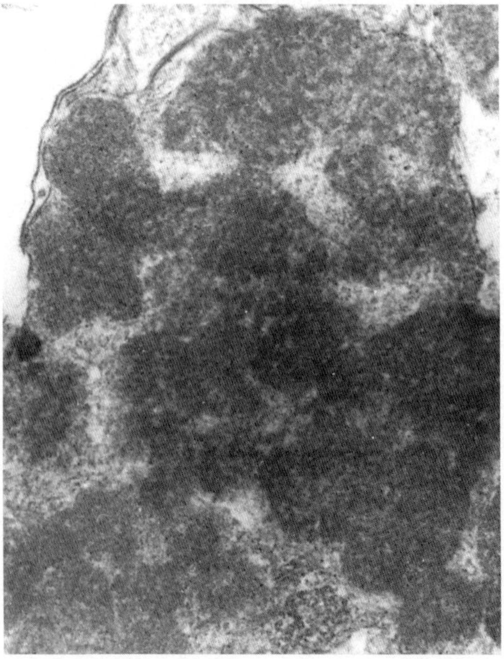

Figure 14.11 Adult NCL: accruing lipopigments in retinal cells show a granular ultrastructure, ×54,000.

inner and outer nuclear layers contained granular storage material (Goebel et al., 1998).

POSSIBLE VARIANT OF ANCL

A peculiar leukoencephalopathy in a 52-year-old woman has been associated with ANCL (Gille and al., 1995). Clinical features and symptoms included partial complex epileptic seizures followed by dementia, cerebellar ataxia, a pyramidal syndrome associated with akinesia-rigidity. The disease duration was 6 years. Histology was limited to a few stereotactic samples.

There was a severe diffuse gliosis without obvious demyelination, and accumulation of autofluorescent inclusions in nerve and glial cells. The cerebrocortical neurons contained increased amounts of autofluorescent material and ultrastructure was of the granular type. Osmiophilic dense bodies showing lamellar structures with curvilinear and mainly rectilinear profiles as well as fingerprint patterns were seen in glial cells of the frontal subcortical white matter. Incomplete genetic data indicate that this might be an autosomal dominant familial disorder. In addition, mononuclear peripheral blood cells (without electron microscopic study) contained vacuoles in 22% and 36% respectively in one of the patient's children and in her sister with dementia. This combination of features suggests a peculiar variant of ANCL or, more likely, a disorder different from ANCL altogether.

MORPHOLOGICAL DIFFERENTIAL DIAGNOSTIC ASPECTS

Since the striking morphological features of NCL, including ANCL, consist of loss of neurons and abnormal storage of a lipofuscin-like material, the differential diagnosis must address both these aspects.

Loss of neurons, especially of the cortex in adult and elderly people is typical of ageing as well as a number of progressive neurodegenerative diseases, particularly Alzheimer's disease. Many of the progressive neurodegenerative disorders are marked by additional disease-specific features, neurofibrillary tangles, senile plaques, Lewy bodies, Pick bodies, and other intracellular inclusions, providing differential diagnostic identification. In Alzheimer's disease lipopigment formation appears to be reduced (Drach, 1996, Snyder et al., 1998).

Apart from the age-related accumulation of normal lipofuscin in ANCL, suggested by the ultrastructural appearance of a granular matrix coincident with NCL-specific curvilinear and fingerprint profiles within ANCL storage material, other morphological hallmarks of ageing may also be seen occasionally, i.e. senile plaques (Wisniewski and al., 1992) as well as neurofibrillary tangles (Constantinidis et al., 1992). Whether they indicate ANCL-related and accelerated ageing or whether they are non-specific features, requires additional studies particularly as they are inconspicuous and rare. In conclusion, since accumulation of storage material with the staining characteristics of lipofuscin, both abnormal in volume as well as in ultrastructure, represents a prerequisite for recognizing ANCL (and other forms of NCL), the mere presence of lipofuscin granules by light microscopy, even in extracerebral cells, is not sufficient to diagnose ANCL even if a clinical pattern in a familial setting might suggest ANCL (Annunziata et al., 1986).

Increased amounts of lipopigment may be seen in neurons and in myofibres in vitamin E deficiency (Larnaout et al., 1997), but the ultrastructure of the lipopigment is finely granular, quite dissimilar to that seen in NCL. In certain biochemically well-defined lysosomal storage disorders (Elleder et al., 1997), there is a secondary increase of SCMAS associated with the presence of 'lipopigment' in the neurons affected by primary storage, usually in patients with a chronic form of the respective lysosomal disorder. Increased accumulation of SCMAS in extracerebral tissues was not observed. Among patients with the pigment variant of ANCL (Goebel et al., 1995a), an adult type has rarely been identified. Here, lipopigment formation occurs intracellularly as well as extracellularly in subcortical regions. Fingerprint profiles inside lipopigments have been reported in eccrine sweat glands in two unrelated patients affected by a progressive degenerative disorder (Goebel et al., 1995b). Granular inclusions with rectilinear profiles as well as fingerprints (Figure 14.12) and vacuolar structures with submembranous fingerprints (Figure 14.13) were found in eccrine sweat glands in a 63-year-old male patient with a progressive dementia and a definitive autopsy diagnosis of Alzheimer's disease (unpublished observation by Ceuterick-de Groote, cited in Goebel et al., 1995b). In pigmentary orthochromatic

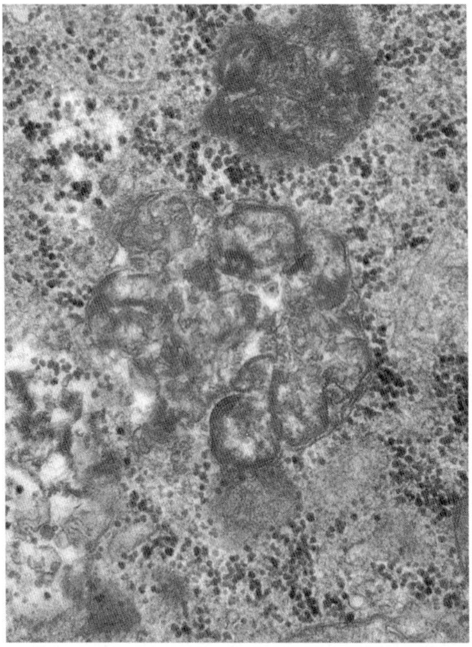

Figure 14.12 Adult patient with a definitive autopsy diagnosis of Alzheimer's disease: skin. Mixed inclusion with rectilinear and fingerprint profiles in eccrine sweat gland epithelial cells, ×36,800.

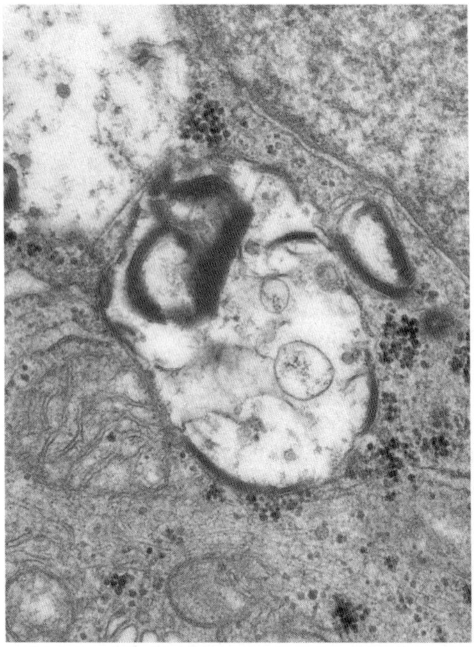

Figure 14.13 Adult patient with a definitive autopsy diagnosis of Alzheimer's disease: skin. Vacuolar inclusion with submembranous fingerprints in eccrine sweat gland epithelial cells, ×36,800.

leukodystrophy, an adult onset progressive neurodegenerative disorder, autofluorescent lipopigments which display lamellar, curved, and occasional fingerprint profiles accumulate within oligodendrocytes, astrocytes, and macrophages of the white matter, but not in glial and neuronal cells of the cerebral cortex (Gray et al., 1987). Hence, a different location, a different involvement of cell types, and an ultrastructure not typical for ANCL distinguish this disorder from ANCL. Moreover, no abnormal lipopigments were observed in biopsied skeletal muscle and peripheral nerve.

Molecular genetics and cell biology

To date, the genetic defect underlying most cases of adult onset NCL is unknown. Exceptions are those that carry mutations in NCL genes that delay onset until late teenage years or adulthood: *CLN1/PPT1* (van Diggelen et al., 2001b, Ramadan et al., 2007), *CLN5* (Sleat et al., 2009, Xin et al., 2010), *CLN10/CTSD* (R. Steinfeld, unpublished data), and possibly *CLCN6* (Poët et al., 2006). It is quite likely that, in time, mutations in other NCL genes will be described that are associated with late onset, including those that have been found to cause late onset disease in animals, for example *ARSG* (Abitbol et al., 2010). There may also be cases diagnosed as ANCL that in reality are milder late onset cases of lysosomal storage disorders or other diseases, and are caused by mutations in genes such as *SGSH*, more usually associated with the more severe and unrelated disease MPSIIIA (Sleat et al., 2009).

The varying phenotypes associated with adult onset NCL cases in which mutations have not been described suggests that mutations in multiple genes may underlie their disease, which complicates genetic linkage studies. In general, insufficient families with adult onset NCL of similar phenotype have been available for classic genetic linkage studies. However, technological advances in genomics, such as high-throughput screening platforms such as single-nucleotide polymorphism arrays and next generation sequencing, offer a comprehensive and increasingly cost effective approach to disease gene identification. Ideally, mutations in known or candidate NCL loci, for example, the genes associated with causing NCL in animal models, will be considered first.

Genes encoding cathepsins and chloride channels that are mutated in mouse models for NCL remain candidates that have yet to be evaluated in most adult onset cases.

Several of the known NCL genes are expressed in the lysosome lumen. The same novel strategy used to identify *CLN2* (Sleat et al., 1997), that is, comparison of the profile of mannose 6-phosphate labelled enzymes destined for the lysosome, may reveal further lysosomal enzymes implicated in adult onset NCL. There was an elevation in two mannose 6-phosphate glycoproteins in one adult NCL patient (Sleat et al., 1998) suggesting that there is indeed a perturbation in lysosomal function. However, at this time it was not possible to identify a missing glycoprotein. The same two glycoproteins, along with CLN2/TPP1 protein, were also considerably elevated in CLN3 disease, juvenile, linking this phenotype, caused by mutations in the CLN3 membrane protein and at least one type of adult onset NCL. Very recently, this updated approach was successfully used to identify mutations in *CLN5* and *SGSH*, in two cases diagnosed with adult onset NCL disease (Sleat et al., 2009).

JUVNEILE ONSET NCL: 'CLN9'

Introduction

NCL has been described in patients with clinical features identical to those seen in CLN3 disease, juvenile (Schulz et al., 2004) but who do not carry mutations in *CLN3*. This is known as the 'CLN9' type. The cell biology of CLN9 disease differs from other known NCLs.

Molecular genetics

CLN9 disease has been diagnosed in four patients from two different families. One family is German and without history of known consanguinity. The other family is Serbian and has no history of close consanguinity but both great-grandmothers originate from the same small village. In both families, pedigrees suggest an autosomal recessive mode of inheritance. Enzyme screening and sequencing of CLN3, CLN6, CLN7, and CLN8 NCL genes did not reveal an underlying mutation in these patients. From biological observations, the CLN9 protein is thought to be a regulator of dihydroceramide synthase, but the *CLN9* gene and protein remain unknown.

Cell biology

CLN9-deficient patient fibroblasts have a distinctive phenotype. Cell bodies are small and rounded, they grow rapidly, are sensitive to apoptosis, and manifest a cell adhesion defect. Their gene expression pattern is significantly different from that reported in other NCL forms. Expression of genes involved in the cell cycle, cell adhesion, and apoptosis is significantly perturbed.

Sphingolipid metabolism is abnormal in CLN9-deficient cells (Schulz et al., 2006): ceramide, dihydroceramide, sphingomyelin, lactosylceramide, gangliosides, ceramide trihexoside and globoside, galactosylceramide, and glucosylceramide mass levels are abnormal. Low ceramide levels suggest a defect in *de novo* ceramide synthesis. Activity of serine palmitoyltransferase (SPT), the key enzyme of *de novo* ceramide synthesis, is increased fourfold, placing the step involved in *de novo* ceramide synthesis in this disease beyond the SPT step. Activity of dihydroceramide synthase, the enzyme generating ceramide from dihydroceramide, is decreased in CLN9-deficient cells.

Expression of CLN8 corrects the CLN9 phenotype with regard to growth and apoptosis. The CLN8 protein contains a Lag1 motif similar to other TLC proteins (TRAM–Lag1p–CLN8) (Winter and Ponting, 2002). The Lag1 motif imparts dihydroceramide synthase activity to yeast cells. The ability of CLN8 to correct the CLN9 phenotype suggests that human Lag1 homologues or their activators could be candidate genes for *CLN9*. Transfection with human Lag1 homologues (*LASS1–LASS6*), except *LASS3*, partially correct ceramide levels, growth, and apoptosis in CLN9-deficient cells. Nevertheless, all Lag homologues have normal sequences in CLN9-cells. *LASS2* expression levels are normal, and *LASS1, 3, 4*, and *6* expression levels are increased in CLN9-deficient cells as measured by reverse transcriptase-polymerase chain reaction (RT-PCR).

4-HPR or fenretinide, a dihydroceramide synthase activator, corrects growth and apoptosis and increases dihydroceramide synthase activity in CLN9-deficient cells. Fumonisin B_1, a dihydroceramide synthase inhibitor, exaggerates the CLN9-deficient phenotype further accelerating growth, decreasing ceramide, and increasing apoptosis. This is neutralized by 4-HPR. This implies that the CLN9 protein is likely to function as a regulator of dihydroceramide synthase. Normal Lag1 homologue sequences, elevated levels of expression of human *LASS* genes by RT-PCR, and increases in dihydroceramide levels in response to 4-HPR give further credence to the idea that the CLN9 protein is an activator of dihydroceramide synthase, should the mutation in the *CLN9* gene result in loss of function. Likewise, a gain of mutation function, as in duplication of a gene, or a mutation resulting in tighter binding of the inhibitor to dihydroceramide synthase, could suggest that the mutated CLN9 protein is an inhibitor of dihydroceramide synthase activity at the protein level.

Clinical data

The clinical course of patients with CLN9 disease is quite similar to that in CLN3 disease, juvenile: the first symptom, declining vision, starts at the age of about 4 years, followed by seizures and cognitive decline by the age of 6 years. Ataxia and rigidity are apparent by the age of 9 years. Patients develop dysarthria and scanning speech between the ages of 10–12 years. They become bedridden and have difficulty swallowing during the course of the illness leading to early death between the ages of 15–20 years.

Fundoscopy shows pigmentary changes, thinned vessels and optic nerve pallor. *ERGs* reveal diminished wave amplitudes. Patient *EEGs* display slowing of the background with frequent polyspike–wave discharges. *Cerebral MRI* of CLN9 disease patients demonstrates progressive cerebral and cerebellar atrophy, predominantly involving grey matter. Abnormal signal intensity is documented in the periventricular white matter.

Morphology

Gross pathology: macroscopically, the brain shows cerebral and cerebellar atrophy. Brain weight at autopsy of one patient was 1140g.

Histopathology: neurons appear ballooned with fine granular material. Dilatation of large neurons is seen in the cerebral cortex, basal ganglia, thalamus, and cerebellar cortex, and to a lesser extent in the red nucleus, locus ceruleus, and the lower olive. Cerebellar Purkinje cells appear dilated by storage material. Lipopigment material is seen in neurons in Ammon's horn. Storage material stains grey with Sudan black and has a yellow autofluorescence. Atrophic changes with moderate- to high-grade astrogliosis have been detected in the nuclei of the thalamus and in the substantia nigra. Moderate subependymal astrogliosis is seen in brain and spinal cord.

Electron microscopy: electron micrographs of brain sections of CLN9 disease patients demonstrate the presence of lysosomal inclusions. They are a combination of membrane-bound granular and curvilinear bodies (Figure 14.14). Electron micrographs of patient lymphocytes show numerous membrane-bound lysosomal vacuoles with some being empty and some containing electron-dense storage material with a fingerprint pattern that is typical for CLN3 disease, juvenile.

Immunohistochemistry: neurons stain positively with an antibody to SCMAS. Positive TUNEL staining demonstrates the presence of apoptotic neurons.

Diagnosis

The diagnosis of CLN9 disease should be considered in a patient with typical clinical symptoms and histological indications of CLN3 disease, juvenile, with normal TTP1, PPT1, and CTSD enzyme activities (Boustany and Zucker, 2006), and electron microscopy shows storage material characterized by a fingerprint pattern in lymphocytes, as well as granular or curvilinear bodies in other tissues. Fibroblasts in culture may have a distinct appearance with small, round cell bodies and grow rapidly as in the known patients. A useful diagnostic test for ascertainment of new CLN9 disease cases may be the determination of dihydroceramide levels and dihydroceramide synthase enzyme activities by tandem mass spectrometry. Low dihydroceramide levels and low dihydroceramide synthase activities are characteristic for the diagnosis of CLN9 disease.

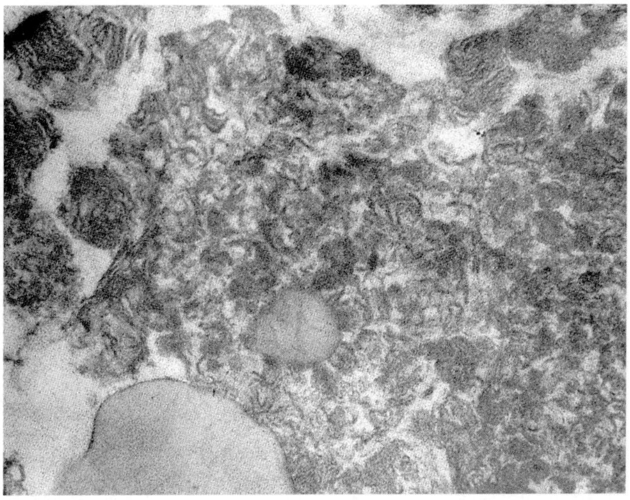

Figure 14.14 CLN9 disease: electron micrograph of brain tissue from a German patient demonstrating the presence of secondary lysosomes containing curvilinear bodies. ×20,000.

Clinical management and experimental therapy

Clinical management of CLN9 disease patients does not differ from patients with CLN3 disease, juvenile (see Chapter 8). Strategies for specific experimental therapy may be developed from the relationship of CLN9 to low dihydroceramide synthase activity. The oral drug 4-HPR, a dihydroceramide synthase activator, may be contemplated as a potential treatment option for CLN9 disease. 4-HPR is already in use as a ceramide-modulating chemotherapeutic agent in clinical trials in children with neuroblastoma and women with breast cancer. There have been no trials of 4-HPR in children with NCL.

OTHER NCL VARIANTS

Introduction

It is clear that patients exist outside of the CLN4 and CLN9 disease variants that remain genetically undefined, although it is difficult to estimate the percentage of patients falling into this category, and this probably varies from country to country. These particularly include patients with onset in late infancy that have disease that resembles that caused by mutations in *CLN5*, *CLN6*, *CLN7*, and *CLN8*, but also NCL with younger and older ages of onset. In time it should be possible to genetically define all these.

This section particularly, but briefly, concentrates on genes that cause disease that overlaps with NCL in humans or animal models, although this may not be the disease that they are most closely associated with.

SGSH

Several of the known NCL genes are expressed in the lysosome lumen. Comparison of the profile of soluble proteins in the lysosome was recently used to identify the genetic defect underlying one case diagnosed with ANCL. Surprisingly, this patient was found to have two mutations in the gene *SGSH*, which encodes the enzyme N-sulphoglucosamine sulphohydrolase, also known as sulphamidase or heparan sulfate sulfatase, and which more usually causes the childhood lysosomal storage disorder mucopolysaccharidosis type IIIA (MPSIIIA) (Sleat et al., 2009). So although this patient is really an adult onset case of MPIIIA, probably with increased amounts of lipopigments, it raises the possibility that other adult onset cases may exist that carry mild mutations in *SGSH*, or indeed in other genes that usually cause more severe childhood onset disease.

To date, all known NCL disease genes, let alone genes that cause other lysosomal storage disorders, or PMEs, have not been excluded from most cases of adult onset NCL and therefore it is a possibility that some late onset cases are caused by 'milder' mutations in such genes. These cases illustrate the necessity of NCL classification requiring genetic data as well as age at onset.

ARSG

A missense mutation in the lysosomal enzyme arylsulphatase G (ARSG) has recently been identified as causing late onset disease in American Staffordshire Terriers (Abitbol et al., 2010). ARSG is one of a number of enzymes that catalyse hydrolysis of sulphate esters and sulphamates that are present in many substrates. Affected dogs suffer from locomotor disabilities with static and dynamic ataxia but no obvious visual impairment. MRI reveals significant cerebellar atrophy, also detectable at necroscopy. Mutation analyses are currently being performed on DNA from human adult onset cases of NCL to determine whether any of them are associated with mutations in *ARSG*.

Chloride channels: Cl^-/H^+-exchangers

Chloride channels or Cl–/H+-exchangers are a highly conserved gene family of chloride channels and transporters with orthologues from bacteria to man. Several have been identified underlying NCL-like disease in mouse models (see Chapter 17). Their connection with NCL has been excellently reviewed (Jalanko and Braulke, 2009, and references therein).

CLCN7

CLCN7 is an 805-amino acid non-glycosylated polytopic membrane protein encoded by the *CLCN7* gene that is localized in late endosomes/lysosomes and the ruffled membrane of osteclasts. CLCN7 is stabilized and protected from degradation by binding to a small membrane protein, OSTM1. The role of the CLCN7 complex is unknown, although thought to be important for lysosomal acidification as well as acidification prior to bone resorption. However, lysosomal pH was not changed in the absence of CLCN7 or OSTM1. CLCN7 is ubiquitously expressed with high expression levels in the pyramidal cell layer in the hippocampus and in Purkinje and granule cells in the cerebellum.

Mutations in *CLCN7* cause a severe autosomal recessive infantile malignant osteopetrosis in children (MIM#259700), and more than 30 disease-causing mutations have been reported. These affect osteoclast function, and cause deficits in bone resorption and osteopetrosis. However, other clinical manifestations include cerebral atrophy, macroencephaly, autism, deafness, and blindness. The osteopetrosis has been successfully treated in a small number of patients by bone marrow transplantation, but these children still develop blindness and severe CNS degeneration, suggesting that the CNS abnormalities are directly related to *CLCN7* mutations. This is supported by recent observations in one CLCN7 mouse model that lacked osteopetrosis via the presence of an alternative spliced CLCN7 transcript in bone that provided function (Rajan et al., 2010). If cases of NCL do exist that are caused by mutations in this gene, these mutations are likely to preserve functional CLCN7 in the bone. Variation in this gene may contribute to neurodegeneration.

CLCN6

In mice *Clcn6* is predominantly expressed in neurons of the central and peripheral nervous system and is localized in late endosomes. Mice mutated in this gene have a progressive lysosomal storage at 4 weeks of age associated with accumulation of lipofuscin and SCMAS. The lysosomal pH was normal, there was no visual impairment, and no loss of neurons was observed. Thus, this gene could underlie clinically mild forms of NCL.

Out of 75 patients sequenced with late onset NCL, two patients were identified who carried a single missense mutation in *CLCN6* on one chromosome only (Poët et al., 2006). The carrier parent was unaffected. This suggests that variation in this gene could affect the disease course of NCL caused by other mutations. One of these patients was subsequently found to be heterozygous for mutations in *CLN5* (Xin et al., 2010).

CLCN3

In mice, CLCN3 is localized in endosomal membranes and synaptic vesicles and functions as vesicular Cl^-/H^+-exchanger. Disruption of *Clcn3* leads to a loss of cells in the hippocampus,

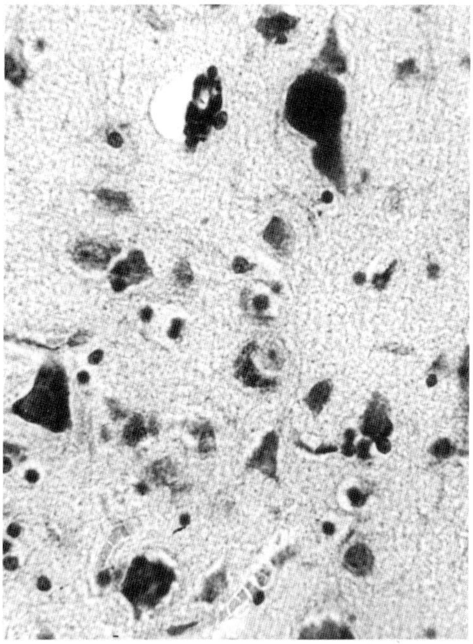

Figure 14.15 Pigment variant of NCL: cerebral neurons are loaded with granular material, Klüver–Barrera stain, ×450.

accumulation of SCMAS, and skeletal and metabolic abnormalities. Given the skeletal involvement, it is probably unlikely that any cases of NCL will be caused by mutations in this gene, although variation in this gene may contribute to neurodegeneration. No human disease has been identified with mutations in this gene.

Pigment variant of NCL

In a so-called pigment variant of NCL, which exists among several clinical types of NCL including a juvenile form (Goebel et al., 1995a), inclusions of a granular type are stored not only in cerebral cortical and subcortical neurons, but also in the subcortical grey matter neuropil (Figures 14.15 and 14.16) and in extracerebral visceral tissues (Goebel et al., 1995a). Extraneuronal storage material shows a rather complex ultrastructure, not identical to that found in classic childhood forms such as CLN1, CLN2, or CLN3 diseases. The ultrastructure of the subcortical storage was also different from that of the subcortical protein-type 'myoclonus' bodies, also called 'spheroids', which in classic CLN2 disease consist of condensed curvilinear profiles (Elleder and Tyynelä, 1998). SCMAS (Figure 14.17) was also scantily

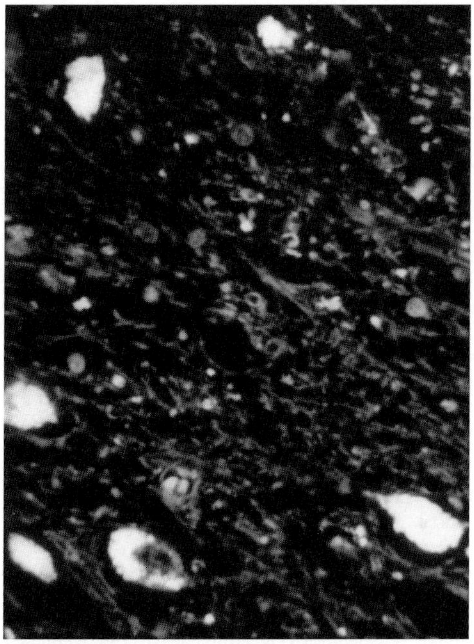

Figure 14.16 Pigment variant of NCL: the intracellular granular material, lipopigments, displays strong autofluorescence, ×350.

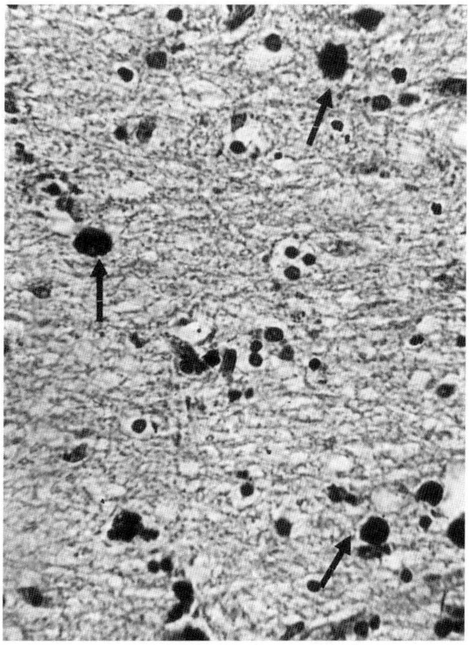

Figure 14.17 Pigment variant of NCL: the lipopigments contain SCMAS (arrows), ×330.

associated with the storage in the pigment variant, in contrast to the rather intense and abundant presence in CLN2 disease, classic late infantile and CLN3 disease, classic juvenile. The scarcity of axonal spheroids in the facial nucleus (Goebel et al., 1995a), but not in other subcortical areas was in striking contrast to the subcortical neuropathology in Hallervorden–Spatz disease (HSD). These HSD-related 'spheroids' differ from those of the 'myoclonus' body type, because the former contain mitochondria and dense bodies, the latter curvilinear bodies.

REFERENCES

Abitbol M, Thibaud JL, Olby NJ, Hitte C, Puech JP, Maurer M, Pilot-Storck F, Hedan B, Dreano S, Brahimi S, Delattre D, Andre C, Gray F, Delisle F, Caillaud C, Bernex F, Panthier JJ, Aubin-Houzelstein G, Blot S, & Tiret L (2010) A canine arylsulfatase G (ARSG) mutation leading to a sulfatase deficiency is associated with neuronal ceroid lipofuscinosis. *Proc Natl Acad Sci U S A*, 107, 14775–14780.

Annunziata P, Pero G, Ibba L, Federico A, Bardelli AM, Sabatelli P, & Guazzi GC (1986) Adult dementia in three siblings: ceroid-lipofuscinosis. *Acta Neurol (Napoli)*, 8, 528–534.

Anzai Y, Hayashi M, Fueki N, Kurata K, & Ohya T (2006) Protracted juvenile neuronal ceroid lipofuscinosis—an autopsy report and immunohistochemical analysis. *Brain Dev*, 28, 462–465.

Baker M, Mackenzie IR, Pickering-Brown SM, Gass J, Rademakers R, Lindholm C, Snowden J, Adamson J, Sadovnick AD, Rollinson S, Cannon A, Dwosh E, Neary D, Melquist S, Richardson A, Dickson D, Berger Z, Eriksen J, Robinson T, Zehr C, Dickey CA, Crook R, McGowan E, Mann D, Boeve B, Feldman H, & Hutton M (2006) Mutations in progranulin cause tau-negative frontotemporal dementia linked to chromosome 17. *Nature*, 442, 916–919.

Barthez-Carpentier MA, Billard C, Maheut J, Santini JJ, & Ruchoux MM (1991) A case of childhood Kufs' disease. *J Neurol Neurosurg Psychiatry*, 54, 655–657.

Berkovic SF, Carpenter S, Andermann F, Andermann E, & Wolfe LS (1988) Kufs' disease: a critical reappraisal. *Brain*, 111 (Pt 1), 27–62.

Boehme DH, Cottrell JC, Leonberg SC, & Zeman W (1971) A dominant form of neuronal ceroid-lipofuscinosis. *Brain*, 94, 745–760.

Boustany RM & Zucker A (2006) Degenerative diseases primarily of gray matter. In Swaiman KF, Ashwal S, Ferriero DM (Eds.) *Pediatric Neurology: Principles and Practice*, 4th edn, pp. 1315–1344. Philadelphia, PA, Mosby.

Braak H & Braak E (1987) Projection neurons of basolateral amygdaloid nuclei develop meganeurites in juvenile and adult human neuronal ceroid lipofuscinosis. *Clin Neuropathol*, 6, 116–119.

Braak H & Braak E (1993) Pathoarchitectonic pattern of iso- and allocortical lesions in juvenile and adult neuronal ceroid-lipofuscinosis. *J Inherit Metab Dis*, 16, 259–262.

Brück W & Goebel HH (1998) Microglia activation in neuronal ceroid-lipofuscinosis. *Clin Neuropathol*, 5, 276 (poster P29).

Burneo JG, Arnold T, Palmer CA, Kuzniecky RI, Oh SJ, & Faught E (2003) Adult-onset neuronal ceroid lipofuscinosis (Kufs disease) with autosomal dominant inheritance in Alabama. *Epilepsia*, 44, 841–846.

Callagy C, O'Neill G, Murphy SF, & Farrell MA (2000) Adult neuronal ceroid lipofuscinosis (Kufs' disease) in two siblings of an Irish family. *Clin Neuropathol*, 19, 109–118.

Ceuterick C & Martin J-J (1998) Extracerebral biopsy in lysosomal and peroxisomal disorders: ultrastructural finding. *Brain Pathol*, 8, 121–132.

Charles N, Vighetto A, Pialat J, Confavreux C, & Aimard G (1990) [Dementia and psychiatric disorders in Kufs disease]. *Rev Neurol (Paris)*, 146, 752–756.

Constantinidis J, Wisniewski KE, & Wisniewski TM (1992) The adult and a new late adult forms of neuronal ceroid lipofuscinosis. *Acta Neuropathol*, 83, 461–468.

Cruts M, Gijselinck I, van der Zee J, Engelborghs S, Wils H, Pirici D, Rademakers R, Vandenberghe R, Dermaut B, Martin JJ, van Duijn C, Peeters K, Sciot R, Santens P, De Pooter T, Mattheijssens M, Van den Broeck M, Cuijt I, Vennekens K, De Deyn PP, Kumar-Singh S, & Van Broeckhoven C (2006) Null mutations in progranulin cause ubiquitin-positive frontotemporal dementia linked to chromosome 17q21. *Nature*, 442, 920–924.

Dawson WW, Armstrong D, Greer M, Maida TM, & Samuelson DA (1985) Disease-specific electrophysiological findings in adult ceroid-lipofuscinosis (Kufs disease). *Doc Ophthalmol*, 60, 163–171.

van Diggelen OP, Keulemans JL, Kleijer WJ, Thobois S, Tilikete C, & Voznyi YV (2001a) Pre- and postnatal enzyme analysis for infantile, late infantile and adult neuronal ceroid lipofuscinosis (CLN1 and CLN2). *Eur J Paediatr Neurol*, 5 Suppl A, 189–192.

van Diggelen OP, Thobois S, Tilikete C, Zabot MT, Keulemans JL, van Bunderen PA, Taschner PE, Losekoot M, & Voznyi YV (2001b) Adult neuronal ceroid lipofuscinosis with palmitoyl-protein thioesterase deficiency: first adult-onset patients of a childhood disease. *Ann Neurol*, 50, 269–272.

Dom R, Brucher JM, Ceuterick C, Carton H, & Martin JJ (1979) Adult ceroid-lipofuscinosis (Kufs' disease) in two brothers. Retinal and visceral storage in one; diagnostic muscle biopsy in the other. *Acta Neuropathol*, 45, 67–72.

Donnet A, Habib M, Pellissier JF, Regis H, Farnarier G, Pelletier J, Gosset A, Roger J, & Khalil R (1992) Kufs' disease presenting as progressive dementia with late-onset generalized seizures: a clinicopathological and electrophysiological study. *Epilepsia*, 33, 65–74.

Drach LM (1996) Meeting report: Dementia with Lewy bodies - Tower of Babel tumbled down? *Clin Neuropathol*, 15, 248.

Dyken P & Wisniewski K (1995) Classification of the neuronal ceroid-lipofuscinoses: expansion of the atypical forms. *Am J Med Genet*, 57, 150–154.

Elleder M, Sokolova J, & Hrebicek M (1997) Follow-up study of subunit c of mitochondrial ATP synthase (SCMAS) in Batten disease and in unrelated lysosomal disorders. *Acta Neuropathol*, 93, 379–390.

Elleder M & Tyynelä J (1998) Incidence of neuronal perikaryal spheroids in neuronal ceroid lipofuscinoses (Batten disease). *Clin Neuropathol*, 17, 184–189.

Fealey ME, Edwards WD, Grogan M, & Orszulak TA (2009) Neuronal ceroid lipofuscinosis in a 31-year-old woman presenting as biventricular heart failure with restrictive features. *Cardiovasc Pathol*, 18, 44–48.

Ferrer I, Arbizu T, Peña J, & Serra JP (1980) A golgi and ultrastructural study of a dominant form of Kufs' disease. *J Neurol*, 222, 183–190.

Gelot A, Maurage CA, Rodriguez D, Perrier-Pallisson D, Larmande P, & Ruchoux MM (1998) In vivo diagnosis of Kufs' disease by extracerebral biopsies. *Acta Neuropathol*, 96, 102–108.

Gille M Brucher JM, Indekeu P, Bis-teau M, & Kollmann P (1995) Maladie de Kufs avec leucoencéphalopathie. *Rev Neurol (Paris)*, 151, 392–397.

Goebel HH & Braak H (1989) Adult neuronal ceroid-lipofuscinosis. *Clin Neuropathol*, 8, 109–119.

Goebel HH, Gullotta F, Bajanowski T, Hansen FJ, & Braak H (1995a) Pigment variant of neuronal ceroid-lipofuscinosis. *Am J Med Genet*, 57, 155–159.

Goebel HH, Jaynes M, Gutmann L, & Schochet S (1997) Diagnostic biopsy of extracerebral tissue in adult neuronal ceroid-lipofuscinosis. *Neuropathol Appl Neurobiol*, 23, 167–168.

Goebel HH, Schochet SS, Jaynes M, & Gutmann L (1998) Ultrastructure of the retina in adult neuronal ceroid lipofuscinosis. *Acta Anat (Basel)*, 162, 127–132.

Goebel HH, Warlo I, Klockgether T, & Harzer K (1995b) Significance of lipopigments with fingerprint profiles in eccrine sweat gland epithelial cells. *Am J Med Genet*, 57, 187–190.

Gray F, Destee A, Bourre JM, Gherardi R, Krivosic I, Warot P, & Poirier J (1987) Pigmentary type of orthochromatic leukodystrophy (OLD): a new case with ultrastructural and biochemical study. *J Neuropathol Exp Neurol*, 46, 585–596.

Hall NA, Lake BD, Dewji NN, & Patrick AD (1991) Lysosomal storage of subunit c of mitochondrial ATP synthase in Batten's disease (ceroid-lipofuscinosis). *Biochem J*, 275 (Pt 1), 269–272.

Ikeda K, Kosaka K, Oyanagi S, & Yamada K (1984) Adult type of neuronal ceroid-lipofuscinosis with retinal involvement. *Clin Neuropathol*, 3, 237–239.

Iseki E, Amano N, Yokoi S, Yamada Y, Suzuki K, & Yazaki M (1987) A case of adult neuronal ceroid-lipofuscinosis with the appearance of membranous cytoplasmic bodies localized in the spinal anterior horn. *Acta Neuropathol*, 72, 362–368.

Ivan CS, Saint-Hilaire MH, Christensen TG, & Milunsky JM (2005) Adult-onset neuronal ceroid lipofuscinosis type B in an African-American. *Mov Disord*, 20, 752–754.

Jakob H & Kolkmann FW (1973) [Pigment variant of the adult type of amaurotic idiocy (Kufs) (author's transl)]. *Acta Neuropathol*, 26, 225–236.

Jalanko A & Braulke T (2009) Neuronal ceroid lipofuscinoses. *Biochim Biophys Acta*, 1793, 697–709.

Josephson SA, Schmidt RE, Millsap P, McManus DQ, & Morris JC (2001) Autosomal dominant Kufs' disease: a cause of early onset dementia. *J Neurol Sci*, 188, 51–60.

Kufs H (1925) Über eine Spätform der amaurotischen Idiotie und ihre heredofamiliären Grundlagen. *Z Ges Neurol Psychiatr*, 95, 168–188.

Kufs H (1927) Über die Bedeutung der optischen Komponente der amaurotischen Idiotie in diagnostischer und erbbiologischer Beziehung und über die Existenz 'spätester' Fälle bei dieser Krankheit. *Z Ges Neurol Psychiatr*, 109, 453–487.

Kufs H (1929) Über einen Fall von Spätform der amaurotischen Idiotie mit atypischem Verlauf und mit terminalen schweren Störungen des Fettstoffwechsels im Gesamtorganismus. *Z Ges Neurol Psychiatr*, 122, 395–415.

Kufs H (1931) Über einen Fall von spätester Form der amaurotische Idiotie mit dem Beginn im 42 und Tod im 59. Lebensjahre in klinischer, histologischer und vererbungspathologischer Beziehung. *Z Ges Neurol Psychiatr*, 137, 432–448.

Larnaout A, Belal S, Zouari M, Fki M, Ben Hamida C, Goebel HH, Ben Hamida M, & Hentati F (1997) Friedreich's ataxia with isolated vitamin E deficiency: a neuropathological study of a Tunisian patient. *Acta Neuropathol*, 93, 633–637.

Leonberg SCJ, Armstrong D, & Boehme D (1982) A century of Kufs disease in an American family. In Armstrong, D., Koppang, N., Rider, J.A. (Eds) *Ceroid-lipofuscinosis (Batten disease)*, pp87-93. Amsterdam, Elsevier Biomedical Press.

Loiseau P, Chedru F, Habib M, & Pellissier JF (1990) [Conference at the Salpetriere. November 1988. Progressive dementia and generalized epilepsy in a young woman]. *Rev Neurol (Paris)*, 146, 383–389.

Martin JJ (1991) Adult type of neuronal ceroid lipofuscinosis. *Dev Neurosci*, 13, 331–338.

Martin JJ (1993) Adult type of neuronal ceroid-lipofuscinosis. *J Inherit Metab Dis*, 16, 237–240.

Martin JJ & Ceuterick C (1997) Adult neuronal ceroid-lipofuscinosis—personal observations. *Acta Neurol Belg*, 97, 85–92.

Martin JJ, Libert J, & Ceuterick C (1987) Ultrastructure of brain and retina in Kufs' disease (adult type-ceroid-lipofuscinosis). *Clin Neuropathol*, 6, 231–235.

Mole SE, Williams RE, & Goebel HH (2005) Correlations between genotype, ultrastructural morphology and clinical phenotype in the neuronal ceroid lipofuscinoses. *Neurogenetics*, 6, 107–126.

Nardocci N, Verga ML, Binelli S, Zorzi G, Angelini L, & Bugiani O (1995) Neuronal ceroid-lipofuscinosis: a clinical and morphological study of 19 patients. *Am J Med Genet*, 57, 137–141.

Nijssen PC, Brekelmans GJ, & Roos RA (2009) Electroencephalography in autosomal dominant adult neuronal ceroid lipofuscinosis. *Clin Neurophysiol*, 120, 1782–1786.

Nijssen PC, Brusse E, Leyten AC, Martin JJ, Teepen JL, & Roos RA (2002) Autosomal dominant adult neuronal ceroid lipofuscinosis: parkinsonism due to both striatal and nigral dysfunction. *Mov Disord*, 17, 482–487.

Nijssen PC, Ceuterick C, van Diggelen OP, Elleder M, Martin JJ, Teepen JL, Tyynelä J, & Roos RA (2003) Autosomal dominant adult neuronal ceroid lipofuscinosis: a novel form of NCL with granular osmiophilic deposits without palmitoyl protein thioesterase 1 deficiency. *Brain Pathol*, 13, 574–581.

O'Neill G, Murphy SF, Moran H, Burke H, & Farrell MA (1993) Kufs disease - a clinicopathologic study in two siblings. *J Neuropathol Exp Neurol*, 52, 300.

Pasquinelli G, Cenacchi G, Piane EL, Russo C, & Aguglia U (2004) The problematic issue of Kufs disease diagnosis as performed on rectal biopsies: a case report. *Ultrastruct Pathol*, 28, 43–48.

Poët M, Kornak U, Schweizer M, Zdebik AA, Scheel O, Hoelter S, Wurst W, Schmitt A, Fuhrmann JC,

Planells-Cases R, Mole SE, Hubner CA, & Jentsch TJ (2006) Lysosomal storage disease upon disruption of the neuronal chloride transport protein ClC-6. *Proc Natl Acad Sci U S A*, 103, 13854–13859.

Rajan I, Read R, Small DL, Perrard J, & Vogel P (2010) An alternative splicing variant in Clcn7-/- mice prevents osteopetrosis but not neural and retinal degeneration. *Vet Pathol.* May 13. [Epub].

Ramadan H, Al-Din AS, Ismail A, Balen F, Varma A, Twomey A, Watts R, Jackson M, Anderson G, Green E, & Mole SE (2007) Adult neuronal ceroid lipofuscinosis caused by deficiency in palmitoyl protein thioesterase 1. *Neurology*, 68, 387–388.

Reif A, Schneider MF, Hoyer A, Schneider-Gold C, Fallgatter AJ, Roggendorf W, & Pfuhlmann B (2003) Neuroleptic malignant syndrome in Kufs' disease. *J Neurol Neurosurg Psychiatry*, 74, 385–387.

Reske-Nielsen E, Baandrup U, Bjerregaard P, & Bruun I (1981) Cardiac involvement in juvenile amaurotic idiocy—a specific heart muscle disorder. Histological findings in 13 autopsied patients. *Acta Pathol Microbiol Scand A*, 89, 357–365.

Reznik M, Arrese-Estrada J, Sadzot B, & Franck G (1995) Un cas anatomo-clinique de la maladie de Kufs familiale. *Rev Neurol (Paris)*, 151, 597.

Robertson T, Tannenberg AE, Hiu J, & Reimers J (2008) 53-year-old man with rapid cognitive decline. *Brain Pathol*, 18, 292–294.

Rowan SA & Lake BD (1995) Tissue and cellular distribution of subunit c of ATP synthase in Batten disease (neuronal ceroid-lipofuscinosis). *Am J Med Genet*, 57, 172–176.

Ruchoux MM, Gelot A, Perrier D, & Larmande P (1996) Two families with Kufs disease, contribution of extracerebral biopsies for diagnosis. Vth European Congress of Neuropathology, Paris. *Neuropathol Appl Neurobiol*, 22, 118.

Rumbach L, Warter JM, Coquillat G, Marescaux C, Collard M, Rohmer F, Bieth R, & Zawislak R (1983) [Anomalies in fatty acids distribution and superoxide dismutase activity in lymphocytes of an adult with atypical ceroid lipofuscinosis]. *Rev Neurol (Paris)*, 139, 269–276.

Sadzot B, Reznik M, Arrese-Estrada JE, & Franck G (2000) Familial Kufs' disease presenting as a progressive myoclonic epilepsy. *J Neurol*, 247, 447–454.

Sakajiri K, Matsubara N, Nakajima T, Fukuhara N, Makifuchi T, Wakabayashi M, Oyanagi S, & Kominami E (1995) A family with adult type ceroid lipofuscinosis (Kufs' disease) and heart muscle disease: report of two autopsy cases. *Intern Med*, 34, 1158–1163.

Schreiner R, Becker I, & Wiegand MH (2000) [Kufs-disease; a rare cause of early-onset dementia]. *Nervenarzt*, 71, 411–415.

Schulz A, Dhar S, Rylova S, Dbaibo G, Alroy J, Hagel C, Artacho I, Kohlschutter A, Lin S, & Boustany RM (2004) Impaired cell adhesion and apoptosis in a novel CLN9 Batten disease variant. *Ann Neurol*, 56, 342–350.

Schulz A, Mousallem T, Venkataramani M, Persaud-Sawin DA, Zucker A, Luberto C, Bielawska A, Bielawski J, Holthuis JC, Jazwinski SM, Kozhaya L, Dbaibo GS, & Boustany RM (2006) The CLN9 protein, a regulator of dihydroceramide synthase. *J Biol Chem*, 281, 2784–2794.

Sinha S, Satishchandra P, Santosh V, Gayatri N, & Shankar SK (2004) Neuronal ceroid lipofuscinosis: a clinicopathological study. *Seizure*, 13, 235–240.

Sleat DE, Ding L, Wang S, Zhao C, Wang Y, Xin W, Zheng H, Moore DF, Sims KB, & Lobel P (2009) Mass spectrometry-based protein profiling to determine the cause of lysosomal storage diseases of unknown etiology. *Mol Cell Proteomics*, 8, 1708–1718.

Sleat DE, Donnelly RJ, Lackland H, Liu CG, Sohar I, Pullarkat RK, & Lobel P (1997) Association of mutations in a lysosomal protein with classical late-infantile neuronal ceroid lipofuscinosis. *Science*, 277, 1802–1805.

Sleat DE, Sohar I, Pullarkat PS, Lobel P, & Pullarkat RK (1998) Specific alterations in levels of mannose 6-phosphorylated glycoproteins in different neuronal ceroid lipofuscinoses. *Biochem J*, 334 (Pt 3), 547–551.

Snyder CK, Ho K-C, & Antuono PG (1998) Comparison of neuronal lipofuscin deposition and neuronal size in the hippocampus of normal aging and Alzheimer's disease population. *J Neuropathol Exp Neurol*, 57, 471.

Tobo M, Mitsuyama Y, Ikari K, & Itoi K (1984) Familial occurrence of adult-type neuronal ceroid lipofuscinosis. *Arch Neurol*, 41, 1091–1094.

Tominaga I, Hattori M, Kaihou M, Takazawa H, Kato Y, Kasahara M, Onaya M, Nojima T, Kashima H, & Iwabuchi K (1994) [Dementia and amyotrophy in Kufs disease. The adult type of neuronal ceroid lipofuscinosis]. *Rev Neurol (Paris)*, 150, 413–417.

Trillet M, Bady B, Kopp N, & Girard PF (1973) [Neuronal ceroid-lipofuscinosis. Apropos of 3 familial cases, one with pathological examination]. *Rev Neurol (Paris)*, 129, 233–250.

Tyynelä J, Suopanki J, Baumann M, & Haltia M (1997a) Sphingolipid activator proteins (SAPs) in neuronal ceroid lipofuscinoses (NCL). *Neuropediatrics*, 28, 49–52.

Vadlamudi L, Westmoreland BF, Klass DW, & Parisi JE (2003) Electroencephalographic findings in Kufs disease. *Clin Neurophysiol*, 114, 1738–1743.

Vercruyssen A, Martin JJ, Ceuterick C, Jacobs K, & Swerts L (1982) Adult ceroid-lipofuscinosis: diagnostic value of biopsies and of neurophysiological investigations. *J Neurol Neurosurg Psychiatry*, 45, 1056–1059.

Vital A, Vital C, Orgogozo JM, Mazeaux JM, Pautrizel B, & Lariviere JM (1991) Adult dementia due to intraneuronal accumulation of ceroidlipofuscinosis (Kufs' disease): ultrastructural study of two cases. *J Geriatr Psychiatry Neurol*, 4, 110–115.

Winter E & Ponting CP (2002) TRAM, LAG1 and CLN8: members of a novel family of lipid-sensing domains? *Trends Biochem Sci*, 27, 381–383.

Wisniewski KE, Kida E, Patxot OF, & Connell F (1992) Variability in the clinical and pathological findings in the neuronal ceroid lipofuscinoses: review of data and observations. *Am J Med Genet*, 42, 525–532.

Wisniewski KE, Kida E, Gordon-Majszak W, & Saitoh T (1990a) Altered amyloid beta-protein precursor processing in brains of patients with neuronal ceroid lipofuscinosis. *Neurosci Lett*, 120, 94–96.

Wisniewski KE, Maslinska D, Kitaguchi T, Kim KS, Goebel HH, & Haltia M (1990b) Topographic heterogeneity of amyloid B-protein epitopes in brains with various forms of neuronal ceroid lipofuscinoses suggesting defective processing of amyloid precursor protein. *Acta Neuropathol*, 80, 26–34.

Xin W, Mullen TE, Kiely R, Min J, Feng X, Cao Y, O'Malley L, Shen Y, Chu-Shore C, Mole SE, Goebel HH, & Sims K (2010) CLN5 mutations are frequent in juvenile and late-onset non-Finnish patients with NCL. *Neurology*, 74, 565–571.

Zini A, Cenacchi G, Nichelli P, Zunarelli E, Todeschini A, & Meletti S (2008) Early-onset dementia with prolonged occipital seizures: an atypical case of Kufs disease. *Neurology*, 71, 1709–1712.

Chapter 15

Unicellular Models

S. Codlin and R.L. Haines

INTRODUCTION

Unicellular eukaryotes have many advantages as model organisms since they are easy to grow and maintain, have short cell cycles, and there are many tools and approaches available to assist analysis. Two such organisms, the budding yeast *Saccharomyces cerevisiae* and the fission yeast *Schizosaccharomyces pombe*, have been utilized in the study of NCLs, since several NCL genes and their gene products are conserved in these species. Both have orthologues for the proteins CLN3, designated Btn1p, and cathepsin D, designated Pep4p in *S. cerevisiae* or Sxa1p in *S. pombe*. The fission yeast, *S. pombe*, also has a CLN1 orthologue, designated Ppt1p.

SACCHAROMYCES CEREVISIAE

The budding yeast, *Saccharomyces cerevisiae*, has been popular as a model organism for over half a century. It was the first eukaryote to have its genome sequenced, and this is now highly annotated and known to consist of approximately 6000 open reading frames on 16 chromosomes, including at least 4850 verified protein coding genes. As a single-celled organism, with a short generation time, which can exist in haploid and diploid forms, *S. cerevisiae* is particularly amenable to genetic analysis. Haploid strains of opposite mating types can fuse and the resulting diploid strain has the ability to sporulate, generating four haploid offspring, allowing for complementation and haplo-insufficiency studies, and the deletion of essential genes. This yeast also readily takes up, recombines, and expresses DNA, allowing the study of gene deletions and genomically tagged proteins, in addition to overexpression studies. Indeed a library of strains deleted for all non-essential genes is commercially available, as are several libraries containing almost all genes with green fluorescent protein (GFP), glutathione-S-transferase, or tandem affinity purification tags that are widely used for localization and biochemical analyses.

CLN3

Since approximately 50% of yeast proteins have some similarity with mammalian proteins, *S. cerevisiae* has regularly been used as a model to study human disease, with varying degrees of success. *CLN3*, the gene mutated in CLN3 disease, juvenile, has an orthologue in *S. cerevisiae*, originally designated *YHC3* but now more commonly referred to as *BTN1*, which encodes a 408-amino acid putative integral membrane protein that is 59% similar and 39% identical to the human protein (see Chapter 19, Figure 19.4). Like CLN3p, overexpressed and tagged Btn1p has been localized to the vacuole membrane (the yeast equivalent of the mammalian lysosome) when N-terminally tagged with GFP, while it has been seen within the vacuole as well as in punctate cytoplasmic structures that may be endoplasmic reticulum or Golgi related compartments when tagged at the C-terminus (Croopnick et al., 1998, Golabek et al., 1999, Pearce et al., 1999a, Kyttälä et al., 2004). More recent data suggest a primary location in the Golgi complex (J. Gerst unpublished data). CLN3p complements many of the phenotypes of strains deleted for *BTN1* (see below), indicating that these proteins are functional orthologues. All residues associated with disease-causing missense mutations in CLN3p are conserved across species (http://www.ucl.ac.uk/ncl/mutation.shtml), and some of these mutations have been modelled in Btn1p in order to assess their impact on function. Evidence suggests that disease severity may correlate with degree of complementation (Pearce and Sherman, 1998, Kim et al., 2003).

A number of groups generated strains that are deleted for all or part of the yeast *BTN1* gene, and investigated the impact of loss of this gene on yeast growth under a variety of conditions. No significant differences between growth of wild-type and *btn1*-Δ cells were observed, despite varying over 100 different growth and media conditions. However, in the absence of Btn1p, cells are slightly more sensitive to combined heat and alkaline stress (39°C, pH 8.5), and are resistant to the chemical D-(–)-threo-2-amino-t-[p-nitrophenyl]-1,3-propanediol (ANP), a chloramphenicol base (see below) (Pearce and Sherman, 1997, Croopnick et al., 1998, Pearce and Sherman, 1998, Guo et al., 1999, Barwell and Broom, 2001). In addition to the lack of an obvious growth defect, cells deleted for *BTN1* have no defects in mitochondrial function or degradation of Atp9p (equivalent to mitochondrial ATP synthase subunit c), in contrast to the situation in human patients where subunit c is a major component of the storage material found in lysosomes (Haltia et al., 1973, Hall et al., 1991, Kominami et al., 1992, Palmer et al., 1995, Pearce and Sherman, 1997). Further investigations have revealed that Btn1p is involved in maintenance of pH regulation, basic amino acid transport/homeostasis, and possibly nitric oxide signalling, and deletion of *BTN1* results in the upregulation of two yeast genes, *HSP30* and *BTN2* (Pearce et al., 1999a, Kim et al., 2003, Padilla-Lopez and Pearce, 2006, Phillips et al., 2006).

PH REGULATION/HOMEOSTASIS

S. cerevisiae deleted for *BTN1* have a slightly more acidic vacuole pH (pH 5.8) compared with wild-type cells (pH 6.15) (Pearce et al., 1999a). This is in contrast to the *Schizosaccharomyces pombe* model, and importantly to cells from patients, where the pH of vacuoles/lysosomes is less acidic in the absence of Btn1p or CLN3p activity respectively (Holopainen et al., 2001, Gachet et al., 2005). Although the opposite vacuole pH phenotype has been observed in *S. cerevisiae* compared to other model systems, it is clear that a defect in pH regulation is present in the absence of Btn1p (and CLN3p), and much effort has been put into characterizing a pH homeostasis phenotype in this system. Pearce and colleagues, who first reported the more acidic vacuole pH phenotype, have shown that during growth the vacuoles of *btn1*-Δ cells increase in pH, being indistinguishable from wild-type after 25 hours of growth in normal YPD growing medium (Pearce et al., 1999a). The vacuole pH of these cells is affected by extracellular medium; when grown in YNB medium at pH 4 *btn1*-Δ cells have decreased vacuole pH compared to wild-type, but when grown at pH 7.5 the vacuole pH is initially indistinguishable from wild-type, and becomes slightly more alkaline after 24 hours of growth (Padilla-Lopez and Pearce, 2006). During early growth (6 hours) the activity of both the plasma membrane and vacuolar H^+ ATPases is increased compared to wild-type cells, and this may act as a buffering effect, since by 25 hours the activities of both H^+ ATPases are similar to wild-type, and the pH of the vacuole is also indistinguishable (Pearce et al., 1999b, Chattopadhyay et al., 2000). The increased activity of the plasma membrane H^+ ATPase results in an increased rate of media acidification during early growth, and this probably confers the reported resistance to ANP. The pH of media significantly affects ANP toxicity: below pH 6.5 ANP is less toxic, while above this pH the toxicity increases. Therefore, the increased rate of media acidification observed in *btn1*-Δ cells may reduce the toxicity of ANP, allowing *btn1*-Δ cells to grow. Importantly, the ANP phenotype can be complemented by ectopic expression of Btn1p or human CLN3p, and the degree of complementation by various disease-causing missense mutations partially correlates with disease severity, suggesting that the pH phenotype is relevant to CLN3p function (Pearce and Sherman, 1998). In addition, in the presence of chloroquine, a lysosomotropic agent that raises the pH of acidic compartments (Slater, 1993), the rate of media acidification and the activity of the plasma membrane H^+ ATPase are returned to wild-type levels, and *btn1*-Δ cells are no longer resistant to ANP (Pearce et al., 1999c). The latest work suggests that Btn1p is required for tight regulation of vacuolar pH (Padilla-Lopez and Pearce, 2006), but more work is required to identify the precise role of Btn1p in this process, particularly since this phenotype does not clearly mimic that of human patient cells.

BASIC AMINO ACID TRANSPORT AND OXIDATIVE STRESS

Investigation into potential vacuole dysfunction in *btn1*-Δ cells suggested that Btn1p may be involved in the transport of basic amino acids into the vacuole. The vacuole in *S. cerevisiae* is known to act as a storage compartment for amino acids within the cell (Weimken and Dürr, 1974, Kitamoto et al., 1988), so the observed decreases in vacuolar arginine and lysine levels and ATP-dependent vacuolar arginine uptake in *S. cerevisiae* cells deleted for *BTN1* are potentially interesting. Arginine transport into the vacuole requires a functioning vacuolar H^+ ATPase, though the decrease in arginine transport into the vacuole of vacuolar H^+ ATPase mutant cells such as *cup5*-Δ and *vma13*-Δ is not as great as the decrease in *btn1*-Δ cells. Therefore, there may be an additional defect in basic amino acid transport in cells lacking *BTN1* on top of the pH/vacuolar H^+ ATPase defects described above. Both *S. cerevisiae* Btn1p and CLN3p complemented the arginine transport defect, suggesting a potential role for these proteins in transport, or regulation of transport, to the vacuole (Kim et al., 2003). A similar phenotype was reported in cells from human patients, in that reduced levels of arginine and decreased arginine (but not lysine) uptake into the lysosome were observed when compared to age- and gender-matched control cells (Ramirez-Montealegre and Pearce, 2005).

More recently it has been shown that the decreased intracellular arginine in *btn1*-Δ is not a result of altered arginine uptake, arginine efflux, or incorporation into peptides (Vitiello et al., 2007). The absence of Gcn4p, a transcription factor involved in the regulation of amino acid synthesis, transport, and storage, causes an increase in expression of genes involved in amino acid transport and synthesis, but a decrease in *BTN1* mRNA was observed. Taken together, these results suggest that Btn1p is not an arginine transporter itself. In *btn1*-Δ cells, overexpression of Can1p, a plasma membrane basic amino acid transporter, caused cell swelling and death, though no increase in intracellular arginine following overexpression of this protein was observed. Indeed, growth of these cells in media lacking arginine did not rescue the cell death phenotype, suggesting that perhaps defective intracellular protein transport, exacerbated by overexpression of this membrane protein, rather than amino acid uptake contributes to cell death.

The decreased levels of L-arginine in *btn1*-Δ cells limit the synthesis of nitric oxide (NO) in both physiological and oxidative stress conditions (Osório et al., 2007). This defect in NO synthesis suppresses the signalling required for yeast menadione-induced apoptosis, causing an increased resistance to this chemical. It may be that in juvenile CLN3 disease, a limited capacity to synthesize NO contributes to the pathology of the disease.

INTERACTIONS

Efforts to identify interactors and compensators for Btn1p have focused on two methods: a yeast two-hybrid screen with full length or sections of Btn1p, and a microarray on *btn1*-Δ cells (Pearce et al., 1999a, Cottone et al., 2001, Vitiello et al., 2010). It was not possible to identify any interacting partners of full-length Btn1p by the two-hybrid system, perhaps because of the hydrophobic nature of this protein. However, an interaction between the C-terminus of CLN3p with SBDSp, a protein associated with an inherited paediatric disorder Shwach–Bodian–Diamond syndrome that is characterized by bone marrow and pancreatic dysfunction, mild mental retardation, and haematological abnormalities with an increased risk of leukaemia, was identified using this system (Vitiello et al., 2010). This interaction was conserved between Btn1p and Sdo1p in fractions enriched with endosomes and Golgi in *S. cerevisiae*. SBDS is thought to play a role in ribosomal maturation, and the yeast protein Sdo1p contributes to export of the ribosome from the nucleus. Vacuole function, particularly acidification, appears to be influenced by Sdo1p. Whether Sdo1p regulates vacuole function or *vice versa* via Btn1p requires further investigation. A link between CLN3 function and RNA binding has been reported in *Drosophila* (Tuxworth et al., 2009).

Microarray analysis revealed that at later stages of growth the expression of two genes, *HSP30* and *BTN2*, was increased at the mRNA level compared to wild-type. Hsp30p is a plasma membrane small heat shock protein, which is known to downregulate the plasma membrane H+ ATPase in response to the induction of stress response (Piper et al., 1997). Deletion of either *HSP30* or *BTN2* on a wild-type or *btn1*-Δ background does not alter vacuolar or cytosolic pH. However, this does diminish the ability of *S. cerevisiae* cells to grow on acidic media and results in increased plasma membrane and vacuolar H+ ATPase activity at later growth stages, which is not caused by increased expression of either ATPase. Neither *HSP30* nor *BTN2* confer the ANP resistance phenotype; deletion of either of these genes on a *btn1*-Δ background does not affect the ability of these cells to grow on ANP (Chattopadhyay et al., 2000).

Btn2p is a novel 410-amino acid protein that is 38% similar to human and *Drosophila* HOOK1p, a coiled coil protein that interacts with the cytoskeleton in mammalian cells and is involved in endocytosis of membrane receptors and sorting to multi-vesicular bodies (MVBs) in *Drosophila*. *S. cerevisiae* Btn2p has been shown by yeast two-hybrid and co-immunoprecipitation studies to interact with Rgs1p, a downregulator of the Can1p arginine and lysine permease, Yif1p, a component of a Golgi protein complex involved in endoplasmic reticulum to Golgi transport, and Ist2p, a plasma membrane protein that may have a function in salt tolerance. In the absence of Btn2p in *S. cerevisiae*, all of these interacting proteins are mislocalized (Chattopadhyay and Pearce, 2002, Chattopadhyay et al., 2003, Kim et al., 2005). Btn2p has now been shown to localize to a late endosome-like compartment, to interact with components of the endocytic SNARE complex, retromer, and Snx4 the sorting nexin, and to be involved in facilitating specific protein retrieval from the late endosome to the Golgi (Kama et al., 2007). Since this protein is upregulated in *btn1*-Δ cells, a role for Btn1p (and therefore CLN3p) in trafficking between the endocytic system and the Golgi apparatus may be inferred, but whether this is true, and how this might relate to CLN3 disease, remains to be discovered.

CLN10

The *S. cerevisiae* lysosomal aspartic protease Pep4p shares 43% identity and 58% similarity with the human protease cathepsin D, encoded by the gene mutated in some CLN10 disease, congenital and late infantile patients (see Chapter 19, Figure 19.1). Pep4p and the *pep4*-Δ strain are well characterized, with Pep4p being required for activation of other vacuole proteases and glucose-induced vacuolar degradation of peroxisomes, and its absence resulting in accumulation of vacuolar protease precursors and aberrant vacuolar morphology (Van Den Hazel et al., 1996, Phillips et al., 2006). Therefore, there is potential to use this yeast as a model for NCL, at least when investigating basic function.

SCHIZOSACCHAROMYCES POMBE

S. pombe, or fission yeast as it is commonly known, is a small, free-living, rod-shaped eukaryote that divides by medial fission. Fission yeast exists stably in both the haploid and diploid states and has a fast cell cycle of 2–4 hours. The fission yeast genome was fully sequenced in 2002. There are just under 5000 genes annotated, with over 5020 predicted, organized onto three chromosomes. Genes can be readily deleted, mutated, and tagged, allowing for deletion/mutation characterization and localization studies. An expression library containing almost all the genes tagged with GFP and a deletion library of all nonessential genes are available. In addition, cDNA and genomic libraries exist that allow for powerful suppressor screen studies. It is a popular model organism that over the past 50 years has greatly influenced the understanding of cell cycle control, cell polarity, and other highly conserved intracellular processes. Importantly, for the study of lysosomal storage disorders, fission yeast cells have a large number of small vacuoles, the yeast equivalent of the lysosome (Bone et al., 1998). Fission yeast has recently been developed as a model system to study two NCL disease genes, namely *CLN1* and *CLN3*, which are both conserved in *S. pombe*. Their conservation suggests an important basic biological function for these particular genes.

CLN1

The fission yeast orthologue of *CLN1* encodes palmitoyl protein thioesterase 1 (Vesa et al., 1995). However, the protein, Ppt1p, is found fused to dolichol pyrophosphate phosphatase 1, Dolpp1p. The entire coding region is denoted *pdf1* and the resulting propeptide is cleaved into its two distinct proteins, probably by a kex-related protease (Cho and Hofmann, 2004). Through deletion and complementation of *pdf1*, Cho and Hofmann observed that Ppt1p is not required for viability, whereas Dolpp1p is. However, Ppt1p is required for growth in media containing sodium orthovanadate and of basic pH. Importantly, expression of human *PPT1* complemented this phenotype suggesting that the primordial function of the protein is conserved. This study links CLN1 disease and perhaps other NCLs with pH alteration phenotypes and supports the use of fission yeast to study the NCLs.

CLN3

The fission yeast orthologue of human *CLN3*, *btn1* encodes the protein Btn1p, which is a predicted transmembrane protein of 396 amino acids that is 30% identical and 48% similar to CLN3 (see Chapter 19, Figure 19.4). Importantly, the same residues that are mutated in JNCL patients are conserved in Btn1p, suggesting that they are important for the function of both genes. Initial studies performed focused on vacuole function and cell morphology in a strain deleted for the *btn1* gene, *btn1*Δ. This strain is viable, but shows subtle and reproducible defects in all stages of cell cycle progression, with a 25% increase in cell length, an increased number of mitotic and dividing cells, and an overall increase in cell cycle length (Gachet et al., 2005).

PH REGULATION/HOMEOSTASIS

Alterations in vacuole dynamics are evident in this strain. First, vacuoles from *btn1*Δ are larger than those of wild-type cells with a mean diameter of 1.3μm compared to 0.9μm, and show a broader vacuole size distribution, suggesting an inherent defect in the regulation of vacuole size. Second, *btn1*Δ cells have an elevation in vacuole pH of one pH unit over that of wild-type cells, (pH 5.1 compared to pH 4.1 for wild-type cells). A positive correlation between increased vacuole size and increased vacuole pH is known in fission yeast (Iwaki et al., 2004) and growth of *btn1*Δ in acidic media (pH 4) was found to restore vacuolar pH and size to wild-type level. Thus, increased vacuole size is a reflection of the increased pH of the vacuole in *btn1*Δ cells. In support of this, cells deleted for either *vma1* or *vma3* (V-type H^+ ATPase (v-ATPase) subunits A and c, respectively), which are severely defective in vacuole acidification (vacuole pH >6 indicated by lack of fluorescence of the fluorophore LysoSensor® Green D189), have a few grossly enlarged vacuoles. However, a genetic interaction between *btn1* and the v-ATPase, with cells deleted for both *vma1* and *btn1* exhibiting slow growth at 25°C and synthetic lethality at 30°C, whereas parental strains grew well under these conditions, indicates that Btn1p does not solely affect vacuole pH. *btn1*Δ cells were also found to be sensitive for growth on media containing the chloramphenicol base ANP (1mM). Although the mechanism for this sensitivity in fission yeast remains to be determined, growth of *btn1*Δ on plates containing 1mM ANP was restored when this media was at pH 4 (S. Codlin, unpublished observation). Thus, ANP sensitivity of *btn1*Δ cells appears to be related to pH homeostatic mechanisms.

The increased vacuole pH and ANP sensitivity in *S. pombe btn1*Δ cells is in contrast to

S. cerevisiae btn1Δ, which was reported to have reduced vacuole pH and show resistance to ANP. Intracellular pH in many yeast species, including *S. cerevisiae* and *S. pombe*, is reported to be similar (Haworth and Fliegel, 1993, Karagiannis and Young, 2001), but few studies have focused on vacuole pH. There is a clear difference in wild-type vacuolar pH of growing cells between these species with *S. pombe* having a vacuole pH near 4 and *S. cerevisiae* a reported vacuole pH above 6. Studies performed by Gachet et al., made use of the fluorophore LysoSensor® Green D189 which vividly fluoresces at the vacuole in growing fission yeast cells. This compound fails to fluoresce above pH 6, supporting vacuole pH of wild-type *S. pombe* being much less than pH 6 (Gachet et al., 2005). Together, these observations suggest that budding and fission yeast set their vacuole pH at different levels and the phenotypic variation between the *btn1Δ* strains of the two yeast species presumably reflects differences in homeostatic mechanisms, and illustrate the validity of using more than one model system in the study of a disease gene. The vacuole pH of *S. pombe* is very similar to that of mammalian cells which are also highly acidic (Holopainen et al., 2001). The *S. pombe* pH observations are in agreement with observations made in patient cells from most types of NCL, including juvenile CLN3 disease, which showed elevated lysosomal pH. CLN3 overexpression studies in HEK293 cells revealed an opposite effect on pH (Golabek et al., 2000), suggesting that the pH effect may be cell type specific; however, all studies clearly demonstrate a dysregulation of vacuole/lysosome homeostasis.

Expression of an N-terminally fused GFP-Btn1p construct in fission yeast deleted for *btn1* rescues the vacuole pH defect and complements the vacuole size phenotype, as well as the subtle cell growth defects associated with *btn1Δ* cells (Gachet et al., 2005). Vacuole defects of *btn1Δ* cells were also rescued by heterologous expression of GFP-CLN3, proving that Btn1p and CLN3 are functional homologues. In addition, a correlation between disease severity and vacuole pH was shown by the expression of GFP-Btn1p containing CLN3 disease, juvenile, associated mutations (p.Gly187Ala, p.Glu295Lys and p.Val330Phe) in a *btn1Δ* strain. Expression of p.Gly187Ala, a mutation causing a severe disease progression, retained elevated vacuole pH, whereas expression of p.Glu295Lys, associated with a milder disease progression, and p.Val330Phe, also associated with a more protracted disease course, had lower vacuole pH, demonstrating that elevated vacuole/lysosome pH contributes to the disease process.

LOCATION AND TRAFFICKING

Both Btn1p and CLN3p traffic to the vacuole membrane via FM4-64 stained prevacuolar compartments, suggesting an endomembrane trafficking route for Btn1p (Gachet et al., 2005). Localization of Btn1p to the vacuole membrane was dependent on the Rab GTPase Ypt7p, with Btn1p being held in prevacuolar compartments in *ypt7Δ*,cells. Cells deleted for both *ypt7* and *btn1* showed synthetic lethality at 36°C and vacuoles in these cells were larger than those of cells deleted for *ypt7* alone and again showed reduced pH. The authors conclude that the presence of Btn1p in the prevacuolar compartments impacts on vacuole homeostasis. Consistently, Btn1p was later shown to be primarily located in the Golgi apparatus at steady-state (Codlin and Mole, 2009). Whether Btn1p normally exerts its function solely from this location, or also from locations en route to the vacuole, remain to be determined.

METABOLISM

S. pombe cells deleted for *btn1* were examined for changes in their metabolism which may give clues to disease mechanism. A metabolomics approach based on high resolution ^{1}H and ^{13}C nuclear magnetic resonance spectroscopy was used (Pears et al., 2010). These cells have a decrease in extracellular glucose and increases in the concentration of extracellular ethanol and alanine labelling. There are also changes in amino acids, including an increase in glutamate and decreases in basic amino acids such as arginine. The increased glycolytic flux and the amino acid changes may arise from vacuole impairment. Supplying glucose, sucrose, sorbitol, and glycerol, but not methylpyruvate, rescues the growth defect of *btn1Δ* cells. An increased glycolytic flux in animals may cause brain impairment due to the high energy requirements of brain cells and of neurotransmission. Depletion of CLN3 activity in mammalian cells causes an increase in glycogen storage (Pears et al., 2010), and uptake of glutamate is coupled to Na^+, K^+ ATPase, whose endocytic recycling is impaired in neurons from a CLN3 disease mouse model (Uusi-Rauva et al., 2008). Such changes represent the first documented metabolic changes associated with deletion of *btn1* and advocate the use of a metabolomic-based approach to analyse other yeast models of NCL disease to better understand the function of the disease genes.

BTN1P AFFECTS MULTIPLE PATHWAYS

*btn1*Δ cells were found to exhibit severe media-dependent growth defects at 37°C (Codlin et al., 2008a, Codlin et al., 2008b). *btn1*Δ cells grown at 37°C in the rich growth media YES, exhibited severe cytokinesis defects, passed through no more than three cell cycles and subsequently lost rod-shaped morphology, resulting in swollen and rounded cells and eventual cell lysis. The swelling phenotype and cell lysis were completely rescued by the addition of 1M sorbitol, an osmolyte, to the media, suggesting that these defects are caused by aberrant cell wall in *btn1*Δ cells. Indeed, electron microscopy revealed grossly thickened cell walls and septum regions, suggesting defects in deposition of cell wall components, the α- and β-glucans. Further characterization revealed progressive defects in polarity maintenance with aberrant F-actin patch formation and polarization and coupled with early endocytic defects, loss of Myo1p localization, and spreading of sterol-rich membrane domains. Intriguingly these defects did not appear to be linked to vacuole pH and were not rescued by growth in acidic media.

In addition, *btn1*Δ cells were found to be sensitive to the lytic enzyme zymolyase, a β-glucanase, perhaps due to an imbalance of cell wall glucans. This defect could be rescued by expression of Btn1p or CLN3p, and correlated with disease severity. In contrast to the temperature sensitive phenotype, the zymolyase sensitivity and vacuole defects appear linked by a common pH-dependent mechanism since they are suppressed by growth in acidic pH. Additionally, a similar glucan defect is also apparent in V-type H+ ATPase (v-ATPase) mutants, *vma1* and *vma3*. Significantly, Btn1p acts as a multicopy suppressor of the cell wall and other vacuole-related defects of v-ATPase null cells.

Thus, *btn1* impacts two independent processes, suggesting that Batten disease is more than a pH-related lysosome disorder. Most recently, data have shown that *btn1* acts upstream of the lysosome, at the Golgi, and affects post-Golgi vacuole protein sorting pathways. This study (Codlin and Mole, 2009) showed that the vacuole hydrolase carboxypeptidase 1 (Cpy1p) is missorted and is, instead, secreted by *btn1*Δ cells. This is probably due to an effect on its major sorting receptor Vps10p/Pep1p since this does not traffic beyond the Golgi in these cells, rather than reaching the TGN (where Cpy1p sorting normally occurs) in wild-type cells. Therefore, the underlying defect in *btn1*Δ cells may be one at the Golgi apparatus, affecting Golgi function, since *btn1*Δ cells have reduced Golgi numbers that have strikingly aberrant morphology, as observed by electron microscopy. This would explain the multiple phenotypes observed in *btn1*Δ cells, since the Golgi, with the *trans* Golgi network, is a major trafficking sorting centre of the cell. Work defining the molecular basis for this Golgi morphological defect should give clues to the function of Btn1p and CLN3.

DISEASE SEVERITY CORRELATES WITH BTN1P FUNCTION

A comprehensive analysis of the effect of CLN3 disease missense, deletion, and targeted mutations in Btn1p on its trafficking, location, and ability to rescue four marker phenotypes of *btn1*Δ cells, revealed that the severity of disease mutations correlated with their effect on Btn1p function (Haines et al., 2009). Some C-terminal mutations caused mutant Btn1p to be internalized into the vacuole, rather than remain on the vacuole membrane, and mutations in the lumenal loops of Btn1p, especially that containing a predicted amphipathic helix (Nugent et al., 2008), had the most significant effect on Btn1p function, indicating that these domains of CLN3 are functionally important. This approach also led to the discovery that the common 1kb deletion carried by juvenile CLN3 disease patients does not completely abolish Btn1p or CLN3 function (Kitzmüller et al., 2008), indicating that CLN3 disease, juvenile, is a mutation-specific phenotype. These findings further support the relevance of study of Btn1p in fission yeast to CLN3 disease.

CLN10

Fission yeast is also a potential model for CLN10 disease, as it has a homologue to cathepsin D, which is implicated in CLN10 disease with congenital and later ages of onset (Siintola et al., 2006) (Steinfeld et al., 2006). The *S. pombe* protein Sxa1p is 22% similar and 40% identical in amino acid sequence to human cathepsin D (see Chapter 19, Figure 19.1). Sxa1p is an aspartyl protease and is involved in the mating pathway (Imai and Yamamoto, 1992). Fission yeast has proved to be a valid model for several NCLs, and will be a valuable tool in the understanding of the molecular basis and progression of CLN10 disease.

CONCLUDING REMARKS

Unicellular eukaryotic model organisms clearly have great potential for informing research into the NCLs by assisting the identification of functions of NCL-related proteins. Defective pH homeostasis, vacuole function, and protein trafficking result from the loss of orthologues of CLN3, providing clues to the potential function of this protein that can be investigated more thoroughly in higher organisms. While CLN3 research has so far benefited most from this work, there is evidently scope for further modelling of the other NCLs, perhaps when potential pathways are identified that may be relevant to multiple forms of the disease. Another organism that may provide useful clues in the future is *Dictyostelium discoideum*, an amoeba which grows as separate, independent cells, but which can interact to form multicellular structures when challenged by adverse conditions. This organism has orthologues for PPT1, TPP1, CLN3, CLN5, and cathepsin D, and therefore could also become a powerful tool in NCL research.

REFERENCES

Barwell KJ & Broom MF (2001) A yeast model for classical juvenile Batten disease (CLN3). *Eur J Paediatr Neurol*, 5 Suppl A, 127–129.

Bone N, Millar JB, Toda T, & Armstrong J (1998) Regulated vacuole fusion and fission in Schizosaccharomyces pombe: an osmotic response dependent on MAP kinases. *Curr Biol*, 8, 135–144.

Chattopadhyay S, Muzaffar NE, Sherman F, & Pearce DA (2000) The yeast model for Batten disease: mutations in BTN1, BTN2, and HSP30 alter pH homeostasis. *J Bacteriol*, 182, 6418–6423.

Chattopadhyay S & Pearce DA (2002) Interaction with Btn2p is required for localization of Rsglp: Btn2p-mediated changes in arginine uptake in Saccharomyces cerevisiae. *Eukaryot Cell*, 1, 606–612.

Chattopadhyay S, Roberts PM, & Pearce DA (2003) The yeast model for Batten disease: a role for Btn2p in the trafficking of the Golgi-associated vesicular targeting protein, Yif1p. *Biochem Biophys Res Commun*, 302, 534–538.

Cho SK & Hofmann SL (2004) pdf1, a palmitoyl protein thioesterase 1 Ortholog in Schizosaccharomyces pombe: a yeast model of infantile Batten disease. *Eukaryot Cell*, 3, 302–310.

Codlin S, Haines RL, Burden JJ, & Mole SE (2008a) Btn1 affects cytokinesis and cell-wall deposition by independent mechanisms, one of which is linked to dysregulation of vacuole pH. *J Cell Sci*, 121, 2860–2870.

Codlin S, Haines RL, & Mole SE (2008b) btn1 affects endocytosis, polarization of sterol-rich membrane domains and polarized growth in Schizosaccharomyces pombe. *Traffic*, 9, 936–950.

Codlin S & Mole SE (2009) S. pombe btn1, the orthologue of the Batten disease gene CLN3, is required for vacuole protein sorting of Cpy1p and Golgi exit of Vps10p. *J Cell Sci*, 122, 1163–1173.

Cottone CD, Chattopadhyay S, & Pearce DA (2001) Searching for interacting partners of CLN1, CLN2 and Btn1p with the two-hybrid system. *Eur J Paediatr Neurol*, 5 Suppl A, 95–98.

Croopnick JB, Choi HC, & Mueller DM (1998) The subcellular location of the yeast Saccharomyces cerevisiae homologue of the protein defective in the juvenile form of Batten disease. *Biochem Biophys Res Commun*, 250, 335–341.

Gachet Y, Codlin S, Hyams JS, & Mole SE (2005) btn1, the Schizosaccharomyces pombe homologue of the human Batten disease gene CLN3, regulates vacuole homeostasis. *J Cell Sci*, 118, 5525–5536.

Golabek AA, Kaczmarski W, Kida E, Kaczmarski A, Michalewski MP, & Wisniewski KE (1999) Expression studies of CLN3 protein (battenin) in fusion with the green fluorescent protein in mammalian cells in vitro. *Mol Genet Metab*, 66, 277–282.

Golabek AA, Kida E, Walus M, Kaczmarski W, Michalewski M, & Wisniewski KE (2000) CLN3 protein regulates lysosomal pH and alters intracellular processing of Alzheimer's amyloid-beta protein precursor and cathepsin D in human cells. *Mol Genet Metab*, 70, 203–213.

Guo WX, Mao C, Obeid LM, & Boustany RM (1999) A disrupted homologue of the human CLN3 or juvenile neuronal ceroid lipofuscinosis gene in Saccharomyces cerevisiae: a model to study Batten disease. *Cell Mol Neurobiol*, 19, 671–680.

Haines RL, Codlin S, & Mole SE (2009) The fission yeast model for the lysosomal storage disorder Batten disease predicts disease severity caused by mutations in CLN3. *Dis Model Mech*, 2, 84–92.

Hall NA, Lake BD, Dewji NN, & Patrick AD (1991) Lysosomal storage of subunit c of mitochondrial ATP synthase in Batten's disease (ceroid-lipofuscinosis). *Biochem J*, 275 (Pt 1), 269–272.

Haltia M, Rapola J, & Santavuori P (1973) Infantile type of so-called neuronal ceroid-lipofuscinosis. Histological and electron microscopic studies. *Acta Neuropathol*, 26, 157–170.

Haworth RS & Fliegel L (1993) Intracellular pH in Schizosaccharomyces pombe—comparison with Saccharomyces cerevisiae. *Mol Cell Biochem*, 124, 131–140.

Holopainen JM, Saarikoski J, Kinnunen PK, & Jarvela I (2001) Elevated lysosomal pH in neuronal ceroid lipofuscinoses (NCLs). *Eur J Biochem*, 268, 5851–5856.

Imai Y & Yamamoto M (1992) Schizosaccharomyces pombe sxa1+ and sxa2+ encode putative proteases involved in the mating response. *Mol Cell Biol*, 12, 1827–1834.

Iwaki T, Goa T, Tanaka N, & Takegawa K (2004) Characterization of Schizosaccharomyces pombe mutants defective in vacuolar acidification and protein sorting. *Mol Genet Genomics*, 271, 197–207.

Kama R, Robinson M, & Gerst JE (2007) Btn2, a Hook1 ortholog and potential Batten disease-related protein, mediates late endosome-Golgi protein sorting in yeast. *Mol Cell Biol*, 27, 605–621.

Karagiannis J & Young PG (2001) Intracellular pH homeostasis during cell-cycle progression and growth state transition in Schizosaccharomyces pombe. *J Cell Sci*, 114, 2929–2941.

Kim Y, Chattopadhyay S, Locke S, & Pearce DA (2005) Interaction among Btn1p, Btn2p, and Ist2p reveals potential interplay among the vacuole, amino acid levels, and ion homeostasis in the yeast Saccharomyces cerevisiae. *Eukaryot Cell*, 4, 281–288.

Kim Y, Ramirez-Montealegre D, & Pearce DA (2003) A role in vacuolar arginine transport for yeast Btn1p and for human CLN3, the protein defective in Batten disease. *Proc Natl Acad Sci U S A*, 100, 15458–15462.

Kitamoto K, Yoshizawa K, Ohsumi Y, & Anraku Y (1988) Dynamic aspects of vacuolar and cytosolic amino acid pools of Saccharomyces cerevisiae. *J Bacteriol*, 170, 2683–2686.

Kitzmüller C, Haines RL, Codlin S, Cutler DF, & Mole SE (2008) A function retained by the common mutant CLN3 protein is responsible for the late onset of juvenile neuronal ceroid lipofuscinosis. *Hum Mol Genet*, 17, 303–312.

Kominami E, Ezaki J, Muno D, Ishido K, Ueno T, & Wolfe LS (1992) Specific storage of subunit c of mitochondrial ATP synthase in lysosomes of neuronal ceroid lipofuscinosis (Batten's disease). *J Biochem*, 111, 278–282.

Kyttälä A, Ihrke G, Vesa J, Schell MJ, & Luzio JP (2004) Two motifs target Batten disease protein CLN3 to lysosomes in transfected nonneuronal and neuronal cells. *Mol Biol Cell*, 15, 1313–1323.

Nugent T, Mole SE, & Jones D (2008) The transmembrane topology of Batten disease protein CLN3 determined by consensus computational prediction constrained by experimental data. *FEBS Letters*, 582, 1019–1024.

Osório NS, Carvalho A, Almeida AJ, Padilla-Lopez S, Leao C, Laranjinha J, Ludovico P, Pearce DA, & Rodrigues F (2007) Nitric oxide signaling is disrupted in the yeast model for Batten disease. *Mol Biol Cell*, 18, 2755–2767.

Padilla-Lopez S & Pearce DA (2006) Saccharomyces cerevisiae lacking Btn1p modulate vacuolar ATPase activity to regulate pH imbalance in the vacuole. *J Biol Chem*, 281, 10273–10280.

Palmer DN, Bayliss SL, & Westlake VJ (1995) Batten disease and the ATP synthase subunit c turnover pathway: raising antibodies to subunit c. *Am J Med Genet*, 57, 260–265.

Pearce DA, Ferea T, Nosel SA, Das B, & Sherman F (1999a) Action of BTN1, the yeast orthologue of the gene mutated in Batten disease. *Nat Genet*, 22, 55–58.

Pearce DA, Nosel SA, & Sherman F (1999b) Studies of pH regulation by Btn1p, the yeast homolog of human Cln3p. *Mol Genet Metab*, 66, 320–323.

Pearce DA, Carr CJ, Das B, & Sherman F (1999c) Phenotypic reversal of the btn1 defects in yeast by chloroquine: a yeast model for Batten disease. *Proc Natl Acad Sci U S A*, 96, 11341–11345.

Pearce DA & Sherman F (1997) BTN1, a yeast gene corresponding to the human gene responsible for Batten's disease, is not essential for viability, mitochondrial function, or degradation of mitochondrial ATP synthase. *Yeast*, 13, 691–697.

Pearce DA & Sherman F (1998) A yeast model for the study of Batten disease. *Proc Natl Acad Sci U S A*, 95, 6915–6918.

Pears MR, Codlin S, Haines RL, White IJ, Mortishire-Smith RJ, Mole SE, & Griffin JL (2010) Deletion of btn1, an orthologue of CLN3, increases glycolysis and perturbs amino acid metabolism in the fission yeast model of Batten disease. *Mol Biosyst*, 6, 1093–1102.

Phillips SN, Muzaffar N, Codlin S, Korey CA, Taschner PE, de Voer G, Mole SE, & Pearce DA (2006) Characterizing pathogenic processes in Batten disease: use of small eukaryotic model systems. *Biochim Biophys Acta*, 1762, 906–919.

Piper PW, Ortiz-Calderon C, Holyoak C, Coote P, & Cole M (1997) Hsp30, the integral plasma membrane heat shock protein of Saccharomyces cerevisiae, is a stress-inducible regulator of plasma membrane H(+)-ATPase. *Cell Stress Chaperones*, 2, 12–24.

Ramirez-Montealegre D & Pearce DA (2005) Defective lysosomal arginine transport in juvenile Batten disease. *Hum Mol Genet*, 14, 3759–3773.

Siintola E, Partanen S, Stromme P, Haapanen A, Haltia M, Maehlen J, Lehesjoki AE, & Tyynelä J (2006) Cathepsin D deficiency underlies congenital human neuronal ceroid-lipofuscinosis. *Brain*, 129, 1438–1445.

Slater AF (1993) Chloroquine: mechanism of drug action and resistance in Plasmodium falciparum. *Pharmacol Ther*, 57, 203–235.

Steinfeld R, Reinhardt K, Schreiber K, Hillebrand M, Kraetzner R, Bruck W, Saftig P, & Gartner J (2006) Cathepsin D deficiency is associated with a human neurodegenerative disorder. *Am J Hum Genet*, 78, 988–998.

Uusi-Rauva K, Luiro K, Tanhuanpaa K, Kopra O, Martin-Vasallo P, Kyttala A, & Jalanko A (2008) Novel interactions of CLN3 protein link Batten disease to dysregulation of fodrin-Na+, K+ ATPase complex. *Exp Cell Res*, 314, 2895–2905.

Van Den Hazel HB, Kielland-Brandt MC, & Winther JR (1996) Review: biosynthesis and function of yeast vacuolar proteases. *Yeast*, 12, 1–16.

Vesa J, Hellsten E, Verkruyse LA, Camp LA, Rapola J, Santavuori P, Hofmann SL, & Peltonen L (1995) Mutations in the palmitoyl protein thioesterase gene causing infantile neuronal ceroid lipofuscinosis. *Nature*, 376, 584–587.

Vitiello SP, Benedict JW, Padilla-Lopez S, & Pearce DA (2010) Interaction between Sdo1p and Btn1p in the Saccharomyces cerevisiae model for Batten disease. *Hum Mol Genet*, 19, 931–942.

Vitiello SP, Wolfe DM, & Pearce DA (2007) Absence of Btn1p in the yeast model for juvenile Batten disease may cause arginine to become toxic to yeast cells. *Hum Mol Genet*, 16, 1007–1016.

Weimken A & Dürr M (1974) Characterization of amino acid pools in the vacuolar compartment of Saccharomyces cerevisiae. *Arch Microbiol*, 101, 45–57.

Chapter 16

Simple Animal Models

G. de Voer, C.A. Korey, L. Myllykangas, P.E.M. Taschner, and R.I. Tuxworth

INTRODUCTION

Biomedical researchers use simple animal models to obtain information about the function of proteins and the cellular processes they are involved in. The evolutionary conservation of gene function allows the extrapolation of this knowledge to more complex higher organisms to help unravel the mechanisms of human disease. Popular simple animal models are the nematode worm *Caenorhabditis elegans* and the fruit fly *Drosophila melanogaster*, which pair a well-studied nervous system with sophisticated genetics. In most cases, the biological function of the NCL proteins and how a mutation in these proteins causes disease remain unclear. Therefore, simple animal models may help to increase our understanding of the pathways important for development of NCL if the corresponding homologous genes have been identified. Of the human NCL proteins, only homologues to PPT1, CTSD, CLN3, and MFSD8/CLN7 are found in *C. elegans* and *D. melanogaster* (Chapter 19), making them important models for understanding the underlying molecular aetiology of CLN1, CLN10, CLN3, and CLN7 diseases (Taschner et al., 1997, Phillips et al., 2006). Studies of natural or genetically modified *Clcn3*, *Clcn6*, *Clcn7*, *Ctsf*, *Ctsb*, *Ctsl*, and *Ostm1* mouse mutants suggest that disruption of these genes might also result in lysosomal accumulation of ceroid or lipofuscin, and these are, therefore, candidates for so far unidentified NCL genes (see Chapter 17). Homologues of these genes can also be found in worms and flies.

THE NEMATODE WORM *CAENORHABDITIS ELEGANS*

C. elegans models of human disease

The nematode worm *Caenorhabditis elegans* is a relatively simple multicellular eukaryotic organism of approximately one millimetre in length, which normally lives in soil (Brenner, 1974). These worms develop from egg to adult in approximately 3 days and live about 2–3 weeks. The six chromosomes of the *C. elegans* genome have been completely sequenced, and contain approximately 19,000 genes (Waterston and Sulston, 1995). The worm has two sexes, males and hermaphrodites, which easily yield homozygous offspring by self-fertilization after a cross of two different mutant strains. For this reason, and because it is possible to grow large numbers of worms for investigations, *C. elegans* is now a popular model for genetic research (Jorgensen and Mango, 2002). Much is known about the anatomy and development of the nematode: a complete map of all 959 somatic cells and a full understanding of their cell lineage are available. The invariably wired nervous system of the worm comprises 302 neuronal cells with approximately 7600 synaptic junctions (Sulston et al., 1983). The well-studied nervous system combined with its genetic power makes the worm a very suitable organism to investigate the molecular mechanisms underlying neuronal disorders. Comparison of the human and worm genomes confirmed that many protein sequences are conserved across species. This suggests that many genes involved in human hereditary disease have worm homologues, which may provide further information about their function (Culetto and Sattelle, 2000). There are different approaches used to generate worm models for human disease (Kaletta and Hengartner, 2006). *C. elegans* has already been used to investigate genes involved in lysosomal storage disorders, e.g. mucolipidosis type IV (Fares and Greenwald, 2001b, Hersh et al., 2002), Niemann–Pick type C (Sym et al., 2000, Li et al., 2004), and Danon disease (Kostich et al., 2000). The worm homologues of human genes involved in lysosomal function and disease has been reviewed recently (de Voer et al., 2008).

The *cln* genes of *C. elegans*

Comparison of known human CLN protein sequences with the predicted proteins of the worm indicated that *C. elegans* has homologues of the *CTSD/CLN10*, *PPT1/CLN1*, *MFSD8/CLN7*, and *CLN3* genes only (see Chapter 19). Models for two diseases have been generated by out-crossing worms with deletion mutations identified by the *C. elegans* knock-out consortium.

THE *CTSD* HOMOLOGUE *ASP-4*

Human cathepsin D, the protein involved in CLN10 disease (Siintola et al., 2006), has significant homology with a group of 20 worm proteins (Syntichaki et al., 2002). The human enzyme shares most homology with the worm aspartyl protease Asp-4 (58% identity and 73% similarity) (see Chapter 19). C-terminal fusions of the GFP gene to *asp-4* suggest that this gene is strongly expressed in intestinal cells and at lower levels in muscle, hyperdermis, and neurons (Syntichaki et al., 2002). Although the Asp-4 protein lacks the conserved Asp71 N-glycosylation site necessary for the lysosomal targeting of cathepsin D enzymes (Tcherepanova et al., 2000), punctate Asp-4-GFP fluorescence was observed in vesicles, which are considered to be lysosomes. No worm strains carrying deleterious *asp-4* mutations are available, but RNAi knockdown suggests that Asp-4 mediates necrotic cell death and is required for neurodegeneration (Syntichaki et al., 2002). Additional work on this worm homologue of cathepsin D may provide more insight in the molecular mechanism underlying CLN10 disease, congenital.

THE *PPT-1* WORM MODEL FOR CLN1 DISEASE

Mutations in *ppt-1*, the worm homologue of the *PPT1* gene mutated in CLN1 disease patients, were isolated from a nematode mutant library generated by chemical mutagenesis (Jansen et al., 1997). Two different *ppt-1* mutations, both deleting at least two exons, are predicted to lead to truncation of the protein (Porter et al., 2005). Although both *ppt-1* deletion mutants displayed no morphological, locomotor, or neuronal defects, the onset of egg-laying was delayed by approximately 4 hours. The *ppt-1* mutants carry more embryos than wild-type worms, and 18% of them displayed a reproductive phenotype called 'bagging', where eggs hatch inside the parent. Since not all of the mutant worms with delayed egg-laying displayed the 'bagging' phenotype, the effect of the mutation varies in severity, but is more than the 1.6% found in normal worms. Lifespan and brood size of the *ppt-1* mutants were similar to wild-type, when worms with the bagging phenotype are not taken into account. Furthermore, *ppt-1* mutants show a decreased 'health span', appearing to age faster and becoming less motile earlier than wild-type worms. Neuronal cells contain many enlarged mitochondria with less cristae and whorling inner membranes in electron micrographs of *ppt-1* mutant nematodes. The *ppt-1* mutants had 26–29% more mitochondria than wild-type, and average mitochondrial size was severely decreased in 6-day-old adult *ppt-1* mutant worms. It is unclear what causes this phenotype, but it is too mild to be used in genetic screens for mutations in other genes that may enhance or suppress the mitochondrial effect. The *ppt-1* mutants, however, did not display neuronal degeneration or accumulation of storage material, two of the main characteristics of CLN1 disease. The abnormalities observed in the *ppt-1* mutants support previous suggestions that mitochondria are involved in NCL pathogenesis (Boriack et al., 1995, Majander et al., 1995, Dawson et al., 1996, Das et al., 1999, Cho and Dawson, 2000, Cho et al., 2000, Cho et al., 2001, Das et al., 2001, Bertoni-Freddari et al., 2002, Chattopadhyay et al., 2002, Jolly et al., 2002, Heine et al., 2003, Fossale et al., 2004) and have prompted further investigation into the integrity of mitochondria in CLN1 disease patients as well as other CLN1 disease model organisms.

THE *CLN-3* GENES

In contrast to most other organisms, *C. elegans* has three *CLN3* homologues, designated *cln-3.1*, *cln-3.2*, and *cln-3.3*. The presence of three *CLN3* homologues in *Caenorhabditis briggsae*, a nematode species closely related to *C. elegans* suggests that the three genes have evolved before the separation of the two species, some 100 million years ago (Stein et al., 2003). If it is assumed that the three genes result from ancient duplications of a common ancestor, their genomic sequences have diverged beyond recognition, but the encoded protein sequences show considerable homology (de Voer et al., 2001), albeit exon structure is not identical (Mitchell et al., 2001). Probably all three genes are functional, since they are conserved across their complete protein sequences, and what appear to be spliced transcripts from each can be detected. This suggests that none of them is an expressed pseudogene, which has lost most of its original function, as was shown for the *elt-4* gene (Fukushige et al., 2003). The biological reason for the existence of multiple *cln-3* genes in the worm is unknown.

EXPRESSION PATTERNS OF THE *CLN-3* GENES

The expression of the *cln-3* genes has been analysed by generating transgenic worms carrying one of the *cln-3* promoters driving the expression of the green fluorescent protein (GFP) gene. The development of the green fluorescent signal in the transgenic worms at different points during their life cycle and at different locations indicates that these genes differ in their temporal and spatial expression patterns. Expression of *cln-3.1* is restricted to cells of the intestine in transgenic hermaphrodite and male worm embryos, larvae and adults (de Voer et al., 2005). The *cln-3.2* gene is expressed in cells of the hypoderm only in adult worms of both sexes. The *cln-3.3* gene is expressed in the intestinal muscle cells and hypoderm of adult hermaphrodite and male worms and also in posterior diagonal muscle cells of males. Although the *cln-3.2* and *cln-3.3* genes are coexpressed in hypodermal cells of adult worms, none of the *cln-3* genes is expressed at detectable levels in all cells. This does not indicate that the *cln-3* genes are not expressed at all, but merely that expression levels in other cell types (neurons) do not cross the threshold of GFP detection by fluorescence microscopy.

Are the cln-3.2 and cln-3.3 genes part of operons?

Apart from the number of *CLN3* homologues, *C. elegans* also differs from other organisms in the organization and regulation of some of its genes. *C. elegans* is one of the few multicellular eukaryotic organisms in which genes can be organized in an operon, a gene structure used by many bacteria for coordinated gene expression (Blumenthal and Gleason, 2003). This means that a single promoter is used to generate one transcript for a group of consecutive genes. In worms, this polycistronic transcript is subsequently processed into separate transcripts for each gene by *trans*-splicing to specific spliced leader sequences, for instance, SL2. In some cases, the proteins encoded by operons are functionally related; in others they might be linked to ensure coordinated temporal expression. Two of the *cln-3* genes, *cln-3.2* and *cln-3.3*, have closely located upstream genes and may therefore be organized in operons.

The detection of an SL2 spliced leader on *cln-3.2* mRNA is in accordance with an operon structure. The *cln-3.2* gene is in fourth position in an operon also containing *erm-1*, *dnj-4*, and *dhs-1*. The first gene, *erm-1*, encodes a protein with homology to ezrin, radixin, and moesin proteins of the ERM family of cytoskeletal linkers, which are involved in organism development and positioning of cell-cell contacts (Van Furden et al., 2004). ERM proteins play diverse roles in cell architecture, cell signalling and membrane trafficking (Louvet-Vallee, 2000), and have recently been shown to be important for actin assembly by phagosomes, which may facilitate their fusion with lysosomes (Defacque et al., 2000). The *erm-1* gene is expressed from the two-cell stage onward throughout the entire life of the worm in epithelial cells lining the luminal surfaces of intestine, excretory canal, and gonad, whereas the *cln-3.2* gene is expressed in the hypoderm of adult worms (de Voer et al., 2005). This difference in expression between genes in the same operon could be caused by common errors in operon transcription, of which the probability decreases with increasing distance between the operon genes, or their mRNAs may be subject to differential mRNA destabilization (Lercher et al., 2003). Expression patterns of the two other genes in the operon, *dnj-4* and *dhs-1*, have not been reported, and RNAi knockdown of these genes did not result in obvious phenotypes (Wormbase website: http://www.wormbase.org/). Therefore, the function of these genes can only be derived from protein sequence homology. The DNJ-4 protein has both chaperone and heat shock protein domains, which could indicate a role in protein folding. The DHS-1 protein has dehydrogenase and reductase domains and may have a function in metabolism of short chain alcohols. Although a role in lysosome-phagosome fusion for ERM proteins suggests a functional connection between them and *cln-3.2*, it is unclear whether a functional relationship exists between *cln-3.2* and the other genes in this operon.

In contrast, the *cln-3.3* transcript is associated with an SL1 splice leader (Mitchell et al., 2001), suggesting that it does not form an operon with its upstream gene, ZC190.2. However, the putative *cln-3.3* promoter-GFP fusion construct failed to cause GFP fluorescence in transgenic nematodes (G. de Voer et al., unpublished results), whereas transgenic worms containing a larger upstream sequence including the ZC190.2 promoter and gene in front of the *cln-3.3* promoter-GFP fusion did show GFP fluorescence (de Voer et al., 2005). Both reporter constructs contain an in-frame fusion of GFP to the first three exons of *cln-3.3* and thus are partial translational reporter constructs (Boulin et al., 2006). This suggests that the GFP fluorescence from the longer one can only be caused by the presence of additional cis-acting elements. Currently, it is unclear whether the ZC190.2 promoter drives *cln-3.3* expression or whether other cis-acting elements overlapping the ZC190.2 coding region are responsible for the observed expression pattern.

The cln-3 *worm models for CLN3 disease*

Deletion mutations in the *cln-3.1*, *cln-3.2*, and *cln-3.3* genes have been identified in deletion mutant libraries and have been transferred from the original mutants into wild-type background by out-crossing six times to remove additional mutations (de Voer et al., 2005). The presence of three *cln-3* genes in the worm complicated the generation of a CLN3 disease model, because the wild-type appearance of the *cln-3* single mutant models suggested that one or two of the genes might be functionally redundant. Therefore, the single mutant models were crossed to generate three double and one triple *cln-3* mutant models. The *cln-3* triple mutant model was viable and superficially displayed wild-type behaviour and normal morphology, indicating that the *cln-3* genes are not essential. The *cln-3* triple mutant has a shorter lifespan than wild-type worms. A less prominent lifespan reduction is observed in *cln-3.1* mutants, while *cln-3.2* and *cln-3.3* single mutants have a normal lifespan. The brood size of the *cln-3* triple mutants is decreased more prominently compared with wild-type than that of the *cln-3.2* single mutants, even though the other single mutants do not have a significantly decreased brood size. The *cln-3* triple mutants have been investigated extensively to detect functional aberrations using assays for correct neuronal function and response to a diversity of external cues, such as temperature, touch, presence of other worms, mating behavior (G. de Voer et al., unpublished results). The nervous system of *cln-3* triple mutants visualized by GFP expressed from the *unc-119* promoter in neuronal cells seemed intact and was similar to wild-type in all of the tests. No altered morphology or lysosomal storage material was observed in electron micrographs of *cln-3* triple mutant neurons. The *cln-3* triple mutants could not be distinguished from wild-type worms after staining with organelle or compound specific fluorescent dyes, LysoTracker Red®, acridine orange, and Nile Red® to assess whether lysosomes, acidic organelles and lipid content, respectively, were altered.

It should perhaps be noted that, in line with results from modelling CLN3 mutations in *Schizosaccharomyces pombe* (Haines et al., 2009) (see Chapter 15), mutant CLN-3 protein that retains some activity could arise from *cln-3.2* and *cln-3.3* mutant alleles since these deletions do not completely remove all of the respective *cln-3* gene. If so, the *cln-3* triple mutant would not be completely lacking CLN-3 activity, perhaps explaining its mild phenotype.

No autofluorescent storage material in C. elegans cln-3 *triple mutants*

One of the hallmarks of NCL, the storage of autofluorescent lipopigments, was not observed in *C. elegans cln-3* triple mutant worms, probably due to their short lifespan. It might be possible to induce lipopigment storage in the *cln-3* triple mutant worm model by overexpressing the main component of the storage material found in Batten disease patients, the hydrophobic subunit c of the mitochondrial ATP synthase (Hall et al., 1991, Palmer et al., 1992, Palmer et al., 1995). Although humans have three subunit c genes (*ATP5G1*, *ATP5G2*, and *ATP5G3*), *C. elegans* has one homologue, *atp-9*, only. Overexpression of *atp-9* under the control of a heat shock promoter was deleterious to wild-type animals, causing overall structural impairment, increased transparency, and near paralysis (G. de Voer et al., unpublished data). Damaged mitochondria could be observed on electron micrographs of subunit c overexpressing worms, which is in accordance with the loss of mitochondrial staining with Mitotracker Red® seen in these animals. A mild subunit c overexpression in a wild-type or *cln-3* triple mutant background allowed the worms to survive, but did not result in an obviously different phenotype.

THE *CLN-7* HOMOLOGUES

The human *MFSD8/CLN7* gene belongs to the major facilitator superfamily of transporter protein genes, which is homologous to a gene family with 15 members in the worm (Siintola et al., 2007). Due to the similarity between the proteins within each family, it is difficult to determine the functional equivalent of MFSD8/CLN7 in the worm. Since no mutant phenotypes or substrate-specificity information is available, these homologues will not be discussed in detail.

HOMOLOGUES OF MOUSE GENES INVOLVED IN LYSOSOMAL LIPOFUSCIN ACCUMULATION

Disruption of the mouse genes *Clcn3*, *Clcn6*, *Clcn7*, *Ctsf*, *Ctsb*, *Ctsl*, and *Ostm1* may also result in the lysosomal accumulation of ceroid or lipofuscin (see Chapter 17). In the worm, homologues for these potential NCL candidate genes can be found, although they have not yet been investigated as such. Therefore, not much information is available for some of them. The *clh-5* gene encodes the worm homologue of the highly similar human *CLCN3*, *CLCN4*, and *CLCN5* chloride channels, which are involved in receptor-mediated endocytosis, but no mutants are available and RNAi knockdown did not result in an obvious phenotype (Fares and Greenwald, 2001a). Using *clh-5*::GFP transcriptional fusions, expression of *clh-5* has been observed in many cell types (Nehrke et al., 2000). *CLCN7*, and to a lesser extent *CLCN6*, are highly homologous to the worm chloride channel protein *Clh-6*, which is expressed in a wide variety of cells according to *clh-6*::GFP transcriptional fusions (Nehrke et al., 2000). In contrast, it is reported that *clh-6* gene expression is restricted to the two GABAergic RMEL and RMER head neurons, using both *clh-6*::GFP transcriptional and translational fusions (Bianchi et al., 2001). This discrepancy can be explained by the difference in size between the used putative promoter fragments: 4kb versus the probably too short 0.25kb intergenic stretch between *clh-6* and its upstream gene *pqn-53* in the latter case. Two *clh-6* mutants are available, but uncharacterized, and RNAi knockdown did not result in an obvious phenotype (Wormbase website). Human CLCN7 interacts with OSTM1, encoded by a homologue of the worm gene F42A8.3, for which a deletion mutation has been identified (Lange et al., 2006). This mutation removes the first two exons of F42A8.3 and the first five exons of its neighbouring gene *sdhb-1*, which encodes the B subunit of the enzyme succinate dehydrogenase (Wormbase website). Worms carrying this mutation can only be maintained as heterozygotes, because the homozygotes show growth arrest in larval stage L2. Although the mutants have not been characterized in detail, the observed phenotype resembles the embryonic lethal and larval arrest phenotype of *sdhb-1* RNAi knockdown, whereas F42A8.3 RNAi knockdown does not result in an obvious phenotype. This suggests that disruption of *sdhb-1* contributes most to the larval arrest of the deletion mutants. Similar to the cathepsin *CTSD*, the cathepsin *CTSB*, *CTSF*, and *CTSL* genes have several worm homologues, but they share most similarity with F57F5.1, F41E6.6, and *Cpl-1*, respectively. No mutants are available for the *CTSB* homologue F57F5.1, but RNAi knockdown results in embryonic lethality and larval arrest (Simmer and al., 2003). Four deletion mutations have been identified in the *CTSF* homologue F41E6.6, one of which has a mild uncoordinated phenotype and egg laying defects (Wormbase website). One deletion mutant of *CTSL* homologue *cpl-1* has been identified showing growth arrest at an undefined stage, but RNAi knockdown results in embryonic lethality and slow growth, suggesting a role during development (Hashmi et al., 2002, Simmer and al., 2003). *Cpl-1* expression has been detected near the periphery of the eggshell and in the hypoderm, pharynx, and intestine (Hashmi et al., 2002). From this short overview, we may conclude that disruptions of the worm chloride channel homologues do not result in an obvious phenotype, whereas the cathepsins seem to play important roles during worm development. Further investigation is necessary to determine whether combinations of specific mutations produce NCL-like phenotypes.

THE FRUIT FLY *DROSOPHILA MELANOGASTER*

Drosophila models of human disease

The fly offers all of the cutting edge technology of higher eukaryotic organisms in a more simple, yet sophisticated experimental package. The tools available for the analysis of the *Drosophila* nervous system, down to the single cell level, have made the fly an important model for characterizing the underlying molecular defects associated with several neurological diseases, for example, Huntington's, Parkinson's, and Alzheimer's diseases and several spinocerebellar ataxias (Fortini and Bonini, 2000, Muqit and Feany, 2002). Regarding lysosomal storage disorders in particular, several studies of fly mutations have provided insight into the molecular mechanisms behind this subset of diseases including Niemann–Pick type C (Huang et al., 2005, Fluegel et al., 2006) and sialic acid storage diseases (Nakano et al., 2001, Sweeney and Davis, 2002, Dermaut et al., 2005). Finally, the fly is also becoming a useful drug discovery tool that can be used in conjunction with other assays to screen drug and small molecule libraries for compounds that ameliorate the cellular or whole organism phenotypes associated with a particular disease model (Desai et al., 2006).

Drosophila model development

The development of a *Drosophila* model of a specific human disease can be approached in several ways depending on the disease mechanism under examination. One approach uses forward or reverse genetics to determine if the disease phenotypes are recapitulated in flies bearing mutations similar to those found in human patients. For recessive human diseases like the NCLs, loss of function mutations in the fly *PPT1* or *CTSD* homologues have been produced which show some phenotypic similarity to their human disease counterparts (Myllykangas et al., 2005, Hickey et al., 2006). For diseases which are produced by a dominant gain-of-function mutation flies can be produced that recapitulate certain disease-specific cellular phenotypes by expressing normal and mutated genes within in a particular tissue or stage of development (Brand and Perrimon, 1993), such as neuronal cells (Muqit and Feany, 2002). In both cases, analysis of the resulting phenotypes in the fly gives greater insight into the molecular mechanisms associated with the disease process in humans.

A clearer understanding of the normal cellular role of a gene underlying human disease can be achieved through the clarification of the function of a protein outside the disease context. Over-expression of a protein using the GAL4/UAS system produces an *in vivo* functional assay that can connect the normal function of the protein to specific cellular processes and signalling pathways. For diseases like CLN1 disease, phenotypes associated with overexpression of wild-type *Drosophila* Ppt1 produced using this method have provided insight into the cellular defects produced by the loss of this protein in CLN1 disease patients (Korey and MacDonald, 2003, Buff et al., 2007).

GENETIC MODIFIER SCREENS

The development of fly models using any of these three techniques sets the stage for large-scale second site genetic modifier screens. This approach identifies mutations in other genes that suppress or enhance the particular phenotypes observed in the fly models. These loci are likely to represent genes that are involved in processes that give rise to the cellular defects found in the fly, and thus help to define the cellular function and signalling context of the disease gene under investigation. Often the results of these genetic screens suggest other previously unrelated pathways that can be targeted for therapeutic development to ameliorate the clinical symptoms of the disease. Upon completion of a screen, the modifier genes identified in the *Drosophila* system must then be verified in mouse or human models to confirm their importance to disease pathogenesis. While not all candidate modifiers are relevant, the final group of genes provides a wealth of information for the functional dissection of the mammalian homologues and their role in the human disease phenotype.

To begin a search for modifiers, candidate genes can be tested based on hypotheses of protein function from previous experimental work. A more systematic and unbiased approach uses chemical or insertional mutagenesis to scan the genome with a loss-of-function genetic modifier screen. Gene mapping in *Drosophila* has progressed to the point where even chemically induced point mutations can be localized relatively quickly using single nucleotide polymorphisms (Berger et al., 2001, Hoskins et al., 2001). Finally, a gain-of-function modifier screen asks whether overexpression of particular gene can modify disease-related phenotypes in the fly. This method takes advantage of a collection of enhancer–promoter (EP) lines that have UAS-containing transposable elements inserted randomly throughout the genome (Rorth et al., 1998). These EP lines permit the expression of the associated open reading frame in a GAL4-dependent manner. Taken together, a combination of these approaches allows for the rapid dissection of the function of a disease gene, and the elucidation of all the cellular pathways that are involved in the molecular aetiology of the disease. In the following sections, the progress of research on *Drosophila Ppt1*, *cathD* and *Cln3* will be highlighted. In addition, the utility of different screening approaches will be discussed in relation to both of these fly NCL models.

The *cln* genes of *D. melanogaster*

A search for *cln* genes in the *Drosophila* genome reveals that, like *C. elegans*, there exist homologues for only *PPT1/CLN1*, *CLN3*, and *CTSD/CLN10*. Work has progressed quickly on the development of several different models for CLN1 and CLN10 diseases. The success of this work makes it likely that CLN3 disease will soon be studied in the fly as well.

DROSOPHILA MODELS OF CLN1 DISEASE

The *Drosophila* Ppt1 homologue is approximately 55% identical and approximately 72% similar to the human protein at the amino acid level (Glaser et al., 2003). Like the human gene, the *ppt1* transcript appears to be expressed ubiquitously, although in *Drosophila* it is found at different levels during the stages of fly development. Consistent with the levels of mRNA, assays using the fluorogenic substrate 4-methylumbelliferyl-6-thiopalmitoyl–D-galactopyranoside show that Ppt1 enzymatic activity is present at varying levels in all tissues that have been tested (Glaser et al., 2003). Like the human and mouse proteins, localization studies with a GFP-Ppt1 fusion protein has demonstrated that fly Ppt1 is localized to lysosomes in cultured cells (Bannan et al., 2008). *Ppt1* loss-of-function analysis has shown that mutant flies are viable, with a reduced lifespan. Unlike CLN1 disease patients, adult flies have no visible signs of neurodegeneration (Hickey et al., 2006). In the mouse knockout model of CLN1 disease, neuronal cell death is associated with activation of the endoplasmic reticulum (ER) stress response (Kim et al., 2006). The *Drosophila* model does not show a similar ER stress response suggesting a reason for the lack of cell death in the fly central nervous system (B. Glaser, personal communication). The flies show a central nervous system specific accumulation of autofluorescent storage material characteristic of the NCLs and abnormal cytoplasmic inclusions. However, the inclusions observed in *Drosophila* are different to the typical granular osmiophilic deposits found in CLN1 disease patients (Hickey et al., 2006) (Figure 16.1). Analysis of the neurons within the adult nervous system of *ppt1* mutant flies using electron microscopy reveals the presence of cytoplasmic deposits with some similarities to the multilamellar deposits present in Tay–Sachs patients (Hickey et al., 2006). The specific association of these cytoplasmic deposits with the loss of *ppt1* was confirmed by their absence in the nervous systems of *ppt1* mutants that are expressing a wild-type copy of the *ppt1* gene. The autoflouresence phenotype was rescued in *ppt1* mutant males by using a genetic duplication of the *ppt1* chromosomal region located on the Y chromosome (Hickey et al., 2006).

Targeted overexpression of *ppt1* in the developing *Drosophila* visual system using the eye driver GMR-Gal4 leads to the loss of cells, including neurons, through apoptotic cell death both early in eye development and after the completion of ommatidial differentiation (Korey and MacDonald, 2003). Transmission electron microscopy of *ppt1* overexpressing retinae reveals highly pigmented and vacuolated photoreceptor neurons; a cellular phenotype associated with apoptotic cell death in the fly (Korey and MacDonald, 2003). To ensure that the abnormal eye phenotypes were the result of increased levels of normal *ppt1* enzymatic activity, a serine 123 to alanine catalytic mutant of *ppt1* was also misexpressed. Expression of the catalytic mutant *ppt1* within the retina yielded no observable abnormal phenotypes when analysed with scanning electron micrography confirming that the observed phenotypes were not due to non-specific effects of increased Ppt1 production (Korey and MacDonald, 2003). The over-expression *ppt1* model demonstrates that while recessive mutations that severely decrease PPT1 activity cause neuronal cell death in CLN1 disease patients, increased levels of PPT1 activity may also lead to neurodegeneration. Thus, the precise level of PPT1 activity is likely to be important for neuronal cell survival.

GENETIC MODIFIER SCREENS OF PPT1-INDUCED DEGENERATION

The degenerative phenotype produced by the over-expression of Ppt1 in the adult visual

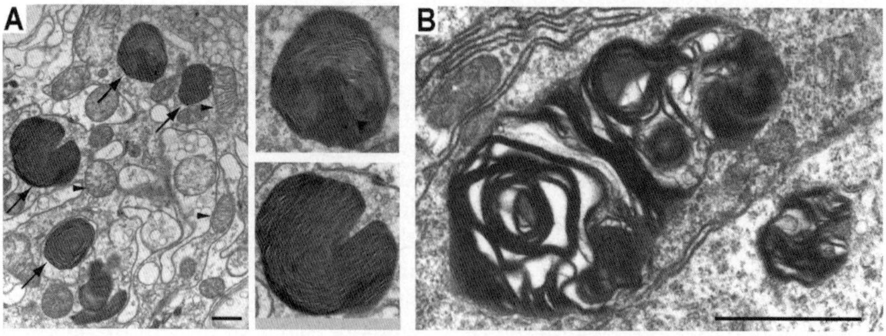

Figure 16.1 PPT1-null flies accumulate abnormal storage material. Tissues from *Df(1)446-20* flies were analysed by electron microscopy (EM). Osmiophilic laminar deposits detected in the brains of 35-day post-eclosion females (A) and 14-day post-eclosion males (B). Enlargements of selected deposits are shown to the right of panel (A). Abnormal storage deposits are indicated by arrows. Mitochondria are indicated by arrowheads. Scale bars represent 1μm. Used with the permission of the Genetics Society of America.

system provides a useful assay to identify other genetic loci that may modify this phenotype. This overexpression system was used as part of a dominant gain-of-function modifier screen of a subset of the EP collections available from the public *Drosophila* stock centres (Buff et al., 2007). This screen combined the previous *GMR:Gal4; UAS:ppt1* phenotype with the EP lines to identify a collection of genes that modify the *ppt1*-induced degeneration when coexpressed in the eye. Suppressing loci were those that could reduce the degeneration and ameliorate the defects in external eye morphology. Those loci termed enhancers increased the observed degeneration as compared to that produced by Ppt1 expression alone. A series of rigorous elimination criteria produced a final collection of ten enhancers and ten suppressors.

A subset of the modifying loci had important roles in neuronal function. The screen identified the synaptic vesicle cycling proteins endophilinA, synaptotagmin, and stonedA and also demonstrated that fasciclin II (NCAM), myospheroid (β-integrin), kayak (dFos), and Hsc70-3 (BiP) all modify the degeneration produced by Ppt1 expression. These genes and several of the other modifiers play a role in the development and remodelling of the synapse in *Drosophila* and other model organisms. The identification of these pathway components provides strong evidence for an important connection between conserved synaptic signalling and Ppt1 function. In addition, several loci, such as the endosomal protein blue cheese and ubiquitination enzymes, suggest connections between Ppt1 and endolysosomal trafficking (Seto et al., 2002, Finley et al., 2003). Finally, palmitoylation regulates several homologues of modifying genes, specifically synaptotagmin and fasciclin II, in other systems and may represent *in vivo* substrates for Ppt1.

A second dominant loss-of-function genetic modifier screen was carried out (Saja et al., 2010). The enhancers and suppressors identified make novel connections between Ppt1 and genes involved in cellular trafficking and the modulation of synaptic growth. In addition, Garland cells from Ppt1 loss-of-function mutants were shown to have defects in endocytic trafficking.

This genetic approach in the fly complements recent work on Ppt1– cells that showed reductions in synaptic vesicle pools in mouse primary neuronal cultures and defects in endosomal trafficking in human fibroblasts (Virmani et al., 2005, Ahtiainen et al., 2007). These data suggest a hypothesis whereby early changes in the trafficking of synaptic vesicles and signalling proteins involved in synaptic structure may lead to a progressive dysfunction of neurons, producing disease symptoms and ultimately widespread cell death. As with all large-scale screens, the modifiers identified must be further validated in Drosophila *ppt1* mutants, higher eukaryotic systems such as the CLN1 disease mouse, and finally in CLN1 disease patient cells. The pathways and processes implicated by results in the fly will be valuable points of entry for future research on CLN1 disease in all other model organisms and patients.

DROSOPHILA MODELS OF CLN10 DISEASE

The *Drosophila* homologue of cathepsin D (cathD) encodes a polypeptide of 392 amino acids, which exhibits approximately 50% identity and approximately 65% similarity with human cathepsin D. A *cathD* loss-of-function model was developed by generating an approximately 1kb deletion in the open reading frame of the *Drosophila cathD* locus (Myllykangas et al., 2005). The *cathD* mutants are viable and fertile and do not show a substantial reduction in lifespan. However, the histological analysis of the brain sections revealed that the *cathD* mutants recapitulate the pathological key features of NCLs: neuronal accumulation of storage material and neurodegeneration.

The storage material closely resembles the granular osmiophilic deposits found in the human CLN10 and CLN1 disease patients. It accumulates progressively with age and appears autofluorescent under a wide range of wavelengths. The ultrastructural analysis of the accumulated material showed that it forms globular membrane-bound structures, is granular with some lamellar elements, but forms no clear fingerprint or curvilinear bodies (Figure 16.2). Furthermore, the storage material is positive in histological periodic acid–Schiff and Luxol fast blue stainings (Myllykangas et al., 2005), similar to that of other forms of NCLs. Although the *cathD* mutants did not show severe neurodegeneration or brain atrophy, a modest neurodegeneration, particularly in the optic lobes, was seen in the aged *cathD* mutants (Myllykangas et al., 2005, Kuronen et al., 2009). When comparing 45-day-old *cathD* mutants and

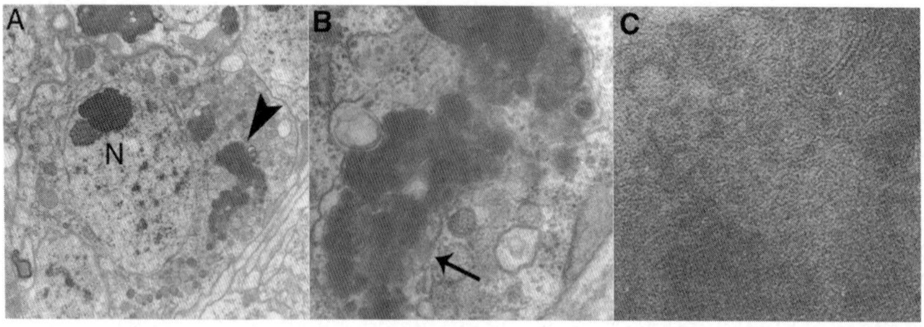

Figure 16.2 Electron micrographs showing granular osmiophilic deposits in a neuron of an aged *cathD* mutant fly. (A, B) The storage material forms globular structures (arrowhead), which are membrane bound (arrow). (C) The ultrastructure is granular with some lamellar structures. No fingerprint or curvilinear bodies were observed. Used with the permission of Elsevier Press.

controls, a significant difference was observed in the number of TUNEL positive neurons and slight vacuolar changes were observed.

An overexpression model for *Drosophila cathD* has also been generated, and the analysis of its phenotype is currently underway.

Candidate modifier gene approach and Drosophila *cathepsin D*

Although the cathD mutants show an NCL-type phenotype, this phenotype is not ideal for genome-wide modifier screens. However, genetic modifiers of the NCL-type pathology can be searched for by the candidate modifier approach. Possible candidate genes are selected based on previous hypotheses or results on other model organisms. *Drosophila* lines carrying transgenes or mutations in the homologues of these candidate genes are crossed with the disease model to investigate the effect on particular disease phenotypes. One study of 17 candidate modifiers of the retinal phenotype found enhancers that support the involvement of endocytosis-, lipid metabolism- and oxidation-related factors in cathepsin D-induced degeneration (Kuronen et al., 2009). None of these enhanced the brain neurodegenerative phenotype. Overexpression of α-synuclein in the cathepsin D deficiency strain caused severe retinal degeneration (Cullen et al., 2009). The possible interaction between cathepsin D and other NCL proteins is also being studied.

DROSOPHILA MODELS OF CLN3 DISEASE

One gene, encoded by the *CG5582* locus, in *Drosophila* is homologous to *CLN3*. There is currently no *cln3*-depleted model for CLN3 disease in the fruit fly but the recent identification of a strain carrying a transposable element within the *CLN3* locus gives scope for mutations to be generated. A gain-of-function approach has been used to express *D. melanogaster* CLN3 ubiquitously throughout the fly or in specific tissues (Tuxworth et al., 2009). Ubiquitous expression of *D. melanogaster cln3* is semi-lethal and surviving adults have roughened eyes, duplicated macrochaetae on the thorax, thickened wing veins, and notches in the wing margins, all phenotypes associated with Notch loss-of-function. Expression of CLN3 in an ectopic domain in the wing imaginal disc inhibits Notch-dependent transcription within that domain providing further evidence of a genetic interaction between CLN3 and Notch signaling.

Expression of either *D. melanogaster cln3* or human *CLN3* in the eye causes a degenerative phenotype, indicating that the function of this protein is conserved between the species, as is the case for the yeast orthologues of *CLN3*. In the developing wing overexpression results in increased apoptosis along with thickening of veins and notching. A genetic screen for modifiers of these phenotypes identified strong interactions with the Jun N-terminal kinase (JNK) signalling pathway that suggests inhibition of Notch by CLN3 may be via activation of JNK.

In cultured cells tagged *D. melanogaster* CLN3 proteins localize to lysosomes, the plasma membrane, and recycling vesicles (Tuxworth et al., 2009) but it is not clear if this reflects the localization of the endogenous protein in the fly. The *D. melanogaster cln3* gene is widely expressed, including in the central nervous system, but generally only at low levels. (R. Tuxworth,

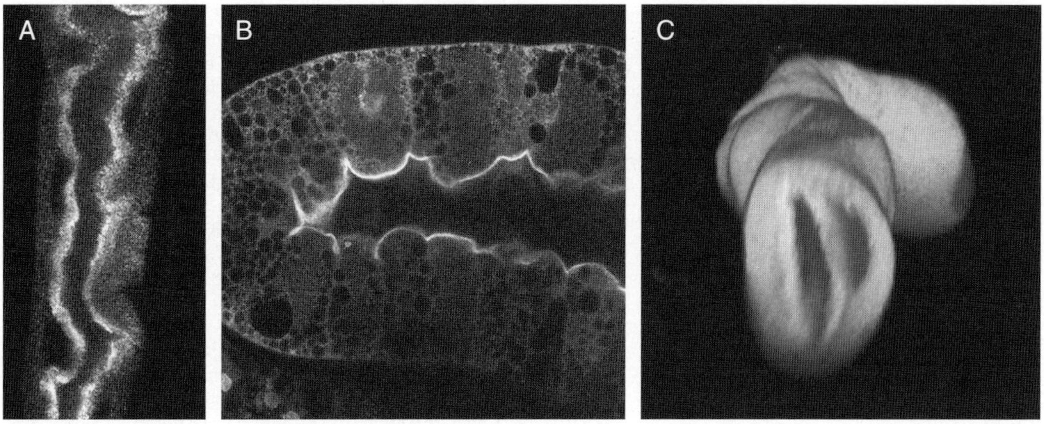

Figure 16.3 Confocal micrographs showing the apical localization of endogenous CLN3 in *Drosophila* secretory tissues. A) Malpighian tubule and B) salivary gland.

unpublished). However, it is highly enriched in Malpighian tubules, the insect excretory and osmoregulatory organ analogous to the kidney. Murine *cln3* is also expressed in the kidney (Eliason et al., 2007) indicating a likely conservation of function. A role for CLN3 in renal control of water and K^+ balance has been suggested (Stein et al., 2010). An antiserum raised to the N-terminus of *D. melanogaster* CLN3 (Tuxworth et al., 2009) reports an unexpected localization of endogenous protein in polarized secretory cells. In both the Malpighian tubule and the salivary gland of *Drosophila* larvae, CLN3 is seen highly enriched in the apical domain adjacent to the lumen (Figure 16.3) although its function there is unknown.

Neuronal functions for CLN3 in the fly remain to be studied but given the powerful neurobiology tools available, *D. melanogaster* is likely to prove an excellent model for further investigations into CLN3 function, including the identification of disease modifiers.

Homologues of mouse genes involved in lysosomal lipofuscin accumulation

Like the worm, the fly is likely to have homologues of *CLN* candidate genes that were first characterized in the mouse (see Chapter 17). Other than annotating their functions using bioinformatic tools, little research has been done on the function of these genes in *Drosophila*. In particular, none have been examined for the lysosomal accumulation of ceroid or lipofuscin that has been observed in mouse mutants. The *CG5284* locus is the probable homologue of *CLCN3*, while *CG8594* represents the fly gene most similar to *CLCN6* and *CLCN7*. The CLCN7 associated protein OSTM1 also has a homologue in the fly encoded by the *CG14969* locus. To date, no mutations have been produced in the fly to examine phenotypes associated with the loss of these chloride channels. An analysis of the genomic region surrounding each gene shows that transposable element insertions are associated with each of these NCL candidates. These insertions will provide a convenient starting point for the production and characterization of mutations to analyse their function in the fly.

In addition to *CTSD*, the fly also has homologues for the cathepsin genes *CTSB*, *CTSF*, and *CTSL*. Like the chloride channel genes, *CG10992* (*CTSB*), *CG12163* (*CTSF*), and *cp1* (*CTSL*) have not been examined for NCL-like phenotypes in the fly and only *cp1* has characterized loss-of-function mutations. Null mutations in the *cp1* gene show female sterility, partial male sterility, wing defects, and pigmentation defects (Gray et al., 1998). The protein has also been localized to lysosomes in haemocyte cells indicating a likely role in degradation of phagocytosed material (Tryselius and Hultmark, 1997). As a group, these enzymes have been associated with autophagic cell death by serial analysis of gene expression (SAGE) studies of *Drosophila* salivary glands during several pre-cell death stages (Gorski et al., 2003). A role for these proteins in autophagy is intriguing given the connection between autophagy and the pathology observed in CLN3 disease knock-in mice (*Cln3*$^{\Delta ex7/8}$) (Cao et al., 2006). Like the chloride channels, *CG10992* and *CG12163* have transposable elements in close proximity that will provide a tool for the genetic analysis of these genes in the fly.

CONCLUSIONS

Small model organisms like the worm and fly will have a strong presence in NCL research for years to come. Future large-scale genetic screens made possible by their well-characterized nervous systems and powerful genetic tools will continue to provide new avenues of inquiry into NCL disease mechanisms. The molecular characterization of these model organism disease homologues will become valuable resources for the future development of therapeutics that aim to prevent the symptoms associated with CTSD, CLN1, CLN3, and CLN7 diseases.

REFERENCES

Ahtiainen L, Kolikova J, Mutka AL, Luiro K, Gentile M, Ikonen E, Khiroug L, Jalanko A, & Kopra O (2007) Palmitoyl protein thioesterase 1 (Ppt1)-deficient mouse neurons show alterations in cholesterol metabolism and calcium homeostasis prior to synaptic dysfunction. *Neurobiol Dis*, 28, 52–64.

Bannan BA, Van Etten J, Kohler JA, Tsoi Y, Hansen NM, Sigmon S, Fowler E, Buff H, Williams TS, Ault JG, Glaser RL, & Korey CA (2008) The Drosophila protein palmitoylome: Characterizing palmitoyl-thioesterases and DHHC palmitoyl-transferases. *Fly (Austin)*, 2.

Berger J, Suzuki T, Senti KA, Stubbs J, Schaffner G, & Dickson BJ (2001) Genetic mapping with SNP markers in Drosophila. *Nat Genet*, 29, 475–481.

Bertoni-Freddari C, Fattoretti P, Casoli T, Di Stefano G, Solazzi M, & Corvi E (2002) Morphometric investigations of the mitochondrial damage in ceroid lipopigment accumulation due to vitamin E deficiency. *Arch Gerontol Geriatr*, 34, 269–274.

Bianchi L, Miller DM, 3rd, & George AL, Jr. (2001) Expression of a ClC chloride channel in Caenorhabditis elegans gamma-aminobutyric acid-ergic neurons. *Neurosci Lett*, 299, 177–180.

Blumenthal T & Gleason KS (2003) Caenorhabditis elegans operons: form and function. *Nat Rev Genet*, 4, 112–120.

Boriack RL, Cortinas E, & Bennett MJ (1995) Mitochondrial damage results in a reversible increase in lysosomal storage material in lymphoblasts from patients with juvenile neuronal ceroid-lipofuscinosis (Batten Disease). *Am J Med Genet*, 57, 301–303.

Boulin T, Etchberger JF, & Hobert O (2006) Reporter gene fusions. In *The C. elegans Research Community (Eds.) WormBook*.doi/10.1895/wormbook.1.106.1,http://www.wormbook.org.

Brand AH & Perrimon N (1993) Targeted gene expression as a means of altering cell fates and generating dominant phenotypes. *Development*, 118, 401–415.

Brenner S (1974) The genetics of Caenorhabditis elegans. *Genetics*, 77, 71–94.

Buff H, Smith AC, & Korey CA (2007) Genetic modifiers of Drosophila palmitoyl-protein thioesterase 1-induced degeneration. *Genetics*, 176, 209–220.

Cao Y, Espinola JA, Fossale E, Massey AC, Cuervo AM, MacDonald ME, & Cotman SL (2006) Autophagy is disrupted in a knock-in mouse model of juvenile neuronal ceroid lipofuscinosis. *J Biol Chem*, 281, 20483–20493.

Chattopadhyay S, Ito M, Cooper JD, Brooks AI, Curran TM, Powers JM, & Pearce DA (2002a) An autoantibody inhibitory to glutamic acid decarboxylase in the neurodegenerative disorder Batten disease. *Hum Mol Genet*, 11, 1421–1431.

Cho S & Dawson G (2000) Palmitoyl protein thioesterase 1 protects against apoptosis mediated by Ras-Akt-caspase pathway in neuroblastoma cells. *J Neurochem*, 74, 1478–1488.

Cho S, Dawson PE, & Dawson G (2000) Antisense palmitoyl protein thioesterase 1 (PPT1) treatment inhibits PPT1 activity and increases cell death in LA-N-5 neuroblastoma cells. *J Neurosci Res*, 62, 234–240.

Cho S, Dawson PE, & Dawson G (2001) Role of palmitoyl-protein thioesterase in cell death: implications for infantile neuronal ceroid lipofuscinosis. *Eur J Paediatr Neurol*, 5 Suppl A, 53–55.

Culetto E & Sattelle DB (2000) A role for Caenorhabditis elegans in understanding the function and interactions of human disease genes. *Hum Mol Genet*, 9, 869–877.

Cullen V, Lindfors M, Ng J, Paetau A, Swinton E, Kolodziej P, Boston H, Saftig P, Woulfe J, Feany MB, Myllykangas L, Schlossmacher MG, & Tyynelä J (2009) Cathepsin D expression level affects alpha-synuclein processing, aggregation, and toxicity in vivo. *Mol Brain*, 2, 5.

Das AM, Jolly RD, & Kohlschutter A (1999) Anomalies of mitochondrial ATP synthase regulation in four different types of neuronal ceroid lipofuscinosis. *Mol Genet Metab*, 66, 349–355.

Das AM, von Harlem R, Feist M, Lucke T, & Kohlschutter A (2001b) Altered levels of high-energy phosphate compounds in fibroblasts from different forms of neuronal ceroid lipofuscinoses: further evidence for mitochondrial involvement. *Eur J Paediatr Neurol*, 5 Suppl A, 143–146.

Dawson G, Kilkus J, Siakotos AN, & Singh I (1996) Mitochondrial abnormalities in CLN2 and CLN3 forms of Batten disease. *Mol Chem Neuropathol*, 29, 227–235.

de Voer G, der Bent P, Rodrigues AJ, van Ommen GJ, Peters DJ, & Taschner PE (2005) Deletion of the Caenorhabditis elegans homologues of the CLN3 gene, involved in human juvenile neuronal ceroid lipofuscinosis, causes a mild progeric phenotype. *J Inherit Metab Dis*, 28, 1065–1080.

de Voer G, Jansen G, van Ommen G-JB, Peters DJM, & Taschner PEM (2001) Caenorhabditis elegans homologues of the CLN3 gene, mutated in juvenile neuronal ceroid lipofuscinosis. *Eur J Paediat Neurol*, **5**, SupplA 115–120.

de Voer G, Peters D, & Taschner PE (2008) Caenorhabditis elegans as a model for lysosomal storage disorders. *Biochim Biophys Acta*, 1782, 433–446.

Defacque H, Egeberg M, Habermann A, Diakonova M, Roy C, Mangeat P, Voelter W, Marriott G, Pfannstiel J, Faulstich H, & Griffiths G (2000) Involvement of ezrin/moesin in de novo actin assembly on phagosomal membranes. *EMBO J*, 19, 199–212.

Dermaut B, Norga KK, Kania A, Verstreken P, Pan H, Zhou Y, Callaerts P, & Bellen HJ (2005) Aberrant lysosomal carbohydrate storage accompanies endocytic defects and neurodegeneration in Drosophila benchwarmer. *J Cell Biol*, 170, 127–139.

Desai UA, Pallos J, Ma AA, Stockwell BR, Thompson LM, Marsh JL, & Diamond MI (2006) Biologically active molecules that reduce polyglutamine aggregation and toxicity. *Hum Mol Genet*, 15, 2114–2124.

Eliason SL, Stein CS, Mao Q, Tecedor L, Ding SL, Gaines DM, & Davidson BL (2007) A knock-in reporter model of Batten disease. *J Neurosci*, 27, 9826–9834.

Fares H & Greenwald I (2001a) Genetic analysis of endocytosis in Caenorhabditis elegans: coelomocyte uptake defective mutants. *Genetics*, 159, 133–145.

Fares H & Greenwald I (2001b) Regulation of endocytosis by CUP-5, the Caenorhabditis elegans mucolipin-1 homolog. *Nat Genet*, 28, 64–68.

Finley KD, Edeen PT, Cumming RC, Mardahl-Dumesnil MD, Taylor BJ, Rodriguez MH, Hwang CE, Benedetti M, & McKeown M (2003) *blue cheese* mutations define a novel, conserved gene involved in progressive neural degeneration. *J Neurosci*, 23, 1254–1264.

Fluegel ML, Parker TJ, & Pallanck LJ (2006) Mutations of a Drosophila NPC1 gene confer sterol and ecdysone metabolic defects. *Genetics*, 172, 185–196.

Fortini ME & Bonini NM (2000) Modeling human neurodegenerative diseases in Drosophila: on a wing and a prayer. *Trends Genet*, 16, 161–167.

Fossale E, Wolf P, Espinola JA, Lubicz-Nawrocka T, Teed AM, Gao H, Rigamonti D, Cattaneo E, MacDonald ME, & Cotman SL (2004) Membrane trafficking and mitochondrial abnormalities precede subunit c deposition in a cerebellar cell model of juvenile neuronal ceroid lipofuscinosis. *BMC Neurosci*, 5, 57.

Fukushige T, Goszczynski B, Tian H, & McGhee JD (2003) The evolutionary duplication and probable demise of an endodermal GATA factor in Caenorhabditis elegans. *Genetics*, 165, 575–588.

Glaser RL, Hickey AJ, Chotkowski HL, & Chu-LaGraff Q (2003) Characterization of Drosophila palmitoyl-protein thioesterase 1. *Gene*, 312, 271–279.

Gorski SM, Chittaranjan S, Pleasance ED, Freeman JD, Anderson CL, Varhol RJ, Coughlin SM, Zuyderduyn SD, Jones SJ, & Marra MA (2003) A SAGE approach to discovery of genes involved in autophagic cell death. *Curr Biol*, 13, 358–363.

Gray YH, Sved JA, Preston CR, & Engels WR (1998) Structure and associated mutational effects of the cysteine proteinase (CP1) gene of Drosophila melanogaster. *Insect Mol Biol*, 7, 291–293.

Haines RL, Codlin S, & Mole SE (2009) The fission yeast model for the lysosomal storage disorder Batten disease predicts disease severity caused by mutations in CLN3. *Dis Model Mech*, 2, 84–92.

Hall NA, Lake BD, Dewji NN, & Patrick AD (1991) Lysosomal storage of subunit c of mitochondrial ATP synthase in Batten's disease (ceroid-lipofuscinosis). *Biochem J*, **275** (Pt 1), 269–272.

Hashmi S, Britton C, Liu J, Guiliano DB, Oksov Y, & Lustigman S (2002) Cathepsin L is essential for embryogenesis and development of Caenorhabditis elegans. *J Biol Chem*, 277, 3477–3486.

Heine C, Tyynelä J, Cooper JD, Palmer DN, Elleder M, Kohlschutter A, & Braulke T (2003) Enhanced expression of manganese-dependent superoxide dismutase in human and sheep CLN6 tissues. *Biochem J*, 376, 369–376.

Hersh BM, Hartwieg E, & Horvitz HR (2002) The Caenorhabditis elegans mucolipin-like gene cup-5 is essential for viability and regulates lysosomes in multiple cell types. *Proc Natl Acad Sci U S A*, 99, 4355–4360.

Hickey AJ, Chotkowski HL, Singh N, Ault JG, Korey CA, MacDonald ME, & Glaser RL (2006) Palmitoyl-protein thioesterase 1 deficiency in Drosophila melanogaster causes accumulation of abnormal storage material and reduced life span. *Genetics*, 172, 2379–2390.

Hoskins RA, Phan AC, Naeemuddin M, Mapa FA, Ruddy DA, Ryan JJ, Young LM, Wells T, Kopczynski C, & Ellis MC (2001) Single nucleotide polymorphism markers for genetic mapping in Drosophila melanogaster. *Genome Res*, 11, 1100–1113.

Huang X, Suyama K, Buchanan J, Zhu AJ, & Scott MP (2005) A Drosophila model of the Niemann-Pick type C lysosome storage disease: dnpc1a is required for molting and sterol homeostasis. *Development*, 132, 5115–5124.

Jansen G, Hazendonk E, Thijssen KL, & Plasterk RH (1997) Reverse genetics by chemical mutagenesis in Caenorhabditis elegans. *Nat Genet*, 17, 119–121.

Jolly RD, Brown S, Das AM, & Walkley SU (2002b) Mitochondrial dysfunction in the neuronal ceroid-lipofuscinoses (Batten disease). *Neurochem Int*, 40, 565–571.

Jorgensen EM & Mango SE (2002) The art and design of genetic screens: Caenorhabditis elegans. *Nat Rev Genet*, 3, 356–369.

Kaletta T & Hengartner MO (2006) Finding function in novel targets: C. elegans as a model organism. *Nat Rev Drug Discov*, 5, 387–398.

Kim SJ, Zhang Z, Hitomi E, Lee YC, & Mukherjee AB (2006) Endoplasmic reticulum stress-induced caspase-4 activation mediates apoptosis and neurodegeneration in INCL. *Hum Mol Genet*, 15, 1826–1834.

Korey CA & MacDonald ME (2003) An over-expression system for characterizing Ppt1 function in Drosophila. *BMC Neurosci*, 4, 30.

Kostich M, Fire A, & Fambrough DM (2000) Identification and molecular-genetic characterization of a LAMP/CD68-like protein from Caenorhabditis elegans. *J Cell Sci*, **113** (Pt 14), 2595–2606.

Kuronen M, Talvitie M, Lehesjoki AE, & Myllykangas L (2009) Genetic modifiers of degeneration in the cathepsin D deficient Drosophila model for neuronal ceroid lipofuscinosis. *Neurobiol Dis*, 36, 488–493.

Lange PF, Wartosch L, Jentsch TJ, & Fuhrmann JC (2006) ClC-7 requires Ostm1 as a beta-subunit to support bone resorption and lysosomal function. *Nature*, 440, 220–223.

Lercher MJ, Blumenthal T, & Hurst LD (2003) Coexpression of neighboring genes in Caenorhabditis elegans is mostly due to operons and duplicate genes. *Genome Res*, 13, 238–243.

Li J, Brown G, Ailion M, Lee S, & Thomas JH (2004) NCR-1 and NCR-2, the C. elegans homologs of the human Niemann-Pick type C1 disease protein, function upstream of DAF-9 in the dauer formation pathways. *Development*, 131, 5741–5752.

Louvet-Vallee S (2000) ERM proteins: from cellular architecture to cell signaling. *Biol Cell*, 92, 305–316.

Majander A, Pihko H, & Santavuori P (1995) Palmitate oxidation in muscle mitochondria of patients with the juvenile form of neuronal ceroid-lipofuscinosis. *Am J Med Genet*, 57, 298–300.

Mitchell WA, Porter M, Kuwabara P, & Mole SE (2001) Genomic structure of three CLN3-like genes in Caenorhabditis elegans. *Eur J Paediatr Neurol*, 5 Suppl A, 121–125.

Muqit MM, & Feany MB (2002) Modelling neurodegenerative diseases in Drosophila: a fruitful approach? *Nat Rev Neurosci*, 3, 237–243.

Myllykangas L, Tyynelä J, Page-McCaw A, Rubin GM, Haltia MJ, & Feany MB (2005) Cathepsin D-deficient Drosophila recapitulate the key features of neuronal ceroid lipofuscinoses. *Neurobiol Dis*, 19, 194–199.

Nakano Y, Fujitani K, Kurihara J, Ragan J, Usui-Aoki K, Shimoda L, Lukacsovich T, Suzuki K, Sezaki M, Sano Y, Ueda R, Awano W, Kaneda M, Umeda M, & Yamamoto D (2001) Mutations in the novel membrane protein spinster interfere with programmed cell death and cause neural degeneration in Drosophila melanogaster. *Mol Cell Biol*, 21, 3775–3788.

Nehrke K, Begenisich T, Pilato J, & Melvin JE (2000) Into ion channel and transporter function. Caenorhabditis elegans ClC-type chloride channels: novel variants and functional expression. *Am J Physiol Cell Physiol*, 279, C2052–2066.

Palmer DN, Bayliss SL, & Westlake VJ (1995) Batten disease and the ATP synthase subunit c turnover pathway: raising antibodies to subunit c. *Am J Med Genet*, 57, 260–265.

Palmer DN, Fearnley IM, Walker JE, Hall NA, Lake BD, Wolfe LS, Haltia M, Martinus RD, & Jolly RD (1992) Mitochondrial ATP synthase subunit c storage in the ceroid-lipofuscinoses (Batten disease). *Am J Med Genet*, 42, 561–567.

Phillips SN, Muzaffar N, Codlin S, Korey CA, Taschner PE, de Voer G, Mole SE, & Pearce DA (2006) Characterizing pathogenic processes in Batten disease: use of small eukaryotic model systems. *Biochim Biophys Acta*, 1762, 906–919.

Porter MY, Turmaine M, & Mole SE (2005) Identification and characterization of Caenorhabditis elegans palmitoyl protein thioesterase1. *J Neurosci Res*, 79, 836–848.

Rorth P, Szabo K, Bailey A, Laverty T, Rehm J, Rubin GM, Weigmann K, Milan M, Benes V, Ansorge W, & Cohen SM (1998) Systematic gain-of-function genetics in Drosophila. *Development*, 125, 1049–1057.

Saja S, Buff H, Smith AC, Williams TS, & Korey CA (2010) Identifying cellular pathways modulated by Drosophila palmitoyl-protein thioesterase 1 function. *Neurobiol Dis*, 40, 135–145.

Seto ES, Bellen HJ, & Lloyd TE (2002) When cell biology meets development: endocytic regulation of signaling pathways. *Genes Dev*, 16, 1314–1336.

Siintola E, Partanen S, Stromme P, Haapanen A, Haltia M, Maehlen J, Lehesjoki AE, & Tyynelä J (2006) Cathepsin D deficiency underlies congenital human neuronal ceroid-lipofuscinosis. *Brain*, 129, 1438–1445.

Siintola E, Topcu M, Aula N, Lohi H, Minassian BA, Paterson AD, Liu XQ, Wilson C, Lahtinen U, Anttonen AK, & Lehesjoki AE (2007) The novel neuronal ceroid lipofuscinosis gene MFSD8 encodes a putative lysosomal transporter. *Am J Hum Genet*, 81, 136–146.

Simmer F, Moorman C, van der Linden AM, Kuijk E, van den Berghe PV, Kamath RS, Fraser AG, Ahringer J, Plasterk RH (2003) Genome-wide RNAi of C. elegans using the hypersensitive rrf-3 strain reveals novel gene functions. *PLoS Biology*, 1, 77–84.

Stein CS, Yancey PH, Martins I, Sigmund RD, Stokes JB, & Davidson BL (2010) Osmoregulation of ceroid neuronal lipofuscinosis type 3 (CLN3) in the renal medulla. *Am J Physiol Cell Physiol*, 298, C1388–C1400.

Stein LD, Bao Z, Blasiar D, Blumenthal T, Brent MR, Chen N, Chinwalla A, Clarke L, Clee C, Coghlan A, Coulson A, D'Eustachio P, Fitch DH, Fulton LA, Fulton RE, Griffiths-Jones S, Harris TW, Hillier LW, Kamath R, Kuwabara PE, Mardis ER, Marra MA, Miner TL, Minx P, Mullikin JC, Plumb RW, Rogers J, Schein JE, Sohrmann M, Spieth J, Stajich JE, Wei C, Willey D, Wilson RK, Durbin R, & Waterston RH (2003) The genome sequence of Caenorhabditis briggsae: a platform for comparative genomics. *PLoS Biol*, 1, E45.

Sulston JE, Schierenberg E, White JG, & Thomson JN (1983) The embryonic cell lineage of the nematode Caenorhabditis elegans. *Dev Biol*, 100, 64–119.

Sweeney ST & Davis GW (2002) Unrestricted synaptic growth in spinster-a late endosomal protein implicated in TGF-beta-mediated synaptic growth regulation. *Neuron*, 36, 403–416.

Sym M, Basson M, & Johnson C (2000) A model for niemann-pick type C disease in the nematode Caenorhabditis elegans. *Curr Biol*, 10, 527–530.

Syntichaki P, Xu K, Driscoll M, & Tavernarakis N (2002) Specific aspartyl and calpain proteases are required for neurodegeneration in C. elegans. *Nature*, 419, 939–944.

Taschner PE, de Vos N, & Breuning MH (1997) Cross-species homology of the CLN3 gene. *Neuropediatrics*, 28, 18–20.

Tcherepanova I, Bhattacharyya L, Rubin CS, & Freedman JH (2000) Aspartic proteases from the nematode Caenorhabditis elegans. Structural organization and developmental and cell-specific expression of asp-1. *J Biol Chem*, 275, 26359–26369.

Tryselius Y & Hultmark D (1997) Cysteine proteinase 1 (CP1), a cathepsin L-like enzyme expressed in the Drosophila melanogaster haemocyte cell line mbn-2. *Insect Mol Biol*, 6, 173–181.

Tuxworth RI, Vivancos V, O'Hare MB, & Tear G (2009) Interactions between the juvenile Batten disease gene,

CLN3, and the Notch and JNK signalling pathways. *Hum Mol Genet*, 18, 667–678.

Van Furden D, Johnson K, Segbert C, & Bossinger O (2004) The C. elegans ezrin-radixin-moesin protein ERM-1 is necessary for apical junction remodelling and tubulogenesis in the intestine. *Dev Biol*, 272, 262–276.

Virmani T, Gupta P, Liu X, Kavalali ET, & Hofmann SL (2005) Progressively reduced synaptic vesicle pool size in cultured neurons derived from neuronal ceroid lipofuscinosis-1 knockout mice. *Neurobiol Dis*, 20, 314–323.

Waterston R & Sulston J (1995) The genome of Caenorhabditis elegans. *Proc Natl Acad Sci U S A*, 92, 10836–10840.

Chapter 17

Small Animal Models

J.D. Cooper, S.E. Mole, C. Russell, and J. Tyynelä

INTRODUCTION

Model systems provide an invaluable tool for investigating the molecular mechanisms that underlie NCL. This review highlights advances made using mice to model NCL, and the potential advantages of zebrafish models, an approach that for NCL is still in its infancy. Mice and zebrafish contain one orthologue of each of the known genes underlying NCL. Therefore, they have great potential for elucidating the roles of these proteins in brain development and function at the molecular and cellular levels, the level of central nervous system (CNS) organization, and at the level of the whole organism. Indeed, the zebrafish not only lends itself to embryology and genetics, but it is also a promising tool for high-throughput screening for therapeutics.

The discovery of the genetic basis of the majority of forms of NCL is a major advance in studying these profoundly disabling disorders. The ongoing process of identifying the genes that are mutated and revealing the specific mutations that are present is the first step towards investigating the underlying disease mechanisms. However, this information is also crucial for developing genetically accurate models of each form of NCL. As reviewed elsewhere in this volume, a wide variety of disease models have been identified or generated experimentally in species that range in scale from unicellular yeasts to large animals such as sheep and cows. Each of these different models has its particular advantages and has revealed new information about the basic neurobiology of different forms of NCL. However, the mainstay for modelling such genetically inherited disorders remains the use of genetically engineered or naturally occurring mutant mouse strains, which bear mutations in the appropriate gene.

MOUSE MODELS

Genetically engineered mutant mice: some general considerations

The advent of homologous recombination techniques and the identification of stem cell lines that can be manipulated experimentally have together led to the development of a vast number of mutant mice that bear genetically engineered mutations. Indeed, following the identification of the mouse homologue of a gene of interest, it is now a relatively routine procedure to generate a null mutant or 'knockout' mouse. This is usually done by disrupting the specific gene by the insertion of an appropriate targeting vector into the correct place in the mouse genome. In some instances, this gene disruption may have devastating effects, resulting in embryonic lethality. However, progressive developments in targeting vector design have made it possible to generate models in which genes can effectively be switched off at different stages of development. There are many different inducible systems via which this goal can be achieved and this is a field that continues to develop rapidly.

Traditionally, characterizing knockout mice is the first step towards identifying the effects of deleting or disrupting a single gene, but may not represent the most accurate model of disease. Indeed, instead of modelling the disease, such knockout mice simply reveal what happens when the gene of interest is absent, which may have consequences that are distinct from a disease-causing mutation in the same gene that modifies gene function. For this reason, it is now commonplace to generate 'knock-in' mouse models in which a specific disease-causing mutation has been introduced into the gene of interest. This methodology often takes advantage of the specific ability of the bacterial Cre recombinase enzyme to recognize and cut at *loxP* sites that have been engineered at appropriate places in the targeting vector. This is a method that can also be used to generate tissue-specific knockout mice, in which the gene of interest is disrupted only in a tissue or cell type of choice. Although dependent on the existence of a suitable mouse strain in which Cre recombinase expression is driven by an appropriate promoter, the ability to control gene expression in a limited subset of tissues or cells is likely to prove a very powerful means to address fundamental questions about disease neurobiology.

The identification of naturally occurring strains of mice that display disease-like phenotypes has also provided many mouse models of disease, and in many cases led to identification of new disease genes. Because these mice are often the result of experimentally-induced mutagenesis in which there is no control over which mutation is present in these strains, these models do not usually recreate a particular disease-causing mutation. Nevertheless, the advantages of such mutant strains lie in avoiding the methodological and financial considerations of first cloning the gene, constructing an appropriate targeting vector, and the uncertainty of homologous recombination that is transmitted into the germ line.

A gene and protein nomenclature convention exists for the mouse, found at http://www.informatics.jax.org/mgihome/nomen/gene.shtml. Gene symbols generally are italicized, with only the first letter in uppercase and the remaining letters in lowercase. Protein designations are the same as the gene symbol, but are not italicized, all letters are in uppercase. Recessive mutant phenotypes in the mouse are known by a symbol in lower cases, e.g. nclf or mnd, which is later incorporated as a specific allele once the gene has been identified (e.g. $Cln6^{nclf}$ or $Cln8^{mnd}$). There are also guidelines for knockout, knock-in, conditional, and other engineered targeted or transgene mutations. Mouse Genome Informatics hosts a searchable database including genes and phenotypes at http://www.informatics.jax.org/.

Mouse models of disease: some words of caution

This genetic tractability of mice, taken together with their relatively rapid generation time, small size, and the wide availability of suitable histological and behavioural methods for their characterization, has seen the development of a plethora of mouse models of disease. Indeed, mouse models of a variety of neurological disorders are now available and have been deposited in commercial repositories such as the Jackson Laboratories (http://www.jax.org) and a repository of knockout mice that is maintained by the US National Institutes of Health (http://www.komp.org/), so that they are now widely available to researchers. One great advantage of these models is the ability to study the phenotype of these mice at different stages of disease progression, something that is not feasible in human patients. In this fashion, it is possible to obtain important information about progressive pathogenesis, especially in the earliest stages of the disease.

Despite these considerable advantages, it is important to recognize that mouse models of disease also have their limitations. Mice may not live long enough to display the entire range of clinical or pathological phenotypes associated with a particular disease and the spiralling cost of keeping mutant mice can be severely limiting. In particular, the cerebral cortex of the mouse is comparatively simple without the extensive folding of the cortical mantle to produce the characteristic 'walnut-like' appearance of gyri and sulci evident on the surface of the human brain. Indeed, this relative simplicity of the mouse CNS and its associated limited range of behaviours make it hard to model many of the complexities of human disease. Another important consideration is that there are many hundreds of strains of laboratory mice, and the background strain upon which a mutant has been made can dramatically modify its disease phenotype. For this reason it is crucial that comparisons between disease models are made in mice that are congenic upon the same strain background. This is particularly important in interpreting data from a newly developed mouse model, which is invariably first characterized on a mixed strain background, necessitating several generations of crossbreeding with an appropriate control strain to produce a congenic disease model. Due to the morphological and behavioural problems associated with 129Sv strains of mice, it is now generally accepted that C57Bl6 strains provide the most suitable background for this purpose.

Mouse models of different forms of NCL

Following the identification of the genes mutated in a variety of forms of NCL (The International Batten Disease Consortium, 1995, Vesa et al., 1995, Sleat et al., 1997, Savukoski et al., 1998, Ranta et al., 1999, Gao et al., 2002, Wheeler et al., 2002, Siintola et al., 2006, Siintola et al., 2007), a series of different gene-specific mutant mice are now available to model the major childhood forms of the disorder (Saftig et al., 1995, Katz et al., 1999, Mitchison et al., 1999, Gupta et al., 2001, Cotman et al., 2002, Kopra et al., 2004, Sleat et al., 2004, Jalanko et al., 2005, Eliason et al., 2007). As described below, the majority of these mouse models were generated via homologous recombination to disrupt or introduce mutations into the gene of interest. However, two naturally occurring mutant mice that bear mutations in *Cln6* and *Cln8* have also been identified as being models of CLN6 and CLN8 diseases, late infantile (Ranta et al., 1999, Gao et al., 2002, Wheeler et al., 2002). The list of available mouse models will continue to grow as new genes are identified and as more refined knock-in or inducible models are generated. Current data is summarized in Table 17.1, and up-to-date information about these different models will continue to appear on the NCL Mouse Model Database (http://www.ucl.ac.uk/nclmodels/).

With systematic efforts underway to discover the results of individually knocking out each gene in the mouse genome, it is inevitable that some of these null mutant mice will display an NCL-like phenotype. In this fashion, mice with mutations in different chloride channels (Kornak et al., 2001, Stobrawa et al., 2001, Dickerson et al., 2002, Yoshikawa et al., 2002, Poët et al., 2006) or lysosomal proteases (Gupta et al., 2001, Gupta et al., 2003, Tang et al., 2006) have been identified as potential models of new forms of NCL. Although no human NCL may yet be associated with these particular genes, analysis of these mice can still be informative about basic disease mechanisms. Indeed, following this rationale, and taking into account a long-studied sheep model of NCL that was found to be deficient in cathepsin D activity (Tyynelä et al., 2000), mutations in cathepsin D were recently identified as underlying certain forms of congenital human NCL (Siintola et al., 2006), now known as congenital CLN10 disease, making the wealth of information already available from cathepsin D deficient mice (see below) directly relevant to understanding this particularly early onset form of the disorder.

Although not a focus of this chapter, mice disrupted in genes that cause NCL, or containing inserted transgenes, are also used to investigate the normal role of the gene.

Detailed observations from each mouse model

The availability of a range of gene-specific mouse models of NCL has proved invaluable

Table 17.1 **Summary of mouse models for human NCL disease**

Human		**Mouse**		
Gene	Protein	Gene	Protein	NCL disease mouse models and alleles*
PPT1 or *CLN1*	PPT1 or CLN1	*Ppt1*	PPT1	$Ppt1^{\Delta ex4} = Ppt1^{tm1Aj}$ $Ppt1^{-/-} = Ppt1^{tm1Hof}$
TPP1 or *CLN2*	TPP1 or CLN2	*Tpp1*	TPP1	$Tpp1^{-/-} = Tpp1^{tm1Plob}$
CLN3	CLN3	*Cln3*	CLN3	$Cln3^{\Delta ex1-6} = Cln3^{tm1Nbm}$ $Cln3^{\Delta ex7/8}$ $Cln3^{\Delta ex7/8neo} = Cln3^{tm1Mkat}$ $Cln3^{lacZ/lacZ}$
CLN5	CLN5	*Cln5*	CLN5	$Cln5^{-/-} = Cln5^{tm1Pltn}$
CLN6	CLN6	*Cln6* (formerly *Nclf*)	CLN6	$Cln6^{nclf}$
MFSD8 or *CLN7*	MFSD8 or CLN7	*Mfsd8*	MFSD8	*None as yet*
CLN8	CLN8	*Cln8* (formerly *Mnd*)	CLN8	$Cln8^{mnd}$
CTSD or *CLN10*	CTSD	*Ctsd*	CTSD	$Ctsd^{-/-}$

Human: http://www.genenames.org/
Mouse: http://www.informatics.jax.org/mgihome/nomen/gene.shtml)
Human gene symbols generally are italicized, with all letters in uppercase. Protein designations are the same as the gene symbol, but are not italicized; all letters are in uppercase. mRNAs and cDNAs use the same formatting conventions as the gene symbol. Mouse gene symbols generally are italicized, with only the first letter in uppercase and the remaining letters in lowercase. Protein designations are the same as the gene symbol, but are not italicized; all letters are in uppercase. Recessive mutant phenotypes in the mouse are known by a symbol in lower cases e.g. nclf or mnd, which is later incorporated as a specific allele with the identified gene name (e.g. $Cln6^{nclf}$ or $Cln8^{mnd}$).
* Other gene alleles, including trangenes may exist, that are not commonly used in NCL research.

for learning fundamental lessons about disease pathogenesis (Mitchison et al., 2004, Cooper et al., 2006). The analysis of these mouse models is providing a wealth of novel data about the onset and progression of many biochemical, behavioural, and morphological phenotypes associated with each form of NCL. As reviewed below, these studies have revealed some unexpected findings about the selective nature of these events, the order in which different brain regions are affected, and the relative timing of glial activation, synaptic pathology, and neuron loss. The recent availability of these mouse models on the same C57Bl6 strain background has made it possible to make meaningful comparisons between these models. Although many of the phenotypic features of these mice are shared, it is also apparent that their relative timing and exact staging display some marked differences between genetically distinct forms of NCL. This section reviews the current state of knowledge successively for each mouse model, starting with the earliest onset form.

CLN10 DISEASE, CTSD; CATHEPSIN D (*Ctsd*) NULL MUTANT MICE

Cathepsin D (CTSD; EC 3.4.23.5) is one of a family of lysosomal proteases, and a lack of its enzyme activity causes particularly early onset and aggressive forms of sheep and human NCL (Tyynelä et al., 2000, Siintola et al., 2006, Fritchie et al., 2009), previously designated as congenital NCL. Mutations in *CTSD* that leave higher residual levels of enzyme activity result in a more delayed onset (even up to adulthood) and slowly progressing form of NCL (Steinfeld et al., 2006, and unpublished), suggesting a direct relationship between the CTSD activity and disease severity. To investigate the functional role of this enzyme a mouse model of cathepsin D deficiency had been generated previously by introducing an insertion mutation to disrupt exon 4 of the *Ctsd* gene to completely abolish CTSD enzyme activity ($Ctsd^{-/-}$; Saftig et al., 1995). As might be expected from human cases (Siintola et al., 2006, Fritchie et al., 2009), this CTSD deficiency in mice results in a pronounced and aggressive NCL-like disease with the development of severe neurological symptoms that starts approximately 2 weeks after birth and culminates in the premature death of these mice before 4 weeks of age (Koike et al., 2000). There are also devastating effects of CTSD deficiency upon the mouse lymphoid system and necrosis of the small intestine (Saftig et al., 1995).

CTSD deficient mice also display the typical neuropathological features of NCL with the progressive accumulation of autofluorescent storage material, widespread brain atrophy, and neuron loss that is accompanied by prominent activation of astrocytes and microglia (Koike et al., 2000, Nakanishi et al., 2001, Haapanen et al., 2007). These activated microglia produce nitric oxide (NO), which may contribute to neuron loss and intestinal necrosis in *Ctsd*$^{-/-}$ mice (Nakanishi et al., 2001), although inhibition of NO synthesis provided only a modest improvement in their lifespan. Apoptosis was originally thought to be the most significant form of neuronal loss in CTSD deficiency (Koike et al., 2000, Nakanishi et al., 2001), however, deleting the proapoptotic molecule Bax in *Ctsd*$^{-/-}$ mice did not significantly abolish neuron loss (Shacka et al., 2007). These findings provide further support for the idea that autophagic stress or aberrant accumulation of autophagosomes is more important in this form of NCL and other types of cathepsin deficiency (Koike et al., 2000). More recently, investigating the sequence of events in the CNS of *Ctsd*$^{-/-}$ mice has shown the thalamus as an important early focus of pathological changes (Partanen et al., 2008), with localized microglial activation, astrocytosis, and neuron loss all beginning within the somatosensory parts of the thalamus. Significantly, the same study also provided evidence for presynaptic alterations at molecular and ultrastructural level (Partanen et al., 2008), some of which may be mediated by astrocytes. These data further implicate the precise nature of localized neuron–glia interactions as important in the early stages of NCL pathogenesis and for the first time revealed the presynaptic compartment to be an important and early pathological target. There are also changes in the structure of myelin in *Ctsd*$^{-/-}$ mice, which suggests that a failure in myelinization may occur within the brains of these mice (Mutka et al., 2010). NO synthesis inhibitors have been considered therapeutically (Nakanishi et al., 2001). Also, early viral delivery of CTSD into brain extended lifespan despite massive ceroid accumulation and microglial activation, and ameliorated both CNS, and visceral symptoms (Shevtsova et al., 2010). This suggests that ceroid and microglial activation are not lethal but can be tolerated in mice.

CLN1 DISEASE, PPT1; PALMITOYL PROTEIN THIOESTERASE 1 (*Ppt1*) MUTANT MICE

Two mouse models of infantile NCL have been generated by slightly different targeting strategies within the *Ppt1* gene to abolish PPT1 enzyme activity. This was achieved either by disruption of exon 9 to produce *Ppt1* null mutant mice (*Ppt1*$^{-/-}$) (Gupta et al., 2001) or complete deletion of exon 4 to produce *Ppt1*$^{\Delta ex4}$ knockout mice (Jalanko et al., 2005). These two mouse models display similar neurological disorders with progressive visual defects, motor and gait abnormalities, and the onset of spontaneous seizures shortly before premature death (Gupta et al., 2001, Griffey et al., 2005, Griffey et al., 2006, Kielar et al., 2007), although this appear to progresses slightly faster in *Ppt1*$^{\Delta ex4}$ knockout mice (Jalanko et al., 2005). Most studies have concentrated upon the effects of PPT1 deficiency upon the mouse brain; however, its consequences in the rest of the body are beginning to emerge (Galvin et al., 2008).

Both models display profound CNS atrophy and neuron loss by the end stages of the disease (Bible et al., 2004, Jalanko et al., 2005). However, even in severely affected *Ppt1*$^{-/-}$ mice, both microglial activation and neuron loss display remarkable regional selectivity, occurring to markedly different extents in cortical regions that serve different functions (Bible et al., 2004). Studying the progressive development of this phenotype has revealed a complex relationship between neuron loss, astrocytosis, and microglial activation within the thalamocortical system of *Ppt1*$^{-/-}$ mice (Kielar et al., 2007). Although widespread late in the disease (Bible et al., 2004), astrocytosis is initially restricted to individual thalamic nuclei and cortical laminae, long before the onset of neuron loss or neurological signs (Kielar et al., 2007), serving as an accurate predictor of where neuron loss subsequently occurs. A similar phenotype is also apparent in the cerebellum, with astrocytosis also evident before the onset of neuron loss (Macauley et al., 2009). Furthermore, astrocytes appear to mediate responses to altered glutamate levels and related events at the synapse in PPT1 deficient mice (Kielar et al., 2009, J. Cooper et al., unpublished observations), suggesting this cell type as central to CLN1 disease pathogenesis.

Surprisingly, the loss of cortical neurons in *Ppt1*$^{-/-}$ mice occurs only after the loss of relay neurons in the corresponding thalamic nucleus (Kielar et al., 2007). This progressive loss of thalamic relay neurons proceeds at different rates, depending on which sensory modality is relayed, and occurs first within the dorsal lateral geniculate nucleus (LGNd) which relays visual information (Kielar et al., 2007), and starts before any overt neurodegeneration or visual dysfunction is evident in the retina or cortex of these mice (Griffey et al., 2005, Lei et al., 2006). The relatively late onset of cortical neuron loss in PPT1 deficient mice follows a similar regional specificity, being most pronounced in the visual cortex before other cortical regions (Kielar et al., 2007). The loss of cortical GABAergic interneurons that is present in both mouse models (Bible et al., 2004, Jalanko et al., 2005) also follows this pattern, and it is only when this reaches a critical threshold that spontaneous seizure activity becomes apparent from 7 months of age onwards (Kielar et al., 2009).

The molecular mechanisms by which PPT1 deficiency leads to this devastating neurological disorder are still poorly understood, but gene profiling studies point towards a significant involvement of inflammatory pathways (Qiao et al., 2007). Furthermore, a combination of endoplasmic reticulum stress, oxidative stress, activation of the unfolded protein response, and RAGE (receptor for advanced glycation end products) activation, may play roles in a disease cascade that culminates in caspase activation and apoptosis (Kim et al., 2006, Zhang et al., 2006, Saha et al., 2008), and it has been suggested that chemical chaperones may be beneficial in alleviating some of these effects (Wei et al., 2008). It has also been proposed that elevated levels of cytosolic phospholipase A2 and the resultant increase in lysophosphatidylcholine act as a signal for the recruitment of lymphocytes into the CNS of *Ppt1* null mutant mice (Zhang et al., 2007). Elevated sterol synthesis is evident early in the pathogenesis of *Ppt1*$^{\Delta ex4}$ knockout mice (Ahtiainen et al., 2007), suggesting that compromised lipid metabolism and trafficking is a common feature of CLN1 disease pathogenesis (Ahtiainen et al., 2007, Lyly et al., 2008). Several lines of evidence also point to effects upon synaptic organization in the mouse as a key event in PPT1 deficiency, with altered synaptic vesicle pool size (Virmani et al., 2005), and significant effects upon the staining for a variety of presynaptic markers apparent in PPT1 deficient mice, similar to findings in *Ctsd*$^{-/-}$ mice (Partanen et al., 2008). More recently, the nature of synaptic defects in *Ppt1* null mutant mice has been defined in more detail, revealing that a lack of depalmitoylating activity hinders synaptic vesicle recycling, leading to abnormal neurotransmission (Kim et al., 2008). Reorganization of the presynaptic compartment is also evident in the thalamocortical system of asymptomatic PPT1 deficient mice and is detectable before axonal pathology or neuron loss (Kielar et al., 2009). Prior to these morphological changes, regionally selective alterations in the expression of proteins involved with synaptic function/stability and cell cycle regulation are evident, occurring first within the thalamus and only later in the cortex (Kielar et al., 2009).

In parallel with these morphological observations, an increasing number of behavioural phenotypes are emerging from PPT1 deficient mice. These have largely emerged from studies investigating the therapeutic impact of gene transfer and neural stem cell transplantation (Griffey et al., 2004, Griffey et al., 2005, Griffey et al., 2006, Tamaki et al., 2009). These phenotypes include progressive impairments in performance on rotarod, pole climbing, ledge tests, and the occurrence of spontaneous seizure activity which is evident in severely affected *Ppt1* mutant mice from 7 months onwards (Kielar et al., 2007).

CLN2 DISEASE, TPP1; TRIPEPTIDYL PEPTIDASE 1 (*Tpp1*) MUTANT MICE

TPP1 deficient mice (*Tpp1*$^{-/-}$) have been generated by insertion of the CLN2-specific Arg447His missense mutation into the *Tpp1* gene in combination with a large intronic insertion (Sleat et al., 2004). These *Tpp1* null mutant mice display a relatively early onset neurological disorder with rapidly progressing motor deficits, spontaneous tremors and seizure activity, and death by 6 months of age (Sleat et al., 2004). Although amounts are elevated, they do not accumulate glial fibrillary acidic protein in their lysosomes (Xu et al., 2010). Consistent with their relatively aggressive phenotype, *Tpp1*$^{-/-}$ mice also display pronounced brain atrophy, marked glial activation, and degeneration within the thalamocortical system and cerebellum (Sleat et al., 2004). Nevertheless, relatively little detailed information is available about the onset and progression of these pathological features, although evidence for progressive degenerative events and characteristic localized glial responses are now emerging (Chang et al., 2008; J. Cooper et al., unpublished observations). In contrast, because gene transfer and enzyme replacement approaches continue to be tested and refined in *Tpp1*$^{-/-}$ mice, there is a wealth of information available regarding the behavioural and neurological consequences of TPP1 deficiency (Passini et al., 2006, Cabrera-Salazar et al., 2007, Sondhi et al., 2007, Chang et al., 2008, Sondhi et al., 2008, Chen et al., 2009). These include rotarod deficits, abnormalities in gait, the progressive decline in grip strength, nesting behaviour, open-field activity, a characteristic resting tremor, and balance beam walking. These quantitative landmarks of disease progression have proved to be sensitive measures to judge the therapeutic efficacy of gene transfer and enzyme replacement (Sondhi et al., 2001, Cabrera-Salazar et al., 2007, Chang et al., 2008, Sondhi et al., 2008, Chen et al., 2009), and will be invaluable for performing similar studies for other therapeutic approaches.

CLN3 DISEASE; *Cln3* MUTANT MICE

CLN3 was the first gene to be identified as being mutated in any form of NCL (The International Batten Disease Consortium, 1995). Since this discovery, four different mouse models have been generated to investigate the role of the CLN3 protein, which nevertheless still remains elusive. The first models to be made were two different *Cln3* null mutant mice (*Cln3*$^{-/-}$) in which the *Cln3* gene was disrupted by the insertion of a neo selection cassette to replace either exons 7–8 (*Cln3*$^{\Delta ex7/8neo}$, (Katz et al., 1999) or exons 1–6 (*Cln3*$^{\Delta ex1-6}$, (Mitchison et al., 1999). There has been debate about whether *Cln3*$^{\Delta ex1-6}$ mice, often referred to as a knockout mouse model, are truly null mutants (Kitzmüller et al., 2008), since cells from patients carrying the common 1kb deletion retain partial CLN3 activity. However, aberrant CLN3 proteins are unlikely to be expressed in these mice (Chan et al., 2008). To mimic the 1kb deletion in *CLN3* that is present in the vast majority of CLN3 disease, juvenile patients, a *Cln3* knock-in mouse (*Cln3*$^{\Delta ex7/8}$) was generated (The International Batten Disease Consortium, 1995, Cotman et al., 2002). This human deletion was recreated in *Cln3*$^{\Delta ex7/8}$ mice by surrounding exons 7 and 8 of *Cln3* in the targeting vector by *loxP* sites so that these exons could be excised by Cre recombinase. Finally, a knock-in reporter mouse (*Cln3*$^{lacZ/lacZ}$) has also been generated, in which most of exon 1 and all of exons 2–8 of the *Cln3* gene have been replaced by the exogenous reporter gene *LacZ* (Eliason et al., 2007). There is no evidence to suggest that any mutant CLN3 protein from this mouse model would be functional (Kitzmüller et al., 2008), although there is a hint that complete loss of CLN3 function is embryonic lethal, since it took a number of backcrosses to generate a mouse homozygous for this mutant *Cln3* gene. To generate this mouse *LacZ* was placed under the endogenous promoter sequences of *Cln3*, not only disrupting this gene, but also providing a simple means to follow where *Cln3* would normally be expressed via immunohistochemical or histochemical detection of β-galactosidase expressed by *LacZ*. This elegant approach, performed in mice heterozygous (*Cln3*$^{lacZ/+}$) for this mutant *Cln3*, overcomes the difficulty in generating specific CLN3 antibodies via conventional methods, and has revealed a number of novel and unexpected sites of *Cln3* expression in respiratory, gastrointestinal epithelia, and kidney, and low level expression in vascular endothelia (Eliason et al., 2007).

The phenotype of these different mouse models of CLN3 disease is broadly similar, with a relatively late onset and slowly progressing neurological disorder that includes visual deficits, impaired motor function and decreased activity, a resting tremor, and increased susceptibility to pharmacologically-induced seizures (Mitchison et al., 1999, Cotman et al., 2002, Kriscenski-Perry et al., 2002, Wendt et al., 2005, Kovács et al., 2006, Eliason et al., 2007, Weimer et al., 2009). Initial pathological characterization of these mice revealed a similarly slow time-course of neurodegeneration, with only minimal effects upon cortical atrophy and a late onset loss of GABAergic interneuron populations (Mitchison et al., 1999, Pontikis et al., 2004). However, it has now become apparent that selective effects upon neuron survival are evident much earlier in disease progression. For example, toxic metabolic intermediates of dopamine accumulate in the striatum of *Cln3*$^{\Delta ex1-6}$ mice, preceding the subsequent progressive loss of substantia nigra neurons (Weimer et al., 2007). This mechanism may involve localized oxidative stress within the striatum, but there is also evidence for more widespread reductions in glutathione and increased expression of manganese superoxide dismutase in these mice with increased age (Benedict et al., 2007), suggesting that progressive oxidative stress contributes to neuron loss.

Early effects on neuron survival are also evident in the cerebellum, with a loss of fastigial deep cerebellar nuclear neurons from 6 months of age, and subsequent progressive loss of Purkinje neurons (Weimer et al., 2009). This loss of Purkinje neurons is accompanied by a localized activation of Bergmann glial cells in both human CLN3 disease, juvenile and mouse CLN3 disease, but no significant effects upon granule neuron survival are reported (Weimer et al., 2009). Another population of neurons to be lost early in disease progression in *Cln3* mutant mice is thalamic relay neurons (Pontikis et al., 2005, Weimer et al., 2006) As in PPT1 deficient mice (Kielar et al., 2007), this cell loss is first evident in the visual relay neurons of LGNd and precedes any overt neurodegeneration within the retina or primary visual cortex of *Cln3*$^{\Delta ex1-6}$ mice (Weimer et al., 2006). This loss of LGNd neurons is accompanied by slowed conduction along the optic nerve and anterograde transport along this pathway (Weimer et al., 2006), and there is morphological evidence for degeneration of the optic nerve of *Cln3*$^{\Delta ex1-6}$ mice with increased age (Sappington et al., 2003). Taken together, these data suggest that visual failure in multiple NCL mouse models is not the result of direct effects upon the retina (Lei et al., 2006, Weimer et al., 2006), but is instead due to a combination of pathological events within the optic nerve and the loss of relay neurons within the thalamus. Because of the marked differences in the relative organization of murine and human visual systems, it will be important to determine whether similar mechanisms contribute to visual failure in human NCL.

As in mouse models of other forms of NCL, neuron loss in CLN3 deficient mice is preceded by evidence of glial activation early in disease progression (Pontikis et al., 2004). However, despite this early upregulation of markers of astrocytosis and microglial activation, both *Cln3*$^{\Delta ex1-6}$ mutant and *Cln3*$^{\Delta ex7/8}$ knock-in mice fail to display evidence for pronounced astrocytic hypertrophy (GFAP) or proliferation (S100β) or significant transformation of microglia into a brain macrophage-like morphology (Pontikis et al., 2004, Pontikis et al., 2005). This is in marked contrast to the pronounced glial responses evident in all other mouse models of NCL (e.g. Bible et al., 2004, Kielar et al., 2007, Partanen et al., 2008, von Schantz et al., 2009), and suggests that neuroimmune responses may be compromised in juvenile CLN3 disease, for which there is now mounting *in vivo* and *in vitro* evidence (J. Cooper et al., unpublished observations).

Further evidence for atypical neuroimmune phenotypes is provided by the presence of an autoimmune response that appears to be specific to this form of NCL. Both human and murine CLN3 disease, juvenile are distinctive in displaying evidence for an autoimmune response that includes functional autoantibodies to GAD65, reduced GAD activity, and elevated glutamate levels in CLN3 deficient mice (Chattopadhyay et al., 2002a, Chattopadhyay et al., 2002b). Metabolomic profiling confirms and extends these findings, providing evidence for altered glutamate/glutamine cycling and reduced levels of GABA within the juvenile CLN3 disease CNS (Pears et al., 2005). The presence of elevated glutamate may be damaging to the CNS, and primary granule cell cultures and cerebellar slice cultures from *Cln3*$^{\Delta ex1-6}$ mice display increased vulnerability to AMPA (α-amino-3-hydroxy-5-methyl-4-isoxazolepropionate) receptor mediated excitotoxicity (Kovács et al., 2006). This has led to the testing of the non-competitive AMPA antagonist EGIS-8332, which results in some attenuation of the motor impairment of these mice (Kovács and Pearce, 2008; Kovács et al., 2010), although it is too early to consider this a complete therapeutic solution (Cooper, 2008).

It is now apparent that the autoimmune response in CLN3 disease, juvenile is not confined to GAD65, but includes immunoglobulins raised against multiple brain autoantigens and can bind to a wide variety of CNS cell types (Lim et al., 2006). These autoantigens are present in the cerebrospinal fluid and are deposited within the CNS in both human and murine CLN3 disease, juvenile (Lim et al., 2007). Furthermore, these immunoglobulins can gain access to the CNS via a size-selective breach in the blood–brain barrier (Lim et al., 2007), a finding that may have significant implications for drug delivery to the CLN3 disease brain. A fundamental issue that will need to be resolved is whether these autoantibodies have a direct pathological role. Recent evidence for altered disease progression in $Cln3^{\Delta ex1-6}$ mutant mice in the absence of an autoimmune response (Seehafer et al., 2010), provides a compelling reason for testing whether immunomodulatory approaches would have any therapeutic benefit in CLN3 disease, juvenile.

Despite these advances in characterizing murine CLN3 disease, very little is known about mechanisms that lead from mutations in *Cln3* to produce this phenotype. As in cathepsin D deficient mice, there is evidence for dysregulated autophagy in $Cln3^{\Delta ex7/8}$ mice (Cao et al., 2006), which may represent a prosurvival feedback response. Deficiency or loss of *Cln3* also leads to an increased expression of lysosomal acid phosphatase and the lysosomal associated membrane protein LAMP2 (Pohl et al., 2007), perhaps as a compensatory mechanism in response to accumulated storage material. An increased sensitivity to Ca^{2+} mediated cell death has been suggested to be the result of a loss of interaction of mutated CLN3 with calsenilin, rendering neurons vulnerable to raised intracellular calcium concentrations (Chang et al., 2007). Additionally, conditionally immortalized cell lines from $Cln3^{\Delta ex7/8}$ mice display a range of membrane trafficking defects, mitochondrial abnormalities, and reduced survival to oxidative stress (Fossale et al., 2004). Profiling of gene expression in primary neuron cultures from $Cln3^{\Delta ex1-6}$ mice has also implicated mitochondrial dysfunction in CLN3 disease, juvenile pathogenesis (Luiro et al., 2006), in addition to evidence for synaptic and cytoskeletal defects. Taken together, these data consistently point to endocytic and vesicular trafficking defects as a consequence of CLN3 deficiency (Fossale et al., 2004, Luiro et al., 2004, Luiro et al., 2006). Some of these effects may be mediated via the loss of reported interactions of CLN3 with the fodrin cytoskeleton (Uusi-Rauva et al., 2008), although other mechanisms and potential interactors of CLN3 are currently under investigation. Recently, based on work in wild-type, $Cln3^{lacZ/+}$, and $Cln3^{lacZ/LacZ}$ mice, an osmoregulated role for CLN3 in renal control of water and potassium balance has been suggested (Stein et al., 2010).

CLN5 DISEASE; *Cln5* MUTANT MICE

A mouse model for Finnish variant late infantile NCL (vLINCL$_{Fin}$/CLN5) has been generated by insertion of a selection cassette into exon 3 of *Cln5* (Kopra et al., 2004). This insertion results in a frameshift mutation to produce a premature stop codon and truncated CLN5 protein, which is predicted to be similar in effect to the p.Glu253Stop mutation in human *CLN5* (Holmberg et al., 2000). Compared to mouse models of other forms of late infantile NCL, CLN5 deficient mice ($Cln5^{-/-}$) display a relatively slowly progressing neurological disorder with severe visual disturbances from 5 months of age onwards, but only moderate effects upon brain atrophy even in aged mutant mice (Kopra et al., 2004). Gene profiling revealed an early upregulation of immune response genes in CLN5 deficient mice (Kopra et al., 2004), consistent with staining for markers of astrocytosis and microglial activation in these mice. More recent microarray studies suggest that common cellular pathways may be affected in CLN5 and PPT1 deficient mouse models (von Schantz et al., 2008), with prominent alterations in protein phosphorylation and cytoskeleton in both mouse models.

In contrast to PPT1 deficient mice, neuron loss is relatively delayed and appears to progress slowly in $Cln5^{-/-}$ mice, with a loss of GABAergic interneuron populations only evident from 6 months of age (Kopra et al., 2004), although this does not result in an obvious spontaneous seizure phenotype. In common with other mouse models of NCL, *Cln5* deficient mice also display a progressive loss of neurons within the thalamocortical system (von Schantz et al., 2009), but the relative timing of these events in the thalamus and cortex appears to be specific to this mouse model. Indeed, in marked contrast to other forms of NCL, neuron loss in *Cln5*$^{-/-}$ mice began in the cortex and only subsequently occurred within thalamic relay nuclei. Nevertheless, as in other NCL mouse models (Weimer et al., 2006, Kielar et al., 2007), this progressive thalamocortical neuron loss occurs first and is most pronounced within the visual system (von Schantz et al., 2009). At present, there are no reports of any attempted therapeutic intervention in CLN5 deficient mice.

CLN6 DISEASE; *Cln6*^{nclf} MUTANT MICE

The *nclf* mutation was first observed in 1991 in a laboratory mouse colony, almost lost by inbreeding, but recovered using frozen embryos and test matings (Bronson et al., 1998). In the new colony, 8-month-old mice developed rear limb paresis that progressed over several months to spastic paralysis and death, possibly due to seizures. Mice also had a slowly progressing retinal degeneration from 4 months. Inclusion material was present in the brain as early as 11 days, and became widespread. Sudanophilic, autofluorescent intraneuronal inclusions in these mice contain subunit c of mitochondrial ATP synthase. There was a reactive gliosis by 6 months that, on further study, was shown to be an early microglial response that closely mimics the phenotype of CLN6 deficient South Hampshire sheep in accurately predicting the distribution of subsequent neurodegeneration (Oswald et al., 2005). It will be important to determine if this reactive phenotype is also evident prenatally in *Cln6*^{nclf} mice, as has been demonstrated in South Hampshire sheep (Kay et al., 2006). It is also now apparent that these CLN6 deficient sheep also display a complex pattern of interneuron loss that is determined by where these cells are located and their connectivity (Oswald et al., 2008), and similar phenotypes are emerging in *Cln6*^{nclf} mice (J. Cooper et al. unpublished observations).

When the human *CLN6* gene was cloned (Gao et al., 2002, Wheeler et al., 2002), it was revealed that *Cln6*^{nclf} mutant mice closely model the corresponding human disease. Indeed, the insertion mutation in exon 4 of *Cln6* present in *Cln6*^{nclf} mice accurately reproduces the frameshift mutation present in CLN6 disease, late infantile patients from Costa Rica (Gao et al., 2002, Wheeler et al., 2002).

Cln6^{nclf} mice remain relatively uncharacterized neuropathologically, although first indications suggest that these mice display many of the characteristic features of other mouse models of NCL (J. Cooper et al., unpublished observations), including synaptic and axonal pathology early in disease progression (Kielar et al., 2009). The phenotype of *Cln6*^{nclf} mice resembles that of *Cln8*^{mnd} mice in some, but not all respects. Both mice display many of the characteristic features of other mouse models of NCL (J. Cooper et al., unpublished observations), including synaptic and axonal pathology early in disease progression (Kielar et al., 2009). The neurological phenotypes of *Cln6*^{nclf} and *Cln8*^{mnd} mice are broadly similar, but are more pronounced and rapidly progressing in *Cln8*^{mnd} mice (Bronson et al., 1998, Cooper et al., 1999), although the microglial response is seen earlier in *Cln6*^{nclf} mice (Oswald et al., 2005).

CLN8 DISEASE; *Cln8*^{mnd} MUTANT MICE

Displaying a profound and progressive motor dysfunction, the *Cln8*^{mnd} mutant mouse was originally thought to be a model of motor neuron disease (Messer and Flaherty, 1986, Messer et al., 1987). However, closer examination of these mice revealed a phenotype that more closely resembled a form of NCL (Bronson et al., 1993, Cooper et al., 1999). These original *Cln8*^{mnd} mutant mice had a progressive retinal atrophy with onset by 5 weeks, and very advanced by 2 months (Bronson et al., 1993, Chang et al., 1994). On a C57BL/6 background there was spastic limb paresis by 6 months, with paralysis by 9 months, and premature death at 10–12 months, probably due to seizures (Bronson et al., 1993).

Neurodegeneration is present in *Cln8*^{mnd} mutant mice, with their motor abnormalities coinciding with degenerative loss and swelling of motor neurons in the spinal cord, loss of Nissl substance and redistribution of neuronal cytoplasmic neurofilaments (Messer et al., 1995, Fujita et al., 1998). Sudanophilic, autofluorescent intraneuronal inclusions that contain subunit c of mitochondrial ATP synthase, are present within a month of birth. Ultrastructurally, cerebral and extracerebral inclusions are of the rectilinear complex and lamellar types. Biochemical analyses have shown that dolichol-linked oligosaccharides also accumulate in the storage bodies in *Cln8*^{mnd} mutant mice (Faust et al., 1994).

Accumulation of the autofluorescent storage material has been extensively studied as a marker of disease progression in *Cln8*^{mnd} mutant mice by several groups (Rodman et al., 1998).

When the *CLN8* gene underlying human variant late infantile NCL was cloned (Ranta et al., 1999), it was revealed that *Cln8*^{mnd} mutant mice closely model the corresponding human disease. The truncation mutation present in the *Cln8*^{mnd} mouse is predicted to completely abolish its function and closely mimics the severe mutation in CLN8 disease, late infantile patients rather than the more slowly progressing clinical presentation of CLN8 disease, EPMR patients (Ranta et al., 1999). The neurological phenotypes of *Cln6*^{nclf} and *Cln8*^{mnd} mice are broadly similar, but are more pronounced and rapidly progressing in *Cln8*^{mnd} mice (Bronson et al., 1998, Cooper et al., 1999).

The neuropathological phenotype of *Cln8*^{mnd} mice has been explored in some detail, with much of the focus understandably falling upon the progression of events within the spinal cord. A variety of mechanisms have been proposed, which can act to shed light on the onset and progression of pathological changes elsewhere in the CNS of these mice. An early glial response and upregulation of pro-inflammatory cytokines was first reported in the spinal cord of *Cln8*^{mnd} mice (Fujita et al., 1998, Mennini et al., 2004), occurring before motor abnormalities and in the absence of motor neuron death. These findings may be related to the altered expression of ionotropic glutamate receptors in spinal cord of these mice (Mennini et al., 2002), which may alter glutamatergic neurotransmission and contribute to neuron loss. In this context, altered levels of glutamate have also been reported in the *Cln8*^{mnd} CNS via metabolomic profiling (Griffin et al., 2002), a finding that is replicated in *Cln3* mutant mice (Pears et al., 2005) and CLN6 deficient sheep (Pears et al., 2007).

Since their identification as an accurate model of CLN8 disease, *Cln8*^{mnd} mice are currently being re-evaluated. Compared to CLN3 deficient mice (Seigel et al., 2002), *Cln8*^{mnd} mice display an earlier onset of cell loss within the retina (Guarneri et al., 2004, Seigel et al., 2005), which may be associated with increased oxidative stress (Guarneri et al., 2004). *Cln8*^{mnd} mice also display many features characteristic of mouse models of other forms NCL including the progressive build-up of autofluorescent storage material, loss of GABAergic interneuron populations (Cooper et al., 1999), but also display regionally selective effects on white matter, neuron survival and pronounced glial activation in the early stages of disease progression (Mennini et al., 2006, J. Cooper et al., unpublished observations). Recently, the onset and progression of behavioural abnormalities has begun to be explored in this mouse model, with evidence for increased activity, poor contextual and cued memory, and heightened aggression early in disease progression (Bolivar et al., 2002) and impaired performance in a T-maze (Wendt et al., 2005). Longitudinal behavioural data of this type will be useful for judging the efficacy of future therapeutic interventions in these and other mouse models of NCL.

CLN7 DISEASE MUTANT MICE

The latest NCL gene to be identified encodes the lysosomal transporter MFSD8, recently identified to be the gene locus mutated in CLN7 disease or Turkish variant late infantile NCL (Siintola et al., 2007). This is one of the few NCLs for which no mouse model is yet available.

OTHER MUTANT MICE THAT DISPLAY AN NCL-LIKE PHENOTYPE

The generation and characterization of a variety of null mutant mice has revealed phenotypes that in some respects are similar to NCL mouse models. Although mutations in these genes may not (yet) have been associated with a human NCL, these mice may nevertheless provide insights into the disease mechanisms that operate in these and related disorders. The first report of *Ppt1* null mutant mice (Gupta et al., 2001), also described the phenotype of mice with a null mutation in the *Ppt2* gene encoding palmitoyl protein thioesterase 2, a lysosomal thioesterase that shares homology with PPT1. The phenotype of these *Ppt2* null mutant mice (*Ppt2*$^{-/-}$) was initially described as a comparatively later onset neurodegenerative disorder that showed some typical NCL-like features (Gupta et al., 2001). However, it is now apparent that unlike the NCLs, there are also distinctive and pronounced visceral manifestations of PPT2 deficiency, which severely affect the bone marrow, spleen and pancreas of these mice (Gupta et al., 2003).

Since the discovery that mutations in cathepsin D underlie some forms of congenital and later onset human NCL (Siintola et al., 2006, Steinfeld et al., 2006), it is now emerging that mutations in other cathepsins may produce a similar phenotype. In addition to bulk protein degradation, cathepsins have been proposed to have diverse range of functions that includes antigen presentation and proteolytic activation of proproteins (Brix et al., 2008). In contrast with more widely expressed lysosomal cysteine proteases, cathepsin F displays a more restricted pattern of expression and has roles in the degradation of lipoproteins (Wang et al., 1998, Lindstedt et al., 2003, Oorni et al., 2004) and antigen processing (Shi et al., 2000). CTSF-deficient mice (*Ctsf*$^{-/-}$) were recently generated by targeted replacement of exons 7–9 by an insertion cassette (Tang et al., 2006), resulting in a slowly progressing neurological disorder that resembles late onset forms of NCL. These *Ctsf*$^{-/-}$ mice display widespread progressive accumulation of autofluorescent storage inclusions in the CNS, significant neuromuscular and motor deficits, and spontaneous seizures in more severely affected animals (Tang et al., 2006). Although analysis of 13 adult onset NCL patients did not reveal any mutations in the human *CTSF* gene (Tang et al., 2006), more detailed analysis of these CTSF deficient mice reveals many reactive and neurodegenerative features characteristic of other mouse models of NCL (J. Cooper et al., unpublished observations).

The family of chloride channel (ClC) proteins are involved in many physiological processes, and act either as channels or voltage dependent exchangers for chloride ions (Cl^-) (Jentsch, 2007). These proteins reside either at the plasma membrane or in intracellular vesicles of the endosomal–lysosomal system and are implicated in the progressive acidification of vesicles along this vesicular pathway or in regulating vesicular chloride concentration (Jentsch, 2007). Mutations in the genes encoding these ClC proteins give rise to a range of conditions, including the formation of kidney stones in Dent disease, or a variety of neurodegenerative and osteopetrotic features (Jentsch, 2007). Amongst these phenotypes mutations in *Clcn7* and *Clcn6* have been reported to share many features in common with the NCLs, but display distinctive features not present in any human NCL. For example, mutations in *Clcn7* produce a CNS phenotype that resembles the NCLs, but also results in pronounced osteopetrosis due to deficient osteoclast function (Frattini et al., 2003, Steward, 2003). However, one CLCN7 mouse model does not exhibit osteopetrosis, due to the presence of an alternative transcript that provides CLCN7 function in the bone, but displays severe neuronal retinal degeneration which closely resembles NCL (Rajan et al., 2010). The normal function of CLCN7 has been shown to be dependent on the presence of its subunit OSTM1 (Chalhoub et al., 2003), with deletion of *Ostm1* producing a phenotype that closely resembles murine CLCN7 deficiency including osteopetrosis (Lange et al., 2006). The CNS phenotype of *Clcn7*$^{-/-}$ or grey lethal mutant mice, which have a spontaneous mutation in *Ostm1*, is of an early onset and rapidly progressive neurodegenerative disorder (Kasper et al., 2005, Kornak et al., 2006; Pressey et al., 2010), which closely resembles that of CTSD deficient mice (Partanen et al., 2008, Pressey et al., 2010). Recent data from mice in which *Clcn7* alone was mutated, suggests that both astrocytes and microglia are activated by factors released by dysfunctional CLCN7 deficient neurons before they die (Wartosch et al., 2009), In contrast, CLCN6 deficient mice display a much later onset and slowly progressing neurodegenerative condition with a characteristic accumulation of storage material that is confined largely to the proximal part of the axon hillock (Poët et al., 2006). However, a more detailed survey of the CLCN6 deficient CNS reveals a phenotype that does not closely resemble NCL mouse models (J. Cooper et al., Pressey et al., 2006 unpublished observations).

As yet, no human form of NCL has been identified with mutations in *CLCN6* or *CLCN7* (Kornak et al., 2006, Poët et al., 2006), but it cannot be excluded that mutations in these genes may yet be identified in novel rare forms of human NCL. Two unrelated patients with NCL have been described who carry a single mutation in *CLCN6* on one chromosome (Poët et al., 2006), and one was subsequently found to be homozygous for mutation in *CLN5* (Xin et al., 2010). Mutations in *Clcn3* also produce a neurodegenerative phenotype (Stobrawa et al., 2001, Dickerson et al., 2002, Yoshikawa et al., 2002). Nevertheless, these events occur in the absence of storage material accumulation (Kasper et al., 2005), although this was initially reported in another strain of CLCN3 deficient mice (Yoshikawa et al., 2002). Indeed, the neurodegenerative phenotype of these mice is distinct quite from the NCLs, with neuron loss so severe in the hippocampal formation to produce complete loss of this structure (Kasper et al., 2005). The continued systematic analysis of mice with mutations in other ClC proteins, or other proteins expressed within the endosomal–lysosomal system is highly likely to provide novel insights in to disease pathogenesis. Whether these represent new forms of NCL, or merely related phenotypes remains to be determined, but direct comparison to established NCL mouse models is likely to be informative.

Summary

With animal models now available in many species, there are many resources available for investigating NCL disease biology, each with their particular advantages and limitations. As reviewed elsewhere in this volume, the powerful genetic tools available for *Drosophila* and zebrafish make them ideally suited for functional screens to finally reveal the pathways in which NCL gene products act. It is also likely that these lower species will prove particularly useful for rapidly and effectively screening potential therapeutic compounds. Nevertheless, the very simplicity of these models also limits their use for understanding events within a much more complex CNS. This can be achieved more easily in larger animal species, but with no reliable methods yet available for homologous recombination in dogs or sheep, we are limited to using spontaneous mutants and have no control of which gene or mutation is present.

This is where mouse models represent a relatively good compromise solution for studying NCL neurobiology. Recent advances in gene targeting strategies have made it possible to target particular genes, to introduce defined mutations that can be induced in specific tissues or times of development in mice. Such more complex approaches are only just beginning in NCL research, but the existence of a wide panel of mutant mice that bear mutations in defined functional pathways provide an invaluable resource for crossing to NCL mouse models. In this fashion, it will be possible to test ideas about pathogenesis by determining if the disease course is altered in the offspring of these crosses.

Although only at the early stages of using such crossbreeding approaches, a great deal of important information has already come from the analysis of existing NCL mouse models. Indeed, despite the relative simplicity of the mouse CNS, especially in the organization of the cortical mantle, significant new findings about disease progression have been made by systematically studying these models, for example, the relatively early involvement of reactive changes before the onset of neuron loss, pronounced effects within the thalamocortical system, and the pathological targeting of synapses. Although generally consistent themes emerge about pathological endpoints, it is becoming clear that the exact sequence in which events occur differs remarkably between different forms of NCL. Moreover some features, such as the autoimmune response present in CLN3 disease, juvenile, appear to be specific to one form of NCL. Some of these differences between forms of NCL are sufficiently striking to raise the question whether the traditional view of these disorders as a related group will need to be reconsidered. Instead, subgroups of NCL types that more closely resemble one another are likely to emerge, with new mutant mice that display NCL-like phenotypes still to be added to this classification.

The wealth of new data about where and when pathological events occur in the NCL brain will be crucial for the efficient targeting of therapeutic approaches to places or times that they can be most effective. Although we now have relatively detailed neuropathological landmarks of disease progression, there remains a pressing need to obtain more detailed data of the behavioural consequences of gene mutation. Indeed, as research moves more towards devising effective therapeutic solutions, it will become increasingly important to be able to judge the relative efficacy of these approaches on all aspects of the disease present in each mouse model.

ZEBRAFISH MODELS

Disease modelling in zebrafish

Small vertebrate models of disease have been developed because many animals can be housed and cared for with ease, at low cost, and with a short generation time. Using these criteria, the zebrafish is far superior to the mouse, the other traditional small vertebrate model organism. The zebrafish is, however, further from humans both in evolutionary time and in anatomy and physiology. Nevertheless, the zebrafish retina is more similar to that of humans than the mouse retina, suggesting that the zebrafish may be particularly useful for studying retinal degeneration in NCL (Pujic and Malicki, 2004). In fact, the zebrafish neurulation process (Lowery and Sive, 2004) and functional neuroanatomy (Mueller and Wulliman, 2005) is closer to that of other vertebrates and humans than was previously thought. Despite this, the anatomy of the zebrafish nervous system is far simpler than that of the mouse (Wulliman et al., 1996, Mueller and Wulliman, 2005), and the lack of a cortex is particularly notable. The simplicity of the zebrafish nervous system, however, means that zebrafish neuroanatomy is well-characterized and relatively easy to study.

The zebrafish does have other advantages over the mouse. Zebrafish embryos and larvae are optically clear and develop externally as large clutches, meaning that the very earliest stages of development can be easily visualized and manipulated without sacrificing the mother, as is necessary with mouse models. Zebrafish are amenable to embryological manipulations such as injections, transplantations, and ablations, and provide a particularly excellent system for studying fluorescently tagged protein localization in real time *in vivo*, rather than in cell culture (Reugels et al., 2006). Such an approach identifies where a protein may act within the cell, organ, or whole organism, and whether this varies between different mutant and morphant animals. Examining a transgenic expressing a fluorescent protein in specific cells (reviewed in Udvadia and Linney, 2003) will therefore be useful for assessing how phenotypes change over time in zebrafish models of NCL.

The zebrafish is best known as a genetic organism and many thousands of mutants have been generated, a great many of which have had their mutations cloned and phenotypes studied. Many such mutants are now considered to be valid disease models. However, some disease-modelling techniques that are possible in the mouse, such as generating mutations that replicate human mutations, are not yet feasible in zebrafish. Disease-modelling technologies that are possible in the zebrafish are described in more detail below.

Perhaps most importantly, the zebrafish is becoming the vertebrate of choice for drug discovery. Compounds can be screened *in vivo* in a high-throughput manner for both toxicity and phenotypic rescue (Zon and Peterson, 2005, Barros et al., 2008). Such screening currently requires a consistent phenotype that lasts for 1 or 2 days, and changes in the phenotype should be easy to assess, ideally using an automated approach. It is likely that video tracking of the swimming pattern, and calculating the distance travelled by zebrafish embryos or larvae in a specific period of time, would be a suitable assay for drug screening, particularly as zebrafish NCL models are likely to have impaired mobility similar to that seen in patients.

The zebrafish is therefore useful for both embryological and genetic manipulations and it is these attributes that have led many researchers to turn to the zebrafish for modelling diseases (Russell, 2003, Guo, 2004). Now NCL researchers are also turning to this organism, as it is possible to study the consequences of NCL protein knockdown, overexpression, and interaction at the level of the whole organism, individual tissues, and within the cell. Several key questions about the nature of NCL may be addressed relatively quickly and easily using the zebrafish: In what order do tissues begin to show defects in NCL models? What is the primary defect and what happens as a consequence? In which tissue(s) or cells are the NCL proteins required? What pathways do the NCL proteins act in? What controls NCL protein localization? Does replacing a NCL protein or a downstream target in one cell result in phenotypic rescue in adjacent cells? Will transient rescue of the nervous system defects result in NCL animals surviving longer and, as a consequence, reveal phenotypes in other tissues?

Assessing gene function in zebrafish

As an experimental organism, zebrafish can be exploited in many ways (reviewed in Nüsslein-Volhard and Dahm, 2002). Zebrafish are amenable to a variety of simple gain- and loss-of-function techniques. Gain-of-function experiments are used to reveal what a gene product can do when expressed in an ectopic position and/or at inappropriate times. The gene is expressed in the whole embryo by mRNA injection into the fertilized egg, where the mRNA and/or exogenous protein may perdure for a couple of days. Alternatively, mRNA can be introduced at specific times and locations either by electroporation (Concha et al., 2003, Hendricks and Jesuthasan, 2007) or via an inducible expression system such as laser-induced heat-shock (Halloran et al., 2000) or the Gal4-UAS system (Asakawa and Kawakami, 2008).

Forward mutagenesis screens are used to generate loss-of-function and other mutations in zebrafish. They produce fish with randomly induced mutations which can be either screened for NCL-like phenotypes, which may help to uncover other genes involved in NCL, or for mutations in genes known to cause NCL (Wienholds et al., 2003, Stemple, 2004). Using this method, known as TILLING, it is possible to uncover not only null alleles but also a series of weaker alleles, which may reveal more about the function(s) of the mutated genes. Alternatively morpholinos, which are modified antisense oligonucleotides that are designed to knockdown the function of target genes such as those that cause NCL, can be injected into the embryo (Ekker and Larson, 2001). Although morpholinos tend to be effective only for a few days in the embryo, this method is nevertheless powerful for providing evidence that NCL can be modelled in zebrafish and for demonstrating the consequences of NCL gene knockdown for the development of the CNS and the animal as a whole. Based on studies in human patients and mouse models of NCL, the possibility remains that early CNS development is incomplete or abnormal in NCL diseases. This view is supported by morpholino knockdown experiments in zebrafish which are beginning to reveal the nature of early CNS defects (C. Russell, unpublished results). In addition, studying the recovery of the zebrafish after the NCL gene morpholino becomes ineffective may shed light on the efficacy of replacement gene therapies.

Some disease-modelling techniques that are possible in the mouse, such as generating mutations that replicate human mutations using knock-in technology, are not yet feasible in zebrafish. To study the effect of a specific human mutation in zebrafish, that mutation can be introduced via mRNA injection into a newly fertilized embryo that is genetically null for the gene. The drawback of this approach compared to the mouse knock-in approach is that there is no temporal and spatial control of mutated gene expression. However, this may not be a problem for the NCLs as most genes are expressed fairly ubiquitously.

When designing therapeutic strategies, it is important to know whether or not a gene product acts cell-autonomously. Chimeric zebrafish can be simply generated by tissue transplantation to answer this question. For example, if a small clone of wild-type cells in a mutant embryo can rescue the phenotype of neighbouring mutant cells, this indicates that there is a secreted factor downstream of the normal NCL gene product that could be of potential therapeutic use. The distance over which rescue is effective is indicative of the distance over which the therapy could work. Analysis of chimeras can also reveal in which tissues a gene product is required, a significant issue in the NCLs, with widely expressed gene products that display tissue-specific phenotypes and selective neuronal vulnerability upon mutation (reviewed in Cooper et al., 2006).

It is similarly important to understand any complications that may arise from delivering a therapy solely to the brain or for only a short period of time. In such cases, although the life of a patient may be extended, the effects of the disease may then be seen in organs other than the nervous system. Transiently rescuing a zebrafish NCL gene mutant with wild-type mRNA injected into the newly fertilized embryo, will allow the effect of such treatments to be recapitulated and the likelihood of late onset symptoms to be assessed. The zebrafish is particularly suited to this approach as the whole embryos can be easily and quickly examined.

Exploring genetic interactions in zebrafish

Epistatic analyses, to reveal whether gene products function in the same or different pathways, are also relatively easy in zebrafish, either by crossbreeding to produce mutants with multiple gene deficits or by combining loss-of-function and gain-of-function techniques. In fact, very little is known about the pathways in which the NCL gene products normally function, and whether or not they function in one or more shared pathways. What is known comes mostly from *in vitro* approaches and it is not yet verified whether the same interactions occur *in vivo*. An epistatic approach in zebrafish is therefore ideal for understanding why mutations in so many diverse genes cause similar NCL phenotypes, albeit with markedly different ages of onset (Mole et al., 2005). Similarly, the zebrafish can be used to test if certain tissues or signalling pathways are necessary for NCL to develop, and whether perturbing a signalling pathway, for example, modifies the NCL phenotype. In fact, screening for randomly induced mutations that modify the NCL phenotype will be a powerful method to uncover interacting loci.

Towards zebrafish models of NCL

Zebrafish have orthologues of many of the genes mutated in different forms of human NCL. One orthologue each of *CLN1/PPT1*, *CLN2/TPP1* (Wlodawer et al., 2003), *CLN3*, *CLN5*, *CLN6*, *CLN7/MFSD8* (Siintola et al., 2007), *CLN8*, and *CLN10/CSTD* are found on the zebrafish Ensembl and ZFIN databases (http://www.ensembl.org/Danio_rerio/index.html and http://www.zfin.org) or identified by BLAST homology searches. The zebrafish genome frequently contains two homologues of each gene found in mice or humans. When this is the case, it is often necessary to knockdown both genes to create a full loss-of-function phenotype. The fact that the zebrafish contains only one orthologue of each gene means it will be relatively simple to create zebrafish NCL models.

The sequence of zebrafish *TPP1* has been published and modelling indicates that the protein shares a similar structure at the active site as that of the human protein (Wlodawer et al., 2003). This suggests a conserved function for the human and zebrafish TPP1 proteins. TPP1 morpholino and mutant experiments, in which *TPP1* gene function is knocked-down in zebrafish embryos, are already underway and these studies are demonstrating that the NCLs can indeed be modelled in this species (C. Russell, unpublished observations), thereby fuelling the search for zebrafish models of other forms of NCL. There is a list of genes for which mutations are being searched by TILLING (http://www.sanger.ac.uk/cgi-bin/Projects/D_rerio/mutres/tracking.pl). To date, this list contains mutations in *CLN1/PPT1* (one allele) and *CLN2/TPP1* (two alleles), with requests to find mutations in *CLN3*, *CLN5*, *CLN6*, *CLN7/MFSD8*, and *CLN8* (no alleles found to date).

The genetics and biology of zebrafish make it the ideal vertebrate for not only addressing basic questions about the functions of the genes that underlie each form of NCL but also for disease modelling and therapeutic agent screening.

REFERENCES

Ahtiainen L, Kolikova J, Mutka AL, Luiro K, Gentile M, Ikonen E, Khiroug L, Jalanko A, & Kopra O (2007) Palmitoyl protein thioesterase 1 (Ppt1)-deficient mouse neurons show alterations in cholesterol metabolism and calcium homeostasis prior to synaptic dysfunction. *Neurobiol Dis*, 28, 52–64.

Asakawa K & Kawakami K (2008) Targeted gene expression by the Gal4-UAS system in zebrafish. *Dev Growth Differ*, 50, 391–399.

Barros TP, Alderton WK, Reynolds HM, Roach AG, & Berghmans S (2008) Zebrafish: an emerging technology for in vivo pharmacological assessment to identify potential safety liabilities in early drug discovery. *Br J Pharmacol*, 154, 1400–1413.

Benedict JW, Sommers CA, & Pearce DA (2007) Progressive oxidative damage in the central nervous system of a murine model for juvenile Batten disease. *J Neurosci Res*, 85, 2882–2891.

Bible E, Gupta P, Hofmann SL, & Cooper JD (2004) Regional and cellular neuropathology in the palmitoyl protein thioesterase-1 null mutant mouse model of infantile neuronal ceroid lipofuscinosis. *Neurobiol Dis*, 16, 346–359.

Bolivar VJ, Scott Ganus J, & Messer A (2002) The development of behavioral abnormalities in the motor neuron degeneration (mnd) mouse. *Brain Res*, 937, 74–82.

Brix K, Dunkhorst A, Mayer K, & Jordans S (2008) Cysteine cathepsins: cellular roadmap to different functions. *Biochimie*, 90, 194–207.

Bronson RT, Donahue LR, Johnson KR, Tanner A, Lane PW, & Faust JR (1998) Neuronal ceroid lipofuscinosis (nclf), a new disorder of the mouse linked to chromosome 9. *Am J Med Genet*, 77, 289–297.

Bronson RT, Lake BD, Cook S, Taylor S, & Davisson MT (1993) Motor neuron degeneration of mice is a model of neuronal ceroid lipofuscinosis (Batten's disease). *Ann Neurol*, 33, 381–385.

Cabrera-Salazar MA, Roskelley EM, Bu J, Hodges BL, Yew N, Dodge JC, Shihabuddin LS, Sohar I, Sleat DE, Scheule RK, Davidson BL, Cheng SH, Lobel P, & Passini MA (2007) Timing of therapeutic intervention determines functional and survival outcomes in a mouse model of late infantile Batten disease. *Mol Ther*, 15, 1782–1788.

Cao Y, Espinola JA, Fossale E, Massey AC, Cuervo AM, MacDonald ME, & Cotman SL (2006) Autophagy is disrupted in a knock-in mouse model of juvenile neuronal ceroid lipofuscinosis. *J Biol Chem*, 281, 20483–20493.

Chalhoub N, Benachenhou N, Rajapurohitam V, Pata M, Ferron M, Frattini A, Villa A, & Vacher J (2003) Grey-lethal mutation induces severe malignant autosomal recessive osteopetrosis in mouse and human. *Nat Med*, 9, 399–406.

Chan CH, Mitchison HM, & Pearce DA (2008) Transcript and in silico analysis of CLN3 in juvenile neuronal ceroid lipofuscinosis and associated mouse models. *Hum Mol Genet*, 17, 3332–3339.

Chang B, Bronson RT, Hawes NL, Roderick TH, Peng C, Hageman GS, & Heckenlively JR (1994) Retinal degeneration in motor neuron degeneration: a mouse model of ceroid lipofuscinosis. *Invest Ophthalmol Vis Sci*, 35, 1071–1076.

Chang JW, Choi H, Kim HJ, Jo DG, Jeon YJ, Noh JY, Park WJ, & Jung YK (2007) Neuronal vulnerability of CLN3 deletion to calcium-induced cytotoxicity is mediated by calsenilin. *Hum Mol Genet*, 16, 317–326.

Chang M, Cooper JD, Sleat DE, Cheng SH, Dodge JC, Passini MA, Lobel P, & Davidson BL (2008) Intraventricular enzyme replacement improves disease phenotypes in a mouse model of late infantile neuronal ceroid lipofuscinosis. *Mol Ther*, 16, 649–656.

Chattopadhyay S, Ito M, Cooper JD, Brooks AI, Curran TM, Powers JM, & Pearce DA (2002a) An autoantibody inhibitory to glutamic acid decarboxylase in the neurodegenerative disorder Batten disease. *Hum Mol Genet*, 11, 1421–1431.

Chattopadhyay S, Kriscenski-Perry E, Wenger DA, & Pearce DA (2002b) An autoantibody to GAD65 in sera of patients with juvenile neuronal ceroid lipofuscinoses. *Neurology*, 59, 1816–1817.

Chen YH, Chang M, & Davidson BL (2009) Molecular signatures of disease brain endothelia provide new sites for CNS-directed enzyme therapy. *Nat Med*, 15, 1215–1218.

Concha ML, Russell C, Regan JC, Tawk M, Sidi S, Gilmour DT, Kapsimali M, Sumoy L, Goldstone K, Amaya E, Kimelman D, Nicolson T, Grunder S, Gomperts M, Clarke JD, & Wilson SW (2003) Local tissue interactions across the dorsal midline of the forebrain establish CNS laterality. *Neuron*, 39, 423–438.

Cooper JD (2008) Moving towards therapies for juvenile Batten disease? *Exp Neurol*, 211, 329–331.

Cooper JD, Messer A, Feng AK, Chua-Couzens J, & Mobley WC (1999) Apparent loss and hypertrophy of interneurons in a mouse model of neuronal ceroid lipofuscinosis: evidence for partial response to insulin-like growth factor-1 treatment. *J Neurosci*, 19, 2556–2567.

Cooper JD, Russell C, & Mitchison HM (2006) Progress towards understanding disease mechanisms in small vertebrate models of neuronal ceroid lipofuscinosis. *Biochim Biophys Acta*, 1762, 873–889.

Cotman SL, Vrbanac V, Lebel LA, Lee RL, Johnson KA, Donahue LR, Teed AM, Antonellis K, Bronson RT, Lerner TJ, & MacDonald ME (2002) $Cln3^{\Delta ex7/8}$ knock-in mice with the common JNCL mutation exhibit progressive neurologic disease that begins before birth. *Hum Mol Genet*, 11, 2709–2721.

Dickerson LW, Bonthius DJ, Schutte BC, Yang B, Barna TJ, Bailey MC, Nehrke K, Williamson RA, & Lamb FS (2002) Altered GABAergic function accompanies hippocampal degeneration in mice lacking ClC-3 voltage-gated chloride channels. *Brain Res*, 958, 227–250.

Ekker SC & Larson JD (2001) Morphant technology in model developmental systems. *Genesis*, 30, 89–93.

Eliason SL, Stein CS, Mao Q, Tecedor L, Ding SL, Gaines DM, & Davidson BL (2007) A knock-in reporter model of Batten disease. *J Neurosci*, 27, 9826–9834.

Faust JR, Rodman JS, Daniel PF, Dice JF, & Bronson RT (1994) Two related proteolipids and dolichol-linked oligosaccharides accumulate in motor neuron degeneration mice (mnd/mnd), a model for neuronal ceroid lipofuscinosis. *J Biol Chem*, 269, 10150–10155.

Fossale E, Wolf P, Espinola JA, Lubicz-Nawrocka T, Teed AM, Gao H, Rigamonti D, Cattaneo E, MacDonald ME, & Cotman SL (2004) Membrane trafficking and mitochondrial abnormalities precede subunit c deposition in a cerebellar cell model of juvenile neuronal ceroid lipofuscinosis. *BMC Neurosci*, 5, 57.

Frattini A, Pangrazio A, Susani L, Sobacchi C, Mirolo M, Abinun M, Andolina M, Flanagan A, Horwitz EM, Mihci E, Notarangelo LD, Ramenghi U, Teti A, Van Hove J, Vujic D, Young T, Albertini A, Orchard PJ, Vezzoni P, & Villa A (2003) Chloride channel ClCN7 mutations are responsible for severe recessive, dominant, and intermediate osteopetrosis. *J Bone Miner Res*, 18, 1740–1747.

Fritchie K, Siintola E, Armao D, Lehesjoki AE, Marino T, Powell C, Tennison M, Booker JM, Koch S, Partanen S, Suzuki K, Tyynelä J, & Thorne LB (2009) Novel mutation and the first prenatal screening of cathepsin D deficiency (CLN10). *Acta Neuropathol*, 117, 201–208.

Fujita K, Yamauchi M, Matsui T, Titani K, Takahashi H, Kato T, Isomura G, Ando M, & Nagata Y (1998) Increase of glial fibrillary acidic protein fragments in the spinal cord of motor neuron degeneration mutant mouse. *Brain Res*, 785, 31–40.

Galvin N, Vogler C, Levy B, Kovacs A, Griffey M, & Sands MS (2008) A murine model of infantile neuronal ceroid lipofuscinosis – ultrastructural evaluation of storage in the central nervous system and viscera. *Pediatr Dev Pathol*, 11, 185–192.

Gao H, Boustany RM, Espinola JA, Cotman SL, Srinidhi L, Antonellis KA, Gillis T, Qin X, Liu S, Donahue LR,

Bronson RT, Faust JR, Stout D, Haines JL, Lerner TJ, & MacDonald ME (2002) Mutations in a novel CLN6-encoded transmembrane protein cause variant neuronal ceroid lipofuscinosis in man and mouse. *Am J Hum Genet*, 70, 324–335.

Griffey M, Bible E, Vogler C, Levy B, Gupta P, Cooper J, & Sands MS (2004) Adeno-associated virus 2-mediated gene therapy decreases autofluorescent storage material and increases brain mass in a murine model of infantile neuronal ceroid lipofuscinosis. *Neurobiol Dis*, 16, 360–369.

Griffey M, Macauley SL, Ogilvie JM, & Sands MS (2005) AAV2-mediated ocular gene therapy for infantile neuronal ceroid lipofuscinosis. *Mol Ther*, 12, 413–421.

Griffey MA, Wozniak D, Wong M, Bible E, Johnson K, Rothman SM, Wentz AE, Cooper JD, & Sands MS (2006) CNS-directed AAV2-mediated gene therapy ameliorates functional deficits in a murine model of infantile neuronal ceroid lipofuscinosis. *Mol Ther*, 13, 538–547.

Griffin JL, Muller D, Woograsingh R, Jowatt V, Hindmarsh A, Nicholson JK, & Martin JE (2002) Vitamin E deficiency and metabolic deficits in neuronal ceroid lipofuscinosis described by bioinformatics. *Physiol Genomics*, 11, 195–203.

Guarneri R, Russo D, Cascio C, D'Agostino S, Galizzi G, Bigini P, Mennini T, & Guarneri P (2004) Retinal oxidation, apoptosis and age- and sex-differences in the mnd mutant mouse, a model of neuronal ceroid lipofuscinosis. *Brain Res*, 1014, 209–220.

Guo S (2004) Linking genes to brain, behavior and neurological diseases: what can we learn from zebrafish? *Genes Brain Behav*, 3, 63–74.

Gupta P, Soyombo AA, Atashband A, Wisniewski KE, Shelton JM, Richardson JA, Hammer RE, & Hofmann SL (2001) Disruption of PPT1 or PPT2 causes neuronal ceroid lipofuscinosis in knockout mice. *Proc Natl Acad Sci U S A*, 98, 13566–13571.

Gupta P, Soyombo AA, Shelton JM, Wilkofsky IG, Wisniewski KE, Richardson JA, & Hofmann SL (2003) Disruption of PPT2 in mice causes an unusual lysosomal storage disorder with neurovisceral features. *Proc Natl Acad Sci U S A*, 100, 12325–12330.

Haapanen A, Ramadan UA, Autti T, Joensuu R, & Tyynelä J (2007) In vivo MRI reveals the dynamics of pathological changes in the brains of cathepsin D-deficient mice and correlates changes in manganese-enhanced MRI with microglial activation. *Magn Reson Imaging*, 25, 1024–1031.

Halloran MC, Sato-Maeda M, Warren JT, Su F, Lele Z, Krone PH, Kuwada JY, & Shoji W (2000) Laser-induced gene expression in specific cells of transgenic zebrafish. *Development*, 127, 1953–1960.

Hendricks M & Jesuthasan S (2007) Electroporation-based methods for in vivo, whole mount and primary culture analysis of zebrafish brain development. *Neural Dev*, 2, 6.

Holmberg V, Lauronen L, Autti T, Santavuori P, Savukoski M, Uvebrant P, Hofman I, Peltonen L, & Jarvela I (2000) Phenotype-genotype correlation in eight patients with Finnish variant late infantile NCL (CLN5). *Neurology*, 55, 579–581.

Jalanko A, Vesa J, Manninen T, von Schantz C, Minye H, Fabritius AL, Salonen T, Rapola J, Gentile M, Kopra O, & Peltonen L (2005) Mice with $Ppt1^{\Delta ex4}$ mutation replicate the INCL phenotype and show an inflammation-associated loss of interneurons. *Neurobiol Dis*, 18, 226–241.

Jentsch TJ (2007) Chloride and the endosomal-lysosomal pathway: emerging roles of CLC chloride transporters. *J Physiol*, 578, 633–640.

Kasper D, Planells-Cases R, Fuhrmann JC, Scheel O, Zeitz O, Ruether K, Schmitt A, Poet M, Steinfeld R, Schweizer M, Kornak U, & Jentsch TJ (2005) Loss of the chloride channel ClC-7 leads to lysosomal storage disease and neurodegeneration. *EMBO J*, 24, 1079–1091.

Katz ML, Shibuya H, Liu PC, Kaur S, Gao CL, & Johnson GS (1999) A mouse gene knockout model for juvenile ceroid-lipofuscinosis (Batten disease). *J Neurosci Res*, 57, 551–556.

Kay GW, Palmer DN, Rezaie P, & Cooper JD (2006) Activation of non-neuronal cells within the prenatal developing brain of sheep with neuronal ceroid lipofuscinosis. *Brain Pathol*, 16, 110–116.

Kielar C, Maddox L, Bible E, Pontikis CC, Macauley SL, Griffey MA, Wong M, Sands MS, & Cooper JD (2007) Successive neuron loss in the thalamus and cortex in a mouse model of infantile neuronal ceroid lipofuscinosis. *Neurobiol Dis*, 25, 150–162.

Kielar C, Wishart TM, Palmer A, Dihanich S, Wong AM, Macauley SL, Chan CH, Sands MS, Pearce DA, Cooper JD, & Gillingwater TH (2009) Molecular correlates of axonal and synaptic pathology in mouse models of Batten disease. *Hum Mol Genet*, 18, 4066–4080.

Kim SJ, Zhang Z, Hitomi E, Lee YC, & Mukherjee AB (2006) Endoplasmic reticulum stress-induced caspase-4 activation mediates apoptosis and neurodegeneration in INCL. *Hum Mol Genet*, 15, 1826–1834.

Kim SJ, Zhang Z, Sarkar C, Tsai PC, Lee YC, Dye L, & Mukherjee AB (2008) Palmitoyl protein thioesterase-1 deficiency impairs synaptic vesicle recycling at nerve terminals, contributing to neuropathology in humans and mice. *J Clin Invest*, 118, 3075–3086.

Kitzmüller C, Haines RL, Codlin S, Cutler DF, & Mole SE (2008) A function retained by the common mutant CLN3 protein is responsible for the late onset of juvenile neuronal ceroid lipofuscinosis. *Hum Mol Genet*, 17, 303–312.

Koike M, Nakanishi H, Saftig P, Ezaki J, Isahara K, Ohsawa Y, Schulz-Schaeffer W, Watanabe T, Waguri S, Kametaka S, Shibata M, Yamamoto K, Kominami E, Peters C, von Figura K, & Uchiyama Y (2000) Cathepsin D deficiency induces lysosomal storage with ceroid lipofuscin in mouse CNS neurons. *J Neurosci*, 20, 6898–6906.

Kopra O, Vesa J, von Schantz C, Manninen T, Minye H, Fabritius AL, Rapola J, van Diggelen OP, Saarela J, Jalanko A, & Peltonen L (2004) A mouse model for Finnish variant late infantile neuronal ceroid lipofuscinosis, CLN5, reveals neuropathology associated with early aging. *Hum Mol Genet*, 13, 2893–2906.

Kornak U, Kasper D, Bosl MR, Kaiser E, Schweizer M, Schulz A, Friedrich W, Delling G, & Jentsch TJ (2001) Loss of the ClC-7 chloride channel leads to osteopetrosis in mice and man. *Cell*, 104, 205–215.

Kornak U, Ostertag A, Branger S, Benichou O, & de Vernejoul MC (2006) Polymorphisms in the CLCN7 gene modulate bone density in postmenopausal women and in patients with autosomal dominant osteopetrosis type II. *J Clin Endocrinol Metab*, 91, 995–1000.

Kovács AD & Pearce DA (2008) Attenuation of AMPA receptor activity improves motor skills in a mouse model of juvenile Batten disease. *Exp Neurol*, 209, 288–291.

Kovács AD, Weimer JM, & Pearce DA (2006) Selectively increased sensitivity of cerebellar granule cells to AMPA receptor-mediated excitotoxicity in a mouse model of Batten disease. *Neurobiol Dis*, 22, 575–585.

Kovács AD, Saje A, Wong A, Szénási G, Kiricsi P, Szabó E, Cooper JD, Pearce DA (2010). Temporary inhibition of AMPA receptors induces a prolonged improvement of motor performance in a mouse model of juvenile Batten disease. Neuropharmacology. 2010 Oct 28. [Epub ahead of print] PMID: 20971125 [PubMed - as supplied by publisher]

Kriscenski-Perry E, Applegate CD, Serour A, Mhyre TR, Leonardo CC, & Pearce DA (2002) Altered flurothyl seizure induction latency, phenotype, and subsequent mortality in a mouse model of juvenile neuronal ceroid lipofuscinosis/Batten disease. *Epilepsia*, 43, 1137–1140.

Lange PF, Wartosch L, Jentsch TJ, & Fuhrmann JC (2006) ClC-7 requires Ostm1 as a beta-subunit to support bone resorption and lysosomal function. *Nature*, 440, 220–223.

Lei B, Tullis GE, Kirk MD, Zhang K, & Katz ML (2006) Ocular phenotype in a mouse gene knockout model for infantile neuronal ceroid lipofuscinosis. *J Neurosci Res*, 84, 1139–1149.

Lim MJ, Alexander N, Benedict JW, Chattopadhyay S, Shemilt SJ, Guerin CJ, Cooper JD, & Pearce DA (2007) IgG entry and deposition are components of the neuroimmune response in Batten disease. *Neurobiol Dis*, 25, 239–251.

Lim MJ, Beake J, Bible E, Curran TM, Ramirez-Montealegre D, Pearce DA, & Cooper JD (2006) Distinct patterns of serum immunoreactivity as evidence for multiple brain-directed autoantibodies in juvenile neuronal ceroid lipofuscinosis. *Neuropathol Appl Neurobiol*, 32, 469–482.

Lindstedt L, Lee M, Oorni K, Bromme D, & Kovanen PT (2003) Cathepsins F and S block HDL3-induced cholesterol efflux from macrophage foam cells. *Biochem Biophys Res Commun*, 312, 1019–1024.

Lowery LA & Sive H (2004) Strategies of vertebrate neurulation and a re-evaluation of teleost neural tube formation. *Mech Dev*, 121, 1189–1197.

Luiro K, Kopra O, Blom T, Gentile M, Mitchison HM, Hovatta I, Tornquist K, & Jalanko A (2006) Batten disease (JNCL) is linked to disturbances in mitochondrial, cytoskeletal, and synaptic compartments. *J Neurosci Res*, 84, 1124–1138.

Luiro K, Yliannala K, Ahtiainen L, Maunu H, Jarvela I, Kyttala A, & Jalanko A (2004) Interconnections of CLN3, Hook1 and Rab proteins link Batten disease to defects in the endocytic pathway. *Hum Mol Genet*, 13, 3017–3027.

Lyly A, Marjavaara SK, Kyttala A, Uusi-Rauva K, Luiro K, Kopra O, Martinez LO, Tanhuanpaa K, Kalkkinen N, Suomalainen A, Jauhiainen M, & Jalanko A (2008) Deficiency of the INCL protein Ppt1 results in changes in ectopic F1-ATP synthase and altered cholesterol metabolism. *Hum Mol Genet*, 17, 1406–1417.

Macauley SL, Wozniak DF, Kielar C, Tan Y, Cooper JD, & Sands MS (2009) Cerebellar pathology and motor deficits in the palmitoyl protein thioesterase 1-deficient mouse. *Exp Neurol*, 217, 124–135.

Mennini T, Bigini P, Cagnotto A, Carvelli L, Di Nunno P, Fumagalli E, Tortarolo M, Buurman WA, Ghezzi P, & Bendotti C (2004) Glial activation and TNFR-I upregulation precedes motor dysfunction in the spinal cord of mnd mice. *Cytokine*, 25, 127–135.

Mennini T, Bigini P, Ravizza T, Vezzani A, Calvaresi N, Tortarolo M, & Bendotti C (2002) Expression of glutamate receptor subtypes in the spinal cord of control and mnd mice, a model of motor neuron disorder. *J Neurosci Res*, 70, 553–560.

Messer A & Flaherty L (1986) Autosomal dominance in a late-onset motor neuron disease in the mouse. *J Neurogenet*, 3, 345–355.

Messer A, Plummer J, MacMillen MC, & Frankel WN (1995) Genetics of primary and timing effects in the mnd mouse. *Am J Med Genet*, 57, 361–364.

Messer A, Strominger NL, & Mazurkiewicz JE (1987) Histopathology of the late-onset motor neuron degeneration (Mnd) mutant in the mouse. *J Neurogenet*, 4, 201–213.

Mitchison HM, Bernard DJ, Greene ND, Cooper JD, Junaid MA, Pullarkat RK, de Vos N, Breuning MH, Owens JW, Mobley WC, Gardiner RM, Lake BD, Taschner PE, & Nussbaum RL (1999) Targeted disruption of the Cln3 gene provides a mouse model for Batten disease. The Batten Mouse Model Consortium [corrected]. *Neurobiol Dis*, 6, 321–334.

Mitchison HM, Lim MJ, & Cooper JD (2004) Selectivity and types of cell death in the neuronal ceroid lipofuscinoses. *Brain Pathol*, 14, 86–96.

Mole SE, Williams RE, & Goebel HH (2005) Correlations between genotype, ultrastructural morphology and clinical phenotype in the neuronal ceroid lipofuscinoses. *Neurogenetics*, 6, 107–126.

Mueller T & Wulliman MF (2005) *Atlas of Early Zebrafish Brain Development: A Tool for Molecular Neurogeneticists*. Amsterdam, Elsevier.

Mutka AL, Haapanen A, Kakela R, Lindfors M, Wright AK, Inkinen T, Hermansson M, Rokka A, Corthals G, Jauhiainen M, Gillingwater TH, Ikonen E, & Tyynelä J (2010) Murine cathepsin D deficiency is associated with dysmyelination/myelin disruption and accumulation of cholesteryl esters in the brain. *J Neurochem*, 112, 193–203.

Nakanishi H, Zhang J, Koike M, Nishioku T, Okamoto Y, Kominami E, von Figura K, Peters C, Yamamoto K, Saftig P, & Uchiyama Y (2001) Involvement of nitric oxide released from microglia-macrophages in pathological changes of cathepsin D-deficient mice. *J Neurosci*, 21, 7526–7533.

Nüsslein-Volhard C & Dahm R (2002) *Zebrafish (A Practical Approach)*. Oxford, Oxford University Press.

Oorni K, Sneck M, Bromme D, Pentikainen MO, Lindstedt KA, Mayranpaa M, Aitio H, & Kovanen PT (2004) Cysteine protease cathepsin F is expressed in human atherosclerotic lesions, is secreted by cultured macrophages, and modifies low density lipoprotein particles in vitro. *J Biol Chem*, 279, 34776–34784.

Oswald MJ, Palmer DN, Kay GW, Barwell KJ, & Cooper JD (2008) Location and connectivity determine GABAergic interneuron survival in the brains of South Hampshire sheep with CLN6 neuronal ceroid lipofuscinosis. *Neurobiol Dis*, 32, 50–65.

Oswald MJ, Palmer DN, Kay GW, Shemilt SJ, Rezaie P, & Cooper JD (2005) Glial activation spreads from specific cerebral foci and precedes neurodegeneration in presymptomatic ovine neuronal ceroid lipofuscinosis (CLN6). *Neurobiol Dis*, 20, 49–63.

Partanen S, Haapanen A, Kielar C, Pontikis C, Alexander N, Inkinen T, Saftig P, Gillingwater TH, Cooper JD, & Tyynelä J (2008) Synaptic changes in the thalamocortical system of cathepsin D-deficient mice: a model of human congenital neuronal ceroid-lipofuscinosis. *J Neuropathol Exp Neurol*, 67, 16–29.

Passini MA, Dodge JC, Bu J, Yang W, Zhao Q, Sondhi D, Hackett NR, Kaminsky SM, Mao Q, Shihabuddin LS, Cheng SH, Sleat DE, Stewart GR, Davidson BL, Lobel P, & Crystal RG (2006) Intracranial delivery of CLN2 reduces brain pathology in a mouse model of classical late infantile neuronal ceroid lipofuscinosis. *J Neurosci*, 26, 1334–1342.

Pears MR, Cooper JD, Mitchison HM, Mortishire-Smith RJ, Pearce DA, & Griffin JL (2005) High resolution 1H NMR-based metabolomics indicates a neurotransmitter cycling deficit in cerebral tissue from a mouse model of Batten disease. *J Biol Chem*, 280, 42508–42514.

Pears MR, Salek RM, Palmer DN, Kay GW, Mortishire-Smith RJ, & Griffin JL (2007) Metabolomic investigation of CLN6 neuronal ceroid lipofuscinosis in affected South Hampshire sheep. *J Neurosci Res*, 85, 3494–3504.

Poët M, Kornak U, Schweizer M, Zdebik AA, Scheel O, Hoelter S, Wurst W, Schmitt A, Fuhrmann JC, Planells-Cases R, Mole SE, Hubner CA, & Jentsch TJ (2006) Lysosomal storage disease upon disruption of the neuronal chloride transport protein ClC-6. *Proc Natl Acad Sci U S A*, 103, 13854–13859.

Pohl S, Mitchison HM, Kohlschutter A, van Diggelen O, Braulke T, & Storch S (2007) Increased expression of lysosomal acid phosphatase in CLN3-defective cells and mouse brain tissue. *J Neurochem*, 103, 2177–2188.

Pontikis CC, Cella CV, Parihar N, Lim MJ, Chakrabarti S, Mitchison HM, Mobley WC, Rezaie P, Pearce DA, & Cooper JD (2004) Late onset neurodegeneration in the $Cln3^{-/-}$ mouse model of juvenile neuronal ceroid lipofuscinosis is preceded by low level glial activation. *Brain Res*, 1023, 231–242.

Pontikis CC, Cotman SL, MacDonald ME, & Cooper JD (2005) Thalamocortical neuron loss and localized astrocytosis in the $Cln3^{\Delta ex7/8}$ knock-in mouse model of Batten disease. *Neurobiol Dis*, 20, 823–836.

Pressey SNR, O'Donnell KJ, Stauber T, Fuhrmann JC, Tyynela J, Jentsch TJ, and Cooper JD (2010). Distinct neuropathological phenotypes after disrupting the chloride transport proteins ClC-6 or ClC-7/Ostm1. *J Neuropath Exp Neurol* (In press).

Pujic Z & Malicki J (2004) Retinal pattern and the genetic basis of its formation in zebrafish. *Semin Cell Dev Biol*, 15, 105–114.

Qiao X, Lu JY, & Hofmann SL (2007) Gene expression profiling in a mouse model of infantile neuronal ceroid lipofuscinosis reveals upregulation of immediate early genes and mediators of the inflammatory response. *BMC Neurosci*, 8, 95.

Rajan I, Read R, Small DL, Perrard J, & Vogel P (2010) An alternative splicing variant in $Clcn7^{-/-}$ mice prevents osteopetrosis but not neural and retinal degeneration. *Vet Pathol*. May 13. [Epub]

Ranta S, Zhang Y, Ross B, Lonka L, Takkunen E, Messer A, Sharp J, Wheeler R, Kusumi K, Mole S, Liu W, Soares MB, Bonaldo MF, Hirvasniemi A, de la Chapelle A, Gilliam TC, & Lehesjoki AE (1999) The neuronal ceroid lipofuscinoses in human EPMR and mnd mutant mice are associated with mutations in CLN8. *Nat Genet*, 23, 233–236.

Reugels AM, Boggetti B, Scheer N, & Campos-Ortega JA (2006) Asymmetric localization of Numb:EGFP in dividing neuroepithelial cells during neurulation in Danio rerio. *Dev Dyn*, 235, 934–948.

Rodman JS, Lipman R, Brown A, Bronson RT, & Dice JF (1998) Rate of accumulation of Luxol Fast Blue staining material and mitochondrial ATP synthase subunit 9 in motor neuron degeneration mice. *Neurochem Res*, 23, 1291–1296.

Russell C (2003) The roles of Hedgehogs and Fibroblast Growth Factors in eye development and retinal cell rescue. *Vision Res*, 43, 899–912.

Saftig P, Hetman M, Schmahl W, Weber K, Heine L, Mossmann H, Koster A, Hess B, Evers M, von Figura K, et al. (1995) Mice deficient for the lysosomal proteinase cathepsin D exhibit progressive atrophy of the intestinal mucosa and profound destruction of lymphoid cells. *EMBO J*, 14, 3599–3608.

Saha A, Kim SJ, Zhang Z, Lee YC, Sarkar C, Tsai PC, & Mukherjee AB (2008) RAGE signaling contributes to neuroinflammation in infantile neuronal ceroid lipofuscinosis. *FEBS Lett*, 582, 3823–3831.

Sappington RM, Pearce DA, & Calkins DJ (2003) Optic nerve degeneration in a murine model of juvenile ceroid lipofuscinosis. *Invest Ophthalmol Vis Sci*, 44, 3725–3731.

Savukoski M, Klockars T, Holmberg V, Santavuori P, Lander ES, & Peltonen L (1998) CLN5, a novel gene encoding a putative transmembrane protein mutated in Finnish variant late infantile neuronal ceroid lipofuscinosis. *Nat Genet*, 19, 286–288.

Seigel GM, Lotery A, Kummer A, Bernard DJ, Greene ND, Turmaine M, Derksen T, Nussbaum RL, Davidson B, Wagner J, & Mitchison HM (2002) Retinal pathology and function in a Cln3 knockout mouse model of juvenile Neuronal Ceroid Lipofuscinosis (Batten disease). *Mol Cell Neurosci*, 19, 515–527.

Seigel GM, Wagner J, Wronska A, Campbell L, Ju W, & Zhong N (2005) Progression of early postnatal retinal pathology in a mouse model of neuronal ceroid lipofuscinosis. *Eye (Lond)*, 19, 1306–1312.

Seehafer SS, Ramirez-Montealegre D, Wong AM, Chan CH, Castaneda J, Horak M, Ahmadi SM, Lim MJ, Cooper JD, Pearce DA (2010). Immunosuppression alters disease severity in juvenile Batten disease mice. *J Neuroimmunol*. 2010 Oct 9. [Epub ahead of print] PMID: 20937531 [PubMed - as supplied by publisher]

Shacka JJ, Klocke BJ, Young C, Shibata M, Olney JW, Uchiyama Y, Saftig P, & Roth KA (2007) Cathepsin D deficiency induces persistent neurodegeneration in the absence of Bax-dependent apoptosis. *J Neurosci*, 27, 2081–2090.

Shevtsova Z, Garrido M, Weishaupt J, Saftig P, Bahr M, Luhder F, & Kugler S (2010) CNS-expressed cathepsin D prevents lymphopenia in a murine model of congenital neuronal ceroid lipofuscinosis. *Am J Pathol*, 177, 271–279.

Shi GP, Bryant RA, Riese R, Verhelst S, Driessen C, Li Z, Bromme D, Ploegh HL, & Chapman HA (2000) Role for cathepsin F in invariant chain processing and major histocompatibility complex class II peptide loading by macrophages. *J Exp Med*, 191, 1177–1186.

Siintola E, Partanen S, Stromme P, Haapanen A, Haltia M, Maehlen J, Lehesjoki AE, & Tyynelä J (2006) Cathepsin D deficiency underlies congenital human neuronal ceroid-lipofuscinosis. *Brain*, 129, 1438–1445.

Siintola E, Topcu M, Aula N, Lohi H, Minassian BA, Paterson AD, Liu XQ, Wilson C, Lahtinen U, Anttonen AK, & Lehesjoki AE (2007) The novel neuronal ceroid lipofuscinosis gene MFSD8 encodes a putative lysosomal transporter. *Am J Hum Genet*, 81, 136–146.

Sleat DE, Donnelly RJ, Lackland H, Liu CG, Sohar I, Pullarkat RK, & Lobel P (1997) Association of mutations in a lysosomal protein with classical late-infantile neuronal ceroid lipofuscinosis. *Science*, 277, 1802–1805.

Sleat DE, Wiseman JA, El-Banna M, Kim KH, Mao Q, Price S, Macauley SL, Sidman RL, Shen MM, Zhao Q, Passini MA, Davidson BL, Stewart GR, & Lobel P (2004) A mouse model of classical late-infantile neuronal ceroid lipofuscinosis based on targeted disruption of the CLN2 gene results in a loss of tripeptidyl-peptidase I activity and progressive neurodegeneration. *J Neurosci*, 24, 9117–9126.

Sondhi D, Hackett NR, Apblett RL, Kaminsky SM, Pergolizzi RG, & Crystal RG (2001) Feasibility of gene therapy for late neuronal ceroid lipofuscinosis. *Arch Neurol*, 58, 1793–1798.

Sondhi D, Hackett NR, Peterson DA, Stratton J, Baad M, Travis KM, Wilson JM, & Crystal RG (2007) Enhanced survival of the LINCL mouse following CLN2 gene transfer using the rh.10 rhesus macaque-derived adeno-associated virus vector. *Mol Ther*, 15, 481–491.

Sondhi D, Peterson DA, Edelstein AM, del Fierro K, Hackett NR, & Crystal RG (2008) Survival advantage of neonatal CNS gene transfer for late infantile neuronal ceroid lipofuscinosis. *Exp Neurol*, 213, 18–27.

Stein CS, Yancey PH, Martins I, Sigmund RD, Stokes JB, & Davidson BL (2010) Osmoregulation of ceroid neuronal lipofuscinosis type 3 (CLN3) in the renal medulla. *Am J Physiol Cell Physiol*, 298, C1388–C1400.

Steinfeld R, Reinhardt K, Schreiber K, Hillebrand M, Kraetzner R, Bruck W, Saftig P, & Gartner J (2006) Cathepsin D deficiency is associated with a human neurodegenerative disorder. *Am J Hum Genet*, 78, 988–998.

Stemple DL (2004) TILLING—a high-throughput harvest for functional genomics. *Nat Rev Genet*, 5, 145–150.

Steward CG (2003) Neurological aspects of osteopetrosis. *Neuropathol Appl Neurobiol*, 29, 87–97.

Stobrawa SM, Breiderhoff T, Takamori S, Engel D, Schweizer M, Zdebik AA, Bosl MR, Ruether K, Jahn H, Draguhn A, Jahn R, & Jentsch TJ (2001) Disruption of ClC-3, a chloride channel expressed on synaptic vesicles, leads to a loss of the hippocampus. *Neuron*, 29, 185–196.

Tamaki SJ, Jacobs Y, Dohse M, Capela A, Cooper JD, Reitsma M, He D, Tushinski R, Belichenko PV, Salehi A, Mobley W, Gage FH, Huhn S, Tsukamoto AS, Weissman IL, & Uchida N (2009) Neuroprotection of host cells by human central nervous system stem cells in a mouse model of infantile neuronal ceroid lipofuscinosis. *Cell Stem Cell*, 5, 310–319.

Tang CH, Lee JW, Galvez MG, Robillard L, Mole SE, & Chapman HA (2006) Murine cathepsin F deficiency causes neuronal lipofuscinosis and late-onset neurological disease. *Mol Cell Biol*, 26, 2309–2316.

The International Batten Disease Consortium (1995) Isolation of a novel gene underlying Batten disease, CLN3. *Cell*, 82, 949–957.

Tyynelä J, Sohar I, Sleat DE, Gin RM, Donnelly RJ, Baumann M, Haltia M, & Lobel P (2000) A mutation in the ovine cathepsin D gene causes a congenital lysosomal storage disease with profound neurodegeneration. *EMBO J*, 19, 2786–2792.

Udvadia AJ & Linney E (2003) Windows into development: historic, current, and future perspectives on transgenic zebrafish. *Dev Biol*, 256, 1–17.

Uusi-Rauva K, Luiro K, Tanhuanpaa K, Kopra O, Martin-Vasallo P, Kyttala A, & Jalanko A (2008) Novel interactions of CLN3 protein link Batten disease to dysregulation of fodrin-Na+, K+ ATPase complex. *Exp Cell Res*, 314, 2895–2905.

Vesa J, Hellsten E, Verkruyse LA, Camp LA, Rapola J, Santavuori P, Hofmann SL, & Peltonen L (1995) Mutations in the palmitoyl protein thioesterase gene causing infantile neuronal ceroid lipofuscinosis. *Nature*, 376, 584–587.

Virmani T, Gupta P, Liu X, Kavalali ET, & Hofmann SL (2005) Progressively reduced synaptic vesicle pool size in cultured neurons derived from neuronal ceroid lipofuscinosis-1 knockout mice. *Neurobiol Dis*, 20, 314–323.

von Schantz C, Kielar C, Hansen SN, Pontikis CC, Alexander NA, Kopra O, Jalanko A, & Cooper JD (2009) Progressive thalamocortical neuron loss in Cln5 deficient mice: Distinct effects in Finnish variant late infantile NCL. *Neurobiol Dis*, 34, 308–319.

von Schantz C, Saharinen J, Kopra O, Cooper JD, Gentile M, Hovatta I, Peltonen L, & Jalanko A (2008) Brain gene expression profiles of Cln1 and Cln5 deficient mice unravels common molecular pathways underlying neuronal degeneration in NCL diseases. *BMC Genomics*, 9, 146.

Wang B, Shi GP, Yao PM, Li Z, Chapman HA, & Bromme D (1998) Human cathepsin F. Molecular cloning, functional expression, tissue localization, and enzymatic characterization. *J Biol Chem*, 273, 32000–32008.

Wartosch L, Fuhrmann JC, Schweizer M, Stauber T, & Jentsch TJ (2009) Lysosomal degradation of endocytosed proteins depends on the chloride transport protein ClC-7. *FASEB J*, 23, 4056–4068.

Wei H, Kim SJ, Zhang Z, Tsai PC, Wisniewski KE, & Mukherjee AB (2008) ER and oxidative stresses are common mediators of apoptosis in both neurodegenerative and non-neurodegenerative lysosomal storage disorders and are alleviated by chemical chaperones. *Hum Mol Genet*, 17, 469–477.

Weimer JM, Benedict JW, Elshatory YM, Short DW, Ramirez-Montealegre D, Ryan DA, Alexander NA, Federoff HJ, Cooper JD, & Pearce DA (2007) Alterations in striatal dopamine catabolism precede loss of substantia nigra neurons in a mouse model of juvenile neuronal ceroid lipofuscinosis. *Brain Res*, 1162, 98–112.

Weimer JM, Benedict JW, Getty AL, Pontikis CC, Lim MJ, Cooper JD, & Pearce DA (2009) Cerebellar defects in a mouse model of juvenile neuronal ceroid lipofuscinosis. *Brain Res*, 1266, 93–107.

Weimer JM, Custer AW, Benedict JW, Alexander NA, Kingsley E, Federoff HJ, Cooper JD, & Pearce DA (2006) Visual deficits in a mouse model of Batten disease are the result of optic nerve degeneration and loss of dorsal lateral geniculate thalamic neurons. *Neurobiol Dis*, 22, 284–293.

Wendt KD, Lei B, Schachtman TR, Tullis GE, Ibe ME, & Katz ML (2005) Behavioral assessment in mouse models of neuronal ceroid lipofuscinosis using a light-cued T-maze. *Behav Brain Res*, 161, 175–182.

Wheeler RB, Sharp JD, Schultz RA, Joslin JM, Williams RE, & Mole SE (2002) The gene mutated in variant late-infantile neuronal ceroid lipofuscinosis (CLN6) and in nclf mutant mice encodes a novel predicted transmembrane protein. *Am J Hum Genet*, 70, 537–542.

Wienholds E, van Eeden F, Kosters M, Mudde J, Plasterk RH, & Cuppen E (2003) Efficient target-selected mutagenesis in zebrafish. *Genome Res*, 13, 2700–2707.

Wlodawer A, Durell SR, Li M, Oyama H, Oda K, & Dunn BM (2003) A model of tripeptidyl-peptidase I (CLN2), a ubiquitous and highly conserved member of the sedolisin family of serine-carboxyl peptidases. *BMC Struct Biol*, 3, 8.

Wulliman MF, Rupp B, & Reichart H (1996) *Neuroanatomy of the Zebrafish Brain: A Topological Atlas*. Basel, Birkhauser Verlag.

Xin W, Mullen TE, Kiely R, Min J, Feng X, Cao Y, O'Malley L, Shen Y, Chu-Shore C, Mole SE, Goebel HH, & Sims K (2010) CLN5 mutations are frequent in juvenile and late-onset non-Finnish patients with NCL. *Neurology*, 74, 565–571.

Xu S, Sleat DE, Jadot M, & Lobel P (2010) Glial fibrillary acidic protein is elevated in the lysosomal storage disease classical late-infantile neuronal ceroid lipofuscinosis, but is not a component of the storage material. *Biochem J*, 428, 355–362.

Yoshikawa M, Uchida S, Ezaki J, Rai T, Hayama A, Kobayashi K, Kida Y, Noda M, Koike M, Uchiyama Y, Marumo F, Kominami E, & Sasaki S (2002) CLC-3 deficiency leads to phenotypes similar to human neuronal ceroid lipofuscinosis. *Genes Cells*, 7, 597–605.

Zhang Z, Lee YC, Kim SJ, Choi MS, Tsai PC, Saha A, Wei H, Xu Y, Xiao YJ, Zhang P, Heffer A, & Mukherjee AB (2007) Production of lysophosphatidylcholine by cPLA2 in the brain of mice lacking PPT1 is a signal for phagocyte infiltration. *Hum Mol Genet*, 16, 837–847.

Zhang Z, Lee YC, Kim SJ, Choi MS, Tsai PC, Xu Y, Xiao YJ, Zhang P, Heffer A, & Mukherjee AB (2006) Palmitoyl-protein thioesterase-1 deficiency mediates the activation of the unfolded protein response and neuronal apoptosis in INCL. *Hum Mol Genet*, 15, 337–346.

Zon LI & Peterson RT (2005) In vivo drug discovery in the zebrafish. *Nat Rev Drug Discov*, 4, 35–44.

Chapter 18

Large Animal Models

D.N. Palmer, I. Tammen,
and C. Drögemüller, G.S. Johnson, M.L. Katz, F. Lingaas

INTRODUCTION

Since the report of 'lipid dystrophic changes' in two English Setter dogs (Hagen, 1953) an extensive literature has arisen reporting cases of NCL in a wide variety of animals, sufficient to suggest that these diseases are common to mammalian species. Cases have been reported in many different dog breeds, and in other species including sheep, cattle, ferrets, cats, horses, goats, pigs (Tables 18.1–18.4), and mice (see Chapter 17). Animal diseases have been described attributable to naturally occurring mutations in many of the NCL-causing genes.

The majority of these animal forms have been found in domesticated production and companion animals, inbred for consistency in production values, character, or appearance and thus susceptible to a strong founder effect. A strong interest in the genetic health status of these populations leads to a thorough veterinary diagnosis and considerable efforts to detect and manage any deleterious mutations. Diagnosis of NCLs in animals is of veterinary interest in its own right, particularly in animals valued as breeding stock or companions, but in many cases veterinary concerns are incidental compared to gains in knowledge of the analogous human diseases and the provision of an animal model to test therapies.

These model studies fall into two categories. A number of passive studies, mainly careful postmortem pathology investigations, have shaped our understanding of the general course of the neuropathology of the diseases. Such work in sheep allowed early molecular characterization of the storage material. This information becomes even more useful with time, as the genetic lesions are determined, allowing a more exact comparison to the human diseases.

Table 18.1 **Molecular characterization of sheep and cattle models of NCL**

	Chromosome*	Gene	DNA change	Protein change & predicted effect	References
Sheep					
South Hampshire	OAR7	CLN6	unknown - reduced mRNA	reduced amount of protein	Broom et al. 1998, Tammen et al. 2006
Swedish Landrace	OAR21***	CTSD	G**>A	Asp**>Asn non-functional protein	Tyynelä et al. 2000
Merino	OAR7	CLN6	c.184C>T	p.Arg62Cys non-functional protein	Tammen et al. 2001, Tammen et al. 2006
Borderdale	OAR10***	CLN5	IVS3+1G>A	splicing variant, truncated protein	Frugier et al. 2007
Cattle					
Devon	BTA12	CLN5	c.662dupG	p.Arg221GlyfsX6 truncated protein	Houweling et al. 2006a,b

*OAR = ovine chromosome, BTA = bovine chromosome.
**corresponding to G934 and Asp295 of corresponding human CTSD sequence.
***location according to the virtual sheep genome (http://www.livestockgenomics.csiro.au/vsheep/).

Active studies utilize colonies containing affected animals deliberately bred and maintained for studies relevant to human disease. All affected animals in a colony have the same mutation and are closely interbred, so individual variations are small. Colonies derived from naturally occurring large domestic animal cases are particularly valuable because the brain size and structure is larger and more human-like than that of rodents. A longer life expectancy allows for investigation of long-term effects of treatments. In general, the clinical progression in larger animals more closely resembles that in humans and animal colonies are maintained free from drugs such as anti-epileptic agents.

Domestic production animals are economic to maintain, have been bred for easy management, and a high-level expertise in reproductive technology and veterinary care is available for them. With good early diagnosis or breeding programmes, experiments can begin at preclinical or early clinical disease, whereas human trials usually focus on the acutely affected patients. Most of the large animal cases reported have been in dogs or ruminants and large animal model studies have focused on these species.

This chapter is organized into sections describing the large animal models including sheep and cattle, with a separate section on dogs.

LARGE ANIMAL MODELS WITH GENETIC ASSIGNMENT

Best characterized of all animal models of NCL is the CLN6 disease form in New Zealand South Hampshire sheep, diagnosed three decades ago (Jolly and West, 1976, Jolly et al., 1980, Jolly et al., 1982), and in a number of ways these sheep are a prototype of the NCLs. Recently another flock of sheep with CLN6 disease caused by a different mutation has been established following diagnosis in Australian Merinos (Cook et al., 2002).

Studies of a congenital NCL diagnosed in White Swedish Landrace lambs led to the discovery of the first NCL caused by a deficiency in a major lysosomal protease, cathepsin D (Järplid and Haltia, 1993, Tyynelä et al., 2000). The value of this model study has been highlighted by the subsequent discovery of CLN10 disease also caused by cathepsin D deficiency, with ages of onset from around birth and later (Siintola et al., 2006, Steinfeld et al., 2006).

More long-standing is a form of NCL in Australian Devon cattle that results in blindness from 14 months (Harper et al., 1988), the cause of which was recently traced to a mutation in bovine *CLN5* (Houweling et al., 2006a). More recently a flock has been established for model studies following diagnosis of CLN5

Table 18.2 **Clinical and pathological features of large animal models for NCL**

Species (Live span*)	Onset	Death	Incidence **	Clinical Signs ***				Atrophy Brain (B) Retina (R)	Storage material ****				Key References
				VI	BC	MD	S		F	US	Subunit c SAPs	D	
Sheep (20)													
South Hampshire	7-12m	25-30m	active EP	yes	yes	yes	yes	B & R	yes	lamellar	subunit c	general.	Jolly et al. 1980; 1982
Swedish Landrace	at birth	<1m	EP	nr	yes	yes	yes	B & nr	yes	GRODs	SAPs	general.	Järplid and Haltia 1993; Tyynelä et al. 1997
Merino	7m	19-27m	active EP	yes	yes	yes	yes	B & R	yes	lamellar	subunit c	general.	Cook et al. 2002
Borderdale	10-11m	24m	active EP	yes	yes	Nr	nr	B & R	yes	lamellar	subunit c	general.	Jolly et al. 2002a; D.N. Palmer *unpublished data*
Rambouillet	8m	24m	EP	yes	yes	yes	nr	B & R	yes	Nr	nr	neuronal	Edwards et al. 1994; Woods et al. 1993
Cattle (20)													
Devon	9m	39m	active EP	yes	yes	yes	no	B & R	yes	lamellar	subunit c	general.	Harper et al. 1988; Jolly et al. 1992
Beefmaster	12m	18m	several	yes	yes	Nr	yes	nr	nr	lamellar	nr	general.	Read and Bridges 1969
Holstein	nr	18m	1	yes	nr	Nr	nr	B & R	yes	lamellar	nr	general.	Hafner et al. 2005
Ferret (12)													
Domestic	> 3y	nr	5	yes	yes	yes	nr	B & R	yes	lamellar	subunit c	general.	France et al. 1999, M. France *personal communication*
Cat (34)													
DSH	8.5m	9m	1	yes	nr	yes	yes	B & nr	yes	lamellar	subunit c	neuronal	Weissenböck and Rössel 1997
Siamese	< 22m	23m	2	yes	yes	yes	yes	nr	nr	lamellar	nr	general.	Green and Little 1974

DSH	15 m	20 m	1	yes	yes	No	yes	B & R	yes	lamellar	nr	neuronal	Bildfell et al. 1995
Japanese	7m	11m	1	nr	nr	yes	yes	B & nr	yes	GRODs	nr	general.	Nakajama et al. 1993
Horse (50)													
Icelandic X Peruvian	6m	24m	3	yes	yes	yes	nr	B	yes	lamellar	subunit c	general.	Url et al. 2001
Goat (20)													
Nubian	10-18m	2-4y	several	nr	yes	yes	nr	nr	yes	lamellar	nr	neuronal#	Fiske and Storts 1988
Pig (20)													
Vietnamese pot-bellied	2y	2.5y	1	no	no	yes	no	B (mild) & nr	yes	lamellar-GRODs	nr	neuronal	Cesta et al. 2006

* maximum life span in years (http://www.demogr.mpg.de/).
** number of sporadic cases or experimental population (EP).
*** VI = visual impairment, BC = behavioural changes, MD = motor deficits, S = seizures.
**** F = fluorescent, US = ultrastructure, D = distribution.
# only central nervous system investigated.
nr = not reported.

disease in New Zealand Borderdale sheep (Jolly et al., 2002a, Frugier et al., 2008).

Several other cases of NCL have been reported in sheep and cattle but not developed into colonies for model studies. The underlying genes and mutations have not been identified in these cases: Rambouillet sheep (Woods et al., 1993, Edwards et al., 1994), Beefmaster cattle (Read and Bridges, 1969), and an American Holstein Friesian steer (Hafner et al., 2005) described later in this chapter.

CLN6 disease in sheep

INTRODUCTION

CLN6 disease in New Zealand South Hampshire sheep has provided the most informative model of the NCLs and a number of general observations have been made in these sheep, before extension to other forms of the diseases in humans and animals. Affected sheep appear to be normal for the first few months of life but at 9–12 months they develop behavioural symptoms (see below) (Jolly et al., 1980, Jolly et al., 1982). They develop clinical symptoms consistent with an NCL, notably blindness, most cells contain characteristic storage bodies, and gross brain atrophy is a defining pathological feature. Heterozygous individuals were identified from breeding records and a flock has been maintained by mating heterozygous carrier ewes with preclinically affected rams.

Another flock of sheep with NCL has been established following diagnosis in Australian Merinos using a similar strategy. Affected sheep develop clinical symptoms between 7 months and a year of age, and show the same progression of symptoms as the New Zealand South Hampshire sheep (Cook et al., 2002). Postmortem examination revealed the same characteristic gross brain atrophy and a similar distribution of fluorescent storage bodies with the same histological and ultrastructural properties.

MOLECULAR GENETICS

The recent unravelling of the molecular lesions in the CLN6 disease sheep closely followed and extended information from humans and other species. The NCL in the South Hampshire sheep was initially thought to fit between the late infantile and juvenile diseases. However, linkage and marker studies excluded the *CLN2* and *CLN3* loci and mapped the gene to sheep chromosome 7q13–15, homologous to human chromosome 15q21–23 which contains the human *CLN6* gene (Broom et al., 1998). Homozygosity mapping followed by linkage analysis located the defect in the affected Australian Merino sheep to the same region (Tammen et al., 2001, Cook et al., 2002). Ovine *CLN6* was sequenced in both these models subsequent to the sequencing of the human and mouse *CLN6* genes and discovery of disease causing mutations in these species (Gao et al., 2002, Wheeler et al., 2002).

These investigations unveiled the mutation responsible for the disease in Merino sheep (c.184C>T; p.Arg62Cys) and three common ovine allelic variants (c.56A>G, c.822G>A and c.933_934insCT) (Tammen et al., 2006). The p.Arg62Cys mutation is at the same place and similar to a human disease-causing mutation, p.Arg62His (Sharp et al., 2003), thus the disease in Merinos is a particularly accurate genetic model of this human form of NCL. A polymerase chain reaction (PCR)-restriction enzyme diagnostic assay has been developed based on the removal of a *Hae*III cleavage site by the base substitution. Affected, heterozygous, and normal animals are identified this way (see below).

Very tight linkage of the disease in South Hampshires to the ovine *CLN6* c.822G>A allelic variation (LOD score of 13.3) established that the disease is caused by a mutation in this gene or extremely close by. No mutation was found in the coding sequence. Real-time PCR studies showed sharply reduced concentrations of *CLN6* mRNA in affected tissues and intermediate concentrations in tissues from heterozygotes, indicating that the mutation is likely to reside in a regulatory region and affect gene expression (Tammen et al., 2006).

The c.822G>A allelic variation is neutral, being the third base of triplets both coding for alanine. However it deletes a *Hae*II restriction site and was the variant found in the affected South Hampshire sheep and is now used as the major diagnostic tool (see below).

CELL BIOLOGY

Discovery of the human *CLN6* gene led to investigations of its function, carried out on cells derived from human patients and also from affected South Hampshire sheep. Two independent studies, using subcellular fractionation and immunocytochemistry indicated that *CLN6* encodes an endoplasmic reticulum resident protein (Heine et al., 2004, Mole et al., 2004). Turnover studies in fibroblasts from the sheep, affected humans, and *nclf* mice indicated that absence of the gene product specifically affects pre-lysosome vesicular transport, indicated by a blockage of arylsulfatase A endocytosis via the plasma membrane 300kDa mannose-6-phosphate receptor. Trafficking of lysosomal enzymes from the endoplasmic reticulum to the lysosomes is not perturbed (Heine et al., 2004).

Neuron cultures have been developed using cells dissociated from prenatal brains of both control and CLN6-affected sheep (Kay et al., 1999, Kay et al., 2006a). Cultured neurons develop a similar range of morphologies and reactions to antibodies to neurotransmitters and calcium binding proteins as neurons display *in situ*. No differences have been detected between control and affected neurons in any of these characteristics, nor in growth or survival. Cultures are stable for a number of weeks and contain a proportion of cells dividing into neurons. Viable cultures can be recovered from frozen stocks of dissociated cells (Kay et al., 2006a).

Cultures also contain glial cells and there are more Sudan black and Luxol fast blue-positive inclusion bodies in cells from affected animals than from controls, but these are relatively sparse, in 1–3% of cells and not generally observed in the high proportion of cells found in the initial experiments (Hughes et al., 1999) (D.N. Palmer, unpublished results). No differences in growth, differentiation, or survival have been noted between affected and control cells, except in the response of 108-day cerebellar neurons to tri-iodothyronine. Treated control cells migrate into clumps over 4 weeks in culture as do normal rodent cells, but affected cells do not (Palmer et al., 2002).

Subunit c reconstituted into black lipid bilayers formed a calcium gated ion pore and it was hypothesized that an overabundance of such pores may have a role in an excitotoxic mechanism of neuronal loss (McGeoch and Palmer, 1999); however, they could not be found in patch clamp electrophysiological experiments on cultured normal and affected neurons (D.N. Palmer and G.W. Kay, unpublished results).

CLINICAL DATA AND DIAGNOSIS

Affected South Hampshire sheep appeared to be normal for the first few months of life but at 9–12 months they developed a tendency to graze away from other members of the flock, lagged behind when the flock was moved, and responded atypically to attempts at control with sheep dogs (Jolly et al., 1980, Jolly et al., 1982). They developed spontaneous episodes of head nodding, champing of jaws, and twitching of ears, eyelids, lips, and muzzle. Postmortem examination revealed gross brain atrophy and the presence of fluorescent storage bodies in a range of cells with histochemical and ultrastructural properties characteristic of a neuronal ceroid lipofuscinosis. Clinical symptoms developed at 10–14 months of age, most notably blindness as a result of atrophy of the occipital cortex and loss of photoreceptors in the retina (Figure 18.1) (Graydon and Jolly, 1984, Mayhew et al., 1985). An early diagnosis was developed, based on the presence of storage bodies in brain biopsy samples

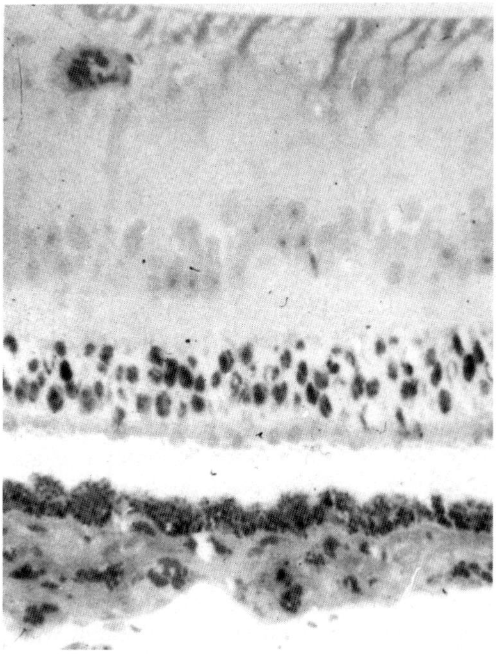

Figure 18.1 Ovine NCL: loss of retinal photoreceptors in South Hampshire sheep, 1μm-thick toluidine blue-stained section, ×460.

taken at 3–5 months of age (Dickson et al., 1989).

More recently the c.822G>A neutral allelic variation that deletes a *Hae*II restriction site (see above) has become the basic diagnostic tool within the flock which is now configured so that all normal sheep are GG and all heterozygotes AG. In the next generation affected animals are AA, with carriers AG and normal sheep GG. This technique allows diagnosis as soon as any DNA samples can be obtained.

The use of this marker has been tested against brain biopsy diagnoses on 213 affected and heterozygous lambs over 4 years with 100% agreement, and it is now used routinely for diagnosis in the South Hampshires (Tammen et al., 2006).

Affected Merino sheep developed clinical symptoms between 7 months and a year of age, and showed the same progression of symptoms as the New Zealand South Hampshire sheep (Cook et al., 2002). A model flock of these sheep has been established using a similar strategy to that used for the South Hampshires. A PCR-restriction enzyme diagnostic assay has been developed based on the removal of a *Hae*III cleavage site by the base substitution (see above), allowing identification of affected, heterozygous, and normal animals.

MORPHOLOGY

Sudan black and Luxol fast blue-positive fluorescent storage bodies accumulate in neurons and most cells throughout the affected sheep, but not in those cells commonly used for cell biology studies, fibroblasts and immortalized lymphocytes in both the affected South Hampshires and Merinos (Jolly et al., 1980, Jolly et al., 1982, Jolly et al., 1988, Jolly et al., 1989, Cook et al., 2002). These electron-dense bodies display a variety of ultrastructures *in situ*; multilamellar, fingerprint, curvilinear, and crystalloid arrays, some being more prominent in some tissues than others (Figures 18.2 and 18.3). For instance, bodies in pancreatic cells are dominantly of the curvilinear type. Storage bodies stained immunohistochemically for subunit c, at both the light and electron microscope level (Westlake et al., 1995a). Some storage bodies in neurons stained solidly while others stained around the periphery leaving a translucent area in the middle (Westlake et al., 1995a, Oswald et al., 2005).

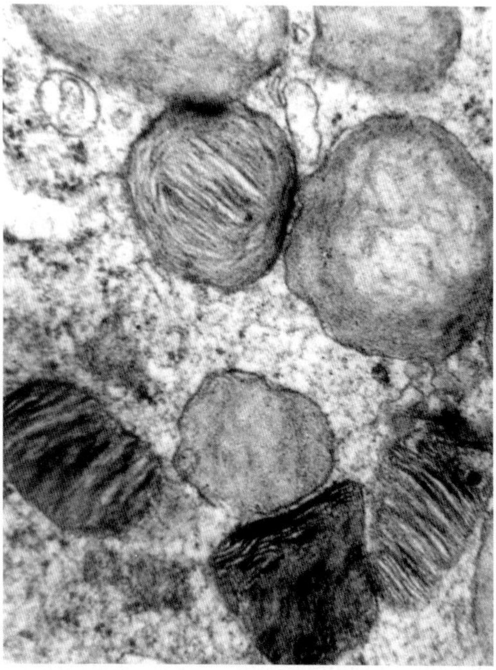

Figure 18.2 Ovine NCL: lamellar inclusions resembling zebra and membranous cytoplasmic bodies in a retinal neuron of South Hampshire sheep, ×95,000.

Storage bodies retain their structure through the heavy sonication used in their purification that fragments all other subcellular organelles composed of lipid bilayers. This suggests that they have a refractory solid structure and is consistent with freeze-fracture electron microscopy (Jolly et al., 1988).

DISEASE MECHANISMS

Understanding of the pathogenesis of the NCLs is still very limited despite considerable effort and a number of hypotheses, some vigorously presented and associated with attempts at treatments. For over two decades, studies based on the South Hampshire sheep were central to testing the veracity of several of these hypotheses.

Lipids and peroxidation

Initial studies concentrated on the structure and composition of the storage bodies and ideas of pathogenesis centred on dysfunctions in lipid metabolism, starting with a possible lack of control of the peroxidation of polyunsaturated fatty acids. These diseases had

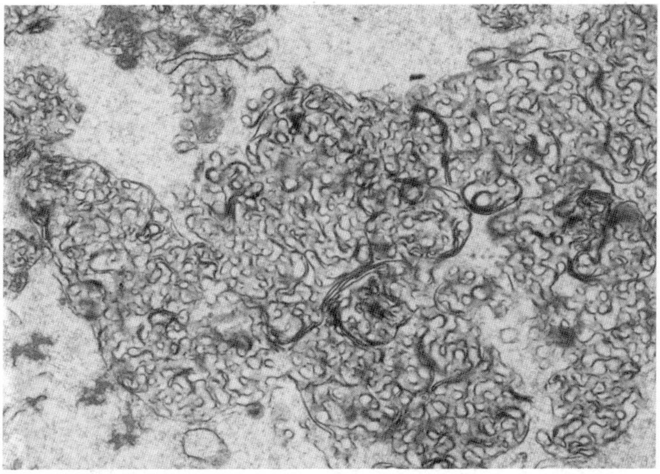

Figure 18.3 Ovine NCL: lamellar and curvilinear profiles of lipopigments isolated from pancreas of South Hampshire sheep (material kindly supplied by Prof. R.D. Jolly) ×34,000.

recently been named neuronal ceroid lipofuscinosis, because of the similarities of the 'highly characteristic autofluorescent' properties of the so-called lipopigment storage bodies to ceroid and lipofuscin, and following the development of the peroxidation hypothesis for the formation of these granules (Chio and Tappel, 1969a, Chio and Tappel, 1969b). This hypothesis was based on the finding that material generated by reacting protein and peroxidized lipids had similar fluorescent spectra to material generated when malonaldehyde reacted with a number of amino acids and in turn was similar to the fluorescence of storage bodies *in situ*.

A 'highly acidic' fluorophor designated to be the Schiff base polymer consequent to lipid peroxidation was found in early studies of storage bodies from human cases and affected English Setter dogs (Siakotos and al., 1972, Siakotos and Koppang, 1973, Elleder, 1981), and a second 'fluorescent polymer' found in the neutral lipids (Siakotos and al., 1972, Siakotos and Koppang, 1973) was designated 'polymalonaldehyde (Gutteridge and al., 1977). It was widely accepted that these diseases were caused by aberrations in the regulation of peroxidation of lipid (Zeman and Dyken, 1969, Zeman, 1974, Zeman, 1976).

This pathogenic mechanism demands the loss of polyunsaturated fatty acids to lipid peroxidation but analyses of brain phospholipids in affected sheep indicated no such loss (Palmer et al., 1985). Methods were developed for the isolation of pure storage body preparations from fresh sheep tissue, in order to analyse storage body composition (Palmer et al., 1986a, Palmer et al., 1986b, Palmer et al., 1988). No 'highly characteristic fluorophor' was found in storage bodies isolated from fresh sheep tissue despite exhaustive analysis (Palmer et al., 1986b, Palmer et al., 1988). Storage body lipids were those expected in lysosome-derived organelles. The phospholipids and their fatty acid profiles were the same as those found in lysosomal membranes, including significant amounts of the lysosomal marker, bis(monoacylglycero)phosphate, also called lysobisphosphatidic acid. A very high proportion of the fatty acids in this phospholipid were polyunsaturated, 69%, indicating that it has a role in the recycling of polyunsaturated fatty acids and denying a significant loss of polyunsaturated fatty acids through peroxidation.

Subsequent studies disproved the existence of any intrinsic fluorophor. Storage bodies dissolve completely in 1% lithium dodecyl sulphate, resulting in solutions that are not fluorescent at all (Palmer et al., 1993, Palmer et al., 2002). This indicates that the microscopically observed fluorescence of storage bodies *in situ* is an array property, confirmed by the reconstitution of fluorescent storage-body like structures from non-fluorescent components. This is consistent with the array spacing found in powder X-ray studies, 10 Å and 4.6Å (Jolly et al., 1988), a spacing likely to cause diffractive scattering responsible for the apparent fluorescence, similar to that exhibited by quantum dots of similar size and now used as antibody tags. In both cases the observed fluorescence is photo-fast, indicating that a chemical fluorophor is not involved.

Measurements of sheep storage body metal contents also supported a lysosomal origin (Palmer et al., 1988) and were not consistent with a role of heavy metal catalysis of lipid peroxidation in the disease, as had been postulated (Gutteridge et al., 1983, Gutteridge, 1985). In the light of the unequivocal nature of these findings, and those below, it is disappointing that supposed antioxidant and lipid-based therapies still play a part in the treatments of clinical NCLs in humans when there is no rationale left for them.

Other studies reporting a retinoid nature of the 'fluorophor' in storage bodies led to the hypothesis of a defect in retinoic acid catabolism (Wolfe et al., 1977), and subsequently of another polyisoprenoid, dolichol (Wolfe and Ng Ying Kin, 1982, Ng Ying Kin et al., 1983). This hypothesis was supported by reports of raised brain dolichol and dolichyl phosphate-linked oligosaccharide concentrations in storage bodies, patients, and affected English Setters (Keller et al., 1984) but not by measurements of dolichol and dolichol-linked oligosaccharide concentrations in the sheep storage bodies, which were consistent with those expected in normal lysosomes (Palmer et al., 1986b, Hall et al., 1989).

Subunit c storage and modification

A series of experiments established that the ovine disease is a lysosomal proteinosis and that a specific protein, the c subunit of mitochondrial ATP synthase, is the abnormally stored component. Elemental analysis, amino acid analysis, and gel electrophoresis, indicated that the major component of storage bodies is protein, specifically a major band with a low apparent molecular weight of 3500Da (Palmer et al., 1986a, Palmer et al., 1986b). Automated Edman degradation sequencing of total storage body proteins gave a clear sequence for the first 40 amino acids of subunit c of mitochondrial ATP synthase (Palmer et al., 1989) and a minor sequence later identified as that of the V_1V_0 ATPase c subunit (Fearnley et al., 1990). The sequence of the major stored protein was completed and found to be that of the complete normal 75 amino acid mitochondrial protein. Another higher-molecular-weight band on gels (14 800 Da) was found to be an oligomer of subunit c.

This single peptide made up over 50% of the storage body mass, calculated by comparing the yield obtained from the sequencer with the amount of protein loaded (Palmer et al., 1989, Fearnley et al., 1990), a much higher proportion of subunit c than is found in its site of action, the inner mitochondrial membrane. Here, subunit c is only one of 16 subunits of the ATP synthase complex (also called F_1F_o ATPase) but none of the other 16 components are stored (Fearnley et al., 1990). Subunit c is highly hydrophobic and insoluble in most solvents, but can be dissolved in chloroform methanol, properties that probably account for its lipid-like histochemical properties. For this reason it is called a proteolipid, sometimes the dicyclohexylcarbodiimide reactive proteolipid, and even the lipid binding subunit of mitochondrial ATP synthase (Palmer et al., 1989, Fearnley et al., 1990).

This finding was almost immediately extended to the late infantile and juvenile human diseases, establishing the sheep as a prototype model of the human diseases (Palmer et al., 1986a, Palmer et al., 1989, Palmer et al., 1992). Sequencing also established subunit c storage in *CLN5* and *CLN8* affected Border Collie and English Setter dogs (Jolly et al., 1994b, Palmer et al., 1997a, Katz et al., 2005a, Melville et al., 2005), *CLN5* cattle (Martinus et al., 1991, Houweling et al., 2006a), *CLN8* (*mnd*) mice (Faust et al., 1994), and in the Finnish *CLN5* late infantile variant form of NCL (Tyynelä et al., 1997). Immunochemical and immunocytochemical studies also implied subunit c storage in *CLN8/mnd* mice (Pardo et al., 1994), horses (Url et al., 2001), and a range of other animals (see Table 18.1) including the affected Australian Merino sheep (Cook et al., 2002), and in the late infantile, juvenile, and adult human forms (Hall et al., 1991, Kominami et al., 1992, Kida et al., 1993, Sakajiri et al., 1995). Subsequent work characterized the stored subunit c as the full functional mitochondrial protein, unmodified in any disease-specific way (Fearnley et al., 1990, Palmer et al., 1992, Palmer et al., 1993, Palmer et al., 1995, Ryan et al., 1996, Chen et al., 2004).

Lack of care about controls resulted in the idea that trimethylation of lysine 43 of the subunit c stored in English Setter dogs was disease associated (Katz et al., 1994, Katz et al., 1995). Trimethyllysine is the carrier in acyl chain transport across the inner mitochondrial membrane and this led to the idea that carnitine imbalance may be a part of the pathological process in the NCLs. Lower than normal carnitine levels were reported in plasma from affected English Setters (Katz and Siakotos, 1995). However, trimethyllysine was found in hydrolysates of normal ovine subunit c (Palmer et al., 1993) and it was established that normal mitochondrial subunit c and the subunit c in Batten disease have the same molecular mass, 42Da greater than that calculated from the primary amino acid sequence (Buzy et al., 1996, Ryan et al., 1996). Subsequent mass spectrometry experiments confirmed that this is due to trimethylation of lysine 43, common to all subunit c in all vertebrate species studied, and confirmed that the subunit c stored in the NCLs is not modified in any disease specific way (Chen et al., 2004), removing the rationale for carnitine therapies.

Storage is specific to subunit c and subunit c storage is specific to the NCLs. This led to the concept of a number of metabolically-related genetic defects affecting a specific turnover pathway for subunit c (Palmer et al., 1995, Palmer et al., 1997a), but there is no mechanistic knowledge of this pathway. Alternatively the highly hydrophobic nature of subunit c and its tendency to form aggregates may favour preferential lysosomal deposition under specific suboptimal turnover conditions. This may be a consequence of disturbed pre-lysosomal membrane trafficking in some forms, as observed in a CLN3 neuron culture model (Fossale et al., 2004). However, no link has been established between subunit c storage and pathogenesis, and recent studies indicate that these two phenomena may be separate manifestations of the gene lesions.

Neuroactive amino acids

Excitotoxicity or excessive stimulation of neurons by excitatory amino acids such as glutamate has been implicated in degenerative neuropathies (Choi, 1988) and postulated to be involved in NCLs (Walkley et al., 1995). A loss of GABAergic neurons in regions of the brain that undergo neurodegeneration in the sheep and a canine model of NCL was associated with apparently disturbed mitochondria (March et al., 1995, Walkley et al., 1995) and possible disturbances in ATP production (Siakotos et al., 1998, Jolly and Walkley, 1999, Jolly et al., 2002b). Other studies determined that populations of GABAergic interneurons are consistently affected in human and mouse NCLs (Williams et al., 1977, Cooper et al., 1999, Mitchison et al., 1999, Bible et al., 2004, Pontikis et al., 2004, Tyynelä et al., 2004, Kielar et al., 2007).

A study of the relative distribution of GABAergic neurons in clinically affected sheep showed a severe loss of parvalbumin-positive neurons in those areas of the brain most affected by neurodegeneration and a lesser loss of calretinin-positive cells. However, no differences were found in the proportion of parvalbumin-positive cells in neurons cultured from control and affected prenatal brains (Oswald et al., 2001).

These findings prompted a systematic study of the distribution and onset of GABAergic interneuron loss in affected sheep brains, starting from 12 days of age (Oswald et al., 2008). The first differences were noted at 4 months of age, and paralleled but did not precede other degenerative changes. Parvalbumin-positive interneurons were affected earlier and more profoundly than somatostatin-, calbindin-, and calretinin-positive interneurons. Interneuron loss displayed a remarkable regional variation, starting and progressing fastest in those areas first associated with neurodegeneration and clinical symptoms; the primary visual and parieto-occipital cortices. This study revealed that cellular location is a more important determinant of neuron survival than phenotypic identity, and that changes in interneuron populations follow pathogenesis and so cannot be its cause.

A metabolomic study of the relative concentrations of GABA, glutamate, and other brain metabolites in various regions of the brain and the cerebrospinal fluid confirmed these findings (Pears et al., 2007). Concentrations changed in parallel to or in consequence of neurodegeneration and there was no evidence of an imbalance in the ratios of glutamate and GABA or any other metabolic disturbance leading to the onset of neurodegeneration. There were also no disease-related changes in cerebrospinal fluid concentrations of the neuroactive amino acids aspartate, glutamate, glycine, taurine, and GABA, nor in the levels of the proteins enolase, S-100b, glial fibrillary acidic protein (GFAP), or myelin basic protein (MBP) (Kay et al., 2009), which have been observed in other diseases affecting the brain.

Glial activation

Recent studies suggest that glial activation plays a primary role in pathogenesis. A precocious activation of glial cells, long before any apparent neurodegeneration and while the brain is being formed, was a surprising finding in a study of presymptomatic affected sheep (Oswald et al., 2005), beginning prenatally (Kay et al., 2006b). Enlarged proliferating perivascular macrophages were found in affected brains 20 days before birth. Activated astrocytes with shorter thicker processes were present in the developing brain 40 days before birth and activated microglia in grey matter at birth, 150 days of gestation, and MHC II activated glia only 12 days after birth. Activated astrocytes and focal clusters of activated microglia were clearly evident in cortical regions at this age (Oswald et al., 2005, Kay et al., 2006b).

Astrocytic activation and the transformation of microglia to brain macrophages were progressive, regionally defined, and preceded the degeneration of different cortical layers and brain areas, starting in outer layers of visual and somatosensory cortex. Activation spread to different cortical areas in the order of development of associated symptoms. Generalized neurodegeneration followed (Oswald et al., 2005). Upregulation of manganese superoxide dismutase (Mn-SOD) found in both Merino and South Hampshire sheep and human tissue and cells affected with CLN6 NCL (Heine et al., 2003) may be part of the activation cascade.

This perinatal onset of a complex cascade of glial activation suggests that glia are central to NCL pathogenesis but it is not clear when this cascade becomes fatally damaging to neurons. Given that glial responses are evident as early as 40 days before birth it is surprising how long the development of the affected sheep brains follows a normal path. In contrast, storage body accumulation was more evenly spread across regions at all ages, suggesting that neurodegeneration and storage body accumulation are independent manifestations of the disease (Oswald et al., 2005).

A role for mitochondrially-related apoptosis has also been postulated in the South Hampshire sheep (Lane et al., 1996), but again definitive evidence has not been forthcoming and it is possible that any apoptosis is part of a wider activation cascade.

Glial activation in other neurodegenerative conditions including multiple sclerosis, Alzheimer's disease, Parkinson's disease, HIV-associated dementia, scrapie, trauma, and ischaemia (Neumann, 2001, Hunot and Hirsch, 2003) has been assumed to be initiated by dying neurons or some ligand such as abnormally deposited β-amyloid protein (Stoll and Jander, 1999, Minagar et al., 2002), but there is mounting evidence that inflammation plays a pathogenic role in other storage diseases. For instance, suppression of microglial activation, as a side effect of bone marrow transplantation, suppressed neurodegeneration in a mouse model of Sandhoff disease (Wada et al., 2000). Deletion of a macrophage inflammatory protein, MIP-1α, had the same effect, directly implicating inflammation in pathogenesis (Wu and Proia, 2004).

EXPERIMENTAL THERAPY

Bone marrow transplantation has been advocated as a possible therapy in the NCLs and this possibility was tested by haematopoietic cell transplantation of fetal cells to CLN6-affected South Hampshire fetuses. Despite a good engraftment of transplanted normal cells into affected fetuses, no amelioration of the symptoms was detected, nor was there any less storage in visceral tissues, suggesting a poor prognosis for bone marrow transplantation, even when carried out prenatally (Westlake et al., 1995b). No other possible therapies have been tested in these sheep models.

CLN5 disease in cattle and sheep

INTRODUCTION

A form of NCL observed in Australian Devon cattle is caused by a mutation in the bovine equivalent of *CLN5*, providing a domestic ruminant model of CLN5 disease, which was defined over the last two decades (Houweling et al., 2006a). Clinical signs are observed in these cattle from 9 months. They become blind, collide with obstacles, tend to walk or trot in a circle when disturbed, and die about 2 years later (Harper et al., 1988). Extensive pedigree information over several generations indicates an autosomal recessive mode of inheritance but a single founder animal could not be identified. Enough heterozygous and affected animals were obtained to establish a small model herd maintained at the University of Sydney. Pathology samples were collected from the herd for over a decade.

Recently an ovine CLN5 disease model was established following diagnosis of an NCL in a flock of New Zealand Borderdale sheep (Jolly et al., 2002a). In this case the pathology and disease course were different enough from those in South Hampshire and Merino to suspect another mutation/gene. DNA parentage analysis identified a carrier ram that was mated to three affected super-ovulated ewes to establish the flock and the number of animals expanded to those required for systematic experimentation. A causative mutation was located in ovine *CLN5* (Frugier et al., 2008).

These models provide an ideal resource for studying CLN5 disease. The weight of evidence now suggests that the *CLN5* gene product is a soluble lysosomal protein and representative of that class. Since the *CLN6* gene product is a membrane protein, both soluble and membrane forms of NCL disease are modelled in large animals.

MOLECULAR GENETICS

The causative mutations have been determined in both the affected Devon cattle and Borderdale sheep. A radiation hybrid study mapped the bovine equivalent of human *CLN5* (Houweling et al., 2006b), to bovine chromosome 12 and the location was confirmed by GenBank annotation. The disease in cattle was linked to this region and only one possible disease-causing mutation was found when the *CLN5* coding sequences of affected and normal cattle were compared, a single base duplication in exon 4, c.662dupG (Houweling et al., 2006a). This duplication is tightly linked to the disease status, there being no recombination between the mutation and the disease phenotype, when tested over a large number of normal, heterozygote and affected cattle ($n=92$, $LOD=11.74$, $\theta=0.00$). The mutation is predicted to introduce a frameshift and disrupt the protein by introducing a premature stop codon causing a major truncation. Analogous human mutations cause NCL.

Linkage studies placed *CLN5* as the candidate gene in the Borderdale sheep and the disease-related defect in *CLN5* confirmed by the discovery of alternative splicing (omission of exon 3) in cDNA from affected Borderdale sheep (Frugier et al., 2008). Exon 3 was missing in cDNA from brain, muscle, and blood from affected animals, whereas it was present in cDNA from blood from all tested control animals and heterozygotes tested yielded cDNA with and without exon 3, confirming disease association. Genomic and cDNA sequencing revealed a disease-associated c.571+1G>A at the junction of exon 3 and intron 3 that disrupts the normal splicing consensus sequence at the 5′ end of the intron. A similar omission of exon 3 causes disease in a knockout mouse model of CLN5 disease (Kopra et al., 2004).

CLINICAL DATA AND DIAGNOSIS

The presenting clinical signs in affected cattle are visual impairment beginning at about 9 months of age that leads to blindness associated with the destruction of rod and cone photoreceptors within the eye. Behavioural characteristics include walking in circles and repetitive head tilting motions indicating altered motor responses and animals become ultimately recumbent. Cerebral and cerebellar degeneration recorded within Devon cattle mirrors that described in human patients (Harper et al., 1988, Martinus et al., 1991). Premature death of affected cattle occurs at approximately 2–3 years of age, a similar reduction in life expectancy to human patients affected with Finnish variant NCL, who succumb to the disorder at 8–12 years of age (Tyynelä et al., 1997).

Blindness is also the first clinical sign of the disease in the affected Borderdale sheep, noticeable at 10–11 months of age and the sheep become easily separated from a flock. Provided with good feed and left relatively undisturbed they live peacefully for another year. Observations so far are that the course of the disease is similar to CLN6 disease in South Hampshire sheep, and despite the brain atrophy being more severe they do not develop the circling behaviour characteristic of advanced disease in the South Hampshire sheep.

Original diagnoses in both these animal models were based on the observance of clinical signs and confirmed by the presence of fluorescent Luxol fast blue and Sudan black storage bodies in brain sections taken at postmortem. The disease in Borderdales was also diagnosed by the presence of these storage bodies in brain biopsies taken at 2–4 months.

Subsequent to the discovery of the disease-causing single base duplication in the *CLN5* gene in affected cattle, a direct DNA test was developed. PCR primers are used that yield a single 62bp product from normal cattle, a single 63bp product from affected cattle and both products from heterozygous cattle. Products can be separated on polyacrylamide gels (Houweling et al., 2006a). The disease specific excision of exon 3 in affected Borderdale sheep allows this to be used for a diagnostic test, and sufficient individuals of known genotype have been tested to ensure it is reliable. Messenger RNA is isolated from blood samples and a region of CLN5 amplified that allows easy separation of the products with or without exon 3 (Frugier et al., 2008).

MORPHOLOGY

Most cells in affected Devon cattle and Borderdale sheep contain fluorescent storage bodies with the histochemical properties and ultrastructure characteristic of the NCLs. They stain with periodic acid–Schiff (PAS), Sudan black, and Luxol fast blue, and stain brown to red with haematoxylin and eosin (Harper et al., 1988, Jolly et al., 2002a). Three types of storage body ultrastructure were observed in both sheep and cattle: curvilinear profiles, dense multilamellar stacks with fingerprint-like profiles, and loose membranous whorls. Subunit c storage was confirmed by direct sequencing of storage body proteins in the cattle (Martinus et al., 1991) and immunohistochemistry in the sheep (Jolly et al., 2002a). Mild astrocytosis was noted in the sheep.

Brain atrophy is profound in both species, brain weights being reduced to 64% of normal weights in cattle and in some animals yellow-brown discoloration of the brain was noted (Harper et al., 1988, Jolly et al., 2002a). A mild loss of neurons in the cerebral cortex and cerebellum, and mild gliosis, occurs in cattle. Immunostaining for GFAP reveals strong astrocytosis in the cerebral cortex.

Neurological degradation occurs within the cerebrocortical grey matter of affected cattle and there is substantial atrophy of the cerebral cortex, thinning of the gyri in the occipital area, atrophy of the cerebellum, and dilation of the lateral ventricles as well as atrophy of the hippocampus (Harper et al., 1988, Martinus et al., 1991). Atrophy of the cerebral cortex is severe in affected sheep with thinning of the cerebral gyri and dilation of the lateral ventricles. Blindness in the affected cattle is associated with retinal atrophy, particularly the loss of rods and cones (Harper et al., 1988, Jolly et al., 1992).

CORRELATIONS

Both the ovine and bovine forms of CLN5 disease have significant similarities to the human disease, and potential as models for active study. Their pathology closely resembles that seen in humans. Blindness accompanied by the destruction of rod and cone photoreceptors within the eye are shared symptoms (Harper et al., 1988). Behavioural characteristics in affected sheep and cattle indicate altered motor responses, which also occur in human CLN5 disease patients. Cerebral and cerebellar degeneration mirrors that described in human patients (Goebel et al., 1999, Haltia, 2003).

Analogous human mutations cause CLN5 disease. A 2bp deletion (c.1175delAT; 'Fin major') in exon 4 of *CLN5* results in premature termination and a longer putative product than the bovine mutation while a single base substitution in exon 1 (c.225G>A; 'Fin minor') results in premature termination (p.Trp75X) and a shorter product (www.ucl.ac.uk/ncl). Another single base duplication (c.669dupC) results in a product similar in length to the truncated aberrant bovine protein. A similar omission of exon 3 causes disease in a CLN5 disease mouse model (Kopra et al., 2004), which serves as a small animal model but lacks the severe brain atrophy characteristic of the sheep and human diseases.

Comparison of the bovine and ovine sequences to those of other species clarified some points of interest to the human gene. Homology to the gene in humans, mice, and dogs is high, 88.95%, 82.09%, and 89.55% respectively in cattle (Houweling et al., 2006a) and similar in sheep (Frugier et al., 2008). Exons 2, 3, and 4 align well but the alignment of the GC-rich exon 1 is more variable. The ovine and bovine genes have only one of the four potential (AUG) initiation sites found in the human gene sequence (Isosomppi et al., 2002). Original computer modelling predicted that the *CLN5* gene product would be a membrane protein, based on initiation from the first available ATG in the human sequence (Savukoski et al., 1998). A careful alignment of human, canine, ovine, and bovine *CLN5* indicated that the third human initiation site is that which is evolutionarily conserved, not the fourth as had been suggested from murine studies (Isosomppi et al., 2002, Holmberg et al., 2004). Initiation from this site is predicted to yield a 358-amino acid protein in cattle and sheep, homologous to a 358-amino acid lysosomally targeted glycoprotein in humans (Houweling et al., 2006a).

Development of the Borderdale sheep model of CLN5 disease continues, and a herd has been established for development of the bovine model. A well-characterized flock of sheep will provide an ideal resource for ongoing model studies, of relevance to this form of NCL and also to soluble lysosomal enzyme forms in general. Hypothetically at least, treatment in these diseases should be easier than for the membrane protein forms, because only a portion of cells need to be repaired which can then secrete enzyme that is taken up by the rest via mannose-6-phosphate receptors on the plasma membrane.

CLN10 disease in sheep

INTRODUCTION

Studies of a congenital NCL diagnosed in White Swedish Landrace lambs that were profoundly affected at birth traced the cause to a mutation in the gene for cathepsin D (Tyynelä et al., 2000). This is the first report of NCL caused by a mutation in a major lysosomal protease. The value of this model study has been highlighted by the subsequent discovery of a congenital human NCL caused by a cathepsin D deficiency (Siintola et al., 2006), as well as disease of later onset. This is the first time that studies of an animal NCL model led to the genetic and biochemical characterization of a human NCL. Milder forms of disease in other animal models are caused by cathepsin D deficiencies in knockout mice (Koike et al., 2000) and a mutation that leaves considerable cathepsin D activity in American Bulldogs (Awano et al., 2006b).

BIOCHEMICAL STUDIES AND MOLECULAR GENETICS

A survey of lysosomal enzyme activities in brain and liver from affected lambs reveal a marked deficiency activity of the aspartyl protease, cathepsin D. Higher concentrations of anti-cathepsin D immunoreactive proteins (Tyynelä et al., 2000) with molecular weights similar to those expected for the single chain and heavy chain forms of this enzyme indicated an active site mutation (Partanen et al., 2003). Sequencing of cathepsin D cDNA from both normal and affected sheep revealed a disease-associated single nucleotide G>A substitution, equivalent to G934>A in the human gene, that codes for a change of the active site aspartic acid, equivalent to human Asp215, to asparagine.

CLINICAL DATA

This disorder occurred in a flock of Swedish sheep on an experimental farm in Northern Sweden (Järplid and Haltia, 1993). Six out of 25 lambs born to carrier parents were affected, consistent with a recessive mode of inheritance. Affected lambs are profoundly affected at birth, being unable to rise to support their bodies, trembling, and weak. They can be kept alive for only a few weeks with bottle feeding and intensive care (Tyynelä et al., 2000).

MORPHOLOGY

Affected brains are only about half the weight of normal at birth. Most affected is the cerebral cortex, the thickness is severely reduced and the white matter throughout the brain is largely devoid of myelin. Deep layers of the cerebral cortex show pronounced neuronal loss, reactive astrocytosis, and infiltration by macrophages. The cerebellum and deeper levels of the brain are less affected, and the visceral organs examined are macroscopically unaffected (Järplid and Haltia, 1993, Tyynelä et al., 2000).

Characteristic storage bodies with a granular osmiophilic ultrastructure are present in neurons and other cells (Järplid and Haltia, 1993, Tyynelä et al., 2000). They stain with PAS, Luxol fast blue, and Sudan black, and are immunohistochemically positive for sphingolipid activator proteins (SAPs) A and D but not for subunit c. Recent biochemistry studies have shown that subunit c is not stored in this disease (D.N. Palmer, M. Baumann, and J. Tyynelä, unpublished results).

LARGE ANIMAL MODELS WITHOUT GENETIC ASSIGNMENT

NCL or NCL-like diseases have been described in a range of species without assignment to a specific genetic locus, and varied levels of information of clinical signs, histopathology, immunohistochemistry, and genetics (Table 18.2). The majority of these reports are individual case studies, which have to be considered with caution as environmental causes of 'ceroid lipofuscin-like' storage with neurological clinical signs have been described in sheep and horses (Hartley et al., 1982, Huxtable et al., 1987). However, in the reports described below on ferrets (France et al., 1999), horses (Url et al., 2001), and a European domestic short-haired cat (Weissenbock and Rossel, 1997), the investigators were able to characterize the storage material as subunit c of mitochondrial ATP synthase, indicating that these cases are NCLs. The substantial clinical and histopathological details provided on Rambouillet sheep (Woods et al., 1993, Edwards et al., 1994, Woods et al., 1994), in combination with the breeding studies (Shelton et al., 1993), confirm these as a model for NCL. Similarly, the disease occurrence in several related Beefmaster cattle (Read and Bridges, 1969) and Nubian goats (Fiske and Storts, 1988), in addition to typical clinical and histopathological findings, strongly supports the NCL diagnoses. More uncertain are the diagnoses of NCLs in two early reports of 'ceroid lipofuscinosis' in a cynomologus monkey (Jasty et al., 1984) and a lovebird (Reece and MacWhirter, 1988).

When considering the information provided on sporadic cases it is important to remember that NCL was diagnosed after necropsy. Animals were often euthanized before full expression of clinical signs, samples for biochemical analysis were often not collected, and in some cases only tissues from the central nervous system were available for pathological investigation. For future reports of sporadic cases it would be advisable to characterize the storage material and where possible attempt to measure enzyme activities for TPP1, PPT1, and CTSD.

In comparison with the experimental research populations with confirmed genetic assignment, described above, these sporadic case studies are less informative for research on NCL. However, the detection and description of these cases is important from a veterinary and agricultural stance and add to our understanding of the range of clinical and histopathological characteristics in this genetically heterogeneous group of diseases. In Rambouillet sheep, some domestic cats, and the Vietnamese pot-bellied pig, the storage material is restricted to neuronal cells (Edwards et al., 1994, Bildfell et al., 1995, Weissenbock and Rossel, 1997, Cesta et al., 2006), whereas the storage is generalized in the other case studies. In most studies visual impairment is one of the characteristic clinical signs, but in goats, ferrets, and pigs (Fiske and Storts, 1988, France et al., 1999, Cesta et al., 2006) hind-limb ataxia appears to be the key clinical finding. Seizures, a key finding in humans suffering from NCL, are most dominant in cats (Green and Little, 1974, Bildfell et al., 1995, Weissenbock and Rossel, 1997). As all these case studies have no genetic assignment it remains unclear if these differences are species specific or due to the involvement of different disease genes.

Rambouillet sheep

Rambouillet sheep with NCL have been reported in four closely related flocks in the USA (Fiske and Storts, 1988, Edwards et al., 1994, Woods et al., 1994), and controlled breeding studies confirmed an autosomal recessive mode of inheritance (Shelton et al. 1993). Detailed clinical signs, computed tomography findings, and pathological findings of animals of different ages have been reported (Woods et al., 1993, Edwards et al., 1994, Woods et al., 1994).

Clinical signs can be identified as early as 4 months by an experienced observer but are more commonly detected at around 8 months of age. They include progressive visual loss, stress-induced circling, decreased cognition (e.g. loss of herding instinct), proprioceptive deficits, poor body condition in later stages of the disease, and premature death at 1–2 years of age. Substantial atrophy of the brain to about half the normal size can be identified at necropsy. Atrophy is more pronounced in the cerebral cortex but also affects the cerebellum and brain stem, and is associated with enlargement of the lateral ventricles. The cerebral cortex is described as firmer when compared with normal brain tissue. Lesions identified by computer tomography of affected sheep aged 4–24 months were limited to the central nervous system and correlated with gross lesions seen at necropsy (Woods et al., 1993). Histological examination identified fluorescent cytoplasmic inclusions limited to neurons in the brain, spinal cord, eye, and dorsal root ganglia which stained with PAS, Sudan black B, Luxol fast blue, and Ziehl–Neelsen acid fast. A wide range of other tissue samples did not contain similar storage material. Progressive neuronal degeneration and fibrillary astrogliosis were evident in the cerebral cortex and to a lesser degree in the cerebellum. Retinal degeneration increased with age, resulting in a pronounced thinning of the retina and a near total loss of rods and cones.

Beefmaster and Holstein Friesian cattle

In addition to the Devon cattle described above, NCL has been reported in a herd of Beefmaster cattle (Read and Bridges, 1969), and more recently in a single Holstein Friesian steer (Hafner et al., 2005). The breeds are not closely related. Devon cattle are an old British beef breed, Beefmasters have been established in the USA by crossing Hereford, Shorthorn, and Brahman in the 1930s, and Holstein Friesians are a dairy breed originating in the Netherlands and the north of Germany.

BEEFMASTERS

A 'neuronal lipodystrophy' with clinical signs and pathology characteristic of an NCL was described in a Beefmaster bull (Read and Bridges, 1969). At about a year of age the bull was noticeably blind and circling intermittently. At about 18 months of age the bull became comatose with periodic clonic convulsions, and died. Similar clinical signs were reported in related animals in the same inbred herd. No gross lesions were reported during necropsy. Histology revealed cytoplasmic granules in neurons in the central nervous system, and the retina that stained with eosin, Luxol fast blue, Oil red O, and Sudan black B, but not with PAS or Ziehl–Neelsen acid fast. Macrophages in the cerebellum, spleen, and lymph nodes were reported to contain eosinophilic granules. Electron microscopy identified the storage material as membrane-bound lamellar and granular structures.

HOLSTEIN FRIESIAN

A single Holstein Friesian steer with NCL has been reported (Hafner et al., 2005). The animal was sent for slaughter at about 15–18 months of age due to progressive visual impairment. Brain atrophy was noted at necropsy, and yellow brown discoloration of the grey matter of the cerebrum. Also noted were potentially unrelated findings of multifocal hepatic abscesses and white foci in the kidney. Histology revealed fluorescent cytoplasmic storage material in neurons, to a lesser degree in macrophages in the brain and retina, and infrequently in cerebral endothelial cells, Kupffer cells in the liver, and the epithelium of cortical tubules in the kidneys. The storage material was PAS, Luxol fast blue, and Sudan black positive, and colourless to moderately eosinophilic. Electron microscopy revealed membrane-bound, electron-dense multilaminar storage bodies. Areas of the cerebrum had increased immunostaining for GFAP compared to controls, and less markedly for synaptophysin, which also stained areas of the retina. Some neuronal necrosis and astrocytosis was noted in the cerebrum, and severe retinal atrophy with total loss of rods and cones. DNA testing for the mutation causing NCL in Devon cattle (Houweling et al., 2006a) excluded this mutation in this animal.

Domestic and Siamese cats

Four independent reports describe case studies of NCLs in different breeds of cats *(Felis catis*), in two unrelated Siamese cats (Green and Little, 1974), a Japanese domestic cat (Nakayama et al., 1993), and two independent cases in domestic shorthaired cats (Bildfell et al., 1995, Weissenbock and Rossel, 1997). Pedigree information was not available for any of the cases, thus the mode of inheritance is unknown.

The onset of disease varied between 7 months and 2 years. In all cases rapid disease progression resulted in premature death or euthanasia within a few months of onset. Clinical signs included behavioural changes (Green and Little, 1974, Bildfell et al., 1995), abnormal reflexes (Bildfell et al., 1995, Weissenbock and Rossel, 1997), visual impairment progressing to blindness, seizures, and/or ataxia (Green and Little, 1974, Nakayama et al., 1993, Bildfell et al., 1995, Weissenbock and Rossel, 1997). Brain atrophy and dilated ventricles were key gross pathological findings (Nakayama et al., 1993, Weissenbock and Rossel, 1997).

Characteristic histopathological findings (cytoplasmic storage material, neuronal loss, gliosis) were restricted to neural tissues except in the Japanese domestic cat, where additional storage material was identified in liver, spleen, and lymph nodes (Nakayama et al., 1993). In all cases the cytoplasmic storage material stained with haematoxylin and eosin, is PAS, Sudan black, and Luxol fast blue positive, and was in general fluorescent, but fluorescence was not mentioned in the Siamese cats (Green and Little, 1974). Differences were found in the ultrastructure of the storage material. That in the Siamese cat was described as 'interwoven pattern with straight and curved elements' (Green and Little, 1974), the material in the domestic cats was membrane-bound and multilamellar (Bildfell et al., 1995, Weissenbock and Rossel, 1997), or aggregates of electron-dense granular material (Nakayama et al., 1993). The storage material was characterized as subunit c of the mitochondrial ATP synthase in one report (Weissenbock and Rossel, 1997) and in all cases the clinical signs and pathology are characteristic of NCLs.

Ferrets

NCL in five domestic pet ferrets (*Mustela putorius furo*) has been discussed as a model for NCL in humans with adult onset (France et al., 1999) (M. France, personal communication). The pedigrees and ages of these animals were unknown but all were fully grown and one was at least 3 years of age at onset of disease.

The initial clinical signs of hind-limb ataxia and paresis progressed to atrophy of hind-limb muscles and incontinence. At this stage behavioural changes and blindness were reported. Repeated clinical examination revealed that the animals were dull and postural responses and proprioceptive positioning of legs were delayed or absent. Patellar reflexes progressed from hypertonic to the development of clonus, whereas pain perception and withdrawal reflexes remained normal. The optic fundi appeared to be normal and pupillary light reflexes intact but menace response was lost at the later stage of the disease.

Gross lesions at necropsy were restricted to diffuse atrophy of grey matter and moderate dilation of cerebral ventricles. Histology revealed cerebrocortical atrophy, reduction in number of neurons, and increase of astrocytes in the brain whereas atrophy of the retina was not significant. Fluorescent intracellular eosinophilic granular material was reported in neurons, macrophages throughout the brain, and to a lesser degree in retinal ganglion cells. The inclusions stained with Luxol fast blue, Sudan black, and PAS but were not acid fast. Storage material was less apparent in other cell types, such as muscle fibres, chondrocytes, and epithelium in a range of organs. Inclusions in these tissues were not noticeable with haematoxylin and eosin staining, but stained with Luxol fast blue and were fluorescent. Immunohistochemistry identified the storage material as predominantly subunit c of mitochondrial ATP synthase and lesser amounts of SAPs. The ultrastructure of the electron-dense, irregular shaped storage material in the brain and retina included a mixture of fingerprint whirls, curvilinear profiles, stacks of membranes, and lipoidal inclusions.

Icelandic/Peruvian Paso horses

Three distantly related Icelandic cross Peruvian Paso horses with NCL were described (Url et al., 2001). The mode of inheritance was considered to be autosomal recessive. Clinical signs included developmental retardation, slow movements, and loss of appetite, which started at about 6 months of age. Neurological signs, such as torticollis, ataxia, head tilt, and abnormal reflexes, became more apparent about 1 year of age; one of the three horses presented with visual failure and the animals were euthanized due to progression of disease at about 2 years.

At necropsy, all three affected horses presented light flattening of gyri, two horses had yellow brownish discoloration of the brain, and one horse had a dilatation of the mesencephalic aqueduct. Light microscopy revealed a massive loss of neurons of all cortical layers of the cerebrum and astrocytosis. Neurons contained coarse granular or homogenous eosinophilic, fluorescent material in the cytoplasm. Similar material was found in neuronal and glial cells in other brain regions, the spinal cord, the myenteric and submucosal ganglia, and trigeminal ganglia. Some retinal cells of neuronal layer III contained storage material but the retinal layers were not atrophied as described in other species with NCL. The storage material stained with Luxol fast blue, Nile blue A, PAS, and Sudan black. Electron microscopy revealed that the storage material in the enlarged lysosomes of neurons, glia, kidney tubular cells, lymphocytes, and macrophages had fingerprint, curvilinear, and rectilinear patterns. Liver cells did not contain abnormal storage bodies. Immunohistochemistry revealed that the storage material was predominantly subunit c of mitochondrial ATP synthase and contained the SAPs A and D.

Nubian goats

NCL has been described in a herd of Nubian goats (Fiske and Storts, 1988) and autosomal recessive inheritance proposed. Two female goats were reported with clinical signs at 10 and 18 months of age, of progressive ataxia, hindquarter paresis, and probable mental retardation. Tissue samples were taken from the central nervous system and the Gasserian ganglia after euthanasia at 2 and 4 years. Some neurons appeared to be swollen. Microscopy revealed cytoplasmic storage material in neurons that was fluorescent, eosinophilic, PAS and acid fast positive, stains black with Sudan black, and dark blue with Luxol fast blue. The material was most abundant in neurons of the ventral horns of the spinal cord and segments of the brain stem. Some macrophages also contained PAS-positive material. The material in the neurons was described ultrastructually as spherical, concentrically-laminated membranous bodies with some occurrence of fingerprint patterns.

Vietnamese pot-bellied pig

NCL has been described in a single Vietnamese pot-bellied pig (Cesta et al., 2006). At about 2 years of age the pig was noticed to have a mild hind-limb ataxia followed by a rapid progression of clinical signs, of tetraparesis, head tilts, stumbling, falling, and intermittent nystagmus over the next month. Mentation and attitude were described as normal and no visual deficits or seizures were reported. The animal ceased to drink and eat and was euthanized after a thorough neurological investigation. No gross lesions were noticed at necropsy and, although a range of tissues were investigated, only central nervous system cells contained characteristic storage material. Neurons, some astrocytes, and microglia contained cytoplasmic fluorescent storage bodies that stained golden brown to deeply pink with haematoxylin and eosin, blue with Luxol fast blue, black with Sudan black B, and were PAS and acid fast positive. Microgliosis and neuronal degeneration were evident. The neuronal loss was most evident in the hippocampus, which also contained the most storage material, but the amount of storage material was not consistently correlated with neuronal loss in other regions of the brain. Electron microscopy was used to characterize the storage bodies as membranous material forming predominantly multilamellar profiles, with some curvilinear profiles and some more granular components.

Uncertain classifications

The following two case studies in lovebirds (Reece and MacWhirter, 1988) and a single, clinically normal cynomolgus monkey (Jasty et al., 1984) were published as possible cases of ceroid lipofuscinosis. However, the fact that a brain tumour was identified in the only lovebird presented for histopathology, which could have been responsible for the clinical signs described, and the lack of neurological disease in the cynomolgus monkey make these cases less convincing than those above.

LOVEBIRD

A 'neuronal ceroid lipofuscinosis' was reported in peach-faced lovebirds, *Agapornis roseicollis* (Reece and MacWhirter, 1988). Several birds in two flocks had similar clinical signs but only one was subject of a detailed clinical and pathological description. The bird presented at 9 months of age with in-coordination, loss of balance, and intermittent convulsive seizures, and died after a seizure. No gross lesions were observed at necropsy but microscopy revealed histological changes to the brain and spinal cord, whereas kidney and liver appeared to be normal. The report does not indicate if the bird had visual problems nor discusses any pathology of the retina.

Histopathology revealed cytoplasmic storage granules in Purkinje cells of the cerebellar cortex, neurons of the brain stem nuclei, and ventral horns in the spinal cord. The storage material was stained yellow gold with haematoxylin and eosin, was acid fast and PAS positive, and fluorescent under ultraviolet light. Many of the neurons with storage material were described as degenerate. A potential Schwann cell tumour of a cranial nerve close to the brain stem was identified, and therefore the underlying cause of the neurological signs in this bird was unclear.

CYNOMOLGUS MONKEY

A single case of 'generalized ceroid lipofuscinosis' was reported in a cynomolgus monkey, *Macaca fascicularis* (Jasty et al., 1984). The monkey was about 7 years of age with normal behaviour and apparently healthy when sacrificed in a drug safety evaluation study. Lesions due to parasite infestations in lungs and caecum, a coarse surface of the right kidney, and a partially healed fracture of radius and ulna were reported.

Surprisingly, microscopic analysis identified cytoplasmic storage bodies in a range of tissues including neuronal cells of the central nervous system and myenteric plexus, cells of the optic nerve, muscle cells, as well as cells of the salivary gland, pancreas, testes, epididymis, bile duct, gall bladder, sweat glands, thyroid, parathyroid, adrenal gland, choroid plexus, liver, and kidney. The round to slightly irregular cytoplasmic granules of approximately 0.5–3μm stained red with haematoxylin and eosin, deep blue with phosphotungstic acid–haematoxilin and toluidine blue, weakly to moderately with Oil red O and Sudan black, and weakly with PAS and acid fast. The material did not react with stains for iron, haemofuscin, or bilirubin pigment. It was fluorescent *in situ*. Only cardiac muscle and a few neuronal cells appeared to be affected by the presence of storage granules. The density of the sarcoplasm was reduced at the poles of the nucleus in cardiac muscle cells and some neurons with abundant storage material appeared to have a degraded nucleus.

Electron micrography revealed that the storage bodies were membrane-bound and that their ultrastructure varied in different tissues. Cardiac muscle cells contained dense osmiophilic material with occasional lamellae formation and ductal cells of the salivary gland bodies contained highly osmiophilic lamellar components. Storage bodies in other tissues appeared to contain several small electron-dense granules. Neuronal cell bodies were more irregular and contained fingerprint-type membranous structures.

It remains unclear if this monkey with 'generalized ceroid lipofuscinosis' represents a preclinical stage of NCL.

DOG MODELS

Introduction

The dog, as a favoured companion of humans, is unique among animal species in providing new insights into human genetic diseases. Naturally occurring NCL-like diseases have been reported in a large number of dog breeds (Table 18.3) (Jolly and Walkley, 1997). The major advantages dogs offer for comparative genetic studies are the high degree of medical surveillance of the dog by veterinary specialists, the structure of dog populations consisting of more than 300 partially inbred genetic isolates (breeds) with genetic disorders predominantly or exclusively in one or a few breeds,

Table 18.3 **Dog breeds diagnosed with NCL. See also 'Neuronal Canine Ceroid Lipofuscinosis Basics' at http://www.caninegeneticdiseases.net/CL_site/basicCL.htm**

American Bulldogs
American Staffordshire Terriers
Australian Cattle Dogs
Australian Shepherds
Blue Heelers
Border Collies
Chihuahuas
Cocker Spaniels
Dachshunds
Dalmatians
English Setters
Golden Retrievers
Japanese Retrievers
Labrador Retrievers
Miniature Schnauzers
Pit Bull Terriers
Polish Owczarek Nizinny (PON) or Polish Lowland Sheepdogs
Salukis
Tibetan Terriers
Welsh Corgis

and the excellent arsenal of dog genome resources (Ostrander et al., 2000). In the past, the limiting step in demonstrating true homology of canine and human diseases at the gene level has been the cloning and characterization of canine disease genes. This changed rapidly. Just after the establishment of the first set of linked canine microsatellite markers (Lingaas et al., 1997) the first meiotic linkage map of the whole dog genome was published (Mellersh et al., 1997). Considerable effort was made by the development of an integrated high quality radiation hybrid map (Guyon et al., 2003) and a high-density resolution dog–human chromosomal comparative map (Breen et al., 2004). Finally, after the availability of a 1.5× Poodle sequence (Kirkness et al., 2003), the first high-quality draft (7.5×) sequence of the Boxer dog was made publicly available in July 2004 (Lindblad-Toh et al., 2005). The recent development of single nucleotide polymorphism (SNP) genotyping arrays with tens of thousands SNPs showed that genome-wide association mapping of Mendelian traits in dog breeds can be achieved with only approximately 20 affected dogs (Karlsson et al., 2007). These outstanding dog genome resources, together with the well-characterized relationship between the human and canine genomes, currently facilitate analyses of well-characterized canine inherited diseases to serve as useful models for the analysis and treatment of corresponding human disorders. The canine disorders have the potential for serving as models for the analogous human diseases. In addition, identification of the mutations responsible for some of the canine NCLs may lead to the discovery of new causes of human NCLs for which the genetic bases remain to be determined.

NCLs are distinguished from other inherited disorders by the unique combination of progressive neurodegeneration and the accumulation of autofluorescent lysosomal storage bodies in neural and other tissues. A diagnosis of NCL is valid only in dogs that exhibit both of these features. In most cases, identification of NCL in a dog breed was first made in clinical case reports in the veterinary literature. For many breeds, these isolated case reports represent the only evidence of NCL and no attempts were made to determine the mode of inheritance or even to establish the existence of affected relatives. There are exceptions, however, and these exceptions have led to the development of canine models of NCL and to the identification of seven specific mutations responsible for NCL disorders in dogs (Table 18.4).

Dog models with identified genes

ENGLISH SETTER (CLN8 DISEASE)

The first canine NCL model to be developed was a group of English Setters in Norway in the 1950s. Nils Koppang, a Norwegian veterinarian, encountered the canine disease in his practice and recognized it as a potential model for human NCL. He had the wisdom to obtain and breed dogs to establish a colony that could be used for research. Dr Koppang and his collaborators performed extensive phenotypic characterization of the English Setter disease and established that it was inherited as an autosomal recessive trait (Koppang, 1966, Koppang, 1988, Koppang, 1992). Subunit c of mitochondrial ATP synthase is stored, with just minor amounts of SAPs A and D deposited (Palmer et al., 1997a). Affected animals show no specific

Table 18.4 **NCLs in dogs for which the causative mutations have been identified**

Dog breed	Age of clinical onset of NCL	Ultrastructure of storage bodies contents	Dog genome location	Affected gene	Mutation	Reference (for mutation)
English Setter	Juvenile (14–16 months)	Fingerprint, membrane-like, granular matrix	CFA37	*CLN8*	p.Leu164Pro	Katz et al., 2005
Border Collie	Juvenile (15 months, varies greatly)	Membranous, fingerprint, crystalloid structures and amorphous matrix	CFA22	*CLN5*	p.Gln206X	Melville et al., 2005
American Bulldog	Later onset (1 and 3 years)	Granular matrices surrounding well-delineated spherical structures	CFA18	*CTSD*	p.Met199Ile	Awano et al., 2006b
Dachshund	Late juvenile (9 months)	Curvilinear	CFA21	*TPP1*	p.Arg109fs	Awano et al., 2006a
Australian Shepherd	Juvenile (17–19 months)	Modified curvilinear	CFA30	*CLN6*	p.Trp277Arg	Katz et al., in press 2010
American Staffordshire Terrier	Adult (3–5 years)	Concentric straight or curved profiles with alternating clear and dense bands	CFA09	*ARSG*	p.Arg299His	Abitbol et al., 2010
Dachshund	Late juvenile (9 months)	Granular and some membrane-like	CFA15	*PPT1*	c.747–748insC, causing a frameshift at residue 245 and a truncated protein	Sanders et al., 2010

symptoms from birth until about 12 months of age. From 12–15 months of age there are progressive symptoms of in-coordination, stiffness, and loss of vision. Mental dullness is also a prominent sign of the disease. From 15–18 months the symptoms are generally distinctive, including loss of bearings, difficulties in localizing sounds, signs of ataxia, and development of a stiff gait. Some dogs may show muscular spasms from about 18 months of age. From the first symptoms to death, usually no later than 24 months of age, convulsions are frequently observed. The dogs often die as the result of an acute severe seizure and very few dogs survive beyond the age of 2 years (Koppang, 1988). The lipopigments show a diversified ultrastructural pattern, including curvilinear, fingerprint, and lamellar contents (Figure 18.4), and they also form extracerebrally, e.g. in circulating lymphocytes (Figures 18.5 and 18.6). Autopsy shows a marked cerebral atrophy, primarily due to a massive neuronal degeneration. In end-stage dogs severely affected by the disease the brain weighs about 60–70% of that of normal control animals. The atrophic brain is firm in consistency, the grey matter areas are reduced in extent and display a yellow-brown discoloration. The ventricular system is dilated with a markedly increased amount of cerebrospinal fluid. In the end-stage disease the neurons are filled

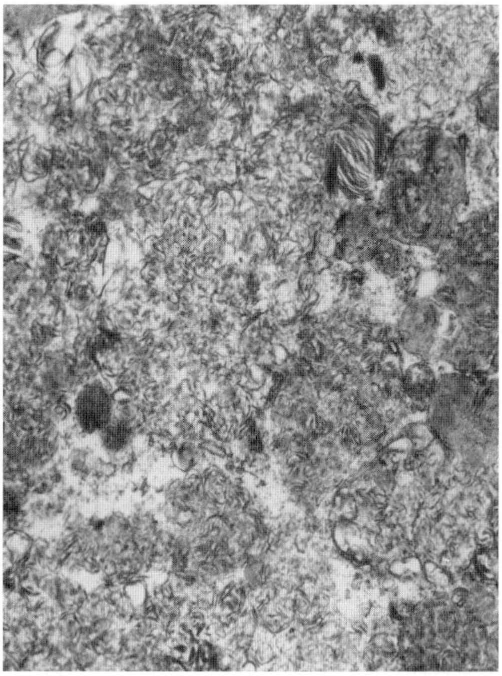

Figure 18.4 Canine NCL: a large aggregate of diversified lamellae make up cerebral lipopigments of an English Setter, ×28,700.

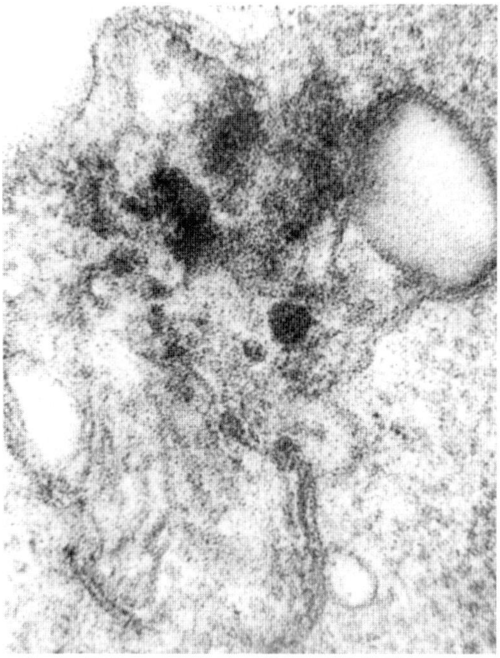

Figure 18.6 Canine NCL: high magnification of complex lamellar lipopigment body in a circulating lymphocyte of an English Setter, ×136,300.

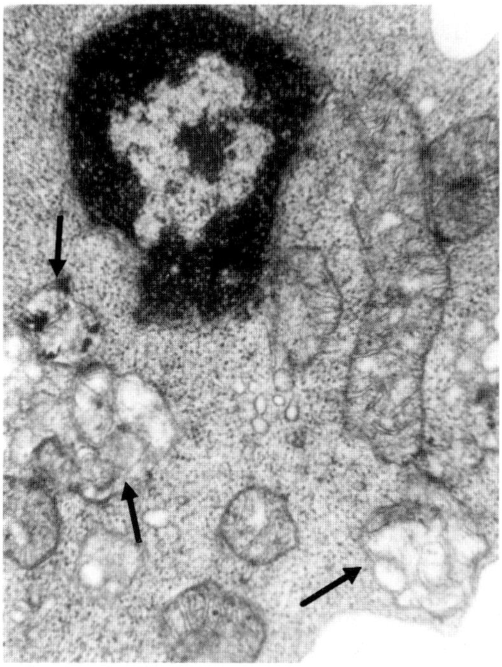

Figure 18.5 Canine NCL: a circulating lymphocyte of an English Setter contains several lipopigments (arrows), ×36,000.

with characteristic dense inclusions. The cerebellum is also affected by atrophic changes.

The first autofluorescent pigments can be detected by conventional light microscopy at around 2–3 months of age in about 30% of the neurons. At 4–5 months, the total amount of autofluorescent intracellular material increases and autofluorescence becomes more intense and stable. Nearly all neurons contain at least a few pigment granules by about 6 months of age. By 12 months these pigment granules occupy most of the cytoplasm in a high percentage of the large neurons. At this time the degenerative changes start, observed as nuclear pyknosis, rounding of soma, and the loss of Nissl substance. A progressive loss of neurons continues, and by age 15–24 months there is a total loss of cells in many grey matter areas, particularly in the cerebellar cortex (Koppang, 1973).

Clinical and morphological findings of the retina in canine NCL of English setters differ from retinal pathology in human NCL. The accumulation of lipopigments does not seem to result in morphological decay of photoreceptor cells (Figure 18.7), a prominent pathological feature in human NCL. Retinal changes in

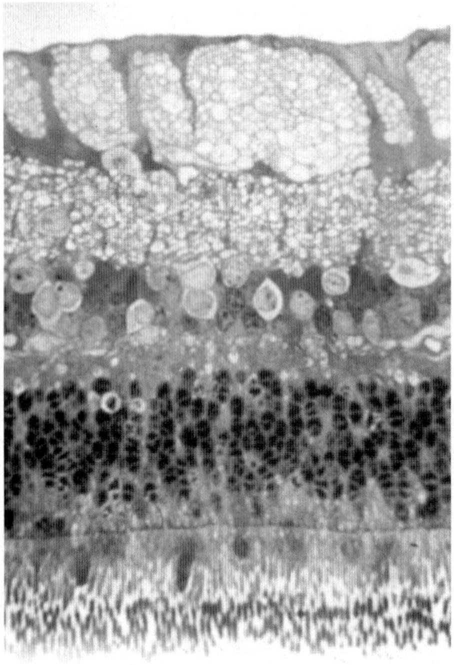

Figure 18.7 Canine NCL: structurally well-preserved retina in an English Setter, 1μm-thick toluidine blue-stained section, ×528.

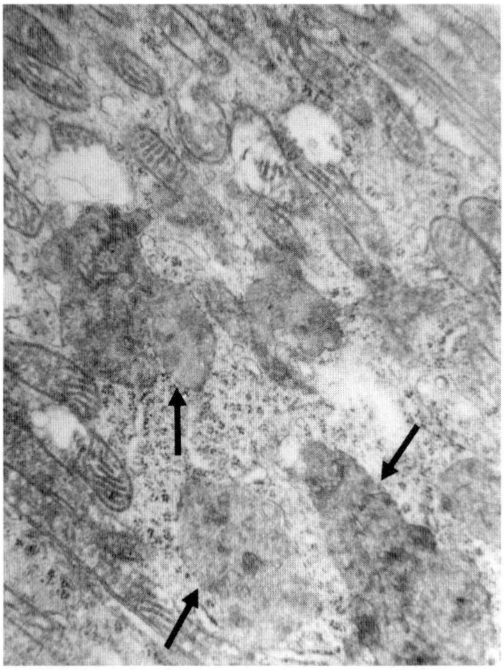

Figure 18.8 Canine NCL: several lipopigments (arrows) in photoreceptor cells of an English Setter, ×29,600.

human patients with NCL occur much earlier and result in a complete loss of photoreceptor elements whereas the dog retina remains relatively intact. Even so, affected dogs have severely reduced vision and are almost blind at the terminal stage of the disease. The loss of vision is probably due to atrophy of the occipital cortex. Electron microscopy of the retina shows that storage material is present in almost every cell type of the retina (Figure 18.8), especially in ganglion cells. The fine structure shows typical curvilinear, fingerprint, membranous, and large complex bodies, resembling the crystalloid inclusions of extraretinal cells. In individual retinal cells only one ultrastructural type occurs (Goebel et al., 1979). Electron microscopic observations on brain biopsies and autopsy material from young puppies show that storage can be detected as early as 2 days of age, and typical membrane bound storage bodies are common in neurons of the spinal cord but rare in cerebral nerve cells at this age. These small bodies frequently show a fingerprint pattern. The storage bodies increase in number and size with advancing age, but no evidence of damage is seen until about 12 months of age. At 12–25 months of age the bodies are very large and there is mounting evidence of neuronal damage (Koppang, 1973). Prof Koppang proposed that English Setter NCL was analogous to what is now known as CLN3 disease, juvenile. However, at the time he was working, no mutations responsible for the human NCLs had been identified.

In 1998, Lingaas and his collaborators (Lingaas et al., 1998) genetically mapped the English Setter NCL locus to canine chromosome 37 (CFA37) by genotyping of microsatellite markers within the established research colony pedigree. At that time the comparative canine/human chromosomal map indicated that CFA37 was completely orthologous to a region of human chromosome 2 (HSA2). Since no known NCL genes map to HSA2, it appeared that the NCL of English Setters was caused by a mutation in an as yet undiscovered NCL gene. In 2004 when the first assembly of the canine genome sequence was released, a sequence-based human–dog comparison revealed that the canine orthologue of human *CLN8* maps to CFA37. Further investigation indicated that although most of CFA37 was orthologous to a segment of HSA2q, canine *CLN8* and other genes in a 1Mb segment at the telomeric end of CFA37, had orthologues on human chromosome 8p (HSA8p) to which CLN8 had been mapped. Therefore, the canine *CLN8* orthologue was evaluated as a candidate gene for the English Setter disease. The coding region of *CLN8* from an affected English Setter was found to contain a T>C transition that predicts a p.Leu164Pro missense mutation which cosegregated with the disease in a small canine family in a pattern consistent with autosomal recessive inheritance (Katz et al., 2005a). Identification of the *CLN8* mutation responsible for English Setter NCL appears to have devalued this animal model in the eyes of funding agencies, as no support could be obtained for maintaining a small research colony. This is probably due to what was thought to be the very low number of human NCL cases caused by *CLN8* mutations. As a result, maintenance of the English Setter colony was discontinued. However, frozen semen and fibroblast cell cultures from affected English Setters are stored at the University of Missouri. In Norway, where the diseases used to be prevalent, the mutation is nearly eradicated from the English setter population through systematic selection of breeders. Carrier dogs from the original research population and frozen seemen is available at the Norwegian School of Veterinary Science for research purposes.

BORDER COLLIE (CLN5 DISEASE)

A second canine NCL mutation was identified in 2005. NCL had been diagnosed in a substantial number of Border Collies in Australia (Taylor and Farrow, 1992). The first clinical sign of ceroid lipofuscinosis in border collies is observed at 16–23 months of age. All dogs develop behaviour changes, motor abnormalities, and blindness. Behavioural changes are often observed as hyperactivity and aimless wandering, fearfulness, continuous barking, and loss of learned behaviour including house training. Blindness or partial visual loss often develops late at about 21 months of age (Studdert and Mitten, 1991). No fundoscopic changes were observed, but ultrastructural studies showed extensive pigment deposition in different cell types of the retina, but preservation of photoreceptors (Taylor and Farrow, 1988). Accumulation of subunit c was reported in the Border Collies (Jolly et al., 1994b) but only minor amounts of SAPs A and D (Palmer et al., 1997a).

Wilton and colleagues collected DNA samples and pedigree information from affected dogs, obligate carriers, and other related dogs from the pet and breeder population (Melville et al., 2005). Using a combination of linkage and candidate gene analyses, they identified a nonsense point mutation in the canine orthologue of *CLN5* on CFA22 which leads to a truncated CLN5 protein (p.Gln206X) as the cause of NCL in this breed. A simple DNA screening test was developed to identify dogs with this mutation. This test is now being employed to eradicate the mutation from the breed. This truncation mutation should result in a protein product of a size similar to that of some mutations identified in human *CLN5* and therefore the Border Collie may make a good model for human NCL. However, no attempt to maintain affected dogs as a possible model for the analogous human disease has been reported. There are currently still a significant number of carrier dogs under private ownership that could potentially be used to establish a research model (A. Wilton, personal communication).

AMERICAN BULLDOG (CLN10 DISEASE)

A progressive neurological disease was observed in a number of American Bulldogs in 2001–2003 (Evans et al., 2005). Clinical signs, first observed at 1–3 years of age, consist primarily of motor abnormalities that included ataxia and hypermetria in all four limbs. Early signs also include delays in conscious proprioception and hopping reactions in the pelvic limbs. Eventually all four limbs become involved and at the end stage of the disease affected dogs have difficulty rising from a recumbent position without assistance. No cognitive abnormalities or personality changes were reported (Evans et al., 2005). Affected dogs were usually euthanized by 5–6 years of age due to the severity of the symptoms. Morphological analyses demonstrated massive accumulations of autofluorescent storage bodies in brain and retinal neurons (Evans et al., 2005), confirming that the disorder in this breed is a form of NCL. Pedigree analysis indicated that the disorder is inherited as an autosomal recessive trait (Evans et al., 2005). DNA from affected American Bulldogs was used to resequence genes that contain NCL-causing mutations in other species. Among these was the gene for cathepsin

D (*CTSD*) that causes congenital NCL in sheep and knockout mice (Koike et al., 2000, Tyynelä et al., 2000). Resequencing canine *CTSD* revealed that American Bulldog NCL is caused by a G>A missense mutation that predicts the replacement of methionine-199 by isoleucine (Awano et al., 2006b). This amino acid change results in a substantial reduction, but not a complete loss, of cathepsin D enzyme activity in the brain (Awano et al., 2006b). The residual cathepsin D activity probably explains why NCL in these dogs is of later onset and less severe than the disease observed in the sheep and mice that lack detectable cathepsin D activity (Koike et al., 2000, Tyynelä et al., 2000). Congenital and later onset forms of human NCL have also been attributed to *CTSD* mutations (Siintola et al., 2006, Steinfeld et al., 2006), also known as CLN10 disease.

The *CTSD* mutation is common among American Bulldogs. At the University of Missouri 640 American Bulldogs, including 23 affected animals, had been genotyped for the *CTSD* mutation by July 2008. All 23 affected American Bulldogs were homozygous for the mutant 'A' allele. The 617 normal American Bulldogs were either homozygous for the wild-type 'G' allele (n=395) or A/G heterozygotes (n=222). Thus, there are a large number of carrier dogs under private ownership and some of them may be available to establish a research model. Several affected dogs underwent observation at the University of Missouri for detailed disease phenotype characterization. However, no affected dogs are currently being maintained in research colonies. Preserved semen and low-passage fibroblast cell cultures from an affected dog are in frozen storage at the University of Missouri.

DACHSHUND (CLN1 AND CLN2 DISEASES)

Reports of NCL in Dachshunds have been published on at least four occasions (Cummings and de Lahunta, 1977, Vandevelde and Fatzer, 1980, Awano et al., 2006a, Sanders et al., 2010). In 1977, a Wirehaired Dachshund was described with a neurodegenerative disease that began with hind-leg weakness at 3 years of age and progressed slowly with marked cerebellar signs and decreased retinal function (Cummings and de Lahunta, 1977). Necropsy findings included cerebellar atrophy, yellow discoloration of cerebellar nuclei and the pontine nuclear area, and enlargement of the lateral and fourth ventricles. There was marked loss of cerebellar Purkinje cells and cerebellar neurons and macrophages contained autofluorescent cytoplasmic granules. Electron microscopy revealed that the storage granules contained membranous forms, often arranged in parallel, forming zebra bodies. No genetic or biochemical analyses were performed on this dog, and no reports of other Dachshunds with similar disease features have appeared.

Related longhaired Dachshunds that exhibited mental deterioration at 5 and 7 years of age have been described (Vandevelde and Fatzer, 1980). Autofluorescent cytoplasmic inclusions were found in neurons throughout the brain. Within the cerebellum, there was marked degeneration of neurons in the granular layer, with relative sparing of the Purkinje cells. Membranous forms were prominent in the ultrastructure of the storage granules; however, fingerprint forms were common and zebra bodies were rare. This Dachshund disease appears to be identical to a more recently reported one of wirehaired Dachshunds that was found to be caused by a 3bp deletion in the canine heparin sulfate sulfamidase gene (*SGSH*), which causes mucopolysaccharidosis IIIA, also known as Sanfilippo syndrome type A (Fischer et al., 1998, Aronovich et al., 2000). Interestingly, a patient diagnosed as adult onset NCL was recently reported to carry mutations in the *SGSH* gene (Sleat et al., 2009).

A male Dachshund with a much earlier onset neurological disorder has also been described (Awano et al., 2006a). Disease symptoms in this pet dog first became apparent at approximately 9 months of age, and included vomiting, mental dullness, loss of housebreaking, and unresponsiveness to previously learned commands. The dullness progressed, and the dog developed ataxia and visual deficits by 10 months of age. Myoclonus of the head appeared at 11 months of age and progressed to generalized myoclonic seizures. The dog exhibited episodes of hyperactivity and howling. He became aggressive and developed a hypermetric gait and circled incessantly. Vomiting became more frequent, diarrhoea developed and progressed to haematochezia, and the dog died at 1 year of age. The owner submitted the refrigerated carcass for necropsy. Autofluorescent cellular inclusions characteristic of NCL were observed in cerebral cortex, cerebellum, and spinal cord. Electron microscopic analysis of these tissues revealed that their contents had the distinctive curvilinear profiles characteristic of human CLN2 disease, late infantile, a disease that results from mutations in the tripeptidyl peptidase 1 (*TPP1*) gene (Awano et al., 2006a). Resequencing of the canine orthologue (*TPP1*) in DNA from the affected dog revealed a single nucleotide deletion in exon 4 which predicted a frameshift after codon 107 and a premature stop codon at position 114. TPP1 enzyme activity was undetectable in brain tissue from this dog. The sire and dam of the affected dog were located, and blood samples were obtained for genetic analyses. Both parents were found to be heterozygous for the *TPP1* mutation. These dogs were donated to the University of Missouri and have been used to establish a research colony that is being investigated as a model for human CLN2 disease (Awano et al., 2006a, Katz et al., 2008) and for evaluating potential therapeutic interventions.

Another male Dachshund that presented at 9 months with NCL-like symptoms was found to have a mutation in the *PPT1* gene (Sanders et al., 2010). Presenting signs included kyphosis and stiffness of gait. The disease progressed over the next 2 months to include uncontrolled rhythmic head movements, loss of peripheral motor control, and vision loss in dim lighting. Fundoscopic analysis revealed diffuse retinal thinning and severe retinal vessel attenuation. By 12 months of age the dog showed complete loss of vision and increased neuropathological signs. The owners reported a progressive increase in nervousness, decreased interactions with other dogs in the household, a severe loss in the ability to recognize or respond to commands or his name, a loss in the ability to recognize the primary owner or other people in the household, an increased sensitivity to loud noises, circling behaviour, increasing inappropriate vocalization, loss of ability to climb stairs or other obstacles, tremors, loss of coordination, severe loss of vision, persistent head movements, and bumping into obstacles. The dog was euthanized at 14 months of age. At necropsy the size and weight of the cerebellum were lower than normal for a dog of that size and age. There was massive accumulation of autofluorescent storage material in neurons of the retina, which was more widely distributed than that in other dogs with different types of NCL, as well as in the cerebellum and cerebral cortex. Ultrastructural examination revealed granular osmiophilic deposits (GRODs) similar to those that occur in CLN1 disease in humans, as well as some more complex structures, in cells from the cerebral cortex and cerebellum. Brain tissue from the affected dog lacked PPT1 enzymatic activity. Sequencing of *PPT1* revealed a single nucleotide insertion in exon 8 (*PPT1* c.747_748insC), upstream of the His289 active site. The affected Dachshund was homozygous for the c.747_748insC mutation, his sire and dam were heterozygotes and 127 unrelated Dachshunds were homozygous for the wild-type allele. This is the first reported instance of canine NCL caused by a mutation in PPT1.

AUSTRALIAN SHEPHERD (CLN6 DISEASE AND UNKNOWN)

Anecdotal reports of NCL in Australian Shepherds have appeared in review articles, but no confirmed cases were described until recently, when the disease was reported in three littermates (O'Brien and Katz, 2008). An 18-month-old, male intact Australian Shepherd presented with a 1-month history of progressive vision loss and tremors. On examination the dog was alert, but nervous and very sensitive to touch or sound. He had a wide-based stance in the hind limbs and mild hypermetria. Menace reflexes were absent, with normal pupillary light reflexes and electroretinograms in each eye. The dog was placed on prednisone 1mg/kg daily with no improvement. The owners elected euthanasia and a necropsy was performed. Two littermates had a similar history. Magnetic resonance imaging (MRI) on one of the dogs showed cerebral atrophy as evidenced by enlarged ventricles and widened sulci. The dogs exhibited massive accumulation of the yellow-emitting autofluorescent pigment characteristic of NCL throughout the central nervous system. Only paraffin-embedded tissue was available, so initially no attempt was made to identify the underlying mutation.

Subsequently, tissues were received from an unrelated Australian Shepherd. This dog also presented with vision loss at 18 months, and within a few months this progressed to complete blindness. The dog exhibited circling behaviour and became progressively ataxic and anxious. In addition, the dog exhibited loss of cognitive ability and developed trouble eating and drinking. This dog was euthanized and a necropsy was performed. Substantial accumulations of the disease-specific autofluorescent storage material were observed in the retina, cerebral cortex, and cerebellum. Partial nucleotide sequence analysis identified a T>C transition mutation in the *CLN6* gene. Only the T allele was observed in 160 clinically normal Australian Shepherds. The mutation predicts in a change of tryptophan-227 to arginine in the CLN6 protein. Tryptophan is conserved across many other species at this position (Katz et al., 2010). These findings make it likely that the *CLN6* T>C transition was responsible for NCL in this dog. Subsequent analysis of the *CLN6* nucleotide sequence in the other three Australian Shepherds with NCL indicated that they were homozygous for the normal allele. Therefore, it appears that there are two genetically distinct forms of NCL in this breed.

AMERICAN STAFFORDSHIRE TERRIER (ARSG DISEASE)

The disease segregating in American Staffordshire Terriers is of late onset, starting in the majority of dogs at 3–5 years of age (Abitbol et al., 2010). There are locomotor disabilities with static and dynamic ataxia that is detected early by the owners. There is no obvious visual impairment. MRI reveals significant cerebellar atrophy, also detectable at necroscopy. There is a marked loss of Purkinje cells. PAS reagent-, Luxol fast blue-, and Sudan black-positive material is present in surviving Purkinje cells, and other cells. Ultrastructural examination of Purkinje cells reveals abnormal lysosomes filled with inclusions of medium electron density, displaying curved, straight, or concentric profiles with alternate clear and dark bands. Unlike other NCL dog models, no lesions or lipofuscin are observed in the retina.

The disease locus was mapped using a cohort of unrelated dogs, including 39 affected dogs, to chromosome 9. A c.296G>A nucleotide change, which causes a predicted missense mutation p.Arg299His, is present in the gene *ARSG*, encoding arylsulphatase G, in homozygous form in affected dogs an in heterozygous form in carrier dogs. This change affects an amino acid conserved between *ARSG* from different species and different aryl sulphatases. ARSG activity is reduced in leucocytes from affected dogs.

A number of cases of adult onset NCL have been reported in humans (Cummings and de Lahunta, 1977, Goebel et al., 1982, Martin et al., 1987, Traboulsi et al., 1987, Carpenter, 1988, Martin, 1991, Sakajiri et al., 1995, Sadzot et al., 2000). For the most part, the loci responsible for human adult onset NCL, including forms known as Kufs disease that does not include visual failure, remain unknown. Some cases of adult onset NCL may result from mutations in the human *ARSG* gene. Mutation analyses are currently being performed on DNA from human adult onset cases of NCL to determine whether any of them are associated with mutations in this gene.

TIBETAN TERRIER (NOVEL NCL DISEASE)

The Tibetan Terrier disease is distinguished from the majority of the described canine NCLs by its late onset. Although there are some conflicting reports on when disease signs first appear (Alroy et al., 1992, Riis et al., 1992, Katz et al., 2005b), health surveys obtained from owners of over 30 dogs with confirmed NCL indicate that disease onset seldom occurs before 5 years of age (M.L. Katz, unpublished data). A report of earlier onset (Riis et al., 1992) may have resulted from a confusion of NCL with progressive retinal atrophy, which also occurs in this breed (Millichamp et al., 1988). The Tibetan Terrier disease progresses slowly, and affected dogs are usually euthanized at 8–10 years of age due to disease-related debility. Clinical signs of NCL in this breed include nervousness or anxiety, aggressiveness, sensitivity to noise, cognitive impairment, ataxia, tremors, loss of coordination, moderate progressive visual impairment, and seizures (Katz et al., 2005b). Symptoms are initially mild but become more severe as the disease progresses. The signs deemed to characterize the disease were reported by owners of dogs that were confirmed upon necropsy to have suffered from NCL (Farias et al., 2010). Substantial accumulation of autofluorescent storage material occurs in the retina and widely throughout the brain (Alroy et al., 1992, Katz et al., 2005b) (Figure 18.9). The storage material exhibits ultrastructural features characteristic of some of the other NCLs (Figure 18.10). The most

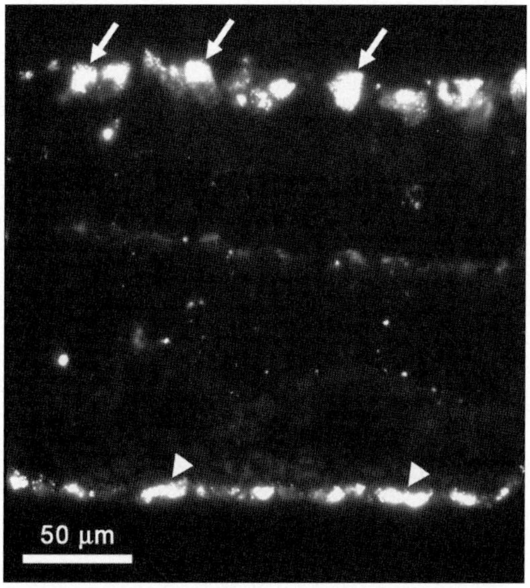

Figure 18.9 Canine NCL: Tibetan Terrier. Fluorescence micrograph of a cryostat section of the retina. Accumulation of autofluorescent inclusions in the ganglion cells (arrows) is diagnostic of NCL in this breed. The retinal pigment epithelium (arrowheads) also exhibits autofluorescent pigment accumulation, but this accumulation occurs as part of the normal aging process.

significant gross pathological finding is a severe reduction in size of the cerebellum. Histologically the retina and cerebellar folia are atrophic. The retina has a massive loss of retinal ganglion cells, cells of the inner and outer nuclear layers and photoreceptors. Extensive loss of neuronal cells is also noted in the cerebellum, while there is a more moderate loss of neurons in the cerebrum. In general viable neurons are enlarged and contain cytoplasmic granules. Ultrastructural studies of the brain revealed perikarya filled with secondary lysosomes containing lamellar material.

Collection of health and pedigree information on affected dogs and their close relatives indicate that Tibetan Terrier NCL is inherited as a simple autosomal recessive trait. Resequencing of NCL candidate genes (*CLN1/PPT1*, *CLN2/TPP1*, *CLN5*, *CLN6*, *CLN8*, *CLN10/CTSD*, and *CLCN3*) failed to identify the mutation responsible for the disorder in this breed (Drögemüller et al., 2005a, Drögemüller et al., 2005b, Wohlke et al., 2005, Wohlke et al., 2006), and recent homozygosity mapping studies exclude all canine chromosome regions harbouring the known comparative NCL genes as potential sites for the Tibetan Terrier disease mutation. These studies located the mutation responsible for the disease to a 1.3 Mb region of canine chromosome 2 (G.S. Johnson, M.L. Katz, and colleagues). This region contains 18 annotated genes. Exon sequencing was performed on a number of genes in this region considered most likely to harbour the NCL mutation based on the known functions of the proteins

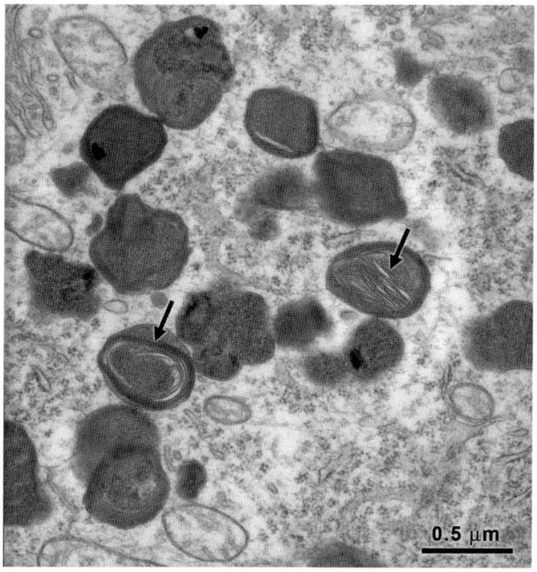

Figure 18.10 Canine NCL: Tibetan Terrier. Electron micrograph of a retinal ganglion cell. Many of the disease-related storage bodies (arrows) contain membrane-like inclusions.

encoded by them. These analyses did not identify any mutations likely to cause the disorder. Initiation of sequence analysis of the entire candidate region resulted in identification of a mutation in a *ATPI3A2*, gene not previously associated with either human or animal NCLs, but rather with a hereditary neurodegenerative disease called Kufor-Rakeb syndrome or PARK9 (Farias et al., 2010). Genotyping of almost 30 affected dogs (confirmed phenotypically and histologically), numerous obligate carriers, and Tibetan Terriers older than 10 years with no phenotypic signs of NCL, indicated that the *ATPI3A2* mutation segregated with the disease in an autosomal recessive pattern with complete penetrance (Farias et al., 2010). A test is now available at the University of Missouri to Tibetan Terrier owners for genotyping their dogs at the disease locus.

In most instances, the loci responsible for human adult onset NCL, including forms known as Kufs disease that does not include visual failure, remain unknown (Cummings and de Lahunta, 1977, Goebel et al., 1982, Martin et al., 1987, Traboulsi et al., 1987, Carpenter, 1988, Martin, 1991, Sakajiri et al., 1995, Sadzot et al., 2000). It is possible that at least some cases of adult onset NCL result from mutations in *ATPI3A2*. In fact, it seems likely that when tissues from subjects with Kufor-Rakeb syndrome are examined, this disease will be found to be a form of NCL.. Nucleotide sequence analyses are currently being performed on genomic DNA from human adult onset cases of NCL to determine whether any of them are associated with mutations in this gene. Unlike human Kufs disease, the Tibetan Terrier NCL mutation appears to be fairly common within both the North American and European Tibetan Terrier populations (M.L. Katz and C. Drögemüller, unpublished). This is likely to change as many Tibetan Terrier breeders are now using the genotyping test in selecting which dogs to mate.

Dog models without genetic assignment

English Setters, Border Collies, American Bulldogs, Dachshunds, Australian Shepherds, and American Staffordshire Terriers are the only breeds exhibiting NCL-like disorders for which the causal mutations are currently known (Table 18.4). Of these breeds, at least two segregate more than one NCL (Dachshunds and Australian Shepherds). In addition, neurological disorders with similarities to the human NCLs have been reported in a number of other dog breeds. Among these are Australian Cattle Dogs, Blue Heelers, Chihuahuas, Cocker Spaniels, Dalmatians, Golden Retrievers, Japanese Retrievers, Labrador Retrievers, Miniature Schnauzers, Pit Bull Terriers, Polish Owczarek Nizinny (PON) or Polish Lowland Sheepdogs, Salukis, Tibetan Terriers, and Welsh Corgis (Table 18.3) (Appleby et al., 1982, Goebel and Dahme, 1985, Umemura et al., 1985, Cho et al., 1986, Goebel et al., 1988, Sisk et al., 1990, Alroy et al., 1992, Riis et al., 1992, Jolly et al., 1994a, Jolly et al., 1994b, Jolly and Palmer, 1995, Narfstrom and Wrigstad, 1995, Wrigstad et al., 1995, Palmer et al., 1997b, Minatel et al., 2000, Kuwamura et al., 2003, Rossmeisl et al., 2003, Siso et al., 2004, Katz et al., 2005b, Narfstrom et al., 2007). The diseases in Polish Lowland Sheepdogs, and Dalmatians have been studied most extensively.

POLISH LOWLAND SHEEPDOG (POLISH OWCZAREK NIZINNY)

NCL was reported in a single Polish Lowland Sheepdog (Polish Owczarek Nizinny, or PON) in 1995, and subsequently in eight additional related dogs of the same breed (Narfstrom and Wrigstad, 1995, Wrigstad et al., 1995, Narfstrom et al., 2007). Among these dogs, the age of onset and pattern of clinical signs of disease was quite variable, even though six of the nine were from the same sire and the others were related (Narfstrom et al., 2007). The age at onset for clinical signs was 6 months for six of the dogs and not until 3–4 years for the remaining animals. Even among dogs with the same age of clinical onset, the pattern of disease signs and rate of disease progression was quite variable (Narfstrom et al., 2007). For example, among dogs that exhibited symptoms starting at 6 months of age, some exhibited severe loss of retinal function, whereas others had only mild alterations in dark adaptation and little degenerative change to the retina. Even though all of the affected dogs displayed neurological signs and autofluorescent storage body accumulation characteristic of NCL, it is not clear that they all suffered from the same disease entity. Alternatively, there may be modifier genes that affect the disease phenotype. Although it appears likely that genetic factors are involved in the NCL-like disorders in the PON dogs, there is currently insufficient information to determine the mode(s) of inheritance or whether the disease(s) is a simple or complex genetic trait. Nevertheless, sequence analysis has been performed on a number of candidate genes using DNA from a single PON dog reported to have a late onset form NCL (Drögemüller et al., 2005a, Drögemüller et al., 2005b, Wohlke et al., 2005, Wohlke et al., 2006). These analyses have not identified a mutation associated with the NCL disorder. There have not been any recent reports of existing cases of NCL in the PON breed, so it is not known whether additional dogs might be available to answer some of the unresolved questions relating to NCL in this breed.

DALMATIAN

In the 1980s Goebel and colleagues identified NCL in a group of inbred Dalmatians (Goebel and Dahme, 1985, Goebel et al., 1988). Clinical symptoms typically started at 6 months of age with visual impairment. By 15 months of age, affected dogs exhibited seizures, signs of self-mutilation, and bruxism. Tremor, ataxia, and clumsiness with staggering became apparent at 20–22 months. Affected dogs exhibited retarded growth and died by age 7–8 years. Autofluorescent storage material accumulation was observed throughout the central nervous system, and the brain showed atrophic changes. Ultrastructural studies showed abnormal inclusions in the central and peripheral nervous system. The inclusions are of a lamellar character that is distinct from curvilinear and fingerprint profiles. There is preservation of photoreceptors in spite of pronounced deposition of disease-specific inclusions in almost every cell type of the retina (Goebel and Dahme, 1985, Goebel et al., 1988), i.e. fingerprint bodies, curvilinear bodies, and more complex membrane-bound lamellar structures, which differs from that observed in the cells of the nervous system. Although the retina exhibited storage body accumulation, retinal degenerative changes were not observed in the affected dogs.

The investigators reported establishment of a research colony to generate affected dogs; however, there are, as yet, no reports of the mode of inheritance of the Dalmatian disorder or the molecular genetic basis of the disease. Due to lack of funding, the research colony was discontinued (H.H. Goebel, personal communication) and it is unknown whether any descendents of the dogs carrying the presumed disease mutation are still in existence.

MINIATURE SCHNAUZER

In this breed signs start with progressive blindness from 3–4 years of age. The dogs show signs of confusion, unawareness of surroundings, loss of memory for normal learned behaviour, trembling, and aimless wandering. Severe photoreceptor degeneration is observed in addition to extensive accumulation of autofluorescent granules in the central nervous tissue, including retina, and in the liver. The storage bodies in the brain are characterized as GRODs (Palmer et al., 1997b). There is accumulation of SAPs A and D in the GRODs. Neither subunit c of mitochondrial ATP synthase nor vacuolar ATP synthase is stored. SAPs A and D storage is detected in human CLN1 and CLN10 diseases, while the Miniature Schnauzer disease had a relatively later clinical onset.

OTHERS

Descriptions of NCL in the remaining breeds of dogs listed above are restricted primarily to isolated case reports. Dogs from these breeds were classified as suffering from NCL on the basis of neurological signs and the presence of autofluorescent storage material in cells of the central nervous system. It will be very difficult to develop disease models in any of these other breeds unless additional affected animals can be identified. In most cases, tissue suitable for molecular genetic analysis has not been preserved and lines of dogs carrying potential NCL mutations have not been maintained. However, due to the relatively high degree of homozygosity in purebred dogs, and based on the number of case reports to date, it appears likely that additional instances of canine NCL will continue to be discovered. Recently available resources including a canine whole genome reference sequence (Lindblad-Toh et al., 2005) and commercially available canine-specific SNP chips with tens of thousands of markers should facilitate the mapping of canine NCL loci and the identification of causative mutations (Karlsson et al., 2007). With appropriate foresight, cooperation, and adequate resources, these spontaneous NCL mutations can be captured and preserved as models for the corresponding human disorders. Such dog models could be valuable resources for evaluating potential therapeutic interventions prior to testing in humans.

REFERENCES

Abitbol M, Thibaud JL, Olby NJ, Hitte C, Puech JP, Maurer M, Pilot-Storck F, Hedan B, Dreano S, Brahimi S, Delattre D, Andre C, Gray F, Delisle F, Caillaud C, Bernex F, Panthier JJ, Aubin-Houzelstein G, Blot S, & Tiret L (2010) A canine arylsulfatase G (ARSG) mutation leading to a sulfatase defi ciency is associated with neuronal ceroid lipofuscinosis. *Proc Natl Acad Sci USA*, 107, 14775–14780.

Alroy J, Schelling SH, Thalhammer JG, Raghavan SS, Natowicz MR, Prence EM, & Orgad U (1992) Adult onset lysosomal storage disease in a Tibetan terrier: clinical, morphological and biochemical studies. *Acta Neuropathol*, 84, 658–663.

Appleby EC, Longstaffe JA, & Bell FR (1982) Ceroid-lipofuscinosis in two Saluki dogs. *J Comp Pathol*, 92, 375–380.

Aronovich EL, Carmichael KP, Morizono H, Koutlas IG, Deanching M, Hoganson G, Fischer A, & Whitley CB (2000) Canine heparan sulfate sulfamidase and the molecular pathology underlying Sanfilippo syndrome type A in Dachshunds. *Genomics*, 68, 80–84.

Awano T, Katz ML, O'Brien DP, Sohar I, Lobel P, Coates JR, Khan S, Johnson GC, Giger U, & Johnson GS (2006a) A frame shift mutation in canine TPP1 (the ortholog of human CLN2) in a juvenile Dachshund with neuronal ceroid lipofuscinosis. *Mol Genet Metab*, 89, 254–260.

Awano T, Katz ML, O'Brien DP, Taylor JF, Evans J, Khan S, Sohar I, Lobel P, & Johnson GS (2006b) A mutation in the cathepsin D gene (CTSD) in American Bulldogs with neuronal ceroid lipofuscinosis. *Mol Genet Metab*, 87, 341–348.

Bible E, Gupta P, Hofmann SL, & Cooper JD (2004) Regional and cellular neuropathology in the palmitoyl protein thioesterase-1 null mutant mouse model of infantile neuronal ceroid lipofuscinosis. *Neurobiol Dis*, 16, 346–359.

Bildfell R, Matwichuk C, Mitchell S, & Ward P (1995) Neuronal ceroid-lipofuscinosis in a cat. *Vet Pathol*, 32, 485–488.

Breen M, Hitte C, Lorentzen TD, Thomas R, Cadieu E, Sabacan L, Scott A, Evanno G, Parker HG, Kirkness EF, Hudson R, Guyon R, Mahairas GG, Gelfenbeyn B, Fraser CM, Andre C, Galibert F, & Ostrander EA (2004) An integrated 4249 marker FISH/RH map of the canine genome. *BMC Genomics*, 5, 65.

Broom MF, Zhou C, Broom JE, Barwell KJ, Jolly RD, & Hill DF (1998) Ovine neuronal ceroid lipofuscinosis: a large animal model syntenic with the human neuronal ceroid lipofuscinosis variant CLN6. *J Med Genet*, 35, 717–721.

Buzy A, Ryan EM, Jennings KR, Palmer DN, & Griffiths DE (1996) Use of electrospray ionization mass spectrometry and tandem mass spectrometry to study binding of F0 inhibitors to ceroid lipofuscinosis protein, a model system for subunit c of mitochondrial ATP synthase. *Rapid Commun Mass Spectrom*, 10, 790–796.

Carpenter S (1988) Morphological diagnosis and misdiagnosis in Batten-Kufs disease. *Am J Med Genet*, 5 Suppl, 85–91.

Cesta MF, Mozzachio K, Little PB, Olby NJ, Sills RC, & Brown TT (2006) Neuronal ceroid lipofuscinosis in a Vietnamese pot-bellied pig (Sus scrofa). *Vet Pathol*, 43, 556–560.

Chen R, Fearnley IM, Palmer DN, & Walker JE (2004) Lysine 43 is trimethylated in subunit C from bovine mitochondrial ATP synthase and in storage bodies associated with Batten disease. *J Biol Chem*, 279, 21883–21887.

Chio KS & Tappel AL (1969a) Inactivation of ribonuclease and other enzymes by peroxidizing lipids and by malonaldehyde. *Biochemistry*, 8, 2827–2832.

Chio KS & Tappel AL (1969b) Synthesis and characterization of the fluorescent products derived from malonaldehyde and amino acids. *Biochemistry*, 8, 2821–2826.

Cho DY, Leipold HW, & Rudolph R (1986) Neuronal ceroidosis (ceroid-lipofuscinosis) in a Blue Heeler dog. *Acta Neuropathol*, 69, 161–164.

Choi DW (1988) Glutamate neurotoxicity and diseases of the nervous system. *Neuron*, 1, 623–634.

Cook RW, Jolly RD, Palmer DN, Tammen I, Broom MF, & McKinnon R (2002) Neuronal ceroid lipofuscinosis in Merino sheep. *Aust Vet J*, 80, 292–297.

Cooper JD, Messer A, Feng AK, Chua-Couzens J, & Mobley WC (1999) Apparent loss and hypertrophy of interneurons in a mouse model of neuronal ceroid lipofuscinosis: evidence for partial response to insulin-like growth factor-1 treatment. *J Neurosci*, 19, 2556–2567.

Cummings JF & de Lahunta A (1977) An adult case of canine neuronal ceroid-lipofuscinosis. *Acta Neuropathol*, 39, 43–51.

Dickson LR, Dopfmer I, Dalefield RR, Graydon RJ, & Jolly RD (1989) A method of cerebro-cortical biopsy in lambs. *N Z Vet J*, 37, 21–22.

Drögemüller C, Wohlke A, & Distl O (2005a) Characterization of candidate genes for neuronal ceroid lipofuscinosis in dog. *J Hered*, 96, 735–738.

Drögemüller C, Wohlke A, & Distl O (2005b) Evaluation of the canine TPP1 gene as a candidate for neuronal ceroid lipofuscinosis in Tibetan Terrier and Polish Owczarek Nizinny dogs. *Anim Genet*, 36, 178–179.

Edwards JF, Storts RW, Joyce JR, Shelton JM, & Menzies CS (1994) Juvenile-onset neuronal ceroid-lipofuscinosis in Rambouillet sheep. *Vet Pathol*, 31, 48–54.

Elleder M (1981) *Chemical characterization of age pigments*. Amsterdam, New York, Elsevier North Holland Biomedical Press.

Evans J, Katz ML, Levesque D, Shelton GD, A. Lahunta, & O'Brien D (2005) Neuronal ceroid lipofuscinosis in the American bulldog: a variant form of the storage disease in a related population. *J Vet Intern Med*, 19, 44–51.

Farias FH, Zeng R; Johnson GS, Wininger FA, Taylor JF, Schnabel RD, McKay SD, Sanders DN; Lohi H, Seppälä EH, Wade CM, Lindblad-Toh K, O'Brien DP, Katz ML (2010) A truncating mutation in ATP13A2 is responsible for adult-onset neuronal ceroid lipofuscinosis in Tibetan Terriers. Submitted.

Faust JR, Rodman JS, Daniel PF, Dice JF, & Bronson RT (1994) Two related proteolipids and dolichol-linked oligosaccharides accumulate in motor neuron degeneration mice (mnd/mnd), a model for neuronal ceroid lipofuscinosis. *J Biol Chem*, 269, 10150–10155.

Fearnley IM, Walker JE, Martinus RD, Jolly RD, Kirkland KB, Shaw GJ, & Palmer DN (1990) The sequence of the major protein stored in ovine ceroid lipofuscinosis is identical with that of the dicyclohexylcarbodiimide-reactive proteolipid of mitochondrial ATP synthase. *Biochem J*, 268, 751–758.

Fischer A, Carmichael KP, Munnell JF, Jhabvala P, Thompson JN, Matalon R, Jezyk PF, Wang P, & Giger U (1998) Sulfamidase deficiency in a family of Dachshunds: a canine model of mucopolysaccharidosis IIIA (Sanfilippo A). *Pediatr Res*, 44, 74–82.

Fiske RA & Storts RW (1988) Neuronal ceroid-lipofuscinosis in Nubian goats. *Vet Pathol*, 25, 171–173.

Fossale E, Wolf P, Espinola JA, Lubicz-Nawrocka T, Teed AM, Gao H, Rigamonti D, Cattaneo E, MacDonald ME, & Cotman SL (2004) Membrane trafficking and mitochondrial abnormalities precede subunit c deposition in a cerebellar cell model of juvenile neuronal ceroid lipofuscinosis. *BMC Neurosci*, 5, 57.

France M, Geraghty F, & Taylor R (1999) Ceroid lipofuscinosis in ferrets. *Annual Conference Australian Society Veterinary Pathology*, 1, 50.

Frugier T, Mitchell NL, Tammen I, Houweling PJ, Arthur DG, Kay GW, van Diggelen OP, Jolly RD, & Palmer DN (2008) A new large animal model of CLN5 neuronal ceroid lipofuscinosis in Borderdale sheep is caused by a nucleotide substitution at a consensus splice site (c.571+1G>>>A) leading to excision of exon 3. *Neurobiol Dis*, 29, 306–315.

Gao H, Boustany RM, Espinola JA, Cotman SL, Srinidhi L, Antonellis KA, Gillis T, Qin X, Liu S, Donahue LR, Bronson RT, Faust JR, Stout D, Haines JL, Lerner TJ, & MacDonald ME (2002) Mutations in a novel CLN6-encoded transmembrane protein cause variant neuronal ceroid lipofuscinosis in man and mouse. *Am J Hum Genet*, 70, 324–335.

Goebel HH, Bilzer T, Dahme E, & Malkusch F (1988) Morphological studies in canine (Dalmatian) neuronal ceroid-lipofuscinosis. *Am J Med Genet Suppl*, 5, 127–139.

Goebel HH, Braak H, Seidel D, Doshi R, Marsden CD, & Gullotta F (1982) Morphologic studies on adult neuronal-ceroid lipofuscinosis (NCL). *Clin Neuropathol*, 1, 151–162.

Goebel HH & Dahme E (1985) Retinal ultrastructure of neuronal ceroid-lipofuscinosis in the dalmatian dog. *Acta Neuropathol*, 68, 224–229.

Goebel HH, Koppang N, & Zeman W (1979) Ultrastructure of the retina in canine neuronal ceroid lipofuscinosis. *Ophthalmic Res*, 11, 65–72.

Goebel HH, Mole SE, & Lake BD (Eds.) (1999) *The Neuronal Ceroid Lipofuscinoses (Batten Disease)*. Amsterdam, IOS Press.

Graydon RJ & Jolly RD (1984) Ceroid-lipofuscinosis (Batten's disease). Sequential electrophysiologic and pathologic changes in the retina of the ovine model. *Invest Ophthalmol Vis Sci*, 25, 294–301.

Green PD & Little PB (1974) Neuronal ceroid-lipofuscin storage in Siamese cats. *Can J Comp Med*, 38, 207–212.

Gutteridge JM (1985) Age pigments and free radicals: fluorescent lipid complexes formed by iron- and copper-containing proteins. *Biochim Biophys Acta*, 834, 144–148.

Gutteridge JM, Heys AD, & Lunec J (1977) Fluorescent malondialdehyde polymers from hydrolysed 1,1,3,3–tetramethoxypropane. *Anal Chim Acta*, 94, 209–211.

Gutteridge JM, Westermarck T, & Santavuori P (1983) Iron and oxygen radicals in tissue damage: implications for the neuronal ceroid lipofuscinoses. *Acta Neurol Scand*, 68, 365–370.

Guyon R, Lorentzen TD, Hitte C, Kim L, Cadieu E, Parker HG, Quignon P, Lowe JK, Renier C, Gelfenbeyn B, Vignaux F, DeFrance HB, Gloux S, Mahairas GG, Andre C, Galibert F, & Ostrander EA (2003) A 1-Mb resolution radiation hybrid map of the canine genome. *Proc Natl Acad Sci U S A*, 100, 5296–5301.

Hafner S, Flynn TE, Harmon BG, & Hill JE (2005) Neuronal ceroid-lipofuscinosis in a Holstein steer. *J Vet Diagn Invest*, 17, 194–197.

Hagen LO (1953) Lipid dystrophic changes in the central nervous system in dogs. *Acta Pathol Microbiol Scand*, 33, 22–35.

Hall NA, Jolly RD, Palmer DN, Lake BD, & Patrick AD (1989) Analysis of dolichyl pyrophosphoryl oligosaccharides in purified storage cytosomes from ovine ceroid-lipofuscinosis. *Biochim Biophys Acta*, 993, 245–251.

Hall NA, Lake BD, Dewji NN, & Patrick AD (1991) Lysosomal storage of subunit c of mitochondrial ATP synthase in Batten's disease (ceroid-lipofuscinosis). *Biochem J*, 275 (Pt 1), 269–272.

Haltia M (2003) The neuronal ceroid-lipofuscinoses. *J Neuropathol Exp Neurol*, 62, 1–13.

Harper PA, Walker KH, Healy PJ, Hartley WJ, Gibson AJ, & Smith JS (1988) Neurovisceral ceroid-lipofuscinosis in blind Devon cattle. *Acta Neuropathol*, 75, 632–636.

Hartley WJ, Kuberski T, LeGonidec G, & Daynes P (1982) The pathology of Gomen disease: a cerebellar disorder of horses in New Caledonia. *Vet Pathol*, 19, 399–405.

Heine C, Koch B, Storch S, Kohlschutter A, Palmer DN, & Braulke T (2004) Defective endoplasmic reticulum-resident membrane protein CLN6 affects lysosomal degradation of endocytosed arylsulfatase A. *J Biol Chem*, 279, 22347–22352.

Heine C, Tyynelä J, Cooper JD, Palmer DN, Elleder M, Kohlschutter A, & Braulke T (2003) Enhanced expression of manganese-dependent superoxide dismutase in human and sheep CLN6 tissues. *Biochem J*, 376, 369–376.

Holmberg V, Jalanko A, Isosomppi J, Fabritius AL, Peltonen L, & Kopra O (2004) The mouse ortholog of the neuronal ceroid lipofuscinosis CLN5 gene encodes a soluble lysosomal glycoprotein expressed in the developing brain. *Neurobiol Dis*, 16, 29–40.

Houweling PJ, Cavanagh JA, Palmer DN, Frugier T, Mitchell NL, Windsor PA, Raadsma HW, & Tammen I (2006a) Neuronal ceroid lipofuscinosis in Devon cattle is caused by a single base duplication (c.662dupG) in the bovine CLN5 gene. *Biochim Biophys Acta*, 1762, 890–897.

Houweling PJ, Cavanagh JA, & Tammen I (2006b) Radiation hybrid mapping of three candidate genes for bovine Neuronal Ceroid Lipofuscinosis: CLN3, CLN5 and CLN6. *Cytogenet Genome Res*, 115, 5–6.

Hughes SM, Kay GW, Jordan TW, Rickards GK, & Palmer DN (1999) Disease-specific pathology in neurons cultured from sheep affected with ceroid lipofuscinosis. *Mol Genet Metab*, 66, 381–386.

Hunot S & Hirsch EC (2003) Neuroinflammatory processes in Parkinson's disease. *Ann Neurol*, 53 Suppl 3, S49–58; discussion S58–60.

Huxtable CR, Chapman HM, Main DC, Vass D, Pearse BH, & Hilbert BJ (1987) Neurological disease and lipofuscinosis in horses and sheep grazing Trachyandra divaricata (branched onion weed) in south Western Australia. *Aust Vet J*, 64, 105–108.

Isosomppi J, Vesa J, Jalanko A, & Peltonen L (2002) Lysosomal localization of the neuronal ceroid lipofuscinosis CLN5 protein. *Hum Mol Genet*, 11, 885–891.

Järplid B & Haltia M (1993) An animal model of the infantile type of neuronal ceroid-lipofuscinosis. *J Inherit Metab Dis*, 16, 274–277.

Jasty V, Kowalski RL, Fonseca EH, Porter MC, Clemens GR, Bare JJ, & Hartnagel RE (1984) An unusual case of generalized ceroid-lipofuscinosis in a cynomolgus monkey. *Vet Pathol*, 21, 46–50.

Jolly RD, Arthur DG, Kay GW, & Palmer DN (2002a) Neuronal ceroid-lipofuscinosis in Borderdale sheep. *N Z Vet J*, 50, 199–202.

Jolly RD, Brown S, Das AM, & Walkley SU (2002b) Mitochondrial dysfunction in the neuronal ceroid-lipofuscinoses (Batten disease). *Neurochem Int*, 40, 565–571.

Jolly RD, Charleston WA, & Hughes PL (2002) Disorders of New Zealand farm dogs. *N Z Vet J*, 50, 115–116.

Jolly RD, Gibson AJ, Healy PJ, Slack PM, & Birtles MJ (1992) Bovine ceroid-lipofuscinosis: pathology of blindness. *N Z Vet J*, 40, 107–111.

Jolly RD, Hartley WJ, Jones BR, Johnstone AC, Palmer AC, & Blakemore WF (1994a) Generalised ceroid-lipofuscinosis and brown bowel syndrome in Cocker spaniel dogs. *N Z Vet J*, 42, 236–239.

Jolly RD, Janmaat A, Graydon RJ, & Clemett RS (1982) *Ceroid-lipofuscinosis: The Ovine Model*. Amsterdam, Elsevier Biomedical Press.

Jolly RD, Janmaat A, West DM, & Morrison I (1980) Ovine ceroid-lipofuscinosis: a model of Batten's disease. *Neuropathol Appl Neurobiol*, 6, 195–209.

Jolly RD & Palmer DN (1995) The neuronal ceroid-lipofuscinoses (Batten disease): comparative aspects. *Neuropathol Appl Neurobiol*, 21, 50–60.

Jolly RD, Palmer DN, Studdert VP, Sutton RH, Kelly WR, Koppang N, Dahme G, Hartley WJ, Patterson JS, & Riis RC (1994b) Canine ceroid-lipofuscinoses: A review and classification. *J Small Anim Pract*, 35, 299–306.

Jolly RD, Shimada A, Craig AS, Kirkland KB, & Palmer DN (1988) Ovine ceroid-lipofuscinosis II: Pathologic changes interpreted in light of biochemical observations. *Am J Med Genet Suppl*, 5, 159–170.

Jolly RD, Shimada A, Dopfmer I, Slack PM, Birtles MJ, & Palmer DN (1989) Ceroid-lipofuscinosis (Batten's disease): pathogenesis and sequential neuropathological changes in the ovine model. *Neuropathol Appl Neurobiol*, 15, 371–383.

Jolly RD & Walkley SU (1997) Lysosomal storage diseases of animals: an essay in comparative pathology. *Vet Pathol*, 34, 527–548.

Jolly RD & Walkley SU (1999) Ovine ceroid lipofuscinosis (OCL6): postulated mechanism of neurodegeneration. *Mol Genet Metab*, 66, 376–380.

Jolly RD & West DM (1976) Blindness in South Hampshire sheep: a neuronal ceroidlipofuscinosis. *N Z Vet J*, 24, 123.

Karlsson EK, Baranowska I, Wade CM, Salmon Hillbertz NH, Zody MC, Anderson N, Biagi TM, Patterson N, Pielberg GR, Kulbokas EJ, 3rd, Comstock KE, Keller ET, Mesirov JP, von Euler H, Kampe O, Hedhammar A, Lander ES, Andersson G, Andersson L, & Lindblad-Toh K (2007) Efficient mapping of mendelian traits in dogs through genome-wide association. *Nat Genet*, 39, 1321–1328.

Katz ML, Christianson JS, Norbury NE, Gao CL, Siakotos AN, & Koppang N (1994) Lysine methylation of mitochondrial ATP synthase subunit c stored in tissues of dogs with hereditary ceroid lipofuscinosis. *J Biol Chem*, 269, 9906–9911.

Katz ML, Coates JR, Cooper JJ, O'Brien DP, Jeong M, & Narfstrom K (2008) Retinal pathology in a canine model of late infantile neuronal ceroid lipofuscinosis. *Invest Ophthalmol Vis Sci*, 49, 2686–2695.

Katz ML, Farias FH, Sanders DN, Zeng R, Khan S, Johnson GS, & O'Brien DP (2010) A missense mutation in CLN6 in an Australian Shepherd with neuronal ceroid lipofuscinosis. *J Biomed Biotech*, in press.

Katz ML, Gao CL, Tompkins JA, Bronson RT, & Chin DT (1995) Mitochondrial ATP synthase subunit c stored in hereditary ceroid-lipofuscinosis contains trimethyl-lysine. *Biochem J*, 310 (Pt 3), 887–892.

Katz ML, Khan S, Awano T, Shahid SA, Siakotos AN, & Johnson GS (2005a) A mutation in the CLN8 gene in English Setter dogs with neuronal ceroid-lipofuscinosis. *Biochem Biophys Res Commun*, 327, 541–547.

Katz ML, Narfstrom K, Johnson GS, & O'Brien DP (2005b) Assessment of retinal function and characterization of lysosomal storage body accumulation in the retinas and brains of Tibetan Terriers with ceroid-lipofuscinosis. *Am J Vet Res*, 66, 67–76.

Katz ML & Siakotos AN (1995) Canine hereditary ceroid-lipofuscinosis: evidence for a defect in the carnitine biosynthetic pathway. *Am J Med Genet*, 57, 266–271.

Kay GW, Hughes SM, & Palmer DN (1999) In vitro culture of neurons from sheep with Batten disease. *Mol Genet Metab*, 67, 83–88.

Kay GW, Oswald MJ, & Palmer DN (2006a) The development and characterisation of complex ovine neuron cultures from fresh and frozen foetal neurons. *J Neurosci Methods*, 155, 98–108.

Kay GW, Palmer DN, Rezaie P, & Cooper JD (2006b) Activation of non-neuronal cells within the prenatal developing brain of sheep with neuronal ceroid lipofuscinosis. *Brain Pathol*, 16, 110–116.

Kay GW, Verbeek MM, Furlong JM, Willemsen MA, & Palmer DN (2009) Neuropeptide changes and neuroactive amino acids in CSF from humans and sheep with neuronal ceroid lipofuscinoses (NCLs, Batten disease). *Neurochem Int*, 55, 783–788.

Keller RK, Armstrong D, Crum FC, & Koppang N (1984) Dolichol and dolichyl phosphate levels in brain tissue from English setters with ceroid lipofuscinosis. *J Neurochem*, 42, 1040–1047.

Kida E, Wisniewski KE, & Golabek AA (1993) Increased expression of subunit c of mitochondrial ATP synthase in brain tissue from neuronal ceroid lipofuscinoses and mucopolysaccharidosis cases but not in long-term fibroblast cultures. *Neurosci Lett*, 164, 121–124.

Kielar C, Maddox L, Bible E, Pontikis CC, Macauley SL, Griffey MA, Wong M, Sands MS, & Cooper JD (2007) Successive neuron loss in the thalamus and cortex in a mouse model of infantile neuronal ceroid lipofuscinosis. *Neurobiol Dis*, 25, 150–162.

Kirkness EF, Bafna V, Halpern AL, Levy S, Remington K, Rusch DB, Delcher AL, Pop M, Wang W, Fraser CM, & Venter JC (2003) The dog genome: survey sequencing and comparative analysis. *Science*, 301, 1898–1903.

Koike M, Nakanishi H, Saftig P, Ezaki J, Isahara K, Ohsawa Y, Schulz-Schaeffer W, Watanabe T, Waguri S, Kametaka S, Shibata M, Yamamoto K, Kominami E, Peters C, von Figura K, & Uchiyama Y (2000) Cathepsin D deficiency induces lysosomal storage with ceroid lipofuscin in mouse CNS neurons. *J Neurosci*, 20, 6898–6906.

Kominami E, Ezaki J, Muno D, Ishido K, Ueno T, & Wolfe LS (1992) Specific storage of subunit c of mitochondrial ATP synthase in lysosomes of neuronal ceroid lipofuscinosis (Batten's disease). *J Biochem*, 111, 278–282.

Koppang N (1966) Familiäre Glykosphingolipoidose des Hundes (Juvenile Amaurotische Idiotie). *Erg Pathol*, 47, 1–43.

Koppang N (1973) Canine ceroid-lipofuscinosis-a model for human neuronal ceroid-lipofuscinosis and aging. *Mech Ageing Dev*, 2, 421–445.

Koppang N (1988) The English setter with ceroid-lipofuscinosis: a suitable model for the juvenile type of ceroid-lipofuscinosis in humans. *Am J Med Genet Suppl*, 5, 117–125.

Koppang N (1992) English setter model and juvenile ceroid-lipofuscinosis in man. *Am J Med Genet*, 42, 599–604.

Kopra O, Vesa J, von Schantz C, Manninen T, Minye H, Fabritius AL, Rapola J, van Diggelen OP, Saarela J, Jalanko A, & Peltonen L (2004) A mouse model for Finnish variant late infantile neuronal ceroid lipofuscinosis, CLN5, reveals neuropathology associated with early aging. *Hum Mol Genet*, 13, 2893–2906.

Kuwamura M, Hattori R, Yamate J, Kotani T, & Sasai K (2003) Neuronal ceroid-lipofuscinosis and hydrocephalus in a chihuahua. *J Small Anim Pract*, 44, 227–230.

Lane SC, Jolly RD, Schmechel DE, Alroy J, & Boustany RM (1996) Apoptosis as the mechanism of neurodegeneration in Batten's disease. *J Neurochem*, 67, 677–683.

Lindblad-Toh K, Wade CM, Mikkelsen TS, Karlsson EK, Jaffe DB, Kamal M, Clamp M, Chang JL, Kulbokas EJ, 3rd, Zody MC, et al. (2005) Genome sequence, comparative analysis and haplotype structure of the domestic dog. *Nature*, 438, 803–819.

Lingaas F, Aarskaug T, Sletten M, Bjerkas I, Grimholt U, Moe L, Juneja RK, Wilton AN, Galibert F, Holmes NG, & Dolf G (1998) Genetic markers linked to neuronal ceroid lipofuscinosis in English setter dogs. *Anim Genet*, 29, 371–376.

Lingaas F, Sorensen A, Juneja RK, Johansson S, Fredholm M, Wintero AK, Sampson J, Mellersh C, Curzon A, Holmes NG, Binns MM, Dickens HF, Ryder EJ, Gerlach J, Baumle E, & Dolf G (1997) Towards construction of a canine linkage map: establishment of 16 linkage groups. *Mamm Genome*, 8, 218–221.

March PA, Wurzelmann S, & Walkley SU (1995) Morphological alterations in neocortical and cerebellar GABAergic neurons in a canine model of juvenile Batten disease. *Am J Med Genet*, 57, 204–212.

Martin JJ (1991) Adult type of neuronal ceroid lipofuscinosis. *Dev Neurosci*, 13, 331–338.

Martin JJ, Libert J, & Ceuterick C (1987) Ultrastructure of brain and retina in Kufs' disease (adult type-ceroid-lipofuscinosis). *Clin Neuropathol*, 6, 231–235.

Martinus RD, Harper PA, Jolly RD, Bayliss SL, Midwinter GG, Shaw GJ, & Palmer DN (1991) Bovine ceroid-lipofuscinosis (Batten's disease): the major component stored is the DCCD-reactive proteolipid, subunit C, of mitochondrial ATP synthase. *Vet Res Commun*, 15, 85–94.

Mayhew IG, Jolly RD, Pickett BT, & Slack PM (1985) Ceroid-lipofuscinosis (Batten's disease): pathogenesis of blindness in the ovine model. *Neuropathol Appl Neurobiol*, 11, 273–290.

McGeoch JE & Palmer DN (1999) Ion pores made of mitochondrial ATP synthase subunit c in the neuronal plasma membrane and Batten disease. *Mol Genet Metab*, 66, 387–392.

Mellersh CS, Langston AA, Acland GM, Fleming MA, Ray K, Wiegand NA, Francisco LV, Gibbs M, Aguirre GD, & Ostrander EA (1997) A linkage map of the canine genome. *Genomics*, 46, 326–336.

Melville SA, Wilson CL, Chiang CS, Studdert VP, Lingaas F, & Wilton AN (2005) A mutation in canine CLN5 causes neuronal ceroid lipofuscinosis in Border collie dogs. *Genomics*, 86, 287–294.

Millichamp NJ, Curtis R, & Barnett KC (1988) Progressive retinal atrophy in Tibetan terriers. *J Am Vet Med Assoc*, 192, 769–776.

Minagar A, Shapshak P, Fujimura R, Ownby R, Heyes M, & Eisdorfer C (2002) The role of macrophage/microglia and astrocytes in the pathogenesis of three neurologic disorders: HIV-associated dementia, Alzheimer disease, and multiple sclerosis. *J Neurol Sci*, 202, 13–23.

Minatel L, Underwood SC, & Carfagnini JC (2000) Ceroid-lipofuscinosis in a Cocker Spaniel dog. *Vet Pathol*, 37, 488–490.

Mitchison HM, Bernard DJ, Greene ND, Cooper JD, Junaid MA, Pullarkat RK, de Vos N, Breuning MH, Owens JW, Mobley WC, Gardiner RM, Lake BD, Taschner PE, & Nussbaum RL (1999) Targeted disruption of the Cln3 gene provides a mouse model for Batten disease. The Batten Mouse Model Consortium [corrected]. *Neurobiol Dis*, 6, 321–334.

Mole SE, Michaux G, Codlin S, Wheeler RB, Sharp JD, & Cutler DF (2004) CLN6, which is associated with a

lysosomal storage disease, is an endoplasmic reticulum protein. *Exp Cell Res*, 298, 399–406.
Nakayama H, Uchida K, Shouda T, Uetsuka K, Sasaki N, & Goto N (1993) Systemic ceroid-lipofuscinosis in a Japanese domestic cat. *J Vet Med Sci*, 55, 829–831.
Narfstrom K & Wrigstad A (1995) Clinical, electrophysiological, and morphological findings in a case of neuronal ceroid lipofuscinosis in the Polish Owczarek Nizinny (PON) dog. *Vet Q*, 17 Suppl 1, S46.
Narfstrom K, Wrigstad A, Ekesten B, & Berg AL (2007) Neuronal ceroid lipofuscinosis: clinical and morphologic findings in nine affected Polish Owczarek Nizinny (PON) dogs. *Vet Ophthalmol*, 10, 111–120.
Neumann H (2001) Control of glial immune function by neurons. *Glia*, 36, 191–199.
Ng Ying Kin NM, Palo J, Haltia M, & Wolfe LS (1983) High levels of brain dolichols in neuronal ceroid-lipofuscinosis and senescence. *J Neurochem*, 40, 1465–1473.
O'Brien DP & Katz ML (2008) Neuronal ceroid lipofuscinosis in 3 Australian shepherd littermates. *J Vet Intern Med*, 22, 472–475.
Ostrander EA, Galibert F, & Patterson DF (2000) Canine genetics comes of age. *Trends Genet*, 16, 117–124.
Oswald MJ, Kay GW, & Palmer DN (2001) Changes in GABAergic neuron distribution in situ and in neuron cultures in ovine (OCL6) Batten disease. *Eur J Paediatr Neurol*, 5 Suppl A, 135–142.
Oswald MJ, Palmer DN, Kay GW, Barwell KJ, & Cooper JD (2008) Location and connectivity determine GABAergic interneuron survival in the brains of South Hampshire sheep with CLN6 neuronal ceroid lipofuscinosis. *Neurobiol Dis*, 32, 50–65.
Oswald MJ, Palmer DN, Kay GW, Shemilt SJ, Rezaie P, & Cooper JD (2005) Glial activation spreads from specific cerebral foci and precedes neurodegeneration in presymptomatic ovine neuronal ceroid lipofuscinosis (CLN6). *Neurobiol Dis*, 20, 49–63.
Palmer DN, Barns G, Husbands DR, & Jolly RD (1986a) Ceroid lipofuscinosis in sheep. II. The major component of the lipopigment in liver, kidney, pancreas, and brain is low molecular weight protein. *J Biol Chem*, 261, 1773–1777.
Palmer DN, Bayliss SL, Clifton PA, & Grant VJ (1993) Storage bodies in the ceroid-lipofuscinoses (Batten disease): low-molecular-weight components, unusual amino acids and reconstitution of fluorescent bodies from non-fluorescent components. *J Inherit Metab Dis*, 16, 292–295.
Palmer DN, Bayliss SL, & Westlake VJ (1995) Batten disease and the ATP synthase subunit c turnover pathway: raising antibodies to subunit c. *Am J Med Genet*, 57, 260–265.
Palmer DN, Fearnley IM, Medd SM, Walker JE, Martinus RD, Bayliss SL, Hall NA, Lake BD, Wolfe LS, & Jolly RD (1989a) Lysosomal storage of the DCCD reactive proteolipid subunit of mitochondrial ATP synthase in human and ovine ceroid lipofuscinoses. *Adv Exp Med Biol*, 266, 211–222; discussion 223.
Palmer DN, Fearnley IM, Walker JE, Hall NA, Lake BD, Wolfe LS, Haltia M, Martinus RD, & Jolly RD (1992) Mitochondrial ATP synthase subunit c storage in the ceroid-lipofuscinoses (Batten disease). *Am J Med Genet*, 42, 561–567.
Palmer DN, Husbands DR, & Jolly RD (1985) Phospholipid fatty acids in brains of normal sheep and sheep with ceroid-lipofuscinosis. *Biochim Biophys Acta*, 834, 159–163.
Palmer DN, Husbands DR, Winter PJ, Blunt JW, & Jolly RD (1986b) Ceroid lipofuscinosis in sheep. I. Bis(monoacylglycero)phosphate, dolichol, ubiquinone, phospholipids, fatty acids, and fluorescence in liver lipopigment lipids. *J Biol Chem*, 261, 1766–1772.
Palmer DN, Jolly RD, van Mil HC, Tyynelä J, & Westlake VJ (1997a) Different patterns of hydrophobic protein storage in different forms of neuronal ceroid lipofuscinosis (NCL, Batten disease). *Neuropediatrics*, 28, 45–48.
Palmer DN, Martinus RD, Barns G, Reeves RD, & Jolly RD (1988) Ovine ceroid-lipofuscinosis. I: Lipopigment composition is indicative of a lysosomal proteinosis. *Am J Med Genet Suppl*, 5, 141–158.
Palmer DN, Oswald MJ, Westlake VJ, & Kay GW (2002) The origin of fluorescence in the neuronal ceroid lipofuscinoses (Batten disease) and neuron cultures from affected sheep for studies of neurodegeneration. *Arch Gerontol Geriatr*, 34, 343–357.
Palmer DN, Tyynelä J, van Mil HC, Westlake VJ, & Jolly RD (1997b) Accumulation of sphingolipid activator proteins (SAPs) A and D in granular osmiophilic deposits in miniature Schnauzer dogs with ceroid-lipofuscinosis. *J Inherit Metab Dis*, 20, 74–84.
Pardo CA, Rabin BA, Palmer DN, & Price DL (1994) Accumulation of the adenosine triphosphate synthase subunit C in the mnd mutant mouse. A model for neuronal ceroid lipofuscinosis. *Am J Pathol*, 144, 829–835.
Partanen S, Storch S, Loffler HG, Hasilik A, Tyynelä J, & Braulke T (2003) A replacement of the active-site aspartic acid residue 293 in mouse cathepsin D affects its intracellular stability, processing and transport in HEK-293 cells. *Biochem J*, 369, 55–62.
Pears MR, Salek RM, Palmer DN, Kay GW, Mortishire-Smith RJ, & Griffin JL (2007) Metabolomic investigation of CLN6 neuronal ceroid lipofuscinosis in affected South Hampshire sheep. *J Neurosci Res*, 85, 3494–3504.
Pontikis CC, Cella CV, Parihar N, Lim MJ, Chakrabarti S, Mitchison HM, Mobley WC, Rezaie P, Pearce DA, & Cooper JD (2004) Late onset neurodegeneration in the $Cln3^{-/-}$ mouse model of juvenile neuronal ceroid lipofuscinosis is preceded by low level glial activation. *Brain Res*, 1023, 231–242.
Read WK & Bridges CH (1969) Neuronal lipodystrophy. Occurrence in an inbred strain of cattle. *Pathol Vet*, 6, 235–243.
Reece RL & MacWhirter P (1988) Neuronal ceroid lipofuscinosis in a lovebird. *Vet Rec*, 122, 187.
Riis RC, Cummings JF, Loew ER, & de Lahunta A (1992) Tibetan terrier model of canine ceroid lipofuscinosis. *Am J Med Genet*, 42, 615–621.
Rossmeisl JH, Jr., Duncan R, Fox J, Herring ES, & Inzana KD (2003) Neuronal ceroid-lipofuscinosis in a Labrador Retriever. *J Vet Diagn Invest*, 15, 457–460.
Ryan EM, Buzy A, Griffiths DE, Jennings KR, & Palmer DN (1996) Electrospray ionisation mass spectrometry (ESI/MS) of ceroid lipofuscin protein; a model system for the study of F0 inhibitor interactions with mitochondrial subunit C. *Biochem Soc Trans*, 24, 289S.
Sadzot B, Reznik M, Arrese-Estrada JE, & Franck G (2000) Familial Kufs' disease presenting as a progressive myoclonic epilepsy. *J Neurol*, 247, 447–454.

Sakajiri K, Matsubara N, Nakajima T, Fukuhara N, Makifuchi T, Wakabayashi M, Oyanagi S, & Kominami E (1995) A family with adult type ceroid lipofuscinosis (Kufs' disease) and heart muscle disease: report of two autopsy cases. *Intern Med*, 34, 1158–1163.

Sanders DN, Farias FH, Johnson GS, Chiang V, Cook JR, O'Brien DP, Hofmann SL, Lu JY, & Katz ML (2010) A mutation in canine PPT1 causes early onset neuronal ceroid lipofuscinosis in a Dachshund. *Mol Genet Metab*, 100, 349–356.

Savukoski M, Klockars T, Holmberg V, Santavuori P, Lander ES, & Peltonen L (1998) CLN5, a novel gene encoding a putative transmembrane protein mutated in Finnish variant late infantile neuronal ceroid lipofuscinosis. *Nat Genet*, 19, 286–288.

Sharp JD, Wheeler RB, Parker KA, Gardiner RM, Williams RE, & Mole SE (2003) Spectrum of CLN6 mutations in variant late infantile neuronal ceroid lipofuscinosis. *Hum Mutat*, 22, 35–42.

Shelton M, Willingham T, Menzine TC, Storts R, & Wood PR (1993) Neuronal ceroid lipofuscinosis, an inherited form of blindness in sheep. *Sheep Res J*, 9, 105–108.

Siakotos AN, Goebel H, Patel V, Watanabe I, & Zeman W (1972) The morphogenesis and biochemical characteristics of ceroid isolated from cases of neuronal ceroid lipofuscinosis. In Volk BW, Aronson SM (Eds.) *Sphingolipids, Sphingolipodoses and Allied Disorders*, pp. 53–61. New York, Plenum Press.

Siakotos AN, Blair PS, Savill JD, & Katz ML (1998) Altered mitochondrial function in canine ceroid-lipofuscinosis. *Neurochem Res*, 23, 983–989.

Siakotos AN, & Koppang N (1973) Procedures for the isolation of lipopigments from brain, heart and liver, and their properties: a review. *Mech Ageing Dev*, 2, 177–200.

Siintola E, Partanen S, Stromme P, Haapanen A, Haltia M, Maehlen J, Lehesjoki AE, & Tyynelä J (2006b) Cathepsin D deficiency underlies congenital human neuronal ceroid-lipofuscinosis. *Brain*, 129, 1438–1445.

Sisk DB, Levesque DC, Wood PA, & Styer EL (1990) Clinical and pathologic features of ceroid lipofuscinosis in two Australian cattle dogs. *J Am Vet Med Assoc*, 197, 361–364.

Siso S, Navarro C, Hanzlicek D, & Vandevelde M (2004) Adult onset thalamocerebellar degeneration in dogs associated to neuronal storage of ceroid lipopigment. *Acta Neuropathol*, 108, 386–392.

Sleat DE, Ding L, Wang S, Zhao C, Wang Y, Xin W, Zheng H, Moore DF, Sims KB, & Lobel P (2009) Mass spectrometry-based protein profiling to determine the cause of lysosomal storage diseases of unknown etiology. *Mol Cell Proteomics*, 8, 1708–1718.

Steinfeld R, Reinhardt K, Schreiber K, Hillebrand M, Kraetzner R, Bruck W, Saftig P, & Gartner J (2006) Cathepsin D deficiency is associated with a human neurodegenerative disorder. *Am J Hum Genet*, 78, 988–998.

Stoll G & Jander S (1999) The role of microglia and macrophages in the pathophysiology of the CNS. *Prog Neurobiol*, 58, 233–247.

Studdert VP & Mitten RW (1991) Clinical features of ceroid lipofuscinosis in border collie dogs. *Aust Vet J*, 68, 137–140.

Tammen I, Cook RW, Nicholas FW, & Raadsma HW (2001) Neuronal ceroid lipofuscinosis in Australian Merino sheep: a new animal model. *Eur J Paediatr Neurol*, 5 Suppl A, 37–41.

Tammen I, Houweling PJ, Frugier T, Mitchell NL, Kay GW, Cavanagh JA, Cook RW, Raadsma HW, & Palmer DN (2006) A missense mutation (c.184C>T) in ovine CLN6 causes neuronal ceroid lipofuscinosis in Merino sheep whereas affected South Hampshire sheep have reduced levels of CLN6 mRNA. *Biochim Biophys Acta*, 1762, 898–905.

Taylor RM & Farrow BR (1988) Ceroid-lipofuscinosis in border collie dogs. *Acta Neuropathol*, 75, 627–631.

Taylor RM & Farrow BR (1992) Ceroid lipofuscinosis in the border collie dog: retinal lesions in an animal model of juvenile Batten disease. *Am J Med Genet*, 42, 622–627.

Traboulsi EI, Green WR, Luckenbach MW, & de la Cruz ZC (1987) Neuronal ceroid lipofuscinosis. Ocular histopathologic and electron microscopic studies in the late infantile, juvenile, and adult forms. *Graefes Arch Clin Exp Ophthalmol*, 225, 391–402.

Tyynelä J, Cooper JD, Khan MN, Shemilts SJ, & Haltia M (2004) Hippocampal pathology in the human neuronal ceroid-lipofuscinoses: distinct patterns of storage deposition, neurodegeneration and glial activation. *Brain Pathol*, 14, 349–357.

Tyynelä J, Sohar I, Sleat DE, Gin RM, Donnelly RJ, Baumann M, Haltia M, & Lobel P (2000) A mutation in the ovine cathepsin D gene causes a congenital lysosomal storage disease with profound neurodegeneration. *EMBO J*, 19, 2786–2792.

Tyynelä J, Suopanki J, Baumann M, & Haltia M (1997a) Sphingolipid activator proteins (SAPs) in neuronal ceroid lipofuscinoses (NCL). *Neuropediatrics*, 28, 49–52.

Tyynelä J, Suopanki J, Santavuori P, Baumann M, & Haltia M (1997b) Variant late infantile neuronal ceroid-lipofuscinosis: pathology and biochemistry. *J Neuropathol Exp Neurol*, 56, 369–375.

Umemura T, Sato H, Goryo M, & Itakura C (1985) Generalized lipofuscinosis in a dog. *Nippon Juigaku Zasshi*, 47, 673–677.

Url A, Bauder B, Thalhammer J, Nowotny N, Kolodziejek J, Herout N, Furst S, & Weissenbock H (2001) Equine neuronal ceroid lipofuscinosis. *Acta Neuropathol*, 101, 410–414.

Vandevelde M & Fatzer R (1980) Neuronal ceroid-lipofuscinosis in older dachshunds. *Vet Pathol*, 17, 686–692.

Wada R, Tifft CJ, & Proia RL (2000) Microglial activation precedes acute neurodegeneration in Sandhoff disease and is suppressed by bone marrow transplantation. *Proc Natl Acad Sci U S A*, 97, 10954–10959.

Walkley SU, March PA, Schroeder CE, Wurzelmann S, & Jolly RD (1995) Pathogenesis of brain dysfunction in Batten disease. *Am J Med Genet*, 57, 196–203.

Weissenbock H & Rossel C (1997) Neuronal ceroid-lipofuscinosis in a domestic cat: clinical, morphological and immunohistochemical findings. *J Comp Pathol*, 117, 17–24.

Westlake VJ, Jolly RD, Bayliss SL, & Palmer DN (1995a) Immunocytochemical studies in the ceroid-lipofuscinoses (Batten disease) using antibodies to subunit c of mitochondrial ATP synthase. *Am J Med Genet*, 57, 177–181.

Westlake VJ, Jolly RD, Jones BR, Mellor DJ, Machon R, Zanjani ED, & Krivit W (1995b) Hematopoietic cell transplantation in fetal lambs with ceroid-lipofuscinosis. *Am J Med Genet*, 57, 365–368.

Wheeler RB, Sharp JD, Schultz RA, Joslin JM, Williams RE, & Mole SE (2002) The gene mutated in variant late-infantile neuronal ceroid lipofuscinosis (CLN6) and in nclf mutant mice encodes a novel predicted transmembrane protein. *Am J Hum Genet*, 70, 537–542.

Williams RS, Lott IT, Ferrante RJ, & Caviness VS, Jr. (1977) The cellular pathology of neuronal ceroid-lipofuscinosis. A Golgi-electronmicroscopic study. *Arch Neurol*, 34, 298–305.

Wohlke A, Distl O, & Drogemuller C (2005) The canine CTSD gene as a candidate for late-onset neuronal ceroid lipofuscinosis. *Anim Genet*, 36, 530–532.

Wohlke A, Distl O, & Drogemuller C (2006) Characterization of the canine CLCN3 gene and evaluation as candidate for late-onset NCL. *BMC Genet*, 7, 13.

Wolfe LS, Kin NM, Baker RR, Carpenter S, & Andermann F (1977) Identification of retinoyl complexes as the autofluorescent component of the neuronal storage material in Batten disease. *Science*, 195, 1360–1362.

Wolfe LS & Ng Ying Kin NM (1982) Batten disease: new research findings on the biochemical defect. *Birth Defects Orig Artic Ser*, 18, 233–239.

Woods PR, Storts RW, Shelton M, & Menzies C (1994) Neuronal ceroid lipofuscinosis in Rambouillet sheep: characterization of the clinical disease. *J Vet Intern Med*, 8, 370–375.

Woods PR, Walker MA, Weir VA, Storts RW, Menzies C, & Shelton M (1993) Computed tomography of Rambouillet sheep affected with neuronal ceroid lipofuscinosis. *Vet Radiol Ultrasound*, 34, 259–262.

Wrigstad A, Nilsson SE, Dubielzig R, & Narfstrom K (1995) Neuronal ceroid lipofuscinosis in the Polish Owczarek Nizinny (PON) dog. *A retinal study. Doc Ophthalmol*, 91, 33–47.

Wu YP & Proia RL (2004) Deletion of macrophage-inflammatory protein 1 alpha retards neurodegeneration in Sandhoff disease mice. *Proc Natl Acad Sci U S A*, 101, 8425–8430.

Zeman W (1974) Presidential address: Studies in the neuronal ceroid-lipofuscinoses. *J Neuropathol Exp Neurol*, 33, 1–12.

Zeman W (1976) The neuronal ceroid lipofuscinoses. In Zimmerman HM (Ed.) Progress in *Neuropathology*, pp. 207–223. New York, Grune and Stratton.

Zeman W & Dyken P (1969) Neuronal ceroid-lipofuscinosis (Batten's disease): relationship to amaurotic family idiocy? *Pediatrics*, 44, 570–583.

Chapter 19

Evolutionary Conservation of NCL Proteins

P.E.M. Taschner

INTRODUCTION

Sequence analysis of DNA from different organisms has revealed that genes and their encoded proteins show more or less similarity depending on the distance between organisms in the tree of life. This similarity is the molecular evidence of the evolution of species from a common ancestor. During evolution, DNA damaging agents and errors during DNA replication have introduced changes, resulting in the variations found between species and also between individuals. In general, DNA variations between the protein-encoding regions of genes show least variation compared to intergenic or intronic sequences. The requirement to maintain the function of essential genes and proteins restrains the number of variations and is considered to be the basis of the evolutionary conservation of proteins. Many aspects of protein evolution have been reviewed recently (Pal et al., 2006). In the context of NCL research, the most important applications of evolutionary protein conservation are: 1) the identification of conserved residues and motifs in genes and proteins, which are considered to be functionally important and can cause disease, when altered, and 2) the identification of homologous genes and proteins in model organisms. Homologous genes and proteins can either be orthologues, which have directly evolved from a common ancestor and are functionally equivalent, or paralogues, which are the result of gene duplications within a species. After gene duplication, the paralogues may have evolved separately to obtain different functionalities.

CLN PROTEIN HOMOLOGUES

Protein homologues in other organisms can be identified by BLAST protein search (Altschul et al., 1990) using human protein sequences. Homologues to the human CLN proteins in dog, cow, mouse, chicken, zebrafish, fly, worm, baker's yeast (*Saccharomyces cerevisiae*) and fission yeast (*Schizosaccharomyces pombe*) were identified using the RefSeq protein sequences retrieved from Entrez Gene searches with human *CLN* gene symbols. The evolutionary conservation between these proteins becomes apparent in the alignments of CLN protein sequences from the different organisms made with Multalin (Corpet, 1988) and GeneDoc (Nicholas and al., 1997) (Figures 19.1–19.8).

```
                    *        20         *        40         *
Human_CTSD --------------------MQPSSLLPL--ALCLLAAPASALVRIPLHK  28
Dog        --------------------MQPPSLLLL--VLGLLAAPAAALVRIPLHK  28
Cow        --------------------MQTPRLLPLLLALGLLAAPAAAVIRIPLHK  30
Mouse      --------------------MKTPGVLLL--ILGLLASSSFAIIRIPLRK  28
Sheep      -----------------------------------------------LHK   3
Chicken    --------------------MAPRGLLVL--LLLALVGPCAALIRIPLTK  28
Zebrafish  -----------------------MRIRFC--CSLLPFSARRRDCRIPLKK  25
Fly        ---------------------------MQKVALLLVAFLAAAVAHPNSQE  23
Worm       ------MNRCILLLLGALLLVQGLHVHKRQQKLRTVSLKKQPTLRETLLQ  44
Baker's    ------MFSLKALLPLALLLVSANQVA----AKVHKAKIYKHELSDEMKE  40
Fission    MKASFFVFAISALQALQASVASAYSEVPGKRSVVLNLQHSQYDHVARKLE  50

                   60         *        80         *       100
Human_CTSD FTSIRRTMSEVGGSVEDLIAKGPVSKYSQAVPAVTEGPIPEVLKNYMDAQ  78
Dog        FTSVRRTMTELGGPVEDLIAKGPISKYAQGAPAVTGGPIPEMLRNYMDAQ  78
Cow        FTSIRRTMSEAMGPVEHLIAKGPISKYATGEPAVRQGPIPELLKNYMDAQ  80
Mouse      FTSIRRTMTEVGGSVEDLILKGPITKYSMQSSPKTTEPVSELLKNYLDAQ  78
Sheep      FTSNRRTMSEAMGPVEHLIAKGPISKYATREPAVRQGPIPELLTNYMDAQ  53
Chicken    FTSTRRMLTEVGSEIPDMNAITQFLKFKLGFADLAE-PTPEILKNYMDAQ  77
Zebrafish  FRTLRRTLSDSGRSLEELVSSSNSLKYNLGFPASND-PTPETLKNYLDAQ  74
Fly        KPGLLRVPLHKFQSARRHFADVG-TELQQLRIRYGGGDVPEPLSNYMDAQ  72
Worm       AGSFETFAKHRHGYKKYLKTNGN-HHFDKYQALNVEGEIDELLRNYMDAQ  93
Baker's    VTFEQHLAHLGQKYLTQFEKANPEVVFSREHPFFTEGGHDVPLTNYLNAQ  90
Fission    RTKVLNKRDSSGYPVLDLEYTDAGGYFANLTLGSNERVYSLTLDTGSPYT 100
                                                   e L ny daq

                    *       120         *       140         *
Human_CTSD YYGEIGIGTPPQCFTVVFDTGSSNLWVPSIHCKLLDIACWIHHKYNSDKS 128
Dog        YYGEIGIGTPPQCFTVVFDTGSSNLWVPSIHCKLLDIACWIHHKYNSGKS 128
Cow        YYGEIGIGTPPQCFTVVFDTGSANLWVPSIHCKLLDIACWTHRKYNSDKS 130
Mouse      YYGDIGIGTPPQCFTVVFDTGSSNLWVPSIHCKILDIACWVHHKYNSDKS 128
Sheep      YYGEIGIGTPPQCFTVVFDTGSANLWVPSIHCKLLDIACWVHHKYNSDKS 103
Chicken    YYGEIGIGTPPQKFTVVFDTGSSNLWVPSVHCHLLDIACLLHHKYDASKS 127
Zebrafish  YYGEIGLGTPVQTFTVVFDTGSSNLWVPSVHCSLTDIACLLHHKYNGGKS 124
Fly        YYGPIAIGSPPQNFRVVFDTGSSNLWVPSKKCHLTNIACLMHNKYDASKS 122
Worm       YFGTISIGTPAQNFTVIFDTGSSNLWIPSKKCPFYDIACMLHHRYDSKSS 143
Baker's    YYTDITLGTPPQNFKVILDTGSSNLWVPSNECG--SLACFLHSKYDHEAS 138
Fission    WVTAKNI-TALSASEIWSDTDGVDAGRSTSDIRTNACTNYTCFDYSSTTA 149
           yyg i igtp q f v fDTgs nlwvps  c    iac  h kY    s

                  160         *       180         *       200
Human_CTSD STYVKNGTSFDIHYGSGS-LSGYLSQDTVSVPCQSASSASALGGVKVERQ 177
Dog        STYVKNGTSFDIHYGSGS-LSGYLSQDTVSVPCKSA--LSGLAGIKVERQ 175
Cow        STYVKNGTTFDIHYGSGS-LSGYLSQDTVSVPCNPS--SSSPGGVTVQRQ 177
Mouse      STYVKNGTSFDIHYGSGS-LSGYLSQDTVSVPCKSD--QSKARGIKVEKQ 175
Sheep      STYVKNGTTFDIHYGSGS-LSGYLSQDTVSVPCNPS--SSSPGGVTVQRQ 150
Chicken    STYVENGTEFAIHYGTGS-LSGFLSQDTVTL-----------GNLKIKNQ 165
Zebrafish  STYVKNGTQFAIQYGSGS-LSGYLSQDTCTI-----------GDIAVEKQ 162
Fly        KTYTKNGTEFAIQYGSGS-LSGYLSTDTVSI-----------AGLDIKDQ 160
Worm       STYKEDGRKMAIQYGTGS-MKGFISKDSVCV-----------AGVCAEDQ 181
Baker's    SSYKANGTEFAIQYGTGS-LEGYISQDTLSI-----------GDLTIPKQ 176
Fission    RRTNSSTIGFLASYGDNTTVLGYNMVDNAYFAGLTL--PGFEFGLATREY 197
           sty  ngt f i YG gs l Gy s Dt                     q
```

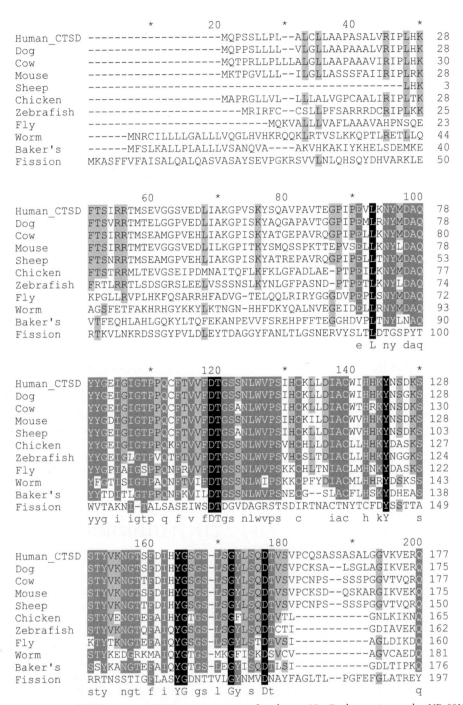

Figure 19.1 Alignment of CTSD proteins. CTSD protein sequences from human (GenBank accession number NP_001900.1), dog (NP_001020792.1), cow (XP_609913.3), sheep (partial sequence AAF80494.1), mouse (NP_034113.1), chicken (NP_990508.1), zebrafish (NP_571785.1), fly (NP_652013.1), worm (NP_510191.1), baker's yeast (*S. cerevisiae*) (NP_015171.1), and fission yeast (*S. pombe*) (P32834.2) were aligned using Multalin. In all alignments, the degree of amino acid conservation is indicated by different background colors (black: 100%, dark grey: 80%, light grey: 60%). The consensus line below the sequences lists residues conserved among all species in uppercase and those conserved in more than 80% in lower case.

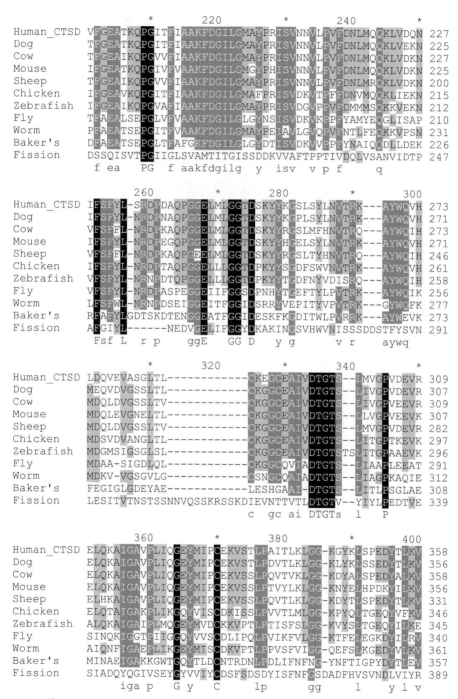

```
                    *         220         *         240         *
Human_CTSD VFGEATKQPGITFIAAKFDGILGMAYPRISVNNVLPVFDNLMQQKLVDQN 227
Dog        TFGEATKQPGITFIAAKFDGILGMAYPRISVNNVLPVFDNLMQQKLVEKN 225
Cow        TFGEAIKQPGVVFIAAKFDGILGMAYPRISVNNVLPVFDNLMQQKLVDKN 227
Mouse      IFGEATKQPGIVFVAAKFDGILGMGYPHISVNNVLPVFDNLMQQKLVDKN 225
Sheep      TFGEAIKQPGVVFIAAKFDGILGMAYPRISVNNVLPVFDNLMRQKLVDKN 200
Chicken    IFGEAVKQPGITFIAAKFDGILGMAFPRISVDKVTPFFDNVMQQKLIEKN 215
Zebrafish  IFGEAIKQPGVAFIAAKFDGILGMAYPRISVDGVPPVFDMMMSQKKVEKN 212
Fly        TFAEALSEPGLVFVAAKFDGILGLGYNSISVDKVKPPFYAMYEQGLISAP 210
Worm       PFAEATSEPGITFVAAKFDGILGMAYPEIAVLGVQPVFNTLFEQKKVPSN 231
Baker's    DFAEATSEPGLTFAFGKFDGILGLGYDTISVDKVVPPFYNAIQQDLLDEK 226
Fission    DSSQISVTPGIIGLSVAMTITGISSDDKVVAFTPPTIVDQLVSANVIDTP 247
            f ea    PG  f aakfdgilg  y  isv  v p f     q

                  260         *         280         *         300
Human_CTSD IFSFYL-SRDPDAQPGGELMLGGTDSKYYKGSLSYLNVTRK---AYWQVH 273
Dog        IFSFYL-NRDPNAQPGGELMLGGTDSKYYKGPLSYLNVTRK---AYWQVH 271
Cow        VFSFFL-NRDPKAQPGGELMLGGTDSKYYRGSLMFHNVTRQ---AYWQIH 273
Mouse      IFSFYL-NRDPEGQPGGELMLGGTDSKYYHGELSYLNVTRK---AYWQVH 271
Sheep      VFSFFL-NRDPKAQPGEELMLGGTDSKYYRGSLTYHNVTRQ---AYWQIH 246
Chicken    IFSFYL-NRDPTAQPGGELLLGGTDPKYYSGDFSWVNVTRK---AYWQVH 261
Zebrafish  VFSFYL-NRNPDTQPGGELLLGGTDPKYYTGDFNYVDISRQ---AYWQIH 258
Fly        VFSFYL-NRDPASPEGGEIIFGGSDPNHYTGEFTYLPVTRK---AYWQIK 256
Worm       LFSFWL-NRNPDSEIGGEITFGGIDSRRYVEPITYVPVTRK---GYWQFK 277
Baker's    RFAFYLGDTSKDTENGGEATFGGIDESKFKGDITWLPVRRK---AYWEVK 273
Fission    AFGIYL------NEDVGELIFGGYDKAKINGSVHWVNISSSDDSTFYSVN 291
            Fsf L  r p    ggE   GG D   y g      v r    aywq

                    *         320         *         340         *
Human_CTSD LDQVEVASGLTL------------CKEGCEAIVDTGTS--LMVGPVDEVR 309
Dog        MEQVDVGSSLTL------------CKGGCEAIVDTGTS--LIVGPVDEVR 307
Cow        MDQLDVGSSLTV------------CKGGCEAIVDTGTS--LIVGPVEEVR 309
Mouse      MDQLEVGNELTL------------CKGGCEAIVDTGTS--LLVGPVEEVK 307
Sheep      MDQLDVGSSLTV------------CKGGCEAIVDTGTS--LMVGPVDEVR 282
Chicken    MDSVDVANGLTL------------CKGGCEAIVDTGTS--LITGPTKEVK 297
Zebrafish  MDGMSIGSGLSL------------CKGGCEAIVDTGTSTSLITGPAAEVK 296
Fly        MDAA-SIGDLQL------------CKGGCQVIADTGTS--LIAAPLEEAT 291
Worm       MDKV-VGSGVLG------------CSNGCQAIADTGTS--LIAGPKAQIE 312
Baker's    FEGIGLGDEYAE------------LESHGAAI-DTGTS--LITLPSGLAE 308
Fission    LESITVTNSTSSNNVQSSKRSSKDIEVNTTVTLDTGTV--YIYLPEDTVE 339
                                   c  gc ai DTGTs   l   P

                  360         *         380         *         400
Human_CTSD ELQKAIGAVPLIQGEYMIPCEKVSTLPAITLKLGG-KGYKLSPEDYTLKV 358
Dog        ELQKAIGAVPLIQGEYMIPCEKVSTLPDVTLKLGG-KLYKLSSEDYTLKV 356
Cow        ELQKAIGAVPLIQGEYMIPCEKVSSLPQVTVKLGG-KDYALSPEDYALKV 358
Mouse      ELQKAIGAVPLIQGEYMIPCEKVSSLPTVYLKLGG-KNYELHPDKYILKV 356
Sheep      ELHKAIGAVPLIQGEYMIPCEKVSSLPQVTLKLGG-KDYTLSPEDYTLKV 331
Chicken    ELQTAIGAKPLIKGQYVISCDKISSLPVVTLMLGG-KPYQLTGEQYVFKV 346
Zebrafish  ALQKAIGAIPLMQGEYMVDCKKVPTLPTISFSLGG-KVYSLTGEQYILKE 345
Fly        SINQKIGGTPIIGGQYVVSCDLIPQLPVIKFVLGG-KTFELEGKDYILRV 340
Worm       AIQNFIGAEPLIKGEYMISCDKVPTLPPVSFVIGG-QEFSLKGEDYVLKV 361
Baker's    MINAEIGAKKGWTGQYTLDCNTRDNLPDLIFNFNG-YNFTIGPYDYTLEV 357
Fission    SIADQYQGIVSEYGYVVIYCDSFSDSDYISFNFGSDADFHVSVNDLVIYR 389
                iga p   G y   C      lp      gg      l    y l v
```

Figure 19.1 Cont'd

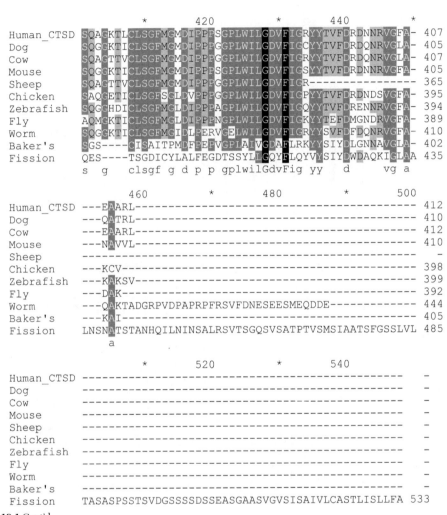

```
                          *        420         *        440         *
Human_CTSD  SQAGKTLCLSGFMGMDIPPPSGPLWILGDVFIGRYYTVFDRDNNRVGFA- 407
Dog         SQGGKTICLSGFMGMDIPPPGGPLWILGDVFIGCYYTVFDRDQNRVGLA- 405
Cow         SQAGTTVCLSGFMGMDIPPPGGPLWILGDVFIGRYYTVFDRDQNRVGLA- 407
Mouse       SQGGKTICLSGFMGMDIPPPSGPLWILGDVFIGSYYTVFDRDNNRVGFA- 405
Sheep       SQAGTTVCLSGFMGMDIPPPGGPLWILGDVFIGR---------------- 365
Chicken     SAQGETICLSGFSGLDVPPPGGPLWILGDVFIGPYYTVFDRDNDSVGFA- 395
Zebrafish   SQGGHDICLSGFMGLDIPPPAGPLWILGDVFIGQYYTVFDRENNRVGFA- 394
Fly         AQMGKTICLSGFMGLDIPPPNGPLWILGDVFIGKYYTEFDMGNDRVGFA- 389
Worm        SQGGKTICLSGFMGIDLPERVGELWILGDVFIGRYYSVFDFDQNRVGFA- 410
Baker's     SGS----CISAITPMDFPEPVGPLAIVGDAFLRKYYSIYDLGNNAVGLA- 402
Fission     QES----TSGDICYLALFEGDTSSYLLGQYFLQYVYSIYDWDAQKIGLAA 435
            s  g   clsgf g d p p gplwilGdvFig yy   d     vg a

                    460        *       480         *       500
Human_CTSD  ---EAARL------------------------------------------ 412
Dog         ---QATRL------------------------------------------ 410
Cow         ---EAARL------------------------------------------ 412
Mouse       ---NAVVL------------------------------------------ 410
Sheep       --------------------------------------------------   -
Chicken     ---KCV-------------------------------------------- 398
Zebrafish   ---KAKSV------------------------------------------ 399
Fly         ---DAK-------------------------------------------- 392
Worm        ---QAKTADGRPVDPAPRPFRSVFDNESEESMEQDDE------------- 444
Baker's     ---KAI-------------------------------------------- 405
Fission     LNSNATSTANHQILNINSALRSVTSGQSVSATPTVSMSIAATSFGSSLVL 485
                a

                          *        520         *        540
Human_CTSD  ------------------------------------------------     -
Dog         ------------------------------------------------     -
Cow         ------------------------------------------------     -
Mouse       ------------------------------------------------     -
Sheep       ------------------------------------------------     -
Chicken     ------------------------------------------------     -
Zebrafish   ------------------------------------------------     -
Fly         ------------------------------------------------     -
Worm        ------------------------------------------------     -
Baker's     ------------------------------------------------     -
Fission     TASASPSSTSVDGSSSSDSSEASGAASVGVSISAIVLCASTLISLLFA   533
```

Figure 19.1 Cont'd

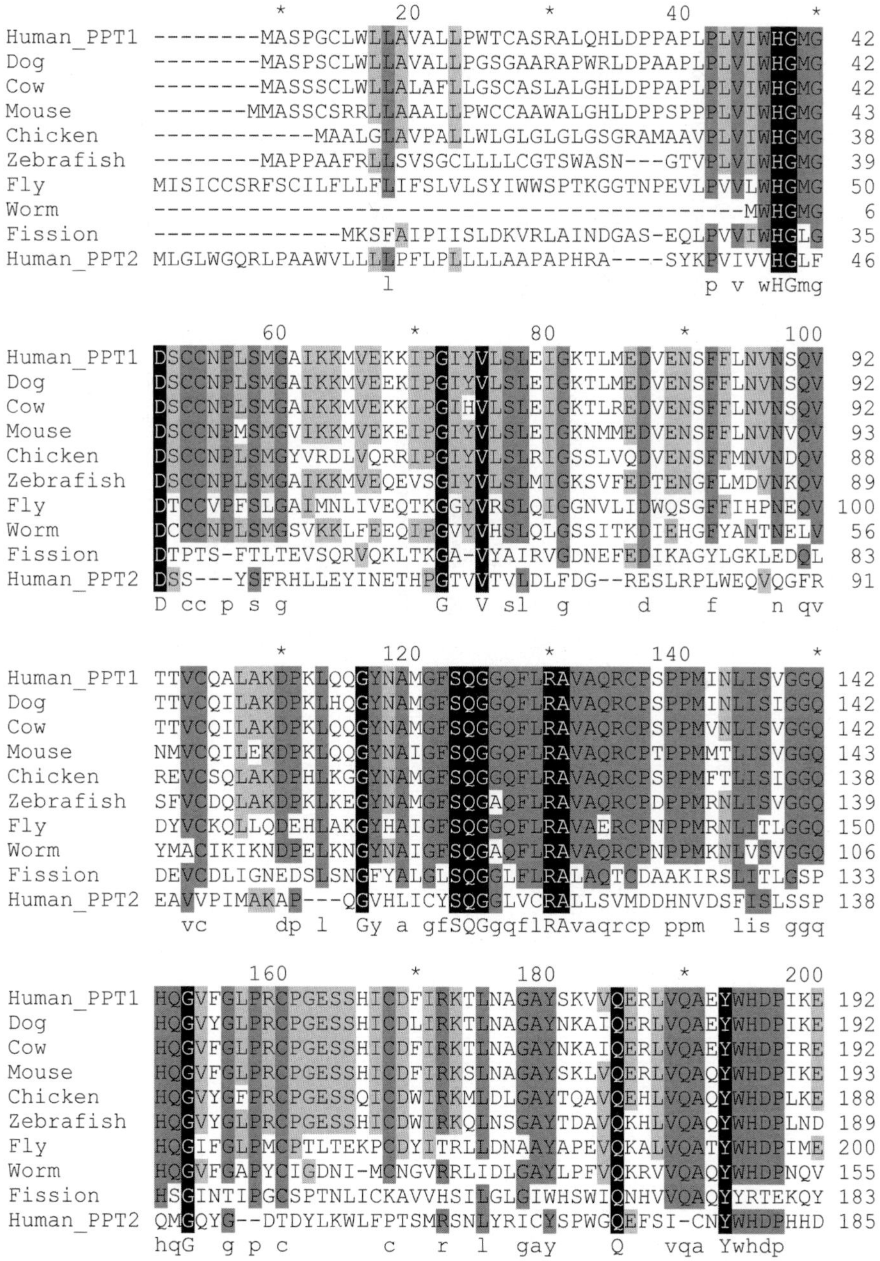

Figure 19.2 Alignment of PPT1 proteins. PPT1 protein sequences from human (GenBank accession number NP_000301.1), dog (NP_001010944.1), cow (NP_776579.1), mouse (NP_032943.2), chicken (NP_001026074.1), zebrafish (NP_998504.1), fly (NP_727284.1), worm (NP_504684.1), and fission yeast (*S. pombe*) (NP_595325.1, first part including the two putative Krp1 cleavage sites) and human PPT2 (NP_005146.3) were aligned using Multalin.

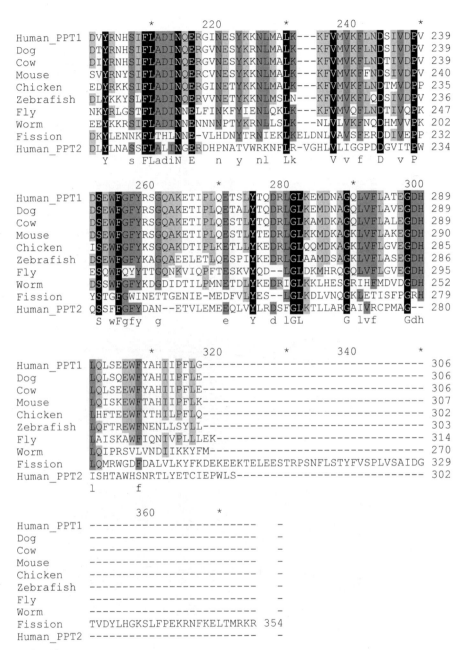

```
                      *        220         *        240         *
Human_PPT1  DVYRNHSIFLADINQERGINESYKKNLMALK---KFVMVKFLNDSIVDPV 239
Dog         DTYRNHSIFLADINQERGVNESYKRNLMALK---KFVMVKFLNDSIVDPV 239
Cow         DIYRNHSIFLADINQERGVNESYKKNLMALK---KFVMVKFLNDTIVDPV 239
Mouse       SVYRNYSIFLADINQERCVNESYKKNLMALK---KFVMVKFFNDSIVDPV 240
Chicken     EDYRKKSIFLADINQERGINETYKKNLMALK---KFVMVKFLNDTMVDPP 235
Zebrafish   DLYKKYSLFLADINQERVVNETYKKNLMSLN---KFVMVKFLQDSIVDPV 236
Fly         NKYRLGSTFLADINNELFINKFYIENLQKLK---KFVMVQFLNDTIVQPK 247
Worm        EEYKKRSIFLADINNENNNNPTYKRNLLSLK---NLVLVKFNQDHMVVPK 202
Fission     DKYLENNKFLTHLNNE-VLHDNYTRNIEKLKELDNLVAVSFERDDIVEPP 232
Human_PPT2  DLYLNASSFLALINGERDHPNATVWRKNFLR-VGHLVLIGGPDDGVITPW 234
              Y   s FLadiN E   n   y  nl  Lk     V v f  D  v P

                    260        *        280         *        300
Human_PPT1  DSEWFGFYRSGQAKETIPLQETSLYTQDRLGLKEMDNAGQLVFLATEGDH 289
Dog         DSEWFGFYRSGQAKETIPLQETALYTQDRLGLKEMDNAGQLVFLAVEGDH 289
Cow         DSEWFGFYRSGQAKETIPLQESTLYTQDRLGLKAMDKAGQLVFLALEGDH 289
Mouse       DSEWFGFYRSGQAKETIPLQESTLYTEDRLGLKKMDKAGKLVFLAKEGDH 290
Chicken     ISEWFGFYKSGQAKDTIPLKETLLYKEDRLGLQQMDKAGKLVFLGVEGDH 285
Zebrafish   DSEWFGFYKAGQAEELETLQESPIYKEDRLGLAAMDSAGKLVFLASEGDH 286
Fly         ESQWFQYYTTGQNKVIQPFTESKVYQD--LGLDKMHRQGQLVFLGVEGDH 295
Worm        DSSWFGFYKDGDIDTILPMNETDLYKEDRIGLKKLHESGRIHFMDVDGDH 252
Fission     YSTGFGWINETTGENIE-MEDFVLYES--LGLKDLVNQGKLETISFPGRH 279
Human_PPT2  QSSFFGFYDAN--ETVLEMEEQLVYLRDSFGLKTLLARGAIVRCPMAG-- 280
             S wFgfy  g          e   Y  d lGL       G lvf    Gdh

                      *        320         *        340         *
Human_PPT1  LQLSEEWFYAHIIPFLG--------------------------------- 306
Dog         LQLSQEWFYAHIIPFLE--------------------------------- 306
Cow         LQLSEEWFYAHIIPFLE--------------------------------- 306
Mouse       LQISKEWFTAHIIPFLK--------------------------------- 307
Chicken     LHFTEEWFYTHILPFLQ--------------------------------- 302
Zebrafish   LQFTREWFNENLLSYLL--------------------------------- 303
Fly         LAISKAWFIQNIVPLLLEK------------------------------- 314
Worm        LQIPRSVLVNDIIKKYFM-------------------------------- 270
Fission     LQMRWGDFDALVLKYFKDEKEEKTELEESTRPSNFLSTYFVSPLVSAIDG 329
Human_PPT2  ISHTAWHSNRTLYETCIEPWLS---------------------------- 302
            l       f

                    360        *
Human_PPT1  -------------------------    -
Dog         -------------------------    -
Cow         -------------------------    -
Mouse       -------------------------    -
Chicken     -------------------------    -
Zebrafish   -------------------------    -
Fly         -------------------------    -
Worm        -------------------------    -
Fission     TVDYLHGKSLFPEKRNFKELTMRKR  354
Human_PPT2  -------------------------    -
```

Figure 19.2 Cont'd

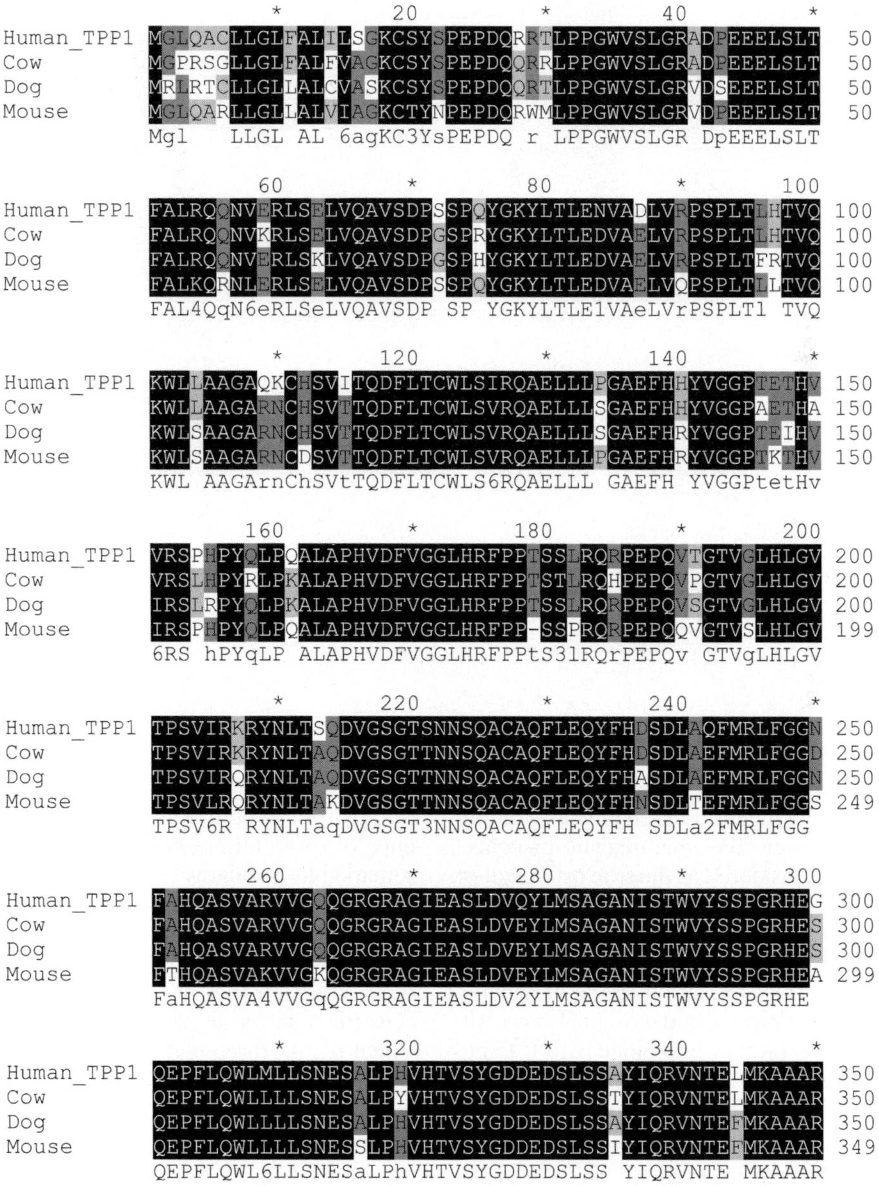

Figure 19.3 Alignment of TPP1 proteins. TPP1 protein sequences from human (GenBank accession number NP_000382.1), dog (NP_001013869.1), cow (NP_001069186.1), and mouse (NP_034036.1) were aligned using Multalin.

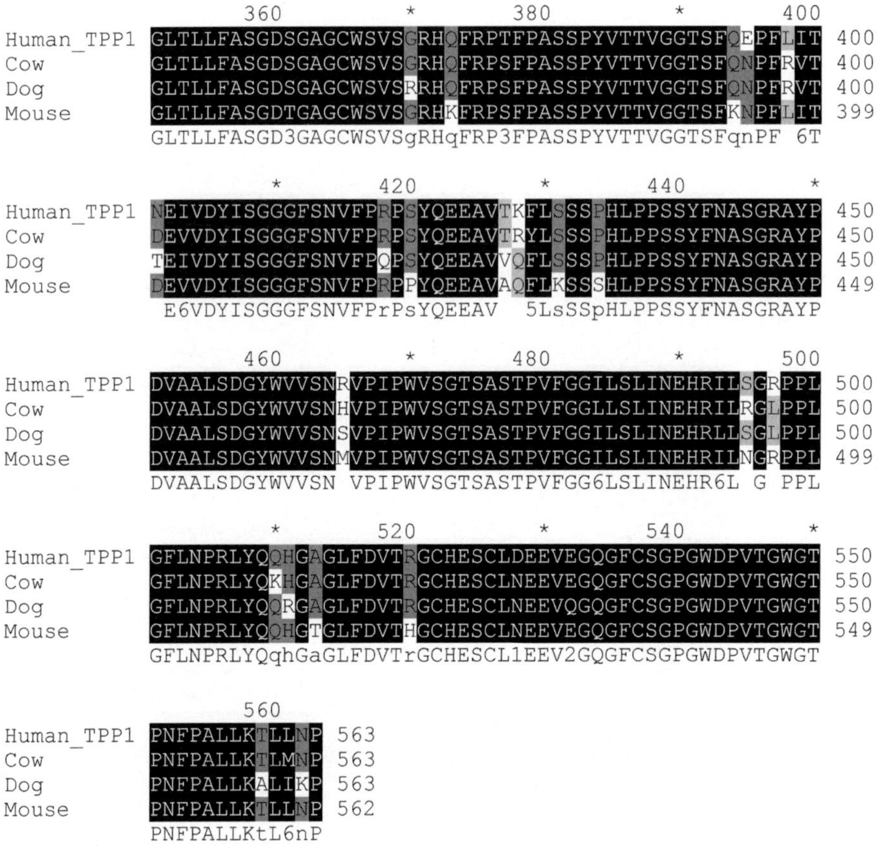

Figure 19.3 Cont'd

As expected, the highest degree of conservation is found between the mammalian proteins, which can be considered as the true orthologues of the human CLN proteins. The absence of conserved genes flanking the *CLN* genes in other organisms makes it difficult to distinguish between an orthologue and a single paralogue remaining after deletion of the original gene. All organisms have protein homologues to CTSD, PPT1, and CLN3, except baker's yeast, which lacks a PPT1 homologue. The chicken TPP1 and CLN3 predicted protein sequences were found to be incomplete and have been excluded from the alignments to prevent interference. The PPT1 protein of fission yeast differs from the others, because it is synthesized as a proprotein, which is probably cleaved by the Krp1 endopeptidase into a palmitoyl protein thioesterase moiety and a dolichol pyrophosphate phosphatase 1 moiety (Cho and Hofmann, 2004). The nematode *Caenorhabditis elegans* differs from all other organisms due to the presence of three CLN3 homologues, which show remarkable similarity despite their separate evolution during the last 100 million years (Figure 19.4). The similarity also suggests that these proteins may still have overlapping functions, although they are expressed in different cells (de Voer et al., 2005). It remains unclear which of the three *cln-3* genes represents the ancestral one. The remaining proteins TPP1, CLN5, CLN6, and CLN8 have homologues in vertebrates only, with the exception of TPP1 in zebrafish, suggesting that these proteins play a role in a process, which is absent in simpler organisms. In general, these proteins show a high homology across the complete protein sequence. The notable exception is CLN5, where only the human protein has four alternative N-terminal sequences (Vesa et al., 2002). The proteins from other organisms correspond to the two shortest CLN5 isoforms, which

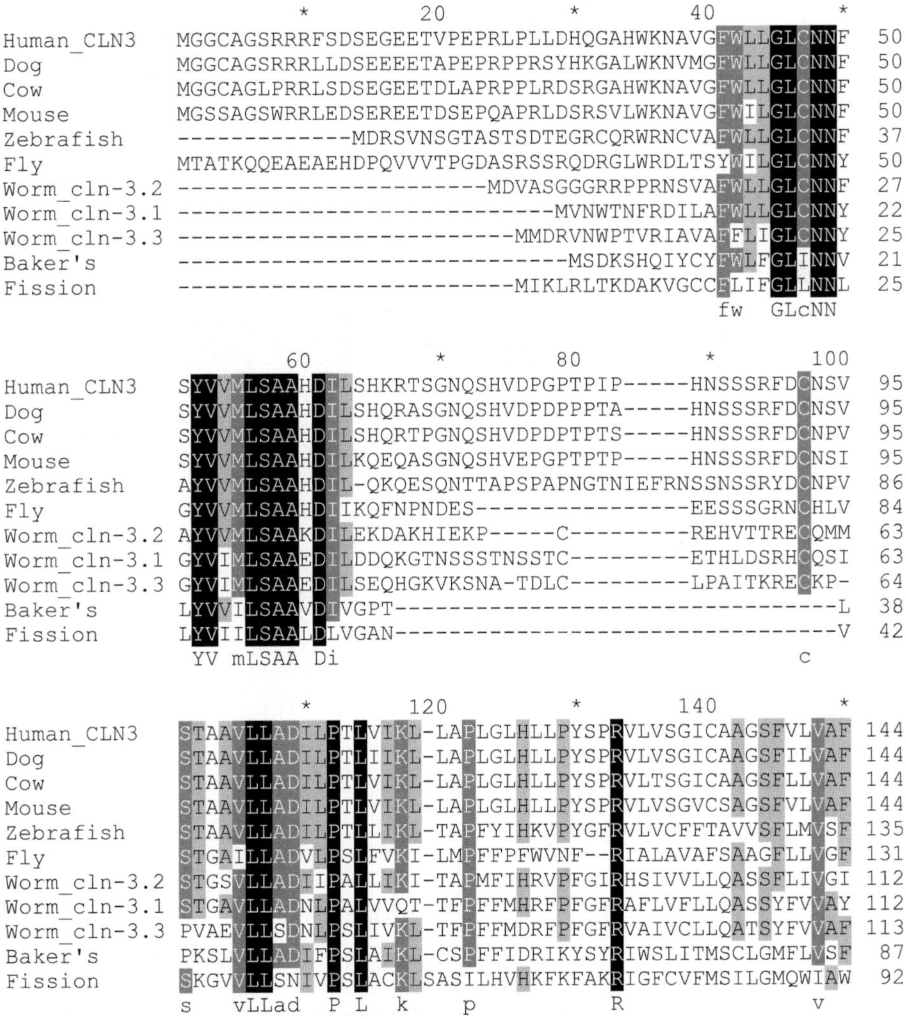

* 20 * 40 *
Human_CLN3 MGGCAGSRRRFSDSEGEETVPEPRLPLLDHQGAHWKNAVGFWLLGLCNNF 50
Dog MGGCAGSRRRLLDSEEEETAPEPRPPRSYHKGALWKNVMGFWLLGLCNNF 50
Cow MGGCAGLPRRLSDSEGEETDLAPRPPLRDSRGAHWKNAVGFWLLGLCNNF 50
Mouse MGSSAGSWRRLEDSEREETDSEPQAPRLDSRSVLWKNAVGFWILGLCNNF 50
Zebrafish -------------MDRSVNSGTASTSDTEGRCQRWRNCVAFWLLGLCNNF 37
Fly MTATKQQEAEAEHDPQVVVTPGDASRSSRQDRGLWRDLTSYWILGLCNNY 50
Worm_cln-3.2 -----------------------MDVASGGGRRPPRNSVAFWLLGLCNNF 27
Worm_cln-3.1 ----------------------------MVNWTNFRDILAFWLLGLCNNY 22
Worm_cln-3.3 -------------------------MMDRVNWPTVRIAVAFFLIGLCNNY 25
Baker's -----------------------------MSDKSHQIYCYFWLFGLINNV 21
Fission -------------------------MIKLRLTKDAKVGCCFLIFGLLNNL 25
fw GLcNN
60 * 80 * 100
Human_CLN3 SYVVMLSAAHDILSHKRTSGNQSHVDPGPTPIP-----HNSSSRFDCNSV 95
Dog SYVVMLSAAHDILSHQRASGNQSHVDPDPPPTA-----HNSSSRFDCNSV 95
Cow SYVVMLSAAHDILSHQRTPGNQSHVDPDPTPTS-----HNSSSRFDCNPV 95
Mouse SYVVMLSAAHDILKQEQASGNQSHVEPGPTPTP-----HNSSSRFDCNSI 95
Zebrafish AYVVMLSAAHDIL-QKQESQNTTAPSPAPNGTNIEFRNSSNSSRYDCNPV 86
Fly GYVVMLSAAHDIIKQFNPNDES----------------EESSSGRNCHLV 84
Worm_cln-3.2 AYVVMLSAAKDILEKDAKHIEKP-----C---------REHVTTRECQMM 63
Worm_cln-3.1 GYVIMLSAAEDILDDQKGTNSSSTNSSTC---------ETHLDSRHCQSI 63
Worm_cln-3.3 GYVIMLSAAEDILSEQHGKVKSNA-TDLC---------LPAITKRECKP- 64
Baker's LYVVILSAAVDIVGPT-------------------------------L 38
Fission LYVIILSAALDLVGAN-------------------------------V 42
YV mLSAA Di c
* 120 * 140 *
Human_CLN3 STAAVLLADILPTLVIKL-LAPLGLHLLPYSPRVLVSGICAAGSFVLVAF 144
Dog STAAVLLADILPTLIIKL-LAPLGLHLLPYSPRVLVSGICAAGSFILVAF 144
Cow STAAVLLADILPTLVIKL-LAPLGLHLLPYSPRVLTSGICAAGSFLLVAF 144
Mouse STAAVLLADILPTLVIKL-LAPLGLHLLPYSPRVLVSGVCSAGSFVLVAF 144
Zebrafish STAAVLLADILPTLLIKL-TAPFYIHKVPYGFRVLVCFFTAVVSFLMVSF 135
Fly STGAILLADVLPSLFVKI-LMPFFPFWVNF--RIALAVAFSAAGFLLVGF 131
Worm_cln-3.2 STGSVLLADIIPALLIKI-TAPMFIHRVPFGIRHSIVVLLQASSFLIVGI 112
Worm_cln-3.1 STGAVLLADNLPALVVQT-TFPFFMHRFPFGFRAFLVFLLQASSYFVVAY 112
Worm_cln-3.3 PVAEVLLSDNLPSLIVKL-TFPFFMDRFPFGFRVAIVCLLQATSYFVVAF 113
Baker's PKSLVLLADIFPSLAIKL-CSPFFIDRIKYSYRIWSLITMSCLGMFLVSF 87
Fission SKGVVLLSNIVPSLACKLSASILHVHKFKFAKRIGFCVFMSILGMQWIAW 92
s vLLad P L k p R v

Figure 19.4 Alignment of CLN3 proteins. CLN3 protein sequences from human (GenBank accession number NP_000077.1), dog (NP_001013435.1), cow (NP_001068642.2), mouse (NP_034037.1), zebrafish (NP_001007307.1), fly (NP_649011.1), worm *cln-3.2* (NP_491556.1), *cln-3.1* (NP_505859.1), *cln-3.3* (NP_505237.1), baker's yeast (*S. cerevisiae*) (NP_012476.1), and fission yeast (*S. pombe*) (NP_593598.1) were aligned using Multalin.

```
                           160         *        180         *        200
Human_CLN3    SHSVGTSLCGVVFASISSGLGEVTFLSLTAFYPRAVISWWSSGTGGAGLL 194
Dog           SHSVGTSLCGVVLASISSGVGEVTFLSLTAFYPRAVISWWSSGTGGAGLM 194
Cow           SHSVTISLCGVVLASISSGLGEVTFLSLTAFYPRAVISCWSSGTGGAGLL 194
Mouse         SQSVGLSLCGVVLASISSGLGEVTFLSLTAFYPSAVISWWSSGTGGAGLL 194
Zebrafish     SSTISMSIIGVIFASVSSGLGELSFLSLSVFFSSDVLSGWGSGTGAAGVA 185
Fly           ANAEWMALLGVIITSASSGIGETTFLAYSSRYNKNVISTWSSGTGGAGVI 181
Worm_cln-3.2  SDSTALALFGVVLASFGSGLGEISYLALSSNYPSTVVASWSSGTGGAGLI 162
Worm_cln-3.1  SKNIAMSLAGVCMASLGQGIGEITFLAMAAHYIPETIASWSSGTGGAGLI 162
Worm_cln-3.3  SVSIPMSLAGVVFVSLGGGLGEITFLGLSAHYQRIAIAGWSSGTGMAGLL 163
Baker's       KNLFVC-LLGISFASISSGFGEVTFLQLTHYYKQISLNGWSSGTGGAGII 136
Fission       SSSVPSKMLGVSLAAISSSFGEISFLHLSSRYHSVSLPCWSSGTGLAGLF 142
              s      l Gv  as  sg GE  fL l   y      WsSGTG AG

                      *       220         *       240         *
Human_CLN3    GALSYLGLTQ---AGLSPQQTLLSMLGIPALLLASYFLLLTSPEA----- 236
Dog           GALSYLGLTQ---AGLSPQHTLLSMLGIPALMLASYFFLLTSPEP----- 236
Cow           GALSYLGLTQ---AGLSPQHTLLSMLGIPALLLASYFLLLTSPGP----- 236
Mouse         GSLSYLGLTQ---AGLSPQHTLLSMLGIPVLLLASYFLLLTSPEP----- 236
Zebrafish     GALLYSALTQ---AGLTPQVTLWIMLVVPVILAVSYFVLLVFPHSFPQWR 232
Fly           GSLSYASLRS---LDFSPRDTMLIMLIFPAIEAFAFWLLLRRPQV----- 223
Worm_cln-3.2  GASAYALLTDSKLLAISPKHTMFIMLTLPALFSVSYWSILKIPHSVQRAH 212
Worm_cln-3.1  GSFSYAFITQ---AGLSPSNTLLVQLFIPVVFAGAYFFLLTIPPTVY-SP 208
Worm_cln-3.3  GSFSYAFLTEPHMANLTPKVALLIQLFIPVLFAFAYFILLKKPESVY-SP 212
Baker's       GGASYMFLTS--IFKVPVKLTLLVFSLLPFAFLFYFKLESNDTNL----- 179
Fission       GASSYLVMTT--WFNFSVRSTLIISSFLPLFLLIMYFFVLPESES----- 185
              G  sY  lt        p  tl   l  P       y  l p

                           260         *        280         *        300
Human_CLN3    ---QDPGGEEEAESAARQPLIRTEAP---ESKPGSS-------SS--LSL 271
Dog           ---QDPGGEEEAETSARQPLIDSETP---ESKPDSS-------SN--LSL 271
Cow           ---QDPGGEADSDTSARQPLINNEAS---ESKPGSG-------SP--LSL 271
Mouse         ---LDPGGENEAETAARQPLIGTETP---ESKPGAS-------WD--LSL 271
Zebrafish     CPEVSQSLSRGLNSEERRALIEEDTDTDEDSEPALEDQDDKHIGP--LTF 280
Fly           ------DILPVTTVESTEVLISDEKP------------------L--VGF 247
Worm_cln-3.2  FLQPSTWLVTGDFIPADDMRREEVEEEEGLLGIREDRENSVDVTSRRRQT 262
Worm_cln-3.1  TIHPSTWIIPKNY---DKDVFEAAEARGDVL-------NTKKVPQRELGP 248
Worm_cln-3.3  TLDPKSWIVPKGY---DDFI----------V-------SEHRVPQRELGP 242
Baker's       ---TYQSLQQIDEAEDDQLVPFPVAFTHTNA-------SQSLYSTRQHIL 219
Fission       ---TSPSINNNYT---------PIESIDLRA-------GHVSFNFVNSLK 216

                      *       320         *       340         *
Human_CLN3    RERWTVFKGLLWYIVPLVVVYFAEYFINQGLFELLFF---WNTSL----- 313
Dog           QERWTVFKGLLWYIVPLVLVYFAEYFINQGLFELLFF---RNTSL----- 313
Cow           QERWTVFKGLLHYIVPLVLVYFAEYFINQGLFELLFF---RNTFL----- 313
Mouse         QERWTVFKGLLWYIIPLVLVYFAEYFINQGLFELLFF---RNTSL----- 313
Zebrafish     TEKKYIIKGLLKFIFPLALVYFAEYFINQGLMELLYF---PDSRL----- 322
Fly           KEKLFYIKHLFKYMLPLCLVYFFEYFINQGLFELVYF---EDIFL----- 289
Worm_cln-3.2  STTLERVLPLLKFMIPLISVYLAEYYINQGLLELLEFDCSHGFSM----- 307
Worm_cln-3.1  LERIKLIGPLLYLMVPLATVYTAEYMINQGLTELIIFNCSQGLSL----- 293
Worm_cln-3.3  SDRLKLILPMIHLMIPLAIVYVGEYMINQGMTQQIVFDCAHGFNL----- 287
Baker's       QTVKRLRRLVFPYMVPLTTVYLFEYLINQAVAPTLLFPINGDERSKSMPF 269
Fission       QTFIFMQPYLLSHMFPQFLVYFSEYTINIGVAPTLLFP---PEKAG---- 259
                       ll    Pl  VY  EY INqg      F
```

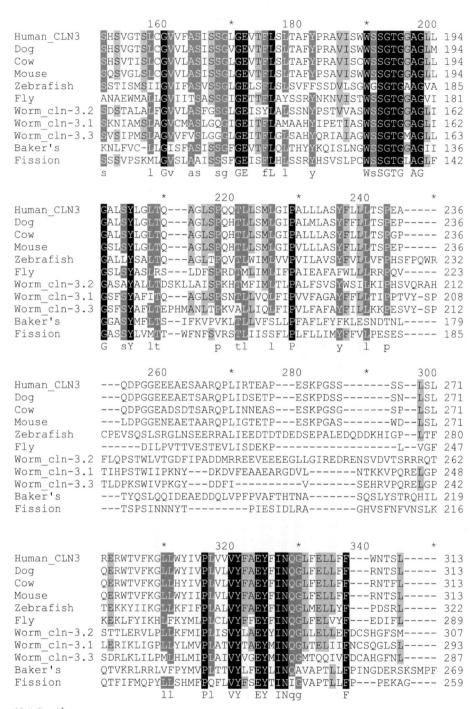

Figure 19.4 Cont'd

```
                         360         *         380         *         400
Human_CLN3     ---SHAQQYRWYQMLYQAGVFASRSSLRCCRIR--FTWALALLQCLNLVF 358
Dog            ---NHAQQYRWYQMLYQAGVFVSRSSLHCCRIR--FTWVLALLQCLNLAF 358
Cow            ---THAEQYRWYQMLYQAGVFASRSSLRCCRIR--HTWVLALLQCLNLAF 358
Mouse          ---SHAQQYRWYQMLYQAGVFASRSSLQCCRIR--FTWVLALLQCLNLAL 358
Zebrafish      ---SHAEQYRWYQTVYQIGVFVSRTSLFCFKIR--KIFLMSLLQCANAVL 367
Fly            ---DKDSQYRWLNVDYQIGVFISRSSVNLFQLD--KIWLMSIFQFVNVVY 334
Worm_cln-3.2   ---SSESQYRWFQVTYQLGVFISRSSSNYVTIPTQYLKSLAVLQIFNAGF 354
Worm_cln-3.1   ---PLSSQYRWYQVLYQLGVFISRSSVKFFEMPLWLIWCLPILQCVNMIF 340
Worm_cln-3.3   ---SLHSQYRWYQVLYQFGVFVSRSSIRLVELPMWMLYLLPFLQLTNMLF 334
Baker's        FFHKYRDIYVTYGTLYQLGVFISRSFGHLMRMR--SLYILAFLQGVNLCI 317
Fission        -FSSFRDFYPTYQTVYQIGVFLSRSSISFFTVP--YLRTLAITQFIILLF 306
                       qYrwyq  YQ GVF SRss              l  lQ  n

                         *         420         *         440         *
Human_CLN3     LLADVWFGFLPSIYLVFLIILYEGLLGGAAYVNTFHNIALETSDEHREFA 408
Dog            LLVDVWFSFLPSIYLVFLIILYEGLLGGAAYVNTFHNIALETSDQHREFA 408
Cow            LLVDVWLSYLPSIYLVFLIIMFEGLLGGAAYVNTFHNIALETSDEHREFA 408
Mouse          LLADVCLNFLPSIYLIFIIILYEGLLGGAAYVNTFHNIALETSDKHREFA 408
Zebrafish      LVFAVYYQFLPNISVVFVIIAFEGLLGGAAYVNTFFFIREESVEREREFA 417
Fly            FLTEVIWWYTPSIWIVFAIVLWEGLLGGGAYVNTFYRMSKEISPERQQFA 384
Worm_cln-3.2   FTITAIYSFLPHILIAFLVILFEGLLGGASYVNTFRAVHKEIPADSREFS 404
Worm_cln-3.1   FFFEAVYWFTPTIIIIFVLIVFEGLLGGSAYVNTYNKIHKKVNPDVREYS 390
Worm_cln-3.3   FFFDALYWFVPQIAIIFALIIFEGLFGGSSYVNTFHKIHNKVEPDVREYC 384
Baker's        TVLQSWFYVTHSPWAVMILIFYEGFLGGASYVNTFLNILEQEDPDETEFA 367
Fission        TILQSALYLTSSYHFVLFLIFVEGLIGGTVYVNVY-HSLQTTESSQRELA 355
                               p i   f  i  EGllGG  YVNtf           re

                         460         *         480         *
Human_CLN3     MAATCISDTLGISLSGLLALPLHDFLCQLS------------ 438
Dog            MAAACISDTLGISLSGLLALPLHDFLCHLS------------ 438
Cow            MATACISDTLGISLSGLLALPLHDFLCQLS------------ 438
Mouse          MEAACISDTLGISLSGVLALPLHDFLCHLP------------ 438
Zebrafish      MATATVGDSLGIAFSAAAAFPVHHYFCSL------------- 446
Fly            MAMVVQSDSYGIALAGFLAIPVHNAICGLPAAARSLVW---- 422
Worm_cln-3.2   MGVVSISDTIGIVFAGFLAMPVHNRICSMPM----------- 435
Worm_cln-3.1   LSAASMGNSLGTNIAAFLSIPLYNWVCTMKAPGR-------- 424
Worm_cln-3.3   LSAASMGDSIGVNFAAGVSIPLHYWMCDQPARL--------- 417
Baker's        MGAVSIADSFGVFLAALLGLGLEPKLCRHQIA-DDRPWCRME 408
Fission        ISTVGSSDSSGIFLASLVSLFLEPSLCHFQAD-RGRDWCALT 396
                      d G          p     C
```

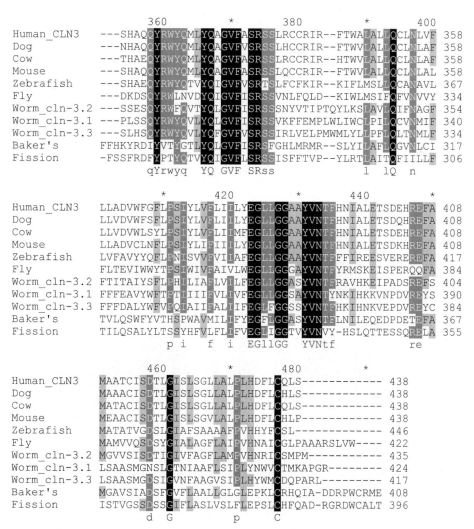

Figure 19.4 Cont'd

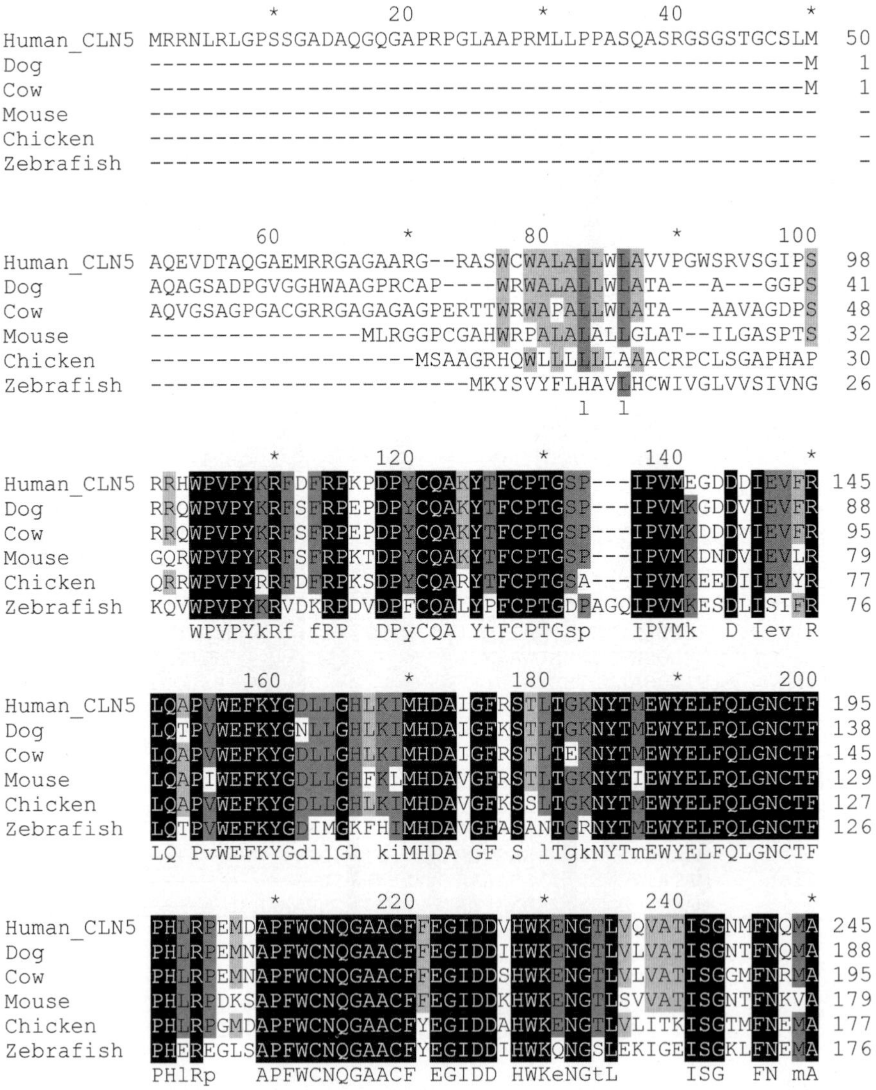

Figure 19.5 Alignment of CLN5 proteins. The CLN5 protein sequences from human (GenBank accession number NP_006484.1), dog (NP_001011556.1), cow (NP_001039764.1), mouse (NP_001028414.1), chicken (XP_417005.2), and zebrafish (XP_697882.1) were aligned using Multalin.

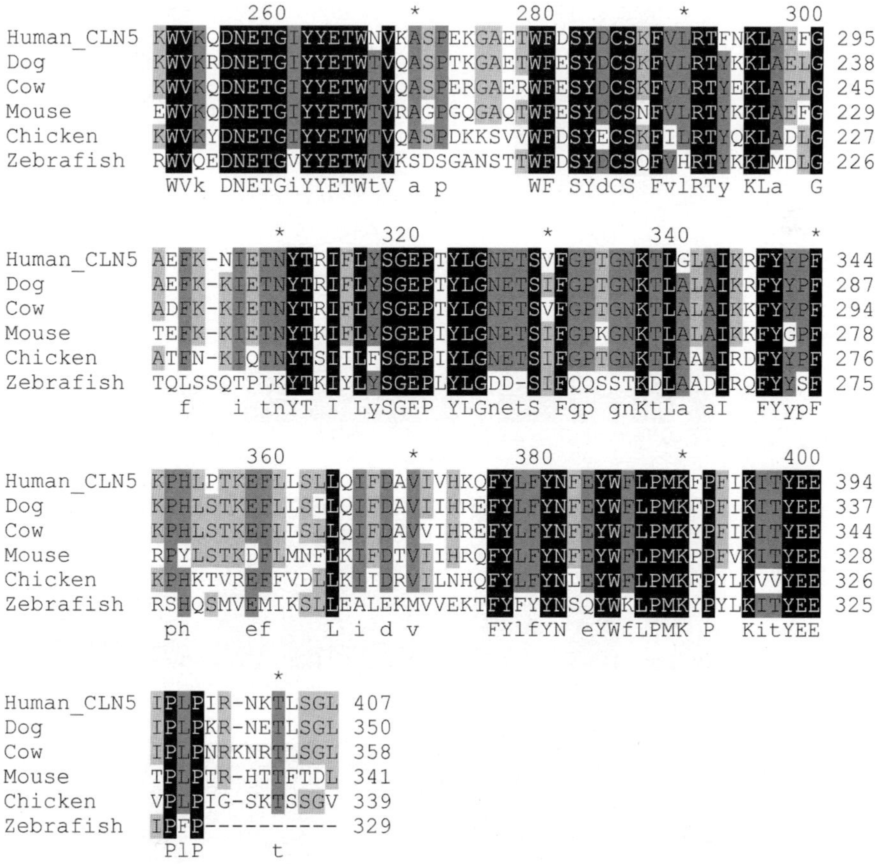
260 * 280 * 300
Human_CLN5 KWVKQDNETGIYYETWNVKASPEKGAETWFDSYDCSKFVLRTFNKLAEFG 295
Dog KWVKRDNETGIYYETWTVQASPTKGAETWFESYDCSKFVLRTYKKLAELG 238
Cow KWVKQDNETGIYYETWTVQASPERGAERWFESYDCSKFVLRTYEKLAELG 245
Mouse EWVKQDNETGIYYETWTVRAGPGQGAQTWFESYDCSNFVLRTYKKLAEFG 229
Chicken KWVKYDNETGIYYETWTVQASPDKKSVVWFDSYECSKFILRTYQKLADLG 227
Zebrafish RWVQEDNETGVYYETWTVKSDSGANSTTWFDSYDCSQFVHRTYKKLMDLG 226
WVk DNETGiYYETWtV a p WF SYdCS FvlRTy KLa G
* 320 * 340 *
Human_CLN5 AEFK-NIETNYTRIFLYSGEPTYLGNETSVFGPTGNKTLGLAIKRFYYPF 344
Dog AEFK-KIETNYTRIFLYSGEPTYLGNETSIFGPTGNKTLALAIKRFYYPF 287
Cow ADFK-KIETNYTRIFLYSGEPTYLGNETSVFGPTGNKTLALAIKKFYYPF 294
Mouse TEFK-KIETNYTKIFLYSGEPIYLGNETSIFGPKGNKTLALAIKKFYGPF 278
Chicken ATFN-KIQTNYTSIILFSGEPIYLGNETSIFGPTGNKTLAAAIRDFYYPF 276
Zebrafish TQLSSQTPLKYTKIYLYSGEPLYLGDD-SIFQQSSTKDLAADIRQFYYSF 275
f i tnYT I LySGEP YLGnetS Fgp gnKtLa aI FYypF
360 * 380 * 400
Human_CLN5 KPHLPTKEFLLSLLQIFDAVIVHKQFYLFYNFEYWFLPMKFPFIKITYEE 394
Dog KPHLSTKEFLLSILQIFDAVIIHREFYLFYNFEYWFLPMKFPFIKITYEE 337
Cow KPHLSTKEFLLSLLQIFDAVVIHREFYLFYNFEYWFLPMKYPFIKITYEE 344
Mouse RPYLSTKDFLMNFLKIFDTVIIHRQFYLFYNFEYWFLPMKPPFVKITYEE 328
Chicken KPHKTVREFFVDLLKIIDRVILNHQFYLFYNLEYWFLPMKFPYLKVVYEE 326
Zebrafish RSHQSMVEMIKSLLEALEKMVVEKTFYFYYNSQYWKLPMKYPYLKITYEE 325
ph ef L i d v FYlfYN eYWfLPMK P KitYEE
*
Human_CLN5 IPLPIR-NKTLSGL 407
Dog IPLPKR-NETLSGL 350
Cow IPLPNRKNRTLSGL 358
Mouse TPLPTR-HTTFTDL 341
Chicken VPLPIG-SKTSSGV 339
Zebrafish IPFP---------- 329
PlP t

Figure 19.5 Cont'd

```
                    *        20          *        40          *
Human_CLN6  -MEATRRRQHLGATGGPGAQLGASFLQARHGSVSADEAARTAPFHLDLWF  49
Dog         MEAAARRRQHPGAAGGAGAQPGASFLQARHSSGKADEAVGTAPFHLDLWF  50
Cow         MEAAARRR-HPGAAGGPGAQPGASFLQARHSSVKADEAAGTAPFHLDLWF  49
Sheep       MEAAARRR-HPGAAGGSGAQPGASFLQARHSSVKADEAAGTAPFHLDLWF  49
Mouse       MEAATRRRQLLGAAGG----PGVAFVQARHGSVKAEDKDRTAPFHLDLWF  46
Chicken     MQGSARRRPFPAAAPGS-PQPSGPLYAGRHGAAKNEDTSKTSPFHLDLWF  49
Zebrafish   ----MRRRPQSATF-------TSAFLRAGSEKTTAAATTR-SQFHTDLWL  38
                 RRR    a  g        f  arh    a     t pFHlDLWf

                   60          *        80          *       100
Human_CLN6  YFTLQNWVLDFGRPIAMLVFPLEWFPLNKPSVGDYFHMAYNVITPFLLLK  99
Dog         YFTLQNWVLDFGRPIAMLVFPLEWFPLNKPSVGDYFHMAYNIITPFLLLK 100
Cow         YFTLQNWVLDFGRPIAMLVFPLEWFPLNKPSVGDYFHMAYNIITPFLLLQ  99
Sheep       YFTLQNWVLDFGRPIAMLVFPLEWFPLNKPSVGDYFHMAYNIITPFLLLK  99
Mouse       YFTLQNWVLDFGRPIAMLVFPIQWFPLNKPSVGDYFHMTYNIITPFLLLK  96
Chicken     YFTLQNWVLDFGRPIAMIILPLEWFPLNKPSAGDYFPMAYNVITPFLLLK  99
Zebrafish   CFTVQNWILDFGRPIAMIIMPLEWFPLNKPSVGDYFHMAYNVITPFLLLK  88
            yFTlQNWvLDFGRPIAM    PleWFPLNKPSvGDYFhMaYN ITPFLLLk

                    *       120          *       140          *
Human_CLN6  LIERSPRTLPRSITYVSIIIFIMGASIHLVGDSVNHRLLFSGYQHHLSVR 149
Dog         LIERSPRTLPRSVIYVSIITFVMGASIHLVGDSVNHRLLFSGYQHHLSVR 150
Cow         LIERCPRTLPRSLIYVSIITFIMGASIHLVGDSVNHRLIFSGYQNHLSVR 149
Sheep       LIERCPRTLPRSLIYVSIITFIMGASIHLVGDSVNHRLIFSGYQNHLSVR 149
Mouse       LIERSPRTLPRSIVYVSIITFIMGASIHLVGDSVNHRLLFSGYQHHLSVR 146
Chicken     LIERSPKTLPRSMVYVSIITFVMGASIHLVGDSVNHRLIFSGYQHHLSVR 149
Zebrafish   LIERSPTALPRSAVYLSIITFVMGASIHLVGDSINHRLILSGYQLHLSVR 138
            LIER P tLPRS  YvSIItF MGASIHLVGDSvNHRL fSGYQ HLSVR

                  160          *       180          *       200
Human_CLN6  ENPIIKNLKPETLIDSFELLYYYDEYLGHCMWYIPFFLILFMYFSGCFTA 199
Dog         ENPIIKNLSPETLIDSFELLYYYDEYLGHCMWYVPFFLILFIYFSGCFTP 200
Cow         ENPIIKNLKPETLIDSFELLYYYDEYLGHSMWYIPFFLILFMYFSSCFTP 199
Sheep       ENPIIKNLKPETLIDSFELLYYYDEYLGHSMWYIPFFLILFMYFSGCFTP 199
Mouse       ENPIIKNLKPETLIDSFELLYYYDEYLGHCMWYIPFFLILFMYFSGCFTT 196
Chicken     ENPIIRNLKPETLIDSFELLYYYDEYLGHSMWYIPFFLILFIYFTGCFTP 199
Zebrafish   ENPIIKDLKPASLIDSFELLYYYDEHLGHSMWYIPFFLIIFLYFTGCFTQ 188
            ENPIIknLkPetLIDSFELLYYYDEyLGH MWYiPFFLIlF YF gCFT
```

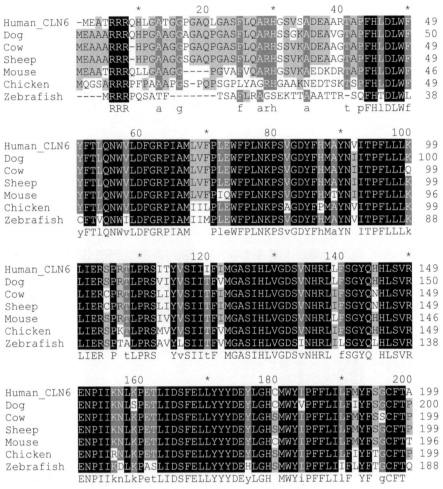

Figure 19.6 Alignment of CLN6 proteins. The CLN6 protein sequences from human (GenBank accession number NP_060352.1), dog (NP_001011888.1), cow (NP_001103454.1), mouse (NP_001028347.1), chicken (XP_413928.2), and zebrafish (NP_001005982.1) were aligned using Multalin.

```
                     *         220          *          240         *
Human_CLN6 SKAESLIPGPALLLVAPSGLYYWYLVTEGQIFILFIFTFFAMLALVLHQK 249
Dog        TKAESSMPGAALLLAMPSGLYYWYLVTEGQIFILFIFTFFAMLALVLHQK 250
Cow        TKAESSMPGAALLLVVPSGLYYWYLVTEGQIFILFIFTSFAMLALVLHQK 249
Sheep      TKAESSMPGAALLLVVPSGLYYWYLVTEGQIFILFIFTSFAMLALVLHQK 249
Mouse      CKAESHMPGPALLLVVPSGLYYWYLVTEGQIFILFIFTFFAMLALVLHQK 246
Chicken    DEDESRMPMSALLLTGPSSLYYWYLVTEGQIFILYIFTFFAMMALVMHQK 249
Zebrafish  VKDEK-MSTSGWLLLGPSAVYYWYLITEGQIFVLYVFTFFAMVATVMRQR 237
            k Es mp  alLL  PS lYYWYLvTEGQIFiL iFT FAM AlV hQk

                   260         *          280         *         300
Human_CLN6 RKRLFLDSNGLFLFSSFALTLLLVALWVAWLWNDPVLRKKYPGVIYVPEP 299
Dog        RKRLFLDSNGLFLFYSFALTLLLVALWVAWLWNDPVLRKKYPGVIYVPEP 300
Cow        RKRLFLDSNGLFLFYSFALTLLLVALWVAWLWNDPVLRKKYPGVIYVPEP 299
Sheep      RKRLFLDSNGLFLFYSFALALLLVALWVAWLWNDPVLRKKYPGVIYVPEP 299
Mouse      RRRLFLDSNGLFLLYSFALTLSLVALWVAWLWNDPVLRKKYPGVIYVPEP 296
Chicken    RKGLVLDSNGLFLFYSFIITLVLIAVWVVWLWNDKTLRKKYPGVIYIPEP 299
Zebrafish  RMGFVLDSNGRFLFYNFIITLGLVLVWVAYLWNDKVLRKKYPGIIYVPEP 287
           R  l LDSNGlFLfysF  tL Lva WVawLWND vLRKKYPGvIYvPEP

                     *
Human_CLN6 WAFYTLHVSSRH------ 311
Dog        WAFYTLHVSSRP------ 312
Cow        WAFYTLHVSSQH------ 311
Sheep      WAFYTLHVSSQ------- 310
Mouse      WAFYTLHVSSQQ------ 308
Chicken    WAFYTLHMSNLHAAKEGL 317
Zebrafish  WSFYTLHIKGS------- 298
           WaFYTLH s
```

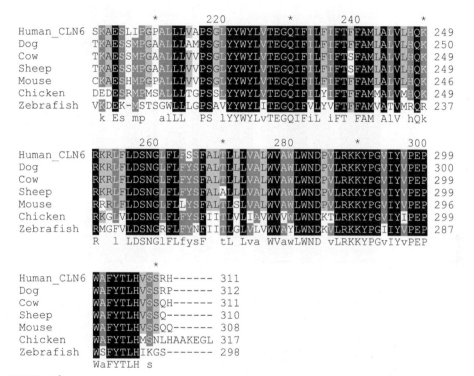

Figure 19.6 Cont'd

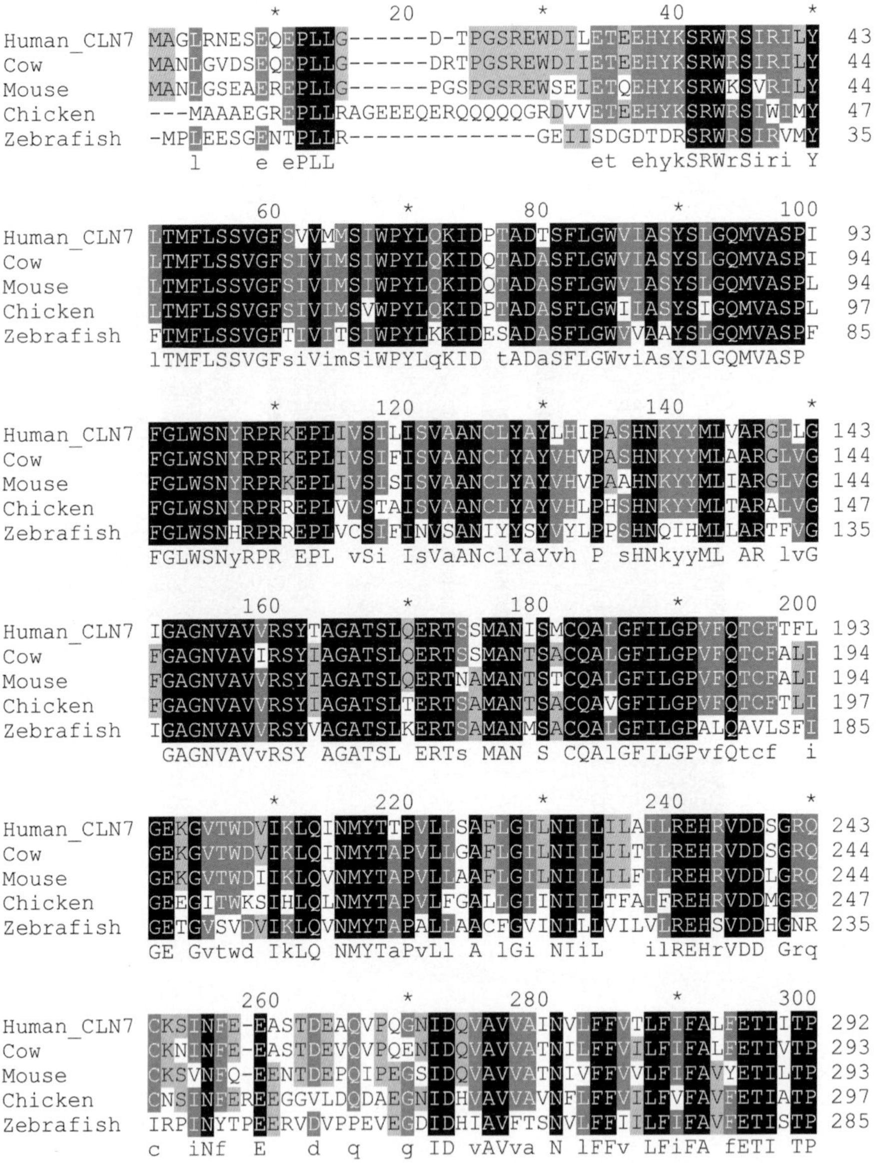

Figure 19.7 Alignment of CLN7 proteins. The CLN7 protein sequences from human (GenBank accession number NP_689991.1), cow (XP_594055.2), mouse (NP_082416.2), chicken (XP_420463.1), and zebrafish (NP_001038513.1), were aligned using Multalin. Due to lack of homology of the 70 N-terminal amino acids of the predicted chicken protein, only the sequence from the second methionine at position 71 has been included in the alignment.

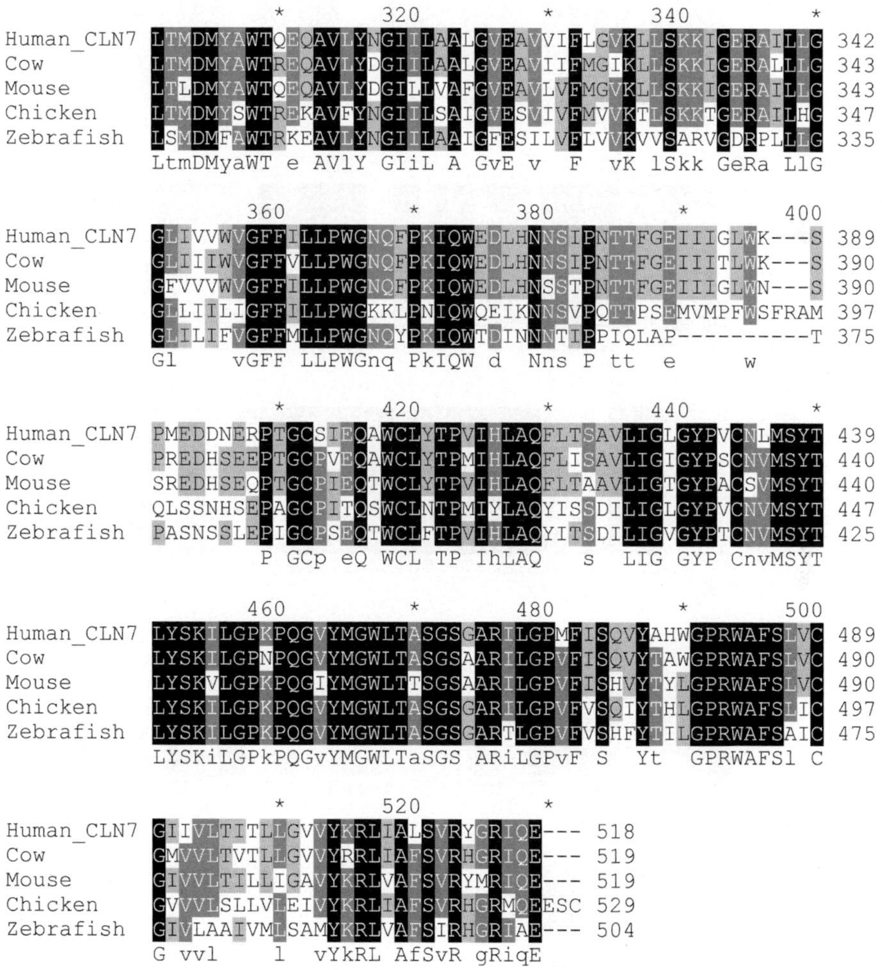
* 320 * 340 *
Human_CLN7 LTMDMYAWTQEQAVLYNGIILAALGVEAVVIFLGVKLLSKKIGERAILLG 342
Cow LTMDMYAWTREQAVLYDGIILAALGVEAVIIFMGIKLLSKKIGERALLIG 343
Mouse LTLDMYAWTQEQAVLYDGILLVAFGVEAVLVFMGVKLLSKKIGERAILLG 343
Chicken LTMDMYSWTREKAVFYNGIILSAIGVESVIVFMVVKTLSKKTGERAILHG 347
Zebrafish LSMDMFAWTRKEAVLYNGIILAAIGFESILVFLVVKVVSARVGDRPLLIG 335
LtmDMyaWT e AVlY GIiL A GvE v F vK lSkk GeRa LlG
360 * 380 * 400
Human_CLN7 GLIVVWVGFFILLPWGNQFPKIQWEDLHNNSIPNTTFGEIIIGLWK---S 389
Cow GLIIIWVGFFVLLPWGNQFPKIQWEDLHNNSIPNTTFGEIIITLWK---S 390
Mouse GFVVVWVGFFILLPWGNQFPKIQWEDLHNSSTPNTTFGEIIIGLWN---S 390
Chicken GLLIILIGFFILLPWGKKLPNIQWQEIKNNSVPQTTPSEMVMPFWSFRAM 397
Zebrafish GLILIFVGFFMLLPWGNQYPKIQWTDINNNTIPPIQLAP----------T 375
Gl vGFF LLPWGnq PkIQW d Nns P tt e w
* 420 * 440 *
Human_CLN7 PMEDDNERPTGCSIEQAWCLYTPVIHLAQFLTSAVLIGLGYPVCNLMSYT 439
Cow PREDHSEEPTGCPVEQAWCLYTPMIHLAQFLISAVLIGIGYPSCNVMSYT 440
Mouse SREDHSEQPTGCPIEQTWCLYTPVIHLAQFLTAAVLIGTGYPACSVMSYT 440
Chicken QLSSNHSEPAGCPITQSWCLNTPMIYLAQYISSDILIGLGYPVCNVMSYT 447
Zebrafish PASNSSLEPIGCPSEQTWCLFTPVIHLAQYITSDILIGVGYPTCNVMSYT 425
P GCp eQ WCL TP IhLAQ s LIG GYP CnvMSYT
460 * 480 * 500
Human_CLN7 LYSKILGPKPQGVYMGWLTASGSGARILGPMFISQVYAHWGPRWAFSLVC 489
Cow LYSKILGPNPQGVYMGWLTASGSAARILGPVFISQVYTAWGPRWAFSLVC 490
Mouse LYSKVLGPKPQGIYMGWLTTSGSAARILGPVFISHVYTYLGPRWAFSLVC 490
Chicken LYSKILGPKPQGVYMGWLTASGSGARILGPVFVSQIYTHLGPRWAFSLIC 497
Zebrafish LYSKILGPKPQGVYMGWLTASGSGARTLGPVFVSHFYTILGPRWAFSAIC 475
LYSKiLGPkPQGvYMGWLTaSGS ARiLGPvF S Yt GPRWAFSl C
* 520 *
Human_CLN7 GIIVLTITLLGVVYKRLIALSVRYGRIQE--- 518
Cow GMVVLTVTLLGVVYRRLIAFSVRHGRIQE--- 519
Mouse GIVVLTILLIGAVYKRLVAFSVRYMRIQE--- 519
Chicken GVVVLSLLVLEIVYKRLIAFSVRHGRMQEESC 529
Zebrafish GIVLAAIVMLSAMYKRLVAFSIRHGRIAE--- 504
G vvl l vYkRL AfSvR gRiqE

Figure 19.7 Cont'd

```
                  *        20         *        40         *
Human_CLN8 MNPASDGGTSESIFDLDYASWGIRSTLMVAGFVFYLGVFVVCHQLSSSLN  50
Dog        MTPMSDGGTSESIFDLDYTSWKIRSTLAVAGFVFYLGVFVVCHQLSSSLN  50
Mouse      MTPVSSHGLAESIFDLDYASWKIRSTLAVAGFVFYLGVFVVCHQLSSSLN  50
Cow        -----MSLLGAGALDLDYTSGRVRGVLVAAGCAFYLGVFVVCHRLSSSLN  45
Chicken    MNPANSNQVFGTIFDWDYLLWEVRLTFIAAGFLIYLGVFLLSHWLSSRMS  50
Zebrafish  ---------------MDYTSLDIQLKITGLGFIFYTFIFFLCHVLSTLLF  35
                          d DY s   r     aGf fYlgvF   cH LSs l

                    60         *        80         *       100
Human_CLN8 ATYRSLVAREKVFWDLAATRAVFGVQSTAAGLWALLGDPVLHADKARGQQ 100
Dog        ATYRSLVAREKVFWNLAATRAVFGVQSTAAGLWALLVDPVLHADKARGQQ 100
Mouse      ATYRSLAAKEKVFWNLAATRAVFGVQSTTAGLWALLGDPVLYADKALGQQ 100
Cow        ATYRSLAAREQVFWNLAATRAVFGIQGTAAGLWALLLDPVLQADKALGQQ  95
Chicken    TTYRALYAKEKVFWNMAVTRGAFGLQSCVAGLWALLIDPVFHADKVYSQQ 100
Zebrafish  QTYRSLSAKEKVFWDLAATRAVFGIQGIVAGLRALMEESVLFSDKILGQE  85
            TYRsL A EkVFW lAaTRavFG Q   AGLwALl dpVl aDK  gQq

                  *       120         *       140         *
Human_CLN8 NWCWFHITTATGFFCFENVAVHLSNLIFRTFDLFLVIHHLFAFLGFLGCL 150
Dog        NWCWFHIATATGFFFFENVAVHLSNVLFRTFDLFLAIHHLFAFLGFLGSV 150
Mouse      NWCWFHITTATGFFFFENVAVHLSNLFFRTFDLFLVVHHLFAFLGFLGSA 150
Cow        DWCWFHITTATGFFFFENLALHVSNALFHTFDGFLAVHHLFAFLGFLGSS 145
Chicken    KWSWFNCLIAAGFFLLENVAVHVSNIVFRTFDVFLGGSSLTCFWWLGWSS 150
Zebrafish  DWSWFNILTSTGFFLFENMALHMSNVVFRSFDLPLAVHHFFALAGFAGAV 135
            W WF i tatGFF fEN A H SN  FrtFD fL  hhlfaf gf g

                   160         *       180         *       200
Human_CLN8 VNLQAGHYLAMTTLLLEMSTPFTCVSWMLLKAGWSESLFWKLNQWLMIHM 200
Dog        VNLGAGHYLAMSTLLLEASTPFTCISWMLLKAGWSESLFWKLNQWLMIHM 200
Mouse      INLRAGHYLAMTTLLLEMSTPFTCISWMLLKAGWSDSLFWKANQWLMIHM 200
Cow        VNLQAGHYLPMVTLLLEMSTPFTCISWMLLKAGCANSRLWRLNQWAMVHL 195
Chicken    NQVKSGHYLPLMGMLLEMSTPATCISWMLLKAGCANTFFWKANQWVMIHL 200
Zebrafish  VWNWQGHFLPMVTLLLEMSTPFTCISWMLLKAGWSKTVFWKVNQWMMIHM 185
                GHyL  m tlLLEmSTPfTCiSWMLLKAG     fWk NQW MiH

                  *       220         *       240         *
Human_CLN8 FHCRMVLTYHMWWVCFWHWDGLVSSLYLPHLTLFLVGLALLTLIINPYWT 250
Dog        FHCRMVLTYHMWWVCFWHWDGLVSSLYLPHLALFLVGLGLLTLVINPYWT 250
Mouse      FHCRMILTYHMWWVCFCHWDALTSSLHLPHWALFLFGLALLTAVINPYWT 250
Cow        FHCRMVLTYHMWWVCLGHWAGLARSLFPPHLALFVVGLALLTLLINPYWT 245
Chicken    FHCRMILTYHMWWVCIFNWNSVVENLGLLHFIVLFSGLFAFTLILNPYWT 250
Zebrafish  FHCRMVVSYYMWWVCLNHWEEMNTHIPLPQRLLFFTGLFLLTFFLNPIWT 235
           FHCRM ltYhMWWVC  hW      l lph  lf  GL llT    NPyWT

                   260         *       280
Human_CLN8 HKKTQQLLNPVDWNFAQPEAKS-RPEG-NGQLLRKKRP- 286
Dog        HKKTQQLLNPVDWNFAQPAPRSSRPAGANGQVPQKKGQ- 288
Mouse      HKKTQQLLHPVDWNFAQEEAKGSRQERTNGQVPRKKRL- 288
Cow        RKKTQQLLNPVDWNFAPGTPNGPAQPKKAR--------- 275
Chicken    YKKTQQLLSPTDWNF---ENKATENGKLNGETSQKKRM- 285
Zebrafish  HKKTLQLLNPVDWNF--HNQSPPENGPLQEQTQQKPHAS 272
            KKTqQLL PvDWNF                   k
```

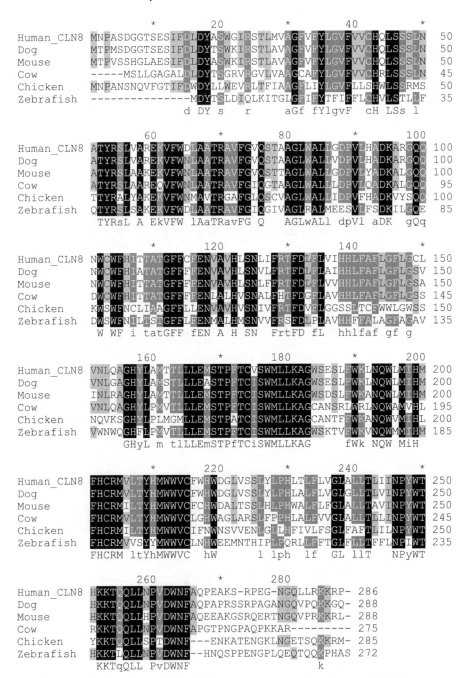

Figure 19.8 Alignment of CLN8 proteins. The CLN8 protein sequences from human (GenBank accession number NP_061764.2), dog (NP_001012343.1), cow (NP_001069409.1), mouse (NP_036130.1), chicken (NP_001026258.1), and zebrafish (NP_001108060.1) were aligned using Multalin.

start at the methionines at positions 50 and 62, respectively. The role of the different human isoforms, if expressed, remains to be established. All vertebrates have protein homologues to MFSD8/CLN7, which belongs to the major facilitator superfamily of transporter proteins (Figure 19.7). More distant homologues to the superfamily are also found in invertebrates. The MFSD8 protein has 15 counterparts in the worm, but the best reciprocal BLAST hit suggests highest homology with the protein encoded by worm gene Y53G8AR.7a, closely followed by ZK550.2 as second best. Which of the invertebrate proteins is the functional equivalent of the human protein still has to be determined.

REFERENCES

Altschul SF, Gish W, Miller W, Myers EW, & Lipman DJ (1990) Basic local alignment search tool. *J Mol Biol*, 215, 403–410.

Cho SK & Hofmann SL (2004) pdf1, a palmitoyl protein thioesterase 1 Ortholog in Schizosaccharomyces pombe: a yeast model of infantile Batten disease. *Eukaryot Cell*, 3, 302–310.

Corpet F (1988) Multiple sequence alignment with hierarchical clustering. *Nucleic Acids Res*, 16, 10881–10890.

de Voer G, der Bent P, Rodrigues AJ, van Ommen GJ, Peters DJ, & Taschner PE (2005) Deletion of the Caenorhabditis elegans homologues of the CLN3 gene, involved in human juvenile neuronal ceroid lipofuscinosis, causes a mild progeric phenotype. *J Inherit Metab Dis*, 28, 1065–1080.

Nicholas KB, Nicholas HB, Jr, & Deerfield DW, II (1997) GeneDoc: analysis and visualization of genetic variation. *EMBNEW NEWS*, 4, 14.

Pal C, Papp B, & Lercher MJ (2006) An integrated view of protein evolution. *Nat Rev Genet*, 7, 337–348.

Vesa J, Chin MH, Oelgeschlager K, Isosomppi J, DellAngelica EC, Jalanko A, & Peltonen L (2002) Neuronal ceroid lipofuscinoses are connected at molecular level: interaction of CLN5 protein with CLN2 and CLN3. *Mol Biol Cell*, 13, 2410–2420.

Chapter 20

Mutations in NCL Genes

S.E. Mole

SUMMARY

SUMMARY

Mutations in ten genes have now been reported in NCL disease (Table 20.1) although there are many families in which the underlying genetic cause has not been defined. Mutations in other genes cause NCL-like disease in animals, and these will continue to suggest candidate genes that can be assessed in such NCL families.

All NCL genes so far identified lie on autosomes and in most cases disease is inherited in a recessive manner, being caused by mutations in both disease gene alleles. Notable exceptions are dominant inheritance for adult onset NCL but in these, as well as most other cases of adult onset NCL the underlying genes(s) have not yet been identified. One patient had complete isodisomy of chromosome 8, leading to homozygosity of a maternally-inherited deletion in *CLN8* (Vantaggiato et al., 2009). This is the first description of uniparental disomy in the NCLs. Two patients have been reported carrying single mutations in the *CLCN6* gene that underlies NCL-like disease in mice. One of these patients was later found to be heterozygous for mutations in *CLN5*. Since the carrier parents did not have the same disease phenotype, this may be the first example in the NCLs of a mutation or specific allele of one gene contributing to or ameliorating the disease phenotype.

For all except one NCL gene there is a known typical disease phenotype associated with complete loss of function. The exception is *CLN3*, where the most common mutation in the *CLN3* gene does not cause total loss of CLN3 function, leading to the hypothesis that disease caused by complete loss of function has not been recognized or is lethal, and that disease associated with mutations in this gene could have a much wider phenotype than currently known (Kitzmüller et al., 2008).

All known mutations and polymorphisms in NCL genes are listed in the NCL Mutation Database (http://www.ucl.ac.uk/ncl) and details of the correlations between genotype, phenotype, and morphological changes in patients can be found in the relevant sections of individual chapters and recent reviews (Mole et al., 2005). More than 260 mutations that cause NCL are currently known. The NCLs exemplify both phenotypic convergence or mimicry, where a similar disease can be caused by mutations in several genes (e.g. late infantile variant NCL—*CLN5*, *CLN6*, *CLN7*, *CLN8*) and also phenotypic divergence, where mutations in a single gene can give rise to different diseases (e.g. *CLN8*—late infantile variant, and EPMR; *SGSH*—ANCL and MPSIIIA (Sleat et al., 2009)). Included in Table 20.1 is *CLCN7*, which causes disease that has similarities to NCL in mice, but in humans is only known to

Table 20.1 **NCL gene mutations and their correlation with phenotype**

Gene	No. mutations	No. polymorphisms	Widespread common mutations	Country-specific mutations	Disease variation*
CTSD/ CLN10	4	0	Not known	Not known	**Congenital**–Late infantile– Adult
CLN1	51	5	p.Arg122Trp p.Arg151X	p.Thr75Pro and p.Leu10X in Scotland	**Infantile**–Late infantile–Juvenile–Adult
CLN2	68	24	c.509-1G>C (p.Val170fs) p.Arg208X	p.Glu284Val in Canada	**Classic late infantile**–Juvenile–Protracted
CLN3	42	5	1kb intragenic deletion in Caucasian populations	1kb deletion in many countries 2.8kb intragenic deletion in Finland	Juvenile–Protracted
CLN5	21	1	None	p.Tyr392X and p.Trp75X in Finland	**Late infantile**–Juvenile–Protracted–Adult
CLN6	41	1	None	p.Ile154del in Portugal	**Late infantile variant**
CLN7	22	2	None	P.Thr294Lys in Roma Gypsies; c.724+2T>A in Eastern Europe	**Late infantile variant-Juvenile/Adult**
CLN8	13	2	None	p.Arg24Gly in Finland causing EPMR p.Arg204Cys and pTrp263Cys in Turkey	**Late infantile variant**–Protracted; EPMR/Northern epilepsy
SGSH	2^	–	N/A	N/A	Adult and MPSIIIA
CLCN6	2[a]	3	Not known	Not known	*Teenage–Adult*[a]
CLCN7	0^^	–	N/A	N/A	**Infantile malignant osteopetrosis**

* bold = phenotype caused by complete loss of gene function.
^ only the mutations that cause NCL are indicated; other mutations cause MPSIIIA.
^^ no mutations have yet been described that cause NCL-like disease in humans.
[a]these mutations in *CLCN6* may modify disease phenotype.

cause the severe autosomal recessive disease infantile malignant osteopetrosis. Since patients develop blindness and central nervous system degeneration even when the osteopetrosis is treated with bone marrow transplantation, specific mutations or alleles in this gene may also cause NCL-like disease or modify that caused by mutations in other genes, as suggested for *CLCN6*.

This chapter serves to summarize mutation data in a readily accessible and useful format. Further details can be found in the chapters describing each gene in more detail.

REFERENCES

Kitzmüller C, Haines RL, Codlin S, Cutler DF, & Mole SE (2008) A function retained by the common mutant CLN3 protein is responsible for the late onset of juvenile neuronal ceroid lipofuscinosis. *Hum Mol Genet*, 17, 303–312.

Mole SE, Williams RE, & Goebel HH (2005) Correlations between genotype, ultrastructural morphology and clinical phenotype in the neuronal ceroid lipofuscinoses. *Neurogenetics*, 6, 107–126.

Sleat DE, Ding L, Wang S, Zhao C, Wang Y, Xin W, Zheng H, Moore DF, Sims KB, & Lobel P (2009) Mass spectrometry-based protein profiling to determine the cause of lysosomal storage diseases of unknown etiology. *Mol Cell Proteomics*, 8, 1708–1718.

Vantaggiato C, Redaelli F, Falcone S, Perrotta C, Tonelli A, Bondioni S, Morbin M, Riva D, Saletti V, Bonaglia MC, Giorda R, Bresolin N, Clementi E, & Bassi MT (2009) A novel CLN8 mutation in late-infantile-onset neuronal ceroid lipofuscinosis (LINCL) reveals aspects of CLN8 neurobiological function. *Hum Mutat*, 30, 1104–1116.

Chapter 21

Therapeutic Strategies

M. Chang, J.D. Cooper, B.L. Davidson, and S.E. Mole

INTRODUCTION

Patients with NCL suffer, and ultimately succumb to, symptoms related to central nervous system (CNS) dysfunction—cognitive decline, progressive visual loss, and motor deficits. Magnetic resonance imaging (MRI) indicates diffuse cerebral and cerebellar atrophy and as such, it is likely that effective therapies for NCL will need to be delivered widely within the CNS. Indeed, with neurological deficits that are not confined to a particular brain region, it is likely that a large percentage of the CNS volume must be treated. However, despite the apparently CNS-specific clinical symptoms in the NCLs, lysosomal storage is also observed in peripheral tissues. Why there should be no peripheral clinical symptoms is not clear, but it is conceivable that they would manifest should the CNS disease be treated and patient lifespan is extended. This is a possibility that researchers and clinicians must be mindful of, and combined targeting of the brain and body are likely to be necessary. Nevertheless, at present the CNS is the primary target for therapeutic strategies in the NCLs, with treating the brain representing a considerable challenge for providing effective therapies.

The first treatments likely to become available are those for NCLs caused by soluble enzyme deficiencies—CLN1/PPT1, CLN2/TPP1, and CTSD/CLN10, and CLN5 diseases are likely to fall into the same category. This chapter focuses largely on these NCLs. Aspects of these disorders are analogous to those of other lysosomal storage disorders caused by enzyme deficiencies. Accordingly, the candidate therapeutic strategies for enzyme deficient NCLs will largely parallel those investigated for these similar disorders. It can also be anticipated that targeted partial treatment, e.g. to prevent visual failure, would be welcome, particularly in CLN3 disease, juvenile but also CLN2 disease and others of late infantile onset, because of the improved quality of life that would result. The principles behind treating forms of NCLs caused by defects in transmembrane proteins, as typified by CLN3 disease, juvenile, are also addressed.

EXPERIMENTAL THERAPY

Introduction

Because what happens downstream of most NCL mutations is not well understood, therapeutic strategies are presently limited to methods that either replenish the missing gene activity or compensate for its function. Expression of the majority of NCL genes does not appear to be localized or enriched in any particular regions of the brain, so successful therapeutic interventions will probably require re-establishing enzyme activities in a large volume of the CNS. This goal may theoretically be achieved by a variety of methods including direct enzyme replacement, or its delivery via gene transfer or cell-based systems.

Enzyme replacement

Enzyme replacement is an obvious therapeutic strategy for metabolic disorders that result from a soluble enzyme deficiency. If decreased enzyme activity leads to disease, it is reasonable to suggest that adding back the enzyme could prevent, or perhaps even reverse, disease. Lysosomal proteases, including newly synthesized palmitoyl protein thioesterase 1 (PPT1), tripeptidyl peptidase I (TPP1), and cathepsin D (CTSD) receive numerous post-translational modifications as they traffic through the rough endoplasmic reticulum (RER) to the Golgi apparatus, and ultimately to the lysosomal compartment. In the RER, the enzymes receive N-linked oligosaccharide side chains, and in the Golgi, some of these oligosaccharide side chains acquire the mannose 6-phosphate (M6P) recognition marker. Enzymes acquiring these modifications are recognized by the mannose 6-phosphate/IGF-II receptor (M6PR) in the *trans*-Golgi network (TGN), which mediates the sorting of lysosomal enzymes either into the endosomal and lysosomal compartments, or into the secretory pathway, via which enzymes are secreted.

Importantly, M6P residues on lysosomal enzymes are also recognized by cell surface M6PRs which mediate the endocytosis and subsequent trafficking of enzymes that have been released to the extracellular space to the lysosomal compartment. This endogenous trafficking system can be exploited for therapeutic purposes, since exogenously applied enzyme, with the appropriate post-translational modifications, can be endocytosed and sorted correctly by diseased cells to the lysosome (Fratantoni et al., 1968). Production of recombinant human TPP1 has been achieved by overexpression in Chinese hamster ovary (CHO) cells, and enzymes produced in this manner can be endocytosed by cultured fibroblasts and cerebellar granule cells, largely via the M6PR. Importantly, recombinant TPP1 can reduce levels of subunit c when applied exogenously to cultured patient fibroblasts (Lin and Lobel, 2001). Although similar studies have not been done for PPT1 or CTSD, recombinant forms of these enzymes can likely be produced and purified in a similar manner, and upon exogenous application, be trafficked and processed appropriately to an active form. The identification of CLN5 as a soluble lysosomal protein that binds to M6PRs (Sleat et al., 2005) suggests that this form of NCL will also be amenable to therapeutic approaches that rely upon the secretion and uptake of this protein to cross-correct deficient neurons in the brain, but this is yet to be demonstrated.

Enzyme replacement studies specifically for CLN10, CLN1, and CLN2 disease patients have not been done, but studies for other metabolic disorders demonstrate its potential and limitations. In recent years, clinical trials have shown that intravenous administration of recombinant enzymes is beneficial for numerous lysosomal storage disorders that affect primarily peripheral tissues. In the non-neuronopathic form of Gaucher disease, intravenous administration of glucocerebrosidase led to decreased distention of the spleen and liver, improvement in haemoglobin and platelet counts, and improvements in skeletal deformities (Barton et al., 1990, Barton et al., 1991). Similar studies for Fabry disease, Pompe disease, and several of the mucopolysaccharidoses (MPSs), have demonstrated significant improvements in peripheral symptoms such as joint pain, joint mobility, organ enlargement, and muscle function (Amalfitano et al., 2001, Kakkis et al., 2001, Schiffmann et al., 2001, Harmatz et al., 2004, Wraith et al., 2004). However, to date, clinical enzyme replacement studies have not reported any benefit for those lysosomal storage disorders with CNS involvement. This is thought to be due to inefficient passage of enzymes across the blood brain–barrier (BBB). Under normal conditions, the BBB is impermeable to most macromolecules—only molecules that are small and lipophilic, or those that have specific transporters or receptors to mediate their entry (e.g. glucose and transferrin), can cross the barrier. The results from the above studies suggest that it is highly unlikely that systemic intravenous administration of recombinant NCL enzymes will have any therapeutic value for CNS disease. In an experimental setting, it is possible to transiently permeabilize the BBB with osmotic or other agents (e.g. mannitol, vascular endothelial growth factor), but this is not a viable option in a clinical setting where repeated enzyme administration is likely to be necessary due to the short half-life of most lysosomal enzymes.

An alternative strategy to deliver enzymes to the CNS is to bypass the BBB completely and deliver the desired enzymes directly to the brain parenchyma or ventricular space. Studies in non-human primates demonstrated that delivery of glucocerebrosidase directly into the brain is feasible. Furthermore, enzyme spread following direct injection can be significantly improved via a technique termed convection-enhanced delivery (Lonser et al., 2005). Studies in a canine model of MPS I demonstrated that delivery of enzyme via the cerebral spinal fluid is also feasible (Kakkis et al., 2004). Intrathecal delivery of human α-L-iduronidase resulted in CNS enzyme activity exceeding physiological levels, and reductions in brain and meningeal glycosaminoglycan levels, as well as histological improvements in lysosomal storage (Kakkis et al., 2004). These studies demonstrate that exogenous enzymes can be endocytosed and trafficked correctly to lysosomes, and suggest that intraparenchymal or intrathecal delivery of PPT1, TPP1, CTSD, or even CLN5, may have therapeutic value in the respective NCLs. This approach has recently been attempted in *TPP1*-deficient mice, with the intracerebroventricular delivery of TPP1 improving the resting tremor, reducing the levels of storage material and glial activation in these mice (Chang et al., 2008). Although these findings are promising, the issues of long-term enzyme delivery, and the associated problem of immunotolerance (see below), plus the logistics of enzyme delivery to a larger brain are yet to be overcome.

An important concern accompanying the administration of any exogenous protein to patients is the possibility of immune responses against the protein. These responses can range from benign generation of non-neutralizing antibodies to severe anaphylactic reactions. The severity of the reaction depends in part on whether the patient retains residual activity of the deficient enzyme. Residual TPP1 activity in CLN2 disease, late infantile leucocytes, as measured by an *in vitro* TPP1 activity assay, ranges from undetectable to around 2% of normal (Sohar et al., 2000). Patients who express some residual enzyme are less likely to have a severe anaphylactic response. However, enzyme replacement studies with Gaucher, Fabry, and MPS types I, II, and VI all reported development of IgG antibodies against the administered enzyme, even when patients retained residual enzyme activity. In some cases, these antibodies can neutralize the activity of the administered enzyme (Richards et al., 1993, Kakkis et al., 2001, Harmatz et al., 2004, Linthorst et al., 2004). However, tolerization regimens to overcome this limitation exist and continue to be developed and improved (Raben et al., 2003, Kakkis et al., 2004).

Gene therapy

Gene therapy refers to the manipulation of gene expression in a diseased organism to achieve a therapeutic goal. In general, the gene therapy strategy for recessive disorders such as NCL is to introduce a functional copy of the recessive gene to the diseased cell population, as opposed to dominant disorders in which stopping or blocking mutant gene expression is necessary. Storage disorders such as the NCLs are excellent candidates for gene therapy for several reasons. First, they are monogenic disorders, so introduction of a single functional gene can potentially rescue the disorder. Second, it is known that in many cases low levels of enzyme activity are sufficient to prevent disease, since heterozygote carriers are disease free, and patients with low levels of enzyme activity can have a protracted disease course (Sleat et al., 1999). Third, soluble lysosomal enzymes can be secreted from the cell in which it is expressed, and subsequently be taken up by a neighbouring cell in a process referred to as cross correction. This phenomenon can facilitate the distribution of lysosomal enzyme beyond the initial region of gene correction, which is essential in difficult-to-target tissues such as the CNS. An advantage that gene therapy has over enzyme replacement therapy is the potential for long-term, endogenous production of the therapeutic enzyme after a single treatment. This is particularly beneficial for disorders like the NCLs that have a pronounced CNS involvement, as it may be undesirable to have repeated invasive procedures to deliver enzyme to the brain. Although transduction by gene transfer may prove to be an effective means to deliver missing enzymes, this approach is less applicable to forms of NCL that are due to defects in transmembrane proteins. These proteins are not released from cells and therefore cannot cross-correct deficient tissue and the likely toxicity associated with their overexpression cannot be overlooked.

Genes can be delivered into a cell by a variety of methods. Although it is possible to introduce genes into cells in the form of plasmid DNA, it is much less efficient than the now widely preferred method of expressing genes from viral vectors. As will be discussed below, viral vectors offer tremendous flexibility in terms of level and longevity of gene expression, as well as tissue specificity. The studies described below all utilize viral vectors as the mode of gene transfer.

TYPES OF VIRAL VECTORS

Numerous viral vectors have been developed and tested for *in vivo* gene transfer to the central nervous system. Among the more prominent viruses are retroviruses, adenoviruses, and adeno-associated viruses (AAVs). Adenoviruses can mediate high levels of protein expression in cells of the CNS, but it is usually transient due to a strong immune response against the vector. Adenoviral vectors that are completely gutted of viral genes can circumvent this disadvantage, making it useful for biological studies. Nonetheless, this type of vector is not commonly used in gene replacement studies, and will not be discussed further.

Retroviruses/lentiviruses

Viruses of the family *Retroviridae* have single-stranded RNA genomes that are reverse transcribed into a double-stranded DNA intermediate. This double-stranded DNA then integrates into host chromosomes and is the template for transcription. Of the retroviruses, those in the *Lentivirus* genus are particularly useful for gene transfer to the CNS because they are able to transduce non-dividing cells, such as mature neurons of the brain. Furthermore, the tissue and cellular tropism of these vectors can be manipulated by expressing envelope proteins from other viruses in a procedure called pseudotyping. For example, viruses pseudotyped with vesicular stomatitis virus glycoprotein (VSV-G) envelope exhibit broad tissue and cellular tropism (Wong et al., 2004). Ross River virus pseudotyped viruses preferentially transduce glial cells over neurons (Kang et al., 2002), and lymphocytic choriomeningitis virus pseudotyped viruses preferentially transduce neural stem cells (Stein et al., 2005). Lentiviral vectors used for gene transfer studies generally do not contain any endogenous viral genes. Viral genes (*gag, pol, env*) necessary for viral replication are provided *in trans* only during production, thus minimizing the risk of immune response against the virus when delivered *in vivo*. Examples of lentiviruses include both primate (human or simian immunodeficiency viruses—HIV, SIV) and non-primate (feline or equine immunodeficiency viruses—FIV, EIAV) viruses.

Immune responses to HIV vectors have been shown to be minimal following delivery into the CNS, and they do not induce systemic immunity to virions (Abordo-Adesida et al., 2005). This is encouraging in that it suggests that repeated administration of virus, if needed, would not induce adverse immune responses. Re-exposure to a particular transgene, however, may still elicit an immune response against the transgene. But as already mentioned with regard to enzyme replacement therapy, NCL patients can retain residual expression of their deficient enzyme, which decreases the risk of adverse immune responses to newly expressed enzyme.

Integration of lentiviruses into the host genome presents a risk in that it could disrupt expression of the transgene or nearby endogenous genes. Lentiviruses tend to integrate into regions of the genome that are transcriptionally active or otherwise prone to strand separation (Kang et al., 2006). A currently active area of research is that of devising ways to target the integration of a lentiviral vector into a benign location in the genome. Feline immunodeficiency virus is capable of directing enzyme expression in neurons of the mouse cerebrum and cerebellum, including Purkinje cells, following direct injection (Haskell et al.,

2003). This type of vector has been used to express TPP1 in the rodent brain (Haskell et al., 2003), but has not been tested in the mouse model (Sleat et al., 2004). Gene therapy studies in CLN1, CLN2 and CLN10 disease animal models have thus far all been done using AAV vectors.

Adeno-associated virus

AAVs are single-stranded DNA viruses in the family *Parvoviridae*. They are small non-enveloped viruses with icosahedral capsids, and are not known to be pathogenic in humans. AAVs are categorized as dependoviruses because they cannot replicate in the absence of a helper virus, which is a virus that is able to supply the protein machinery necessary for viral replication. For example, adenovirus is a common helper virus for AAV. Like lentiviruses, AAVs are able to transduce non-dividing cells, and thus are attractive candidates for gene transfer to the CNS and unlike lentiviruses, AAVs typically do not integrate into the host genome. At least nine serotypes of AAV have been identified, and probably many more exist. Each serotype displays a different pattern of transduction and propensity to spread beyond the initial site of delivery. As with lentiviruses, the viral genome of AAVs can be deleted to minimize risk of adverse immune responses to the vector. Nonetheless, antibodies to capsid proteins can develop after repeated dosing (Mastakov et al., 2002, Zaiss and Muruve, 2005). This may not be a significant concern, however, as AAVs can mediate long-term expression of a transgene, precluding the need for additional doses.

CLN1/PPT1

Expression of PPT1 from AAV vectors has been achieved in the *PPT1*-deficient mouse. Intracranial injections of AAV2-*PPT1* in newborn *Ppt1*-deficient mice resulted in increased PPT1 activity in the brain, decreased storage material in cortical, hippocampal, and cerebellar neurons, and partially rescued the decrease in brain weight and cortical thickness observed in this animal model (Griffey et al., 2004). Behavioural and electroencephalic measures were also improved, but interestingly, seizure frequency and lifespan were not affected by this treatment (Griffey et al., 2006). These findings suggest that AAV-mediated PPT1 expression has therapeutic potential, but the lack of effect on lifespan may indicate a need for wider spread of the enzyme, perhaps to vital regions of the brain such as the brainstem.

In addition to intracranial AAV administration, other routes of delivery have also been demonstrated successfully. Following intravitreal injection of AAV2-*PPT1*, enzyme levels increased in the eye, but interestingly also in distal areas of the brain along visual pathways. Retinal function improved following treatment, and histological improvements were seen in the eye and along the visual pathway, suggesting that PPT1 can be transported along axons of the visual pathways (Griffey et al., 2005). Anterograde axonal transport such as this likely applies to other lysosomal enzymes as well, including TPP1 and CTSD.

CLN2/TPP1

Expression of TPP1 in the rodent brain has been achieved via AAV vectors. AAV5-*TPP1*, when injected into the mouse striatum, transduces primarily neurons, including neurons in the hippocampus, increasing TPP1 activity 3–7-fold (Haskell et al., 2000). AAV2-*TPP1* injected into the rat striatum led to TPP1-positive striatal neurons for the duration of the study. TPP1 was also secreted and spread along CNS white matter tracts to the substantia nigra, thalamus, and cerebral cortex. This same vector, when injected into the CNS of non-human primates, led to TPP1 expression in neurons at 13 weeks post injection (Sondhi et al., 2005). Curiously, in this study TPP1 was not detected in glial cells, suggesting that cross correction of these cells did not occur, or that it occurred at an undetectable level. Although the role of glial dysfunction in the pathogenesis of CLN2 disease, late infantile is not clear, correction of glial cells may be necessary in treatment, given their importance in normal neuronal physiology. While some AAV vectors exhibit considerable spread following injection, convection-enhanced injections can also be used to further expand the area of initial transduction (Hadaczek et al., 2006). Together, these studies demonstrate the feasibility of expressing TPP1 in the mammalian brain.

To test the therapeutic efficacy of gene transfer in CLN2 disease, late infantile, AAV vectors expressing TPP1 have been injected into the brain of *Tpp1*-deficient mice (Passini et al., 2006). TPP1 expressed from AAV2 or 5, when injected into the motor cortex, thalamus, and cerebellum, led to a reduction of autofluorescent storage near the injection sites. This finding was supported by electron microscopy showing a decrease in the number of curvilinear bodies characteristic of CLN2 disease, late infantile, but no increase in survival of the mice was reported (Passini et al., 2006).

A gene transfer vector derived from a rhesus macaque AAV serotype has also been tested for its ability to deliver TPP1 to the *Tpp1*-deficient mouse (Sondhi et al., 2007). AAVrh.10-*TPP1* injected into four locations in each brain hemisphere of 7 week old *Tpp1*$^{-/-}$ mice increased TPP1 activity in the brain. Treated mice displayed a histological decrease in lysosomal storage, and also an improvement in several measures of motor function—gait, balance beam, and grip strength. Importantly, treated mice also displayed an increase in survival over untreated and mock treated mice. This vector was functional in naïve mice, as well as mice pre-immunized with human serotypes of AAV, suggesting that using AAV serotypes derived from non-human primates may be advantageous in avoiding immune responses (Sondhi et al., 2007). Significantly, subsequent studies with this viral vector suggest that treatment in the neonatal period results in increased survival rates in the mouse model (Sondhi et al., 2008). These are exciting studies in that they demonstrate that TPP1 can effectively rescue the phenotype of the *Tpp1*-deficient mice.

More recently, further evidence for the potential of gene transfer in CLN2 disease, late infantile has been provided using a systemically injected AAV2 vector with a modified capsid to target it to the vascular endothelium and cross the BBB (Chen et al., 2009). This vascular targeting was achieved by phage panning to identify a series of peptides enriched on the vascular endothelium, which were inserted into the capsid of a AAV2 vector and shown to deliver enzyme widely within the CNS and improve the disease phenotypes of mouse models of both CLN2 disease, late infantile and MPS VII, another lysosomal storage disorder (Chen et al., 2009). Although, this method may be applicable to other enzyme deficiencies, this study suggested that the molecular signature of the vascular endothelium was disease-specific, meaning that phage panning would need to be performed for each disorder (Chen et al., 2009).

Several other AAV serotypes have been shown to transduce cells of the CNS, and thus may prove to be useful vectors for NCL. AAV serotypes 7, 8, and 9 can transduce neurons in multiple brain regions, and AAV9, in particular, appears to be efficiently transported via axonal pathways in the brain (Cearley and Wolfe, 2006). AAV4 transduces primarily ependymal cells following intraventricular injection, but expression of β-glucuronidase from ependyma results in widespread enzyme distribution, suggesting that the enzyme was distributed via the cerebrospinal fluid. AAV4 delivery in this manner was able to rescue the behavioural and pathological phenotypes of a murine model of MPS VII (Liu et al., 2005), and thus may be useful for delivery of other lysosomal enzymes such as PPT1 and TPP1.

Although few animal studies for CLN2 disease, late infantile gene therapy had been completed, a human gene therapy trial for CLN2 disease was initiated in 2004 (Crystal et al., 2004). Two groups of patients, one with severe disease, the other with moderate disease, received AAV2 vectors expressing human *CLN2/TPP1* by direct injection into 12 sites in the brain, six sites per hemisphere. The outcome measures of the study are based on an evolving CLN2 disease, late infantile clinical rating scale, and MRI of the brain regions that received injections. Treated patients trended towards a reduced rate of decline based on MRI parameters and the neurological rating scale, although the study was not large enough for statistical significance (Worgall et al., 2008). Based on their relative efficacy in *Tpp1*-deficient mice (Sondhi et al., 2007, Sondhi et al., 2008), a second clinical trial using the newer generation of AAVrh.10-*CLN2* vectors is anticipated.

CLN10/CTSD

Expression of AAV vector of mosaic serotype 1/2 was used to express mouse CTSD in the brains of mice deficient for this enzyme. This was found to extend lifespan despite massive ceroid accumulation and microglial activation, and ameliorate both CNS and visceral symptoms of this animal model (Shevtsova et al., 2010).

Eye-targeted gene therapies

While most of the CNS remains a difficult therapeutic target, the eye is a much more accessible organ for gene transfer. This strategy may represent a means to slow down or prevent the degeneration of the retina that is evident in all childhood onset forms of NCL. For this goal to be achieved, effective means for long-lasting gene delivery will need to be developed. Since there are several relatively common inherited disorders in which retinal degeneration occurs, the last decade has seen concerted efforts to develop eye-targeted gene therapies (see review by Smith et al., 2009). Following successful proof of concept studies in both mouse and large animal models (Bennett et al., 1996, Jomary et al., 1997, Acland et al., 2001, Le Meur et al., 2007), clinical trials have been undertaken for Leber congenital amaurosis (LCA) using subretinal delivery of AAV2 vectors (Bainbridge et al., 2008, Hauswirth et al., 2008, Maguire et al., 2008). Despite several technical differences between the protocols and assessment measures employed in these trials, all reported improvements in retinal sensitivity (Bainbridge et al., 2008, Hauswirth et al., 2008, Maguire et al., 2008). Indeed one subject displayed a dramatic improvement in visual mobility in dim light (Bainbridge et al., 2008), but no patients displayed any positive impact upon electroretinogram recordings. Nevertheless, there is optimism that treating younger LCA patients may have greater effects, and other forms of inherited retinal dystrophy are now being considered as candidates for retinal gene therapy (Smith et al., 2009). It remains to be seen whether similar approaches will be successful for any form of NCL, and the potential problems associated with overexpressing transmembrane proteins like CLN3 means these strategies will need to be tested rigorously in animal models. Nevertheless, any positive impact upon visual function would significantly increase the quality of life of CLN3 disease, juvenile and late infantile NCL patients, but it remains to be seen if this potential will be realized.

CELL-BASED THERAPIES

Haematopoietic stem cells

Haematopoietic stem cells (HSCs) are the precursors to numerous types of cells of the immune system, including lymphocytes, neutrophils, macrophages, and with particular importance to NCL, microglial cells in the CNS. Through the migration of microglial cells from the periphery to the CNS, HSCs can act as a vehicle by which enzyme can be delivered to the CNS, thus the rationale for using bone marrow transplants to treat disorders such as CLN1 or CLN2 disease.

Risks of bone marrow transplantation include rejection of the transplant, graft-versus-host disease, and other immunological reactions against the graft. Although the risks of bone marrow transplants are points of concern, tolerizing regimens continue to be developed and improved (Stephan et al., 2006, Markova et al., 2007).

Bone marrow transplants have been successfully performed in lysosomal storage disorders affecting primarily peripheral tissues, such as MPS I, and in these cases it seemed to slow disease progression and improve quality of life (Hopwood et al., 1993). Several reports exist of NCL patients having received bone marrow transplants as an experimental therapy. There are two reports of CLN2 disease, late infantile patients receiving bone marrow transplants (Lake et al., 1997), but this treatment did not appear to be beneficial for the CNS deficits of the patients. The reason for the lack of efficacy is not clear, but may be due to either poor donor cell engraftment, or inefficient cell migration to the CNS. Attempts at bone marrow transplants in infantile CLN1 disease (Lonnqvist et al., 2001) and juvenile CLN3 disease (Lake et al., 1997) have also proven to be of minimal benefit, and this strategy cannot be recommended as therapy currently.

Recent efforts have focused on *ex vivo* gene therapy of HSCs prior to transplant (see below), the rationale being that if bone marrow-derived macrophages repopulate the brain at a relatively slow rate, perhaps overexpressing the desired enzyme in HSCs would enable the few cells that do migrate to the brain to express and secrete a therapeutic level of enzyme.

Ex vivo gene therapy

Ex vivo gene therapy refers to the application of gene transfer techniques to harvested cells, and the subsequent transplantation of the cells back into the patient. Such a strategy offers advantages from both direct gene transfer as well as conventional allogeneic stem cell transplantation in the context of NCL and other similar disorders. Genetically modified cells can overexpress the protein of interest, which, in the case of bone marrow transplant, may be able to compensate for the relative inefficiency by which microglial precursors repopulate the CNS. Furthermore, since the cells to be transplanted can be autologous cells harvested from the patient, there is no risk of graft-versus-host disease.

The effectiveness of this strategy has been demonstrated in several animal models of LSDs with CNS manifestations. In a study with MPS I mice, bone marrow from donor mice was transduced with a retrovirus expressing human iduronidase, and then transplanted into recipient mice. This treatment led to improvements in the pathology of peripheral tissues including liver, spleen, and kidney. Importantly, pathological improvements were also observed within the CNS, specifically within the thalamus and choroid plexus (Zheng et al., 2003). In a mouse model of metachromatic leucodystrophy, bone marrow transplant with cells overexpressing arylsulfatase A led to restoration of enzyme activity and also improvements in learning and motor function (Biffi et al., 2004). In addition to traditional bone marrow transplant procedures, cells transduced *ex vivo* can also be directly delivered to the CNS, thus eliminating the need for transplanted cells to migrate to the CNS from the periphery. In a mouse model of MPS VII, bone marrow stromal cells overexpressing β-glucuronidase were able to improve brain pathology after implantation into the lateral ventricles of the brain (Sakurai et al., 2004). Non-haematopoietic cells have also been used in a similar strategy. MPS VII fibroblasts overexpressing β-glucuronidase, can reduce lysosomal storage when transplanted into the neocortex of MPS VII mice (Taylor and Wolfe, 1997). These types of approaches could all conceivably be adapted to deliver missing enzymes to the NCL brain, but there are no reports of this taking place.

Neuroprogenitor cells

Neuroprogenitor cells (NPCs) are largely undifferentiated cells that retain the potential to develop into neurons or glia. Once introduced into the CNS environment, they also have the potential of developing functional connections with existing cells. NPC implantation has been investigated as an experimental therapy, the rationale being similar to other cell-based studies—the transplanted cells may act as a 'biological factory' from which non-mutant, functional, enzyme can be secreted, leading to cross-correction of adjacent diseased cells. In a mouse model of MPS VII, NPCs expressing β-glucuronidase were injected into the cerebral ventricles of MPS VII mice. A population of donor cells grafted and provided enough enzyme to cause a local decrease in lysosomal storage (Snyder et al., 1995). Similar studies have been performed in models of Tay–Sachs, Niemann–Pick, and Sandhoff diseases, with encouraging results even in symptomatic mice (Lacorazza et al., 1996, Shihabuddin et al., 2004).

This approach has also recently been tested in CLN1 disease, infantile with human neural stem cell (hCNS-SCns) transplants made in immunodeficient *Ppt1-NSCID* mutant mice (Tamaki et al., 2009). When transplanted early in disease progression, these hCNS-SCns migrated widely and persisted within the CNS to deliver sufficient levels of PPT1 to alter host neuropathology. Grafted mice displayed dose-dependent reduction in autofluorescent lipofuscin, significant neuroprotection of host neurons, and delayed loss of motor coordination assessed by rotarod performance (Tamaki et al., 2009). It is not yet clear how these effects are mediated, but very few of transplanted hCNS-SCns appear to become neurons. This may differ between forms of NCL, but suggests that cell transplantation may be limited to the delivery of deficient enzymes and may not be applicable to the types of NCL caused by deficiencies in transmembrane proteins. Nevertheless, it appears that hCNS-SCns can serve as a continuous and long-lasting source of missing lysosomal enzymes and provide some therapeutic benefit (Tamaki et al., 2009). Based upon these data a phase I clinical trial was recently undertaken to determine the safety of neuroprogenitor cell implantation in CLN1 and CLN2 disease patients. Although the outcome of this trial is yet to be published, future trials to assess the efficacy of this approach are under consideration.

SMALL MOLECULE THERAPIES

Chemical chaperones

In some cases, a mutation in a particular enzyme does not completely abolish its activity, but instead leads to a misfolding of the enzyme in the endoplasmic reticulum (ER) following translation. The failure of the mutant enzyme to adopt a functional conformation leads to its degradation via a process termed ER-associated protein degradation (ERAD). Disease in these cases is thus due to mutant enzymes not trafficking correctly to the lysosome. Chemical chaperones are synthetic molecules that act to promote correct protein folding in the ER. These chaperones are commonly active site inhibitors and are thought to provide a structure around which a nascent enzyme can fold. Once the enzyme folds correctly and is trafficked to the lysosome, it is fully functional and is no longer susceptible to ERAD.

The feasibility of this type of approach has been demonstrated in studies with Fabry and Gaucher diseases. Studies with Fabry patient lymphoblasts show that exposure to low doses of 1-deoxygalactonojirimycin (DGJ), a competitive inhibitor of α-galactosidase A can paradoxically lead to increases in enzyme activity. Furthermore, oral administration of DGJ to transgenic mice expressing mutant α-galactosidase A led to elevated enzyme activity in some organs (Fan et al., 1999). A similar phenomenon has been observed in Gaucher patient lymphoblasts using the β-glucosidase inhibitor, N-(n-nonyl)-deoxynojirimycin (Sawkar et al., 2005). Several early phase clinical trials are currently underway testing the effects of chemical chaperones in Fabry and Gaucher diseases.

Although this type of approach might potentially be applied to NCL, the vast majority of mutations result in very little production of enzyme. Nevertheless where mutations do not occur within the active site of the enzyme, the chaperone approach may be applicable. This was first demonstrated for PPT1 containing missense mutations thought to result in a misfolded unstable protein, where residual enzyme activity in patient lymphoblasts was doubled (Dawson et al., 2010). While studies have focused exclusively on rescuing enzyme activity, the chemical chaperone approach could conceivably be applied to other soluble or even membrane bound proteins such as CLN3, CLN6, CLN7, or CLN8. The difficulty lies in screening for a compound that is an effective chaperone and that is easily targeted to the ER where it can exert its action.

Stop codon readthrough

Mammalian cells utilize three mRNA stop codons to terminate protein translation—UAA, UAG, and UGA. Although these termination signals are highly efficient, 'readthrough' of stop codons does occur, and this phenomenon is in part influenced by bases immediately downstream of the stop codon (McCaughan et al., 1995). For genetic disorders resulting from a premature stop codon, inducing readthrough may be a viable strategy to increase expression of functional protein. Several aminoglycoside antibiotics have been show to promote stop codon readthrough, most notably gentamicin. Preclinical studies have demonstrated the feasibility of this approach for several lysosomal disorders, including the NCLs. Exposure of Hurler disease patient fibroblasts to gentamicin resulted in a 2–3% increase in α-L-iduronidase activity, and a reduction in storage of glysosaminoglycans (Keeling et al., 2001). In late infantile CLN2 disease patient fibroblasts with a nonsense mutation, treatment with gentamicin restored TPP1 activity up to 7% of normal (Sleat et al., 2001). This strategy has been extended to clinical trials for lysosomal storage disorders. Similar clinical studies for cystic fibrosis (CF) yielded promising results, with intranasal application of gentamicin leading to histological and functional improvements in patients with premature stop codons (Wilschanski et al., 2003). More recently success has been claimed in preliminary experiments for CF and Duchenne muscular dystrophy using PTC124, a molecule with reportedly fewer side effects (Hirawat et al., 2007, Welch et al., 2007).

A significant percentage of alleles associated with CLN1 disease and CLN2 disease contain premature stop codons. Indeed, in a survey of mutations in 29 US and Canadian families, the p.Arg115X in *CLN1* mutation accounted for 40% of mutant alleles and was associated with severe disease in the homozygous state (Das et al., 1998). A survey of 58 late infantile CLN2 disease families showed that the p.Arg208X mutation in *CLN2/TPP1* accounted for approximately 28% of mutant alleles (Sleat et al., 1999). The prevalence of stop codon mutations indicates that readthrough may have legitimate clinical utility for CLN1 disease and CLN2 disease.

Nevertheless, there are significant limitations to this approach including toxicity of the antibiotic, with the association between aminoglycoside use and neuro- and ototoxicity being well established. Furthermore, successful induction of stop codon readthrough does not guarantee that the correct amino acid will be inserted and a resulting missense mutation may result in an equally inactive enzyme. Off-target effects are also a concern, as the readthrough effects of the antibiotic are not specific to the mutant transcript being rescued. Unintended readthrough of stop codons can potentially cause undesirable side effects. As such, although the readthrough approach may theoretically have some potential, this is yet to be realized.

Immunomodulation

In the absence of any clear functional role for a disease-causing gene or its product, therapeutic interventions are limited to characterizing the downstream effects of gene mutation and investigating whether blocking these effects affords any benefit. With the normal function of CLN3 remaining elusive, this strategy has been applied to juvenile CLN3 disease, with a detailed series of phenotypes documented in *Cln3* deficient mice (Cooper et al., 2006). One of the first phenotypes to emerge was an autoimmune response in both human and murine CLN3 disease (Chattopadhyay et al., 2002), with a range of brain-directed autoantibodies generated that can gain access to the CNS due to size-selective breach in the BBB (Lim et al., 2006, Lim et al., 2007). The early presence of these IgGs within the CNS raised the question of whether blocking the production of autoantibodies would afford any therapeutic benefit. This strategy has been tested by both genetic and pharmacological methods and based on altered disease severity (Seehafer et al., 2010), data, a phase I clinical trial of the immunosuppressant mycophenolate (mycophenolate mofetil, Cellcept®, Myfortic®, mycophenolate sodium or mycophenolic acid) has recently been approved. Given the complexity of the immune system, the choice of drug to target the adaptive and innate immune responses evident in juvenile CLN3 disease is likely to be important for determining their therapeutic efficacy. Administration of the steroid prednisolone to juvenile CLN3 disease patients in Finland reduced the occurrence of antibodies to GAD65, but produced no significant effect on the disease course (Åberg et al., 2008). Indeed, there are significant risks associated with immunomodulation in children who are already seriously ill and the benefit of these approaches will need to be carefully considered against potentially harmful side effects.

Receptor modulation

As more is discovered about changes that occur in the brain in NCL patients or animal models there may be drugs identified that can potentially ameliorate these effects. One class of drugs currently under investigation is glutamate receptor antagonists (Cooper et al., 2006), based on the observations of elevated levels of glutamate (Pears et al., 2005) and the vulnerability of *CLN3* deficient neurons to AMPA (α-amino-3-hydroxy-5-methyl-4-isoxazolepropionate)-mediated neurotoxicity (Kovács et al., 2006). Administration of the non-competitive AMPA antagononist EGIS-8332 improved the rotarod performance of a CLN3 disease mouse model (Kovács and Pearce, 2008). Similar effects have been reported in Cln3 deficient mice after a single intraperitoneal injection of administration of EGIS-8332 (Kovács et al., 2010), but with minimal effects glial activation or neuron loss, and it is unclear what other effects glutamate antagonists may have. Nevertheless, the relative success of drugs such as talampanel (LY300164), which is used to treat seizures and Parkinson's disease, makes it likely that other glutamate antagonists will be assessed in juvenile CLN3 disease, but it remains unclear whether these will reach the clinic (Cooper, 2008).

Storage material degradation

The widespread and progressive accumulation of storage material in all forms of NCL has long been considered a pathological hallmark of these disorders, even giving rise to their naming as neuronal ceroid lipofuscinosis. As such, an approach that helps cells to break down accumulated storage material more efficiently might be beneficial. The drug Cystagon® (cysteamine) reduces the storage load of PPT1 deficient fibroblasts *in vitro* (Zhang et al., 2001), but has not been shown to have positive effects upon the disease phenotype of mouse models of CLN1 disease. Nevertheless, this drug has been tested in children with both classic infantile and later onset CLN1 disease, but the results of these studies are not yet available. Although such strategies have been employed successfully in other lysosomal storage disorders, most notably with miglustat or N-buteromycin (Jeyakumar et al., 2005), the relationship between storage material accumulation and neuron loss has not been clearly established in any form of NCL. Indeed, there appears to be no direct correlation between the build-up of storage material and the onset of neuron loss (Cooper et al., 2006). Moreover, it is possible to significantly reduce the storage burden in CLN1 disease with no positive effect upon disease outcome (Griffey et al., 2006), which questions whether reducing storage material accumulation will prove to have any clinically significant therapeutic benefit.

Inhibition of cell death

As in many neurodegenerative disorders, work to identify the different mechanisms that may cause cell death in the NCLs is underway. The hope is that blocking this process may prevent neuron loss, although the net result of rescuing many dysfunctional neurons may not be as positive as anticipated. Indeed, rather than simply preventing neuron loss the true challenge is instead to restore the function of the mutated disease-causing gene. Nevertheless, from time to time different compounds have been suggested to be of possible therapeutic value. In the last decade one such compound was the non-opioid analgesic flupirtine, which was reported to prevent certain induced forms of NCL cell death in tissue culture (Dhar et al., 2002). On this basis many parents opted to administer flupirtine to their children, but this has not been found to alter the rate of disease progression to any appreciable extent.

DIETARY THERAPIES

Several dietary therapies have been tested for NCL. Based on evidence that antioxidant mechanisms are impaired in juvenile NCL (Westermarck et al., 1997), the efficacy of antioxidant supplementation in NCL was studied, but demonstrated very little effect on disease outcome (Santavuori et al., 1989). The possible reduction in polyunsaturated fatty acids in CLN3 disease, juvenile patients (Bennett et al., 1994), has prompted efforts to normalize these levels by supplementing with omega-3 fatty acids from fish oil extracts. As different dietary supplements are suggested, these approaches are frequently administered to affected children by their parents in the hope of slowing disease progression, but none have produced positive effects. Although dietary therapies can potentially be of clinical benefit in NCL, the current lack of understanding of disease mechanisms precludes the ability to design dietary treatment regimens in a rational manner. As is the case with other modes of therapy, a better understanding of the biology of NCL will eventually facilitate the development of novel and effective therapeutic approaches.

ASSESSMENT OF THERAPY

If the advances that are being made in animal models are to be realized in a clinical setting, it is essential to be able to assess the effect of treatments on the long-term natural history of each type of NCL disease. Towards this there are readily quantifiable scales to score the clinical course of different forms of NCL. Much progress has been made towards this goal in CLN3 disease, juvenile, with the development of the Unified Batten Disease Rating Scale (Marshall et al., 2005). A scale is also in place for CLN2 disease, late infantile (Steinfeld et al., 2002), and in a modified form is now in use in clinical trials of AAV-mediated gene therapy and neural stem cell transplantation. The development of these scales not only provides valuable information about the normal rate of disease progression, but will also prove invaluable for defining specific endpoints in the design of future clinical trials. It is crucial to have detailed clinical information available about affected individuals and to achieve this goal an International NCL Patient Registry is currently being established.

It will also be important to consider if and when to stop providing a treatment that is no longer providing any benefit. For this, measurable outcomes of efficacy will be required to evaluate benefit, as well as discussions prior to starting any therapy to consider this possibility.

CONCLUSIONS

To summarize, several promising therapeutic approaches for the NCLs are being investigated, including enzyme replacement, gene therapy, cell-based therapies, and small molecule therapies. Current evidence suggests that restoration of deficient NCL enzymes and membrane proteins in the CNS would be important for effective treatment, but numerous important questions remain unanswered. Are there particular cell populations within the CNS that must be targeted? At what point along the disease course must treatment be initiated before the disease process becomes irreversible? What are the risks of elevating NCL enzyme or protein activity above physiological levels? Will peripheral disease still develop if CNS disease is treated? Further studies will be necessary to address these and other unanswered questions. Most significantly, the molecular mechanisms underlying pathogenesis have not been elucidated for any form of NCL. As a more detailed understanding of the disease process emerges, so will additional insights into therapy and more mechanistic-based strategies. However, it is likely that therapy will be most effective if begun presymptomatically, and may be particularly valuable for those NCLs in which mild mutations cause a later than usual age of onset, giving a bigger window of opportunity to initiate therapy.

REFERENCES

Åberg L, Talling M, Harkonen T, Lonnqvist T, Knip M, Alen R, Rantala H, & Tyynelä J (2008) Intermittent prednisolone and autoantibodies to GAD65 in juvenile neuronal ceroid lipofuscinosis. *Neurology*, 70, 1218–1220.

Abordo-Adesida E, Follenzi A, Barcia C, Sciascia S, Castro MG, Naldini L, & Lowenstein PR (2005) Stability of lentiviral vector-mediated transgene expression in the brain in the presence of systemic antivector immune responses. *Hum Gene Ther*, 16, 741–751.

Acland GM, Aguirre GD, Ray J, Zhang Q, Aleman TS, Cideciyan AV, Pearce-Kelling SE, Anand V, Zeng Y, Maguire AM, Jacobson SG, Hauswirth WW, & Bennett J (2001) Gene therapy restores vision in a canine model of childhood blindness. *Nat Genet*, 28, 92–95.

Amalfitano A, Bengur AR, Morse RP, Majure JM, Case LE, Veerling DL, Mackey J, Kishnani P, Smith W, McVie-Wylie A, Sullivan JA, Hoganson GE, Phillips JA, 3rd, Schaefer GB, Charrow J, Ware RE, Bossen EH, & Chen YT (2001) Recombinant human acid alpha-glucosidase enzyme therapy for infantile glycogen storage disease type II: results of a phase I/II clinical trial. *Genet Med*, 3, 132–138.

Bainbridge JW, Smith AJ, Barker SS, Robbie S, Henderson R, Balaggan K, Viswanathan A, Holder GE, Stockman A, Tyler N, Petersen-Jones S, Bhattacharya SS, Thrasher AJ, Fitzke FW, Carter BJ, Rubin GS, Moore AT, & Ali RR (2008) Effect of gene therapy on visual function in Leber's congenital amaurosis. *N Engl J Med*, 358, 2231–2239.

Barton NW, Brady RO, Dambrosia JM, Di Bisceglie AM, Doppelt SH, Hill SC, Mankin HJ, Murray GJ, Parker RI, Argoff CE, Grewal RP, Yu K-T, & Collaborators (1991) Replacement therapy for inherited enzyme deficiency—macrophage-targeted glucocerebrosidase for Gaucher's disease. *N Engl J Med*, 324, 1464–1470.

Barton NW, Furbish FS, Murray GJ, Garfield M, & Brady RO (1990) Therapeutic response to intravenous infusions of glucocerebrosidase in a patient with Gaucher disease. *Proc Natl Acad Sci U S A*, 87, 1913–1916.

Bennett J, Tanabe T, Sun D, Zeng Y, Kjeldbye H, Gouras P, & Maguire AM (1996) Photoreceptor cell rescue in retinal degeneration (rd) mice by in vivo gene therapy. *Nat Med*, 2, 649–654.

Bennett MJ, Gayton AR, Rittey CD, & Hosking GP (1994) Juvenile neuronal ceroid-lipofuscinosis: developmental progress after supplementation with polyunsaturated fatty acids. *Dev Med Child Neurol*, 36, 630–638.

Biffi A, De Palma M, Quattrini A, Del Carro U, Amadio S, Visigalli I, Sessa M, Fasano S, Brambilla R, Marchesini S, Bordignon C, & Naldini L (2004) Correction of metachromatic leukodystrophy in the mouse model by transplantation of genetically modified hematopoietic stem cells. *J Clin Invest*, 113, 1118–1129.

Cearley CN & Wolfe JH (2006) Transduction characteristics of adeno-associated virus vectors expressing cap serotypes 7, 8, 9, and Rh10 in the mouse brain. *Mol Ther*, 13, 528–537.

Chang M, Cooper JD, Sleat DE, Cheng SH, Dodge JC, Passini MA, Lobel P, & Davidson BL (2008) Intraventricular enzyme replacement improves disease phenotypes in a mouse model of late infantile neuronal ceroid lipofuscinosis. *Mol Ther*, 16, 649–656.

Chattopadhyay S, Ito M, Cooper JD, Brooks AI, Curran TM, Powers JM, & Pearce DA (2002a) An autoantibody inhibitory to glutamic acid decarboxylase in the neurodegenerative disorder Batten disease. *Hum Mol Genet*, 11, 1421–1431.

Chen YH, Chang M, & Davidson BL (2009) Molecular signatures of disease brain endothelia provide new sites for CNS-directed enzyme therapy. *Nat Med*, 15, 1215–1218.

Cooper JD (2008) Moving towards therapies for juvenile Batten disease? *Exp Neurol*, 211, 329–331.

Cooper JD, Russell C, & Mitchison HM (2006) Progress towards understanding disease mechanisms in small vertebrate models of neuronal ceroid lipofuscinosis. *Biochim Biophys Acta*, 1762, 873–889.

Crystal RG, Sondhi D, Hackett NR, Kaminsky SM, Worgall S, Stieg P, Souweidane M, Hosain S, Heier L, Ballon D, Dinner M, Wisniewski K, Kaplitt M, Greenwald BM, Howell JD, Strybing K, Dyke J, & Voss H (2004) Clinical protocol. Administration of a replication-deficient adeno-associated virus gene transfer vector expressing the human CLN2 cDNA to the brain of children with late infantile neuronal ceroid lipofuscinosis. *Hum Gene Ther*, 15, 1131–1154.

Das AK, Becerra CH, Yi W, Lu JY, Siakotos AN, Wisniewski KE, & Hofmann SL (1998) Molecular genetics of palmitoyl-protein thioesterase deficiency in the U.S. *J Clin Invest*, 102, 361–370.

Dawson G, Schroeder C, & Dawson PE (2010) Palmitoyl:protein thioesterase (PPT1) inhibitors can act as pharmacological chaperones in infantile Batten disease. *Biochem Biophys Res Commun*, 395, 66–69.

Dhar S, Bitting RL, Rylova SN, Jansen PJ, Lockhart E, Koeberl DD, Amalfitano A, & Boustany RM (2002) Flupirtine blocks apoptosis in Batten patient lymphoblasts and in human postmitotic CLN3- and CLN2-deficient neurons. *Ann Neurol*, 51, 448–466.

Fan JQ, Ishii S, Asano N, & Suzuki Y (1999) Accelerated transport and maturation of lysosomal alpha-galactosidase A in Fabry lymphoblasts by an enzyme inhibitor. *Nat Med*, 5, 112–115.

Fratantoni JC, Hall CW, & Neufeld EF (1968) Hurler and Hunter syndromes: mutual correction of the defect in cultured fibroblasts. *Science*, 162, 570–572.

Griffey M, Bible E, Vogler C, Levy B, Gupta P, Cooper J, & Sands MS (2004) Adeno-associated virus 2-mediated gene therapy decreases autofluorescent storage material and increases brain mass in a murine model of infantile neuronal ceroid lipofuscinosis. *Neurobiol Dis*, 16, 360–369.

Griffey M, Macauley SL, Ogilvie JM, & Sands MS (2005) AAV2-mediated ocular gene therapy for infantile neuronal ceroid lipofuscinosis. *Mol Ther*, 12, 413–421.

Griffey MA, Wozniak D, Wong M, Bible E, Johnson K, Rothman SM, Wentz AE, Cooper JD, & Sands MS (2006) CNS-directed AAV2-mediated gene therapy ameliorates functional deficits in a murine model of infantile neuronal ceroid lipofuscinosis. *Mol Ther*, 13, 538–547.

Hadaczek P, Kohutnicka M, Krauze MT, Bringas J, Pivirotto P, Cunningham J, & Bankiewicz K (2006) Convection-enhanced delivery of adeno-associated virus type 2 (AAV2) into the striatum and transport of AAV2 within monkey brain. *Hum Gene Ther*, 17, 291–302.

Harmatz P, Whitley CB, Waber L, Pais R, Steiner R, Plecko B, Kaplan P, Simon J, Butensky E, & Hopwood JJ (2004) Enzyme replacement therapy in mucopolysaccharidosis VI (Maroteaux-Lamy syndrome). *J Pediatr*, 144, 574–580.

Haskell RE, Carr CJ, Pearce DA, Bennett MJ, & Davidson BL (2000) Batten disease: evaluation of *CLN3* mutations on protein localization and function. *Hum Mol Genet*, 9, 735–744.

Haskell RE, Hughes SM, Chiorini JA, Alisky JM, & Davidson BL (2003) Viral-mediated delivery of the late-infantile neuronal ceroid lipofuscinosis gene, TPP-I to the mouse central nervous system. *Gene Ther*, 10, 34–42.

Hauswirth WW, Aleman TS, Kaushal S, Cideciyan AV, Schwartz SB, Wang L, Conlon TJ, Boye SL, Flotte TR, Byrne BJ, & Jacobson SG (2008) Treatment of leber congenital amaurosis due to RPE65 mutations by ocular subretinal injection of adeno-associated virus gene vector: short-term results of a phase I trial. *Hum Gene Ther*, 19, 979–990.

Hirawat S, Welch EM, Elfring GL, Northcutt VJ, Paushkin S, Hwang S, Leonard EM, Almstead NG, Ju W, Peltz SW, & Miller LL (2007) Safety, tolerability, and pharmacokinetics of PTC124, a nonaminoglycoside nonsense mutation suppressor, following single- and multiple-dose administration to healthy male and female adult volunteers. *J Clin Pharmacol*, 47, 430–444.

Hopwood JJ, Vellodi A, Scott HS, Morris CP, Litjens T, Clements PR, Brooks DA, Cooper A, & Wraith JE (1993) Long-term clinical progress in bone marrow transplanted mucopolysaccharidosis type I patients with a defined genotype. *J Inherit Metab Dis*, 16, 1024–1033.

Jeyakumar M, Dwek RA, Butters TD, & Platt FM (2005) Storage solutions: treating lysosomal disorders of the brain. *Nat Rev Neurosci*, 6, 713–725.

Jomary C, Vincent KA, Grist J, Neal MJ, & Jones SE (1997) Rescue of photoreceptor function by AAV-mediated gene transfer in a mouse model of inherited retinal degeneration. *Gene Ther*, 4, 683–690.

Kakkis E, McEntee M, Vogler C, Le S, Levy B, Belichenko P, Mobley W, Dickson P, Hanson S, & Passage M (2004) Intrathecal enzyme replacement therapy reduces lysosomal storage in the brain and meninges of the canine model of MPS I. *Mol Genet Metab*, 83, 163–174.

Kakkis ED, Muenzer J, Tiller GE, Waber L, Belmont J, Passage M, Izykowski B, Phillips J, Doroshow R, Walot I, Hoft R, & Neufeld EF (2001) Enzyme-replacement therapy in mucopolysaccharidosis I. *N Engl J Med*, 344, 182–188.

Kang Y, Moressi CJ, Scheetz TE, Xie L, Tran DT, Casavant TL, Ak P, Benham CJ, Davidson BL, & McCray PB, Jr. (2006) Integration site choice of a feline immunodeficiency virus vector. *J Virol*, 80, 8820–8823.

Kang Y, Stein CS, Heth JA, Sinn PL, Penisten AK, Staber PD, Ratliff KL, Shen H, Barker CK, Martins I, Sharkey CM, Sanders DA, McCray PB, Jr., & Davidson BL (2002) In vivo gene transfer using a nonprimate lentiviral vector pseudotyped with Ross River Virus glycoproteins. *J Virol*, 76, 9378–9388.

Keeling KM, Brooks DA, Hopwood JJ, Li P, Thompson JN, & Bedwell DM (2001) Gentamicin-mediated suppression of Hurler syndrome stop mutations restores a low level of alpha-L-iduronidase activity and reduces lysosomal glycosaminoglycan accumulation. *Hum Mol Genet*, 10, 291–299.

Kovács AD & Pearce DA (2008) Attenuation of AMPA receptor activity improves motor skills in a mouse model of juvenile Batten disease. *Exp Neurol*, 209, 288–291.

Kovács AD, Weimer JM, & Pearce DA (2006) Selectively increased sensitivity of cerebellar granule cells to AMPA receptor-mediated excitotoxicity in a mouse model of Batten disease. *Neurobiol Dis*, 22, 575–585.

Kovács AD, Saje A, Wong A, Szénási G, Kiricsi P, Szabó E, Cooper JD, Pearce DA (2010). Temporary inhibition of AMPA receptors induces a prolonged improvement of motor performance in a mouse model of juvenile Batten disease. *Neuropharmacology*. 2010 Oct 28. [Epub ahead of print] PMID: 20971125 [PubMed - as supplied by publisher]

Lacorazza HD, Flax JD, Snyder EY, & Jendoubi M (1996) Expression of human beta-hexosaminidase alpha-subunit gene (the gene defect of Tay-Sachs disease) in mouse brains upon engraftment of transduced progenitor cells. *Nat Med*, 2, 424–429.

Lake BD, Steward CG, Oakhill A, Wilson J, & Perham TG (1997) Bone marrow transplantation in late infantile Batten disease and juvenile Batten disease. *Neuropediatrics*, 28, 80–81.

Le Meur G, Stieger K, Smith AJ, Weber M, Deschamps JY, Nivard D, Mendes-Madeira A, Provost N, Pereon Y,

Cherel Y, Ali RR, Hamel C, Moullier P, & Rolling F (2007) Restoration of vision in RPE65-deficient Briard dogs using an AAV serotype 4 vector that specifically targets the retinal pigmented epithelium. *Gene Ther*, 14, 292–303.

Lim MJ, Alexander N, Benedict JW, Chattopadhyay S, Shemilt SJ, Guerin CJ, Cooper JD, & Pearce DA (2007) IgG entry and deposition are components of the neuroimmune response in Batten disease. *Neurobiol Dis*, 25, 239–251.

Lim MJ, Beake J, Bible E, Curran TM, Ramirez-Montealegre D, Pearce DA, & Cooper JD (2006) Distinct patterns of serum immunoreactivity as evidence for multiple brain-directed autoantibodies in juvenile neuronal ceroid lipofuscinosis. *Neuropathol Appl Neurobiol*, 32, 469–482.

Lin L & Lobel P (2001) Production and characterization of recombinant human CLN2 protein for enzyme-replacement therapy in late infantile neuronal ceroid lipofuscinosis. *Biochem J*, 357, 49–55.

Linthorst GE, Hollak CE, Donker-Koopman WE, Strijland A, & Aerts JM (2004) Enzyme therapy for Fabry disease: neutralizing antibodies toward agalsidase alpha and beta. *Kidney Int*, 66, 1589–1595.

Liu G, Martins I, Wemmie JA, Chiorini JA, & Davidson BL (2005) Functional correction of CNS phenotypes in a lysosomal storage disease model using adeno-associated virus type 4 vectors. *J Neurosci*, 25, 9321–9327.

Lonnqvist T, Vanhanen SL, Vettenranta K, Autti T, Rapola J, Santavuori P, & Saarinen-Pihkala UM (2001) Hematopoietic stem cell transplantation in infantile neuronal ceroid lipofuscinosis. *Neurology*, 57, 1411–1416.

Lonser RR, Walbridge S, Murray GJ, Aizenberg MR, Vortmeyer AO, Aerts JM, Brady RO, & Oldfield EH (2005) Convection perfusion of glucocerebrosidase for neuronopathic Gaucher's disease. *Ann Neurol*, 57, 542–548.

Maguire AM, Simonelli F, Pierce EA, Pugh EN, Jr., Mingozzi F, Bennicelli J, Banfi S, Marshall KA, Testa F, Surace EM, Rossi S, Lyubarsky A, Arruda VR, Konkle B, Stone E, Sun J, Jacobs J, Dell'Osso L, Hertle R, Ma JX, Redmond TM, Zhu X, Hauck B, Zelenaia O, Shindler KS, Maguire MG, Wright JF, Volpe NJ, McDonnell JW, Auricchio A, High KA, & Bennett J (2008) Safety and efficacy of gene transfer for Leber's congenital amaurosis. *N Engl J Med*, 358, 2240–2248.

Markova M, Barker JN, Miller JS, Arora M, Wagner JE, Burns LJ, MacMillan ML, Douek D, DeFor T, Tan Y, Repka T, Blazar BR, & Weisdorf DJ (2007) Fludarabine vs cladribine plus busulfan and low-dose TBI as reduced intensity conditioning for allogeneic hematopoietic stem cell transplantation: a prospective randomized trial. *Bone Marrow Transplant*, 39, 193–199.

Marshall FJ, de Blieck EA, Mink JW, Dure L, Adams H, Messing S, Rothberg PG, Levy E, McDonough T, DeYoung J, Wang M, Ramirez-Montealegre D, Kwon JM, & Pearce DA (2005) A clinical rating scale for Batten disease: reliable and relevant for clinical trials. *Neurology*, 65, 275–279.

Mastakov MY, Baer K, Symes CW, Leichtlein CB, Kotin RM, & During MJ (2002) Immunological aspects of recombinant adeno-associated virus delivery to the mammalian brain. *J Virol*, 76, 8446–8454.

McCaughan KK, Brown CM, Dalphin ME, Berry MJ, & Tate WP (1995) Translational termination efficiency in mammals is influenced by the base following the stop codon. *Proc Natl Acad Sci U S A*, 92, 5431–5435.

Passini MA, Dodge JC, Bu J, Yang W, Zhao Q, Sondhi D, Hackett NR, Kaminsky SM, Mao Q, Shihabuddin LS, Cheng SH, Sleat DE, Stewart GR, Davidson BL, Lobel P, & Crystal RG (2006) Intracranial delivery of CLN2 reduces brain pathology in a mouse model of classical late infantile neuronal ceroid lipofuscinosis. *J Neurosci*, 26, 1334–1342.

Pears MR, Cooper JD, Mitchison HM, Mortishire-Smith RJ, Pearce DA, & Griffin JL (2005) High resolution 1H NMR-based metabolomics indicates a neurotransmitter cycling deficit in cerebral tissue from a mouse model of Batten disease. *J Biol Chem*, 280, 42508–42514.

Raben N, Nagaraju K, Lee A, Lu N, Rivera Y, Jatkar T, Hopwood JJ, & Plotz PH (2003) Induction of tolerance to a recombinant human enzyme, acid alpha-glucosidase, in enzyme deficient knockout mice. *Transgenic Res*, 12, 171–178.

Richards SM, Olson TA, & McPherson JM (1993) Antibody response in patients with Gaucher disease after repeated infusion with macrophage-targeted glucocerebrosidase. *Blood*, 82, 1402–1409.

Sakurai K, Iizuka S, Shen JS, Meng XL, Mori T, Umezawa A, Ohashi T, & Eto Y (2004) Brain transplantation of genetically modified bone marrow stromal cells corrects CNS pathology and cognitive function in MPS VII mice. *Gene Ther*, 11, 1475–1481.

Santavuori P, Heiskala H, Autti T, Johansson E, & Westermarck T (1989a) Comparison of the clinical courses in patients with juvenile neuronal ceroid lipofuscinosis receiving antioxidant treatment and those without antioxidant treatment. *Adv Exp Med Biol*, 266, 273–282.

Sawkar AR, Adamski-Werner SL, Cheng WC, Wong CH, Beutler E, Zimmer KP, & Kelly JW (2005) Gaucher disease-associated glucocerebrosidases show mutation-dependent chemical chaperoning profiles. *Chem Biol*, 12, 1235–1244.

Schiffmann R, Kopp JB, Austin HA, 3rd, Sabnis S, Moore DF, Weibel T, Balow JE, & Brady RO (2001) Enzyme replacement therapy in Fabry disease: a randomized controlled trial. *JAMA*, 285, 2743–2749.

Seehafer SS, Ramirez-Montealegre D, Wong AM, Chan CH, Castaneda J, Horak M, Ahmadi SM, Lim MJ, Cooper JD, Pearce DA (2010). Immunosuppression alters disease severity in juvenile Batten disease mice. *J Neuroimmunol*. 2010 Oct 9. [Epub ahead of print] PMID: 20937531 [PubMed - as supplied by publisher]

Shevtsova Z, Garrido M, Weishaupt J, Saftig P, Bahr M, Luhder F, & Kugler S (2010) CNS-expressed cathepsin D prevents lymphopenia in a murine model of congenital neuronal ceroid lipofuscinosis. *Am J Pathol*, 177, 271–279.

Shihabuddin LS, Numan S, Huff MR, Dodge JC, Clarke J, Macauley SL, Yang W, Taksir TV, Parsons G, Passini MA, Gage FH, & Stewart GR (2004) Intracerebral transplantation of adult mouse neural progenitor cells into the Niemann-Pick-A mouse leads to a marked decrease in lysosomal storage pathology. *J Neurosci*, 24, 10642–10651.

Sleat DE, Gin RM, Sohar I, Wisniewski K, Sklower-Brooks S, Pullarkat RK, Palmer DN, Lerner TJ, Boustany RM, Uldall P, Siakotos AN, Donnelly RJ, & Lobel P (1999) Mutational analysis of the defective protease in classic late-infantile neuronal ceroid lipofuscinosis, a neurodegenerative lysosomal storage disorder. *Am J Hum Genet*, 64, 1511–1523.

Sleat DE, Lackland H, Wang Y, Sohar I, Xiao G, Li H, & Lobel P (2005) The human brain mannose 6-phosphate glycoproteome: a complex mixture composed of multiple isoforms of many soluble lysosomal proteins. *Proteomics*, 5, 1520–1532.

Sleat DE, Sohar I, Gin RM, & Lobel P (2001) Aminoglycoside-mediated suppression of nonsense mutations in late infantile neuronal ceroid lipofuscinosis. *Eur J Paediatr Neurol*, 5 Suppl A, 57–62.

Sleat DE, Wiseman JA, El-Banna M, Kim KH, Mao Q, Price S, Macauley SL, Sidman RL, Shen MM, Zhao Q, Passini MA, Davidson BL, Stewart GR, & Lobel P (2004) A mouse model of classical late-infantile neuronal ceroid lipofuscinosis based on targeted disruption of the CLN2 gene results in a loss of tripeptidyl-peptidase I activity and progressive neurodegeneration. *J Neurosci*, 24, 9117–9126.

Smith AJ, Bainbridge JW, & Ali RR (2009) Prospects for retinal gene replacement therapy. *Trends Genet*, 25, 156–165.

Snyder EY, Taylor RM, & Wolfe JH (1995) Neural progenitor cell engraftment corrects lysosomal storage throughout the MPS VII mouse brain. *Nature*, 374, 367–370.

Sohar I, Lin L, & Lobel P (2000) Enzyme-based diagnosis of classical late infantile neuronal ceroid lipofuscinosis: comparison of tripeptidyl peptidase I and pepstatin-insensitive protease assays. *Clin Chem*, 46, 1005–1008.

Sondhi D, Hackett NR, Peterson DA, Stratton J, Baad M, Travis KM, Wilson JM, & Crystal RG (2007) Enhanced survival of the LINCL mouse following CLN2 gene transfer using the rh.10 rhesus macaque-derived adeno-associated virus vector. *Mol Ther*, 15, 481–491.

Sondhi D, Peterson DA, Edelstein AM, del Fierro K, Hackett NR, & Crystal RG (2008) Survival advantage of neonatal CNS gene transfer for late infantile neuronal ceroid lipofuscinosis. *Exp Neurol*, 213, 18–27.

Sondhi D, Peterson DA, Giannaris EL, Sanders CT, Mendez BS, De B, Rostkowski AB, Blanchard B, Bjugstad K, Sladek JR, Jr., Redmond DE, Jr., Leopold PL, Kaminsky SM, Hackett NR, & Crystal RG (2005) AAV2-mediated CLN2 gene transfer to rodent and non-human primate brain results in long-term TPP-I expression compatible with therapy for LINCL. *Gene Ther*, 12, 1618–1632.

Stein CS, Martins I, & Davidson BL (2005) The lymphocytic choriomeningitis virus envelope glycoprotein targets lentiviral gene transfer vector to neural progenitors in the murine brain. *Mol Ther*, 11, 382–389.

Steinfeld R, Heim P, von Gregory H, Meyer K, Ullrich K, Goebel HH, & Kohlschutter A (2002) Late infantile neuronal ceroid lipofuscinosis: quantitative description of the clinical course in patients with *CLN2* mutations. *Am J Med Genet*, 112, 347–354.

Stephan L, Pichavant C, Bouchentouf M, Mills P, Camirand G, Tagmouti S, Rothstein D, & Tremblay JP (2006) Induction of tolerance across fully mismatched barriers by a nonmyeloablative treatment excluding antibodies or irradiation use. *Cell Transplant*, 15, 835–846.

Tamaki SJ, Jacobs Y, Dohse M, Capela A, Cooper JD, Reitsma M, He D, Tushinski R, Belichenko PV, Salehi A, Mobley W, Gage FH, Huhn S, Tsukamoto AS, Weissman IL, & Uchida N (2009) Neuroprotection of host cells by human central nervous system stem cells in a mouse model of infantile neuronal ceroid lipofuscinosis. *Cell Stem Cell*, 5, 310–319.

Taylor RM & Wolfe JH (1997) Decreased lysosomal storage in the adult MPS VII mouse brain in the vicinity of grafts of retroviral vector-corrected fibroblasts secreting high levels of beta-glucuronidase. *Nat Med*, 3, 771–774.

Welch EM, Barton ER, Zhuo J, Tomizawa Y, Friesen WJ, Trifillis P, Paushkin S, Patel M, Trotta CR, Hwang S, Wilde RG, Karp G, Takasugi J, Chen G, Jones S, Ren H, Moon YC, Corson D, Turpoff AA, Campbell JA, Conn MM, Khan A, Almstead NG, Hedrick J, Mollin A, Risher N, Weetall M, Yeh S, Branstrom AA, Colacino JM, Babiak J, Ju WD, Hirawat S, Northcutt VJ, Miller LL, Spatrick P, He F, Kawana M, Feng H, Jacobson A, Peltz SW, & Sweeney HL (2007) PTC124 targets genetic disorders caused by nonsense mutations. *Nature*, 447, 87–91.

Westermarck T, Åberg L, Santavuori P, Antila E, Edlund P, & Atroshi F (1997) Evaluation of the possible role of coenzyme Q10 and vitamin E in juvenile neuronal ceroid-lipofuscinosis (JNCL). *Mol Aspects Med*, 18 Suppl, S259–262.

Wilschanski M, Yahav Y, Yaacov Y, Blau H, Bentur L, Rivlin J, Aviram M, Bdolah-Abram T, Bebok Z, Shushi L, Kerem B, & Kerem E (2003) Gentamicin-induced correction of CFTR function in patients with cystic fibrosis and CFTR stop mutations. *N Engl J Med*, 349, 1433–1441.

Wong LF, Azzouz M, Walmsley LE, Askham Z, Wilkes FJ, Mitrophanous KA, Kingsman SM, & Mazarakis ND (2004) Transduction patterns of pseudotyped lentiviral vectors in the nervous system. *Mol Ther*, 9, 101–111.

Worgall S, Sondhi D, Hackett NR, Kosofsky B, Kekatpure MV, Neyzi N, Dyke JP, Ballon D, Heier L, Greenwald BM, Christos P, Mazumdar M, Souweidane MM, Kaplitt MG, & Crystal RG (2008) Treatment of late infantile neuronal ceroid lipofuscinosis by CNS administration of a serotype 2 adeno-associated virus expressing CLN2 cDNA. *Hum Gene Ther*, 19, 463–474.

Wraith JE, Clarke LA, Beck M, Kolodny EH, Pastores GM, Muenzer J, Rapoport DM, Berger KI, Swiedler SJ, Kakkis ED, Braakman T, Chadbourne E, Walton-Bowen K, & Cox GF (2004) Enzyme replacement therapy for mucopolysaccharidosis I: a randomized, double-blinded, placebo-controlled, multinational study of recombinant human alpha-L-iduronidase (laronidase). *J Pediatr*, 144, 581–588.

Zaiss AK & Muruve DA (2005) Immune responses to adeno-associated virus vectors. *Curr Gene Ther*, 5, 323–331.

Zhang Z, Butler JD, Levin SW, Wisniewski KE, Brooks SS, & Mukherjee AB (2001) Lysosomal ceroid depletion by drugs: therapeutic implications for a hereditary neurodegenerative disease of childhood. *Nat Med*, 7, 478–484.

Zheng Y, Rozengurt N, Ryazantsev S, Kohn DB, Satake N, & Neufeld EF (2003) Treatment of the mouse model of mucopolysaccharidosis I with retrovirally transduced bone marrow. *Mol Genet Metab*, 79, 233–244.

Chapter 22

Outlook into the Next Decade

S.E. Mole, R.E. Williams, and H.H. Goebel

CURRENT STATE

Considerable progress in elucidating and understanding the NCLs has been achieved during the last three decades, but they are far from being completely explained. Genetic and biochemical studies suggest that a new and more sensitive classification of NCL is required. It is clear that in many cases the age of onset does not indicate to which classic subdivision a patient's type belongs. The morphology is a good guide, but even here careful interpretation is required to distinguish between subtle variations—many types, particularly within the variant late infantile group, have similar morphology. The distinction between the main protein components of the storage material in different types is still unexplained. Of the NCL genes identified, three are lysosomal lumenal enzymes whereas others are definitely not. A common ground for all the NCLs still appears to be a connection with the lysosome, but this remains a hypothesis, albeit well supported. The NCLs may still eventually be split into further non-overlapping groups just as the original collection of disorders known as the amaurotic family idiocies, which had neuronal storage in common and to which NCL belonged, has been further divided into a number of biochemically and genetically distinct lysosomal disorders. However any such subdivisions of the NCLs should await a full understanding of the molecular basis of these diseases.

Research in the NCLs will continue over the next decade within the areas represented by individual sections and chapters in this book, and considerable progress is anticipated.

NCL COLLECTIONS AND DATABASES

Since there are clearly NCL genes that are unknown, it is important that samples (DNA) and cell lines of rare and atypical cases continue to be deposited with clinical, diagnostic, and research laboratories. There is encouragement that these centres are recognizing the value of these rare samples and are working together to facilitate the identification of the remaining genes through a variety of collaborative genetic and proteomic approaches (e.g. the Rare NCL Gene Consortium).

MOLECULAR GENETICS AND BIOLOGY

Despite the identification of many NCL genes, more genes that cause NCL remain to be identified. The completion of the sequencing of the human genome and many of the animal models has contributed significantly to the identification of the genes underlying rare human clinical subtypes as will recent improvements in high-throughput screening and sequencing technologies.

These advances should help provide insights into the basic biological processes involved in NCL. At the present time there is still no unifying hypothesis that explains the different NCL types, and the function of many of the identified genes remains obscure. It can be anticipated that some hypothesis will emerge which links together the diverse genes involved and the observed biochemical and ultrastructural changes.

Concurrent with the complete identification of NCL genes will be the continued elucidation of NCL gene function. The function of three genes only (*CTSD*, *CLN1*, *CLN2*), all encoding enzymes is known to date, although important details of substrates and interactions have still to be described. The function and role of the chloride channel genes are partially understood, but the function of the remaining NCL genes remains uncertain and, of course, the function of the as yet unidentified genes remains to be explored. During the next few years it is hoped that the complete elucidation of the function of all NCL gene products will be achieved.

NCL CLASSIFICATION AND DIAGNOSIS

The identification of all genes underlying NCL may provide a new and coherent genetic basis for classification. At least eight, possibly up to 11, human genetic loci are known at the present time that cause NCL or NCL-like disease, and more are expected to emerge during the next decade. Clinicians will thus be able to address the issue of clinical variants and will be able to distinguish between cases of classic childhood NCL, those causing the large group of so-called variant late infantile NCL, and those with unusual clinical manifestations. In addition the relationship between adult onset NCL (*CLN4* and perhaps others) and the many childhood forms will be understood.

The improved classification will lead to new methods for accurate diagnosis of NCL type that build on the existing practice of enzymatic testing and electron microscopy morphology and will extend into robust DNA-based methodologies for individual genes. This diagnosis, of necessity, will become more complex with time, but new technological advances should facilitate complete genetic diagnosis of most patients. More complete data on incidence and prevalence should become available.

THERAPY

The most important field of research that will continue to be developed in the next decade will be that of therapy. New experimental forms of treatment are already emerging which are based on increased understanding of the pathological process involved at a molecular level and on experience gained from treating other lysosomal storage and neurological disorders. At the moment treatment for NCL is mainly palliative and supportive as the results of ongoing clinical trials are awaited.

The first improvements in therapy may be aimed at preventing or slowing disease progression, thus being prophylactic and/or disease-modifying rather than curative. For example, therapy may be directed at influencing the rate of formation of the storage material, and more importantly at preventing degeneration and loss of nerve cells, perhaps initially targeting the eye.

The advances made in diagnosis of NCL type combined with advances in therapy will alter the significance of prenatal diagnosis. At the moment such early diagnosis leaves parents with the choice of knowingly accepting the birth of a child who will become very ill or terminating the pregnancy. In the future it is hoped that therapy will allow the correction of the basic biological problem in addition to disease prevention.

MORPHOLOGY

In order to achieve such goals, morphologists and biochemists have to further clarify why storage materials accumulate, a topic somewhat neglected at present. This will include analytical studies of the formation of extracerebral lipopigments and its significance in terms of the function of the host cells and host tissues; the complete chemical composition of the storage material; and whether and how their accumulation is related to neuronal degeneration and death. Although intensive postmortem studies on NCL tissues have been performed for more than 100 years, precise morphometric analysis of the extent and distribution of neuronal cell loss, cortical as well as subcortical, among the different clinical forms of NCL is not available. It may be that this will only be possible in the NCL animal models.

Such morphometric quantitative analysis of neuronal cell death in NCL may provide not only relevant information about neuronal cell death applicable to other human neurodegenerative disorders, but also allow more precise clinicopathological correlations. For example, it may be possible to define the association between parkinsonian clinical symptoms in juvenile NCL with the observed dearth in pigmentation of the substantia nigra, or to explain how neuronal cell loss is related to targets of projecting nigral neurons in NCL. In addition, morphometric quantitative analysis may provide an accurate reflection of the success of novel therapies.

ANIMAL MODELS

The NCLs are among the most frequent neurodegenerative diseases in children, and it is no surprise that numerous spontaneous animal models have been discovered in different species. The identification of the genes underlying mouse and dog models has influenced human research considerably, and mapping of the remaining dog loci may reveal hitherto unsuspected genes whose defects will join the NCL group of disorders. However, all the models, whether naturally occurring or experimentally derived, will contribute to further understanding of the molecular basis of NCL as the full picture of NCL genes is put together. In addition, the results of previous work on many of these models will take on new significance once it is known which type of human NCL is being mimicked. Finally, they will provide an excellent basis for the development of successful therapy.

FINAL STATEMENT

Much work remains to be done on the NCLs. This will require the continued cooperation of families, physicians, researchers, and providers of financial support, in order to fully define the molecular basis of the NCLs and provide effective treatment and therapy for those afflicted by such a devastating disorder.

Chapter 23

Appendix 1: NCL Incidence and Prevalence Data

R.E. Williams

METHOD

International NCL physician experts were contacted directly by email in 2007–2008 and asked to provide data where possible. Some family support groups were also contacted. Using population and live birth statistics, incidence and prevalence rates were calculated where possible for each country. These data were supplemented with published figures for incidence and prevalence rates.

RESULTS

Data were available from 17 countries and Newfoundland. Over 1000 surviving children and young adults with NCL from 14 countries are currently known (Table 23.1). Assuming some under-reporting, the prevalence rates for NCL may vary from 1 per million in some regions to 1:100,000 in Scandinavian countries and incidence rates for NCL may vary from 1:14,000 in Iceland to 1:67,000 in Italy and Germany. Additionally cases have been reported from Japan, Saudi Arabia, and in Arab populations.

The data available for different NCL types are much more limited and Tables 23.2–23.4 provide summaries of the incidence and prevalence data by country for CLN1 disease, CLN2 disease, and CLN3 disease respectively.

CONCLUSIONS AND COMMENTS

- NCL has a worldwide distribution.
- The incidence and prevalence appears to vary between ethnic groups and a genetic founder effect is well documented in some populations.
- So far, cases of congenital and adult NCL are rare.
- Incidence data are probably more robust than prevalence data.
- Prevalence data are likely to be gross underestimates in many countries where there are more than a few centres responsible for the medical/health/social care of affected individuals, and no routine capture of NCL data.
- Prevalence rates for NCL may vary from 1 per million in some regions to 1:100,000 in Scandinavian countries.

Table 23.1 **Incidence and prevalence rates for all NCL by country**

Country	Population (millions)	Estimated number of new NCL diagnoses per year	Estimated NCL incidence/ 100,000 live births	Estimated number of surviving cases known	Estimated NCL prevalence/million population	Source
United States	305,887,000	66	1.6–2.4	420	1.37	L. Johnson, BDSRA[1], 2008
Germany	82,062,200	10–12	1.54	143	1.74	A. Schulz, 2008*
United Kingdom	61,612,300	12–13	1.8	100–150	1.6+	BDFA[2] and BPNA PIND study[3], 2008, Verity et al., 2010
Italy	60,090,400	8	1.5	100–150	1.6+	A. Simonati, M. Santorelli, 2008*
South Africa	47,850,700	No data	No data	4	0.08	L. Johnson, BDSRA, 2008*
Argentina	39,745,613	8.75	1.28	30	0.75	Noher de Halac, 2008*
Canada	33,567,000	No data	No data	25	0.744	L. Johnson, BDSRA, 2008*
Australia	21,597,121	No data	No data	38	1.76	L. Johnson, BDSRA, 2008*
Netherlands	16,499,084	4–5	2.26	50	3	M.C. Niezen-de Boer, 2008*
Portugal	10,631,800	2–3	2.21 1.55	No data	No data	G Ribeiro, 2008* Teixeira et al., 2003
Czech Rep	10,474,600		1.3 2.29			Elleder et al., 1997 Poupetova et al., 2010
Sweden	9,259,000	No data	No data	40	4.6	Uvebrant and Hagberg, 1997
Denmark	5,519,300	No data	2–2.5	30	5.4	J. Ostergaard, 2008*
Finland	5,329,243	2–3	4.82	50	9.4	L. Aberg, M.-L. Punkari, 2008*
Norway	4,808,050	No data	3.9 (1978–1999: Augestad and Flanders, 2006)	41	8.5	I. Helland, 2008*
New Zealand	4,297,537	No data	No data	9	2.09	L. Johnson, BDSRA, 2008*
Iceland	319,326	No data	7	No data	11	Uvebrant and Hagberg, 1997
Newfoundland			13.6			Moore et al., 2008

[1]Batten Disease Support and Research Association (US and others).
[2]Batten Disease Family Association (UK).
[3]Progressive Intellectual and Neurological Deterioration Study Group, British Paediatric Surveillance Unit.
*Personal communication to the author.

Table 23.2 **Incidence and prevalence rates CLN1 disease by country**

Country	Population (millions)	Estimated number of new NCL diagnoses per year	Estimated NCL incidence/ 100,000 live births	Estimated number of surviving cases known	Estimated NCL prevalence/ million population	Source
Germany	82,062,200	4	0.05	3	0.04	A. Schulz, 2008*
United Kingdom	61,612,300	1.7	0.03	10	0.16+	BDFA[1] and BPNA PIND study[2], 2008 Verity et al., 2010
Argentina	39,745,613	0.25	0.04	7	0.17	Noher de Halac, 2008*
Portugal	10,631,800	<1		0.05		G. Ribeiro, 2008*
Sweden	9,259,000		0.06		0.7	Uvebrant and Hagberg, 1997
Denmark	5,519,300	<1		1	0.18	J. Ostergaard, 2008*
Finland	5,329,243		5.0		5.4	Uvebrant and Hagberg, 1997

[1] Batten Disease Family Association (UK).
[2] Progressive Intellectual and Neurological Deterioration Study Group, British Paediatric Surveillance Unit.
* Personal communication to the author

Table 23.3 **Incidence and prevalence rates for CLN2 disease by country**

Country	Population (millions)	Estimated number of new NCL diagnoses per year	Estimated NCL incidence/ 100,000 live births	Estimated number of surviving cases known	Estimated NCL prevalence/ million population	Source
Germany	82,062,200	15–20	0.22	62	0.75	A. Schulz, 2008*
United Kingdom	61,612,300	4.8	0.78	19	0.31+	BDFA[1] and BPNA PIND study[2], 2008 Verity et al., 2010
Argentina	39,745,613	1.75	0.25	4	0.10	Noher de Halac, 2008*
Portugal	10,631,800	1			0.15	G. Ribeiro, 2008*
Sweden	9,259,000			4	0.43	Uvebrant and Hagberg, 1997
Denmark	5,519,300	<1		3	0.54	J. Ostergaard, 2008*
Newfoundland			9.0			Moore et al., 2008

[1] Batten Disease Family Association (UK).
[2] Progressive Intellectual and Neurological Deterioration Study Group, British Paediatric Surveillance Unit.
* Personal communication to the author.

- Incidence rates for NCL may vary from 1:14,000 in Iceland to 1:67,000 in Italy and Germany.
- The most commonly diagnosed types of NCL are CLN2 and CLN3 disease.

Future international collaborations and the development of NCL disease registries may help to provide some additional epidemiological data, although their main objectives are likely to be the detailed description of disease phenotypes and the further elucidation of genotype–phenotype correlations.

Table 23.4 **Incidence and prevalence rates for CLN3 disease by country**

Country	Population (millions)	Estimated number of new NCL diagnoses per year	Estimated NCL incidence/ 100,000 live births	Estimated number of surviving cases known	Estimated NCL prevalence/ million population	Source
United States	305,887,000	30	0.7			L. Johnson, BDSRA 2008*
Germany	82,062,200	15–20	0.25	74	0.90	A. Schulz, 2008*
United Kingdom	61,612,300	3.3	0.47	26	0.42+	BDFA[1] and BPNA PIND study[2], 2008 Verity et al., 2010
Argentina	39,745,613	0.75	0.11	3	0.07+	Noher de Halac, 2008*
Portugal	10,631,800	1	0.09		0.50	G. Ribeiro, 2008*
Sweden	9,259,000		2.2	40	4.6	Uvebrant and Hagberg, 1997
Denmark	5,519,300	1	0.2	27	4.89	J. Østergaard, 2008*
Finland	5,329,243		4.8 4.4	61	12.2 9.2	Uvebrant and Hagberg, 1997 L. Aberg, M.-L. Punkari, 2009*
Norway	4,808,050		3.7	28	6.5	I. Helland, 2008*
Iceland	319,326		7.0	3	11	Uvebrant and Hagberg, 1997

[1]Batten Disease Family Association (UK).
[2]Progressive Intellectual and Neurological Deterioration Study Group, British Paediatric Surveillance Unit.
*Personal communication to the author

REFERENCES

Elleder M, Franc J, Kraus J, Nevsimalova S, Sixtova K, & Zeman J (1997) Neuronal ceroid lipofuscinosis in the Czech Republic: analysis of 57 cases. Report of the 'Prague NCL group'. *Eur J Paediatr Neurol*, 1, 109–114.

Moore SJ, Buckley DJ, MacMillan A, Marshall HD, Steele L, Ray PN, Nawaz Z, Baskin B, Frecker M, Carr SM, Ives E, & Parfrey PS (2008) The clinical and genetic epidemiology of neuronal ceroid lipofuscinosis in Newfoundland. *Clin Genet*, 74, 213–222.

Poupetova H, Ledvinova J, Berna L, Dvorakova L, Kozich V & Elleder M (2010) The birth prevalence of lysosomal storage disorders in the Czech Republic: comparison with data in different populations. *J Inherit Metab Dis*, 33, 387–396.

Teixeira C, Guimaraes A, Bessa C, Ferreira MJ, Lopes L, Pinto E, Pinto R, Boustany RM, Sa Miranda MC, & Ribeiro MG (2003) Clinicopathological and molecular characterization of neuronal ceroid lipofuscinosis in the Portuguese population. *J Neurol*, 250, 661–667.

Uvebrant P & Hagberg B (1997) Neuronal ceroid lipofuscinoses in Scandinavia. Epidemiology and clinical pictures. *Neuropediatrics*, 28, 6–8.

Verity C, Winstone AM, Stellitano L, Will R, & Nicoll A (2010) The epidemiology of progressive intellectual and neurological deterioration in childhood. *Arch Dis Child*, 95, 361–364.

Chapter 24

Appendix 2: Useful Information

S.E. Mole and R.E. Williams

FAMILY SUPPORT GROUPS

There are many groups around the world with an interest in the NCLs. These often have a national focus and may support families or raise the profile of Batten disease or raise money for research or other family needs. Such groups can make a huge difference to rare diseases such as the NCLs. Most have their own web site, and many are now also represented on networking sites such as Facebook which increases their global impact. These groups are kept updated on http://www.ucl.ac.uk/ncl/familysupport.shtml, and are listed here. There are also several foundations or web sites devoted to the story of a single family.

Europe

BELGIUM

Contact: Dr Mattheeuws Stefan, Dalstraat 12, 2400 Mol, Tel: +32 14320666, Fax: +32 14320666, Email: stefan.mattheeuws@skynet.be

THE CZECH REPUBLIC

The Prague NCL Group: Contact: Milan Elleder MD PhD, Email: melleder@cesnet.cz

DENMARK

Dansk Spielmeyer-Vogt Forening: http://www.dsvf.dk/cms.ashx

FINLAND

Family Federation provides genetic counselling: http://www.vaestoliitto.fi/in_english/
Finnish Association on Intellectual and Developmental Disabilities (FAIDD) or Finnish Association on Mental Retardation (FAMR): http://kehitysvammaliitto.fi/en; http://kehitysvammaliitto.fi

Finnish INCL Association: Suomen INCL yhdistys: http://www.incl.fi/
Finnish Federation of the Visually Impaired: http://www.nkl.fi/yleista/english.htm; http://www.nkl.fi/index.htm
NCL consultant: Maria Liisa Punkari, Email: ml.punkari@nkl.fi for Spielmeyer-Jansky Association

FRANCE

Association Vaincre les Maladies Lysosomales: http://www.vml-asso.org/

GERMANY

NCL-Foundation (NCL-Stiftung): http://www.ncl-stiftung.de/englisch/home/index.php
http://www.ncl-stiftung.de/deutsch/home/index.php
German NCL-Group (NCL-Gruppe Deutschland e.V.): http://www.ncl-deutschland.de/
Caring for others Group (Nächstenliebe e.V.): http://www.ncl-naechstenliebe.de/

IRELAND/EIRE

Bee for Battens: http://www.beeforbattens.org/

ITALY

Italian Association for NCL (Associatione Italiana per la NCL): http://www.ceroido-lipofuscinosi.it/
COMETA/A.S.M.E. Associazione Studio Malattie Metaboliche Ereditarie ONLUS: http://www.cometaasmme.org/

THE NETHERLANDS

De Nederlandse Vereniging Batten-Spielmeyer-Vogt (BSV): http://www.bsv-vereniging.nl/
Bartimeus or Bartiméushage - a centre that provides care and services for visual and intellectual disability: http://www.bartimeus.nl/

NORWAY

Norwegian NCL Family Association. Norsk Spielmeyer-Vogt Forening (NCL): http://www.nsvf.org/

PORTUGAL

Associação Portuguesa das Doenças do Lisossoma (APL) Av. Defensores de Chaves, 33 - 5°, 1000 - 111 Lisboa, Portugal. geral@aplisosoma.org

SPAIN

Ceroidolipofuscinosis: http://www.hispataxia.es/ELENA/HOME.htm

SWEDEN

Svenska Spielmeyer-Vogt Föreningen (SSVF) supports the parent group for children with Spielmeyer-Vogt disease (Föräldragruppen för Spielmeyer-Vogt): http://www.ssvf.se/
The Swedish association for the visually impaired (SRF Synskadades Riksförbund): http://www.srfgoteborg.se/

SWITZERLAND

Retina Suisse (formerly Retinitis pigmentosa-Vereinigung Schweiz): http://www.retina.ch/

UNITED KINGDOM

Batten Disease Family Association: http://www.bdfa-uk.org.uk/
British Inherited Metabolic Disease Group: http://www.bimdg.org.uk/
Children living with inherited metabolic diseases (Climb): The National Information Centre for Metabolic Diseases (formerly Research Trust for Metabolic Diseases in Children): http://www.climb.org.uk/
Contact a family - for families with disabled children: http://www.cafamily.org.uk/
Rare Disease UK Alliance: http://www.raredisease.org.uk/index.html/
Seeability: http://www.seeability.org/

Worldwide

AUSTRALIA

The Australian Chapter of the BDSRA: http://www.battens.org.au/

BRAZIL

The Brasilian Chapter of the BDSRA: Associação Brasileira Doença de Batten: http://www.abdb.com.br/index.html

CHILE

Servicio de Neuropsiquiatria Infantil, Hospital Clinico Can Borja Arriaran: http://www.neuroinf.cl/

COSTA RICA

Asociación Pro Niños(as) Con Enfermedades Progresivas (Batten), APRONEP. Contact: Mr Yamileth Chávez Soto, Education Committee Coordinator, 75 metros al sur de la Fábrica Neón Nieto, San Juan de Tibás, San José, Costa Rica, Tel: +506 236 96 20, Fax: +506 236 96 20.

NEW ZEALAND

New Zealand Battens Support Group, care of Lysosomal Diseases of New Zealand (LDNZ): http://www.ldnz.org.nz/

REPUBLIC OF SOUTH AFRICA

South Africa chapter of BDSRA: President: Pam Jooste, Contact: shanty@lantic.net

RUSSIA

Rare disease web site: www.redkiebolezni.ru
Contains information for professionals and patients about interregional patients' society of lysososomal storage disorders. E-mail: LSDrussia@yandex.ru, 115478 Moscow, Moskvorechie st 1, Zakharova E.

UNITED STATES OF AMERICA

Batten Disease Support and Research Association (BDSRA): http://www.bdsra.org/
Children's Brain Diseases Foundation. Parnassus Heights Medical Building, Suite 900, San Fransciso, CA 94117, USA. Contact: Dr Dean Rider; Email: jrider6022@aol.com

VENEZUELA

Contact: Dr Joaquín Peña, Hospital de Especialidades Pediátricas, Maracaibo. Email: juaco949@hotmail.com

ORGANIZATIONS RELEVANT TO NCL

The European Agency for Development in Special Needs Education is an independent and self-governing organization, established by its member countries to act as their platform for collaboration in the field of special needs education. It provides comprehensive lists by country: http://www.european-agency.org/

Genetic Alliance (USA): http://www.geneticalliance.org/
GOLD, the Global Organisation for Lysosomal Diseases: http://www.goldinfo.org/
Lysosomal Disease Network: http://www.lysosomaldiseasenetwork.org/resources/
National Organization for Rare Disorders (NORD): http://www.rarediseases.org/
Online Mendelian Inheritance in Man (OMIM): http://www.ncbi.nlm.nih.gov/sites/entrez?db=omim.
Orphanet. The portal for rare diseases and orphan drugs: http://www.orpha.net/
Society for the Study of Inborn Errors of Metabolism (SSIEM): http://www.ssiem.org.uk/
Specialised Healthcare Alliance (SHCA): http://www.shca.info/

NCL-SPECIFIC WEB SITES

NCL Resource—a gateway for Batten disease

http://ucl.ac.uk/ncl

NCL Mutation Database

http://www.ucl.ac.uk/ncl/mutation.shtml

NCL in mice

http://www.ucl.ac.uk/ncl/mouse.shtml

NCL in dogs

http://www.caninegeneticdiseases.net/CL_site/basicCL.htm

NCL diagnostic algorithms and approaches

http://www.ucl.ac.uk/ncl/algorithms.shtml
http://www.ucl.ac.uk/ncl/diagnostic_approach.shtml

NCL GENE AND MUTATION NOMENCLATURE

Human

http://www.genenames.org/guidelines.html for nomenclature and a searchable database.
For human, gene symbols generally are italicized, with all letters in uppercase. Protein designations are the same as the gene symbol, but are not italicized; all letters are in uppercase. mRNAs and cDNAs use the same formatting conventions as the gene symbol.
http://www.hgvs.org/rec.html.
Human Genome Variation Society guidelines for nomenclature of gene variations including mutations and variation databases.

Mouse

http://www.informatics.jax.org/mgihome/nomen/gene.shtml.
Mouse gene symbols generally are italicized, with only the first letter in uppercase and the remaining letters in lowercase. Protein designations are the same as the gene symbol, but are not italicized, all letters are in uppercase. Recessive mutant phenotypes in the mouse are known by a symbol in lower cases e.g. *nclf* or *mnd*, which is later incorporated as a specific allele once the gene had been identified (e.g. $Cln6^{nclf}$ or $Cln8^{mnd}$). There are also guidelines for knockout, knock-in, conditional, and other engineered targeted or transgene mutations.
Mouse Genome Informatics hosts a searchable database including genes and phenotypes at http://www.informatics.jax.org/.

NCL SCIENTIFIC MEETINGS

International research meetings focusing on the NCLs are currently held every 2 years, usually alternating between Europe and the USA. Occasional or other international or regional meetings may have a partial or full focus on the NCLs. These are listed at http://www.ucl.ac.uk/ncl/meetings.shtml and many are summarized here:

1980 International Symposium on Human and Animal Models of Ceroid-lipofuscinosis, Røros, Norway. 1–4 June 1980
1987 Second Congress on the Neuronal Ceroid Lipofuscinosis, Staten Island, USA. 30 May–1 June 1987
1990 Third International Conference on the Neuronal Ceroid Lipofuscinosis, Indianapolis, USA. 30 May–1 June 1990
1992 4th International Symposium on the Neuronal ceroid-lipofuscinoses, Hamburg, Germany. 10–13 June 1992
1994 Fifth International Conference on Neuronal Ceroid-Lipofuscinoses. Newark, USA. 19–21 May 1994
1996 Workshop: Advances in the neuronal ceroid-lipofuscinoses. Vth European Congress of Neuropathology. European Confederation of Neuropathological Societies. Hôpital de la Salpêtrière, Paris. 23–27 April 1996
1996 The Sixth International Congress on Neuronal Ceroid-lipofuscinoses (NCL-96). Gustavelund, Finland. 8–11 June 1996
1996 Workshop on Diagnostic (clinical and morphological) criteria of adult neuronal ceroid-lipofuscinoses (Kufs'

Disease), Paris, France. 5 December 1996

1997 Workshop on 'Retinopathy in neuronal ceroid-lipofuscinoses in comparison to retinitis pigmentosa'. Bad Horn am Bodensee, Switzerland. 1–2 March 1997.

1997 Concerted Action on Molecular Pathological and Clinical Investigations of Neuronal Ceroid Lipofuscinosis. Workshop on the Genetic and Molecular Basis of the NCLs. London, UK. 14–15 November 1997

1998 The Seventh International Congress on the Neuronal Ceroid-Lipofuscinoses (NCL-98), Dallas, USA. 13–16 June 1998

1998 Workshop on 'Neuronal ceroid-lipofuscinoses'. Mainz, Germany. 27–29 November 1998.

1999 International Workshop: Neuronal Ceroid Lipofuscinoses – Current knowledge and perspectives, Milan, Italy. 11–12 February l999

1999 12th Workshop of the European Study Group on Lysosomal Diseases, Vidago, Portugal. 24–26 September 1999

2000 NCL-2000. The 8th International Congress on Neuronal Ceroid Lipofuscinoses (Batten Disease). Exeter College, Oxford, UK. 20–24 September 2000

2003 9th International Congress on Neuronal Ceroid Lipofuscinosis (Batten Disease). Chicago, USA. 9–13 April 2003

2003 Neuronal ceroid lipofuscinoses and other genetic lysosomal storage disorders: From the clinical to the molecular aspects. Centro de Estudio de las Metabolopatías Congénitas (CEMECO), Córdoba, Argentina. 18–20 September 2003.

2005 NCL-2005. The 10th International Congress on Neuronal Ceroid Lipofuscinoses. Helsinki, Finland. 5–8 June 2005.

2006 First International Education Conference on Batten Disease: Quality of life – Lifelong enrichment. Örebro, Sweden 3–6 May 2006.

2007 NCL2007. 11th International Congress on Neuronal Ceroid Lipofuscinosis (Batten Disease). Rochester, NY, USA. 14–17 July 2007.

2009 NCL2009. 12th International Congress on Neuronal Ceroid Lipofuscinoses. Hamburg, Germany. 3–6 June 2009.

2009 17th European Study Group on Lysosomal Diseases Workshop. Bad Honnef, Germany. 10–13 September 2009.

2010 Progressive myoclonus epilepsies in the new millennium. From Marseille to Venice. Venice, Italy. 28 April–1 May 2010.

2012 13th International Congress on Neuronal Ceroid Lipofuscinoses. To be held in the United Kingdom. March 2012.

SUMMARY TABLE

Table 24.1 **Classification of human neuronal ceroid lipofuscinoses**

Disease	Eponym	OMIM number	Clinical phenotype	Former abbreviated name	Ultrastructural phenotype	Chromosome	Gene	Gene product	Stored protein
CLN1	Haltia–Santavuori	256730	Infantile classic, late infantile, juvenile, adult	INCL	GRODs	1p32	*PPT1/CLN1*	PPT1	SAPs
CLN2	Janský–Bielschowsky	204500	Late infantile classic, juvenile	LINCL	CL	11p15	*TPP1/CLN2*	TPP1	SCMAS
CLN3	Spielmeyer–Sjögren	204200	Juvenile, classic	JNCL	FP (CL, RL)	16p12	*CLN3*	CLN3	SCMAS
Kufs disease	Kufs	204300	Adult 'CLN4'	ANCL	FP, granular	?	?	?	SCMAS
CLN5	Finnish variant late infantile	256731	Late infantile variant, juvenile, adult	vLINCL	RL, CL, FP	13q22	*CLN5*	CLN5	SCMAS
CLN6	Lake–Cavanagh early juvenile variant or Indian variant late infantile	601780	Late infantile variant	vLINCL	RL, CL, FP	15q21–23	*CLN6*	CLN6	SCMAS
CLN7	Turkish variant late infantile	610951	Late infantile variant, juvenile-adult	vLINCL	RL, FP	4q28.1–28.2	*MFSD8/CLN7*	MFSD8	SCMAS
CLN8	Northern epilepsy/ EPMR	610003	EPMR, late infantile variant	vLINCL	CL-like, FP, granular	8p23	*CLN8*	CLN8	SCMAS
Juvenile variant	Juvenile variant	609055	Juvenile variant 'CLN9'	vJNCL	GRODs, CL, FP	?	?	?	SCMAS
CLN10	Congenital	610127	Congenital classic, late infantile, adult	CNCL	GRODs	11p15.5	*CTSD/CLN10*	Cathepsin D	SAPs
Parry	Parry	162350	Adult autosomal dominant	ANCL	GRODs	?	?	?	SAPs

CNCL, INCL, LINCL, vLINCL, JNCL, vJNCL and ANCL, congenital, infantile, late infantile, variant late infantile, juvenile, variant juvenile and adult onset neuronal ceroid lipofuscinosis; EPMR, progressive epilepsy with mental retardation; GRODs, granular osmiophilic deposits; CL, curvilinear profiles; FP, fingerprint bodies; RL, rectilinear profiles; SCMAS, subunit c of mitochondrial ATP synthase; SAPs, sphingolipid activator proteins.

Bibliography

Åberg L, Heiskala H, Vanhanen SL, Himberg JJ, Hosking G, Yuen A, & Santavuori P (1997) Lamotrigine therapy in infantile neuronal ceroid lipofuscinosis (INCL). *Neuropediatrics*, 28, 77–79.

Åberg L, Jarvela I, Rapola J, Autti T, Kirveskari E, Lappi M, Sipila L, & Santavuori P (1998) Atypical juvenile neuronal ceroid lipofuscinosis with granular osmiophilic deposit-like inclusions in the autonomic nerve cells of the gut wall. *Acta Neuropathol*, 95, 306–312.

Åberg L, Kirveskari E, & Santavuori P (1999) Lamotrigine therapy in juvenile neuronal ceroid lipofuscinosis. *Epilepsia*, 40, 796–799.

Åberg L, Liewendahl K, Nikkinen P, Autti T, Rinne JO, & Santavuori P (2000a) Decreased striatal dopamine transporter density in JNCL patients with parkinsonian symptoms. *Neurology*, 54, 1069–1074.

Åberg L, Talling M, Harkonen T, Lonnqvist T, Knip M, Alen R, Rantala H, & Tyynelä J (2008) Intermittent prednisolone and autoantibodies to GAD65 in juvenile neuronal ceroid lipofuscinosis. *Neurology*, 70, 1218–1220.

Åberg LE, Bäckman M, Kirveskari E, & Santavuori P (2000b) Epilepsy and antiepileptic drug therapy in juvenile neuronal ceroid lipofuscinosis. *Epilepsia*, 41, 1296–1302.

Åberg LE, Rinne JO, Rajantie I, & Santavuori P (2001) A favorable response to antiparkinsonian treatment in juvenile neuronal ceroid lipofuscinosis. *Neurology*, 56, 1236–1239.

Åberg LE, Tiitinen A, Autti TH, Kivisaari L, & Santavouri P (2002) Hyperandrogenism in girls with juvenile neuronal ceroid lipofuscinosis. *Eur J Paediatr Neurol*, 6, 199–205.

Abitbol M, Thibaud JL, Olby NJ, Hitte C, Puech JP, Maurer M, Pilot-Storck F, Hedan B, Dreano S, Brahimi S, Delattre D, Andre C, Gray F, Delisle F, Caillaud C, Bernex F, Panthier JJ, Aubin-Houzelstein G, Blot S, & Tiret L (2010) A canine arylsulfatase G (ARSG) mutation leading to a sulfatase deficiency is associated with neuronal ceroid lipofuscinosis. *Proc Natl Acad Sci U S A*, 107, 14775–14780.

Abordo-Adesida E, Follenzi A, Barcia C, Sciascia S, Castro MG, Naldini L, & Lowenstein PR (2005) Stability of lentiviral vector-mediated transgene expression in the brain in the presence of systemic antivector immune responses. *Hum Gene Ther*, 16, 741–751.

Acland GM, Aguirre GD, Ray J, Zhang Q, Aleman TS, Cideciyan AV, Pearce-Kelling SE, Anand V, Zeng Y, Maguire AM, Jacobson SG, Hauswirth WW, & Bennett J (2001) Gene therapy restores vision in a canine model of childhood blindness. *Nat Genet*, 28, 92–95.

Adams H, de Blieck EA, Mink JW, Marshall FJ, Kwon J, Dure L, Rothberg PG, Ramirez-Montealegre D, & Pearce DA (2006) Standardized assessment of behavior and adaptive living skills in juvenile neuronal ceroid lipofuscinosis. *Dev Med Child Neurol*, 48, 259–264.

Ahtiainen L, Kolikova J, Mutka AL, Luiro K, Gentile M, Ikonen E, Khiroug L, Jalanko A, & Kopra O (2007) Palmitoyl protein thioesterase 1 (Ppt1)-deficient mouse neurons show alterations in cholesterol metabolism and calcium homeostasis prior to synaptic dysfunction. *Neurobiol Dis*, 28, 52–64.

Ahtiainen L, Luiro K, Kauppi M, Tyynelä J, Kopra O, & Jalanko A (2006) Palmitoyl protein thioesterase 1 (PPT1) deficiency causes endocytic defects connected to abnormal saposin processing. *Exp Cell Res*, 312, 1540–1553.

Ahtiainen L, Van Diggelen OP, Jalanko A, & Kopra O (2003) Palmitoyl protein thioesterase 1 is targeted to the axons in neurons. *J Comp Neurol*, 455, 368–377.

Aiello C, Terracciano A, Simonati A, Discepoli G, Cannelli N, Claps D, Crow YJ, Bianchi M, Kitzmuller C, Longo D, Tavoni A, Franzoni E, Tessa A, Veneselli E, Boldrini R, Filocamo M, Williams RE, Bertini ES, Biancheri R, Carrozzo R, Mole SE, & Santorelli FM (2009) Mutations in MFSD8/CLN7 are a frequent cause of variant-late infantile neuronal ceroid lipofuscinosis. *Hum Mutat*, 30, E530–540.

Al-Muhaizea MA, Al-Hassnan ZN, & Chedrawi A (2009) Variant late infantile neuronal ceroid lipofuscinosis (CLN6 gene) in Saudi Arabia. *Pediatr Neurol*, 41, 74–76.

Aldahmesh MA, Al-Hassnan ZN, Aldosari M, & Alkuraya FS (2009) Neuronal ceroid lipofuscinosis caused by MFSD8 mutations: a common theme emerging. *Neurogenetics*, 10, 307–311.

Alroy J, Schelling SH, Thalhammer JG, Raghavan SS, Natowicz MR, Prence EM, & Orgad U (1992) Adult onset lysosomal storage disease in a Tibetan terrier: clinical, morphological and biochemical studies. *Acta Neuropathol*, 84, 658–663.

Altschul SF, Gish W, Miller W, Myers EW, & Lipman DJ (1990) Basic local alignment search tool. *J Mol Biol*, 215, 403–410.

Amalfitano A, Bengur AR, Morse RP, Majure JM, Case LE, Veerling DL, Mackey J, Kishnani P, Smith W, McVie-Wylie A, Sullivan JA, Hoganson GE, Phillips JA, 3rd, Schaefer GB, Charrow J, Ware RE, Bossen EH, & Chen YT (2001) Recombinant human acid alpha-glucosidase enzyme therapy for infantile glycogen storage disease type II: results of a phase I/II clinical trial. *Genet Med*, 3, 132–138.

Amrani N, Sachs MS, & Jacobson A (2006) Early nonsense: mRNA decay solves a translational problem. *Nat Rev Mol Cell Biol*, 7, 415–425.

Andersen KJ & McDonald JK (1987) Subcellular distribution of renal tripeptide-releasing exopeptidases active on collagen-like sequences. *Am J Physiol*, 252, F890–898.

Anderson G, Smith VV, Malone M, & Sebire NJ (2005) Blood film examination for vacuolated lymphocytes in the diagnosis of metabolic disorders; retrospective experience of more than 2,500 cases from a single centre. *J Clin Pathol*, 58, 1305–1310.

Anderson GW, Smith VV, Brooke I, Malone M, & Sebire NJ (2006) Diagnosis of neuronal ceroid lipofuscinosis (Batten disease) by electron microscopy in peripheral blood specimens. *Ultrastruct Pathol*, 30, 373–378.

Annunziata P, Pero G, Ibba L, Federico A, Bardelli AM, Sabatelli P, & Guazzi GC (1986) Adult dementia in three siblings: ceroid-lipofuscinosis. *Acta Neurol (Napoli)*, 8, 528–534.

Anzai Y, Hayashi M, Fueki N, Kurata K, & Ohya T (2006) Protracted juvenile neuronal ceroid lipofuscinosis—an autopsy report and immunohistochemical analysis. *Brain Dev*, 28, 462–465.

Aoyagi T, Morishima H, Nishizawa R, Kunimoto S, & Takeuchi T (1972) Biological activity of pepstatins, pepstanone A and partial peptides on pepsin, cathepsin D and renin. *J Antibiot (Tokyo)*, 25, 689–694.

Appleby EC, Longstaffe JA, & Bell FR (1982) Ceroid-lipofuscinosis in two Saluki dogs. *J Comp Pathol*, 92, 375–380.

Arai N (1989) 'Grumose degeneration' of the dentate nucleus. A light and electron microscopic study in nuclear palsy and dentatorubropallidoluysial atrophy. *J Neurol Sci*, 90, 131–145.

Armstrong D, Koppang N, & Rider JA (1982) *Ceroid-lipofuscinosis (Batten's disease). Proceedings of the International Symposium on Human and Animal Models of Ceroid-Lipofuscinosis*. Amsterdam, New York, Oxford, Elsevier Biomedical Press.

Aronovich EL, Carmichael KP, Morizono H, Koutlas IG, Deanching M, Hoganson G, Fischer A, & Whitley CB (2000) Canine heparan sulfate sulfamidase and the molecular pathology underlying Sanfilippo syndrome type A in Dachshunds. *Genomics*, 68, 80–84.

Asakawa K & Kawakami K (2008) Targeted gene expression by the Gal4-UAS system in zebrafish. *Dev Growth Differ*, 50, 391–399.

Autefage H, Albinet V, Garcia V, Berges H, Nicolau ML, Therville N, Altie MF, Caillaud C, Levade T, & Andrieu-Abadie N (2009) Lysosomal serine protease CLN2 regulates tumor necrosis factor-alpha-mediated apoptosis in a Bid-dependent manner. *J Biol Chem*, 284, 11507–11516.

Autti T, Raininko R, Launes J, Nuutila A, & Santavuori P (1992) Janský-Bielschowsky variant disease: CT, MRI, and SPECT findings. *Pediatr Neurol*, 8, 121–126.

Autti T, Raininko R, Santavuori P, Vanhanen SL, Poutanen VP, & Haltia M (1997) MRI of neuronal ceroid lipofuscinosis. II. Postmortem MRI and histopathological study of the brain in 16 cases of neuronal ceroid lipofuscinosis of juvenile or late infantile type. *Neuroradiology*, 39, 371–377.

Autti T, Raininko R, Vanhanen SL, & Santavuori P (1996) MRI of neuronal ceroid lipofuscinosis. I. Cranial MRI of 30 patients with juvenile neuronal ceroid lipofuscinosis. *Neuroradiology*, 38, 476–482.

Awano T, Katz ML, O'Brien DP, Sohar I, Lobel P, Coates JR, Khan S, Johnson GC, Giger U, & Johnson GS (2006a) A frame shift mutation in canine TPP1 (the ortholog of human CLN2) in a juvenile Dachshund with neuronal ceroid lipofuscinosis. *Mol Genet Metab*, 89, 254–260.

Awano T, Katz ML, O'Brien DP, Taylor JF, Evans J, Khan S, Sohar I, Lobel P, & Johnson GS (2006b) A mutation in the cathepsin D gene (CTSD) in American Bulldogs with neuronal ceroid lipofuscinosis. *Mol Genet Metab*, 87, 341–348.

Bäckman ML, Åberg LE, Aronen ET, & Santavuori PR (2001) New antidepressive and antipsychotic drugs in juvenile neuronal ceroid lipofuscinoses—a pilot study. *Eur J Paediatr Neurol*, 5 Suppl A, 163–166.

Bäckman ML, Santavuori PR, Åberg LE, & Aronen ET (2005) Psychiatric symptoms of children and adolescents with juvenile neuronal ceroid lipofuscinosis. *J Intellect Disabil Res*, 49, 25–32.

Bainbridge JW, Smith AJ, Barker SS, Robbie S, Henderson R, Balaggan K, Viswanathan A, Holder GE, Stockman A, Tyler N, Petersen-Jones S, Bhattacharya SS, Thrasher AJ, Fitzke FW, Carter BJ, Rubin GS, Moore AT, & Ali RR (2008) Effect of gene therapy on visual function in Leber's congenital amaurosis. *N Engl J Med*, 358, 2231–2239.

Baker M, Mackenzie IR, Pickering-Brown SM, Gass J, Rademakers R, Lindholm C, Snowden J, Adamson J, Sadovnick AD, Rollinson S, Cannon A, Dwosh E, Neary D, Melquist S, Richardson A, Dickson D, Berger Z, Eriksen J, Robinson T, Zehr C, Dickey CA, Crook R, McGowan E, Mann D, Boeve B, Feldman H, & Hutton M (2006) Mutations in progranulin cause tau-negative frontotemporal dementia linked to chromosome 17. *Nature*, 442, 916–919.

Baldwin SA, Beal PR, Yao SY, King AE, Cass CE, & Young JD (2004) The equilibrative nucleoside transporter family, SLC29. *Pflugers Arch*, 447, 735–743.

Bannan BA, Van Etten J, Kohler JA, Tsoi Y, Hansen NM, Sigmon S, Fowler E, Buff H, Williams TS, Ault JG, Glaser RL, & Korey CA (2008) The Drosophila protein palmitoylome: Characterizing palmitoyl-thioesterases and DHHC palmitoyl-transferases. *Fly (Austin)*, 2.

Barohn RJ, Dowd DC, & Kagan-Hallet KS (1992) Congenital ceroid-lipofuscinosis. *Pediatr Neurol*, 8, 54–59.

Barros TP, Alderton WK, Reynolds HM, Roach AG, & Berghmans S (2008) Zebrafish: an emerging technology for in vivo pharmacological assessment to identify potential safety liabilities in early drug discovery. *Br J Pharmacol*, 154, 1400–1413.

Barthez-Carpentier MA, Billard C, Maheut J, Santini JJ, & Ruchoux MM (1991) A case of childhood Kufs' disease. *J Neurol Neurosurg Psychiatry*, 54, 655–657.

Barton NW, Brady RO, Dambrosia JM, Di Bisceglie AM, Doppelt SH, Hill SC, Mankin HJ, Murray GJ, Parker RI, Argoff CE, Grewal RP, Yu K-T, & Collaborators (1991) Replacement therapy for inherited enzyme deficiency—macrophage-targeted glucocerebrosidase for Gaucher's disease. *N Engl J Med*, 324, 1464–1470.

Barton NW, Furbish FS, Murray GJ, Garfield M, & Brady RO (1990) Therapeutic response to intravenous infusions of glucocerebrosidase in a patient with Gaucher disease. *Proc Natl Acad Sci U S A*, 87, 1913–1916.

Barwell KJ & Broom MF (2001) A yeast model for classical juvenile Batten disease (CLN3). *Eur J Paediatr Neurol*, 5 Suppl A, 127–129.

Batten FE (1903) Cerebral degeneration with symmetrical changes in the maculae in two members of a family. *Trans Ophthalmol Soc UK*, 23, 386–390.

Batten FE (1914) Family cerebral degeneration with macular change (so-called juvenile form of family amaurotic idiocy). *Q J Med*, 7, 444–454.

Batten FE & Mayou MS (1915) Family cerebral degeneration with macular changes. *Proc R Soc Med*, 8, 70–90.

Beaudoin D, Hagenzieker J, & Jack R (2004) Neuronal ceroid lipofuscinosis: what are the roles of electron microscopy, DNA, and enzyme analysis in diagnosis. *J Histotechnol*, 27, 237–243.

Bellizzi JJ, 3rd, Widom J, Kemp C, Lu JY, Das AK, Hofmann SL, & Clardy J (2000) The crystal structure of palmitoyl protein thioesterase 1 and the molecular basis of infantile neuronal ceroid lipofuscinosis. *Proc Natl Acad Sci U S A*, 97, 4573–4578.

Benedict JW, Getty AL, Wishart TM, Gillingwater TH, & Pearce DA (2009) Protein product of CLN6 gene responsible for variant late-onset infantile neuronal ceroid lipofuscinosis interacts with CRMP-2. *J Neurosci Res*, 87, 2157–2166.

Benedict JW, Sommers CA, & Pearce DA (2007) Progressive oxidative damage in the central nervous system of a murine model for juvenile Batten disease. *J Neurosci Res*, 85, 2882–2891.

Benes P, Vetvicka V, & Fusek M (2008) Cathepsin D—many functions of one aspartic protease. *Crit Rev Oncol Hematol*, 68, 12–28.

Bennett J, Tanabe T, Sun D, Zeng Y, Kjeldbye H, Gouras P, & Maguire AM (1996) Photoreceptor cell rescue in retinal degeneration (rd) mice by in vivo gene therapy. *Nat Med*, 2, 649–654.

Bennett MJ, Gayton AR, Rittey CD, & Hosking GP (1994) Juvenile neuronal ceroid-lipofuscinosis: developmental progress after supplementation with polyunsaturated fatty acids. *Dev Med Child Neurol*, 36, 630–638.

Bensaoula T, Shibuya H, Katz ML, Smith JE, Johnson GS, John SK, & Milam AH (2000) Histopathologic and immunocytochemical analysis of the retina and ocular tissues in Batten disease. *Ophthalmology*, 107, 1746–1753.

Benuck M, Grynbaum A, & Marks N (1978) Breakdown of somatostatin and substance P by cathepsin D purified from calf brain by affinity chromatography. *Brain Res*, 143, 181–185.

Berger J, Suzuki T, Senti KA, Stubbs J, Schaffner G, & Dickson BJ (2001) Genetic mapping with SNP markers in Drosophila. *Nat Genet*, 29, 475–481.

Berkovic SF, Carpenter S, Andermann F, Andermann E, & Wolfe LS (1988) Kufs' disease: a critical reappraisal. *Brain*, 111 (Pt 1), 27–62.

Berkovic SF, So NK, & Andermann F (1991) Progressive myoclonus epilepsies: clinical and neurophysiological diagnosis. *J Clin Neurophysiol*, 8, 261–274.

Bernardini F & Warburton MJ (2001) The substrate range of tripeptidyl-peptidase I. *Eur J Paediatr Neurol*, 5 Suppl A, 69–72.

Bernardini F & Warburton MJ (2002) Lysosomal degradation of cholecystokinin-(29-33)-amide in mouse brain is dependent on tripeptidyl peptidase-I: implications for the degradation and storage of peptides in classical late-infantile neuronal ceroid lipofuscinosis. *Biochem J*, 366, 521–529.

Berry-Kravis E, Sleat DE, Sohar I, Meyer P, Donnelly R, & Lobel P (2000) Prenatal testing for late infantile neuronal ceroid lipofuscinosis. *Ann Neurol*, 47, 254–257.

Bertoni-Freddari C, Fattoretti P, Casoli T, Di Stefano G, Solazzi M, & Corvi E (2002) Morphometric investigations of the mitochondrial damage in ceroid lipopigment accumulation due to vitamin E deficiency. *Arch Gerontol Geriatr*, 34, 269–274.

Bessa C, Teixeira CA, Dias A, Alves M, Rocha S, Lacerda L, Loureiro L, Guimaraes A, & Ribeiro MG (2008) CLN2/TPP1 deficiency: the novel mutation IVS7-10A>G causes intron retention and is associated with a mild disease phenotype. *Mol Genet Metab*, 93, 66–73.

Bessa C, Teixeira CA, Mangas M, Dias A, Sa Miranda MC, Guimaraes A, Ferreira JC, Canas N, Cabral P, & Ribeiro MG (2006) Two novel CLN5 mutations in a Portuguese patient with vLINCL: insights into molecular mechanisms of CLN5 deficiency. *Mol Genet Metab*, 89, 245–253.

Bi HY, Yao S, Bu DF, Wang ZX, Zhang Y, Qin J, Yang YL, & Yuan Y (2006) [Two novel mutations in palmitoyl-protein thioesterase gene in 2 Chinese babies with infantile neuronal ceroid lipofuscinosis]. *Zhonghua Er Ke Za Zhi*, 44, 496–499.

Bianchi L, Miller DM, 3rd, & George AL, Jr. (2001) Expression of a CIC chloride channel in Caenorhabditis elegans gamma-aminobutyric acid-ergic neurons. *Neurosci Lett*, 299, 177–180.

Bible E, Gupta P, Hofmann SL, & Cooper JD (2004) Regional and cellular neuropathology in the palmitoyl protein thioesterase-1 null mutant mouse model of infantile neuronal ceroid lipofuscinosis. *Neurobiol Dis*, 16, 346–359.

Bielschowsky M (1913) Über spätinfantile familiäre amaurotische Idiotie mit Kleinhirnsymptonen. *Deutsche Zeitschrift für Nervenheilkunde*, 50, 7–29.

Bielschowsky M (1920) Zur Histopathologie und Pathogenese der amaurotischen Idiotie mit besonderer Berücksichtigung der zerebellaren Veränderungen. *J Psychol Neurol (Leipzig)*, 26, 123–99.

Bielschowsky M (1928) Amaurotische Idiotie und lipoidzellige Splenohepatomegalie. *J Psychol Neurol (Leipzig)*, 36, 103–123.

Bielschowsky M (1932) Review on 'Revision in der Pathobiologie und Pathogenese der Infantil-amaurotischen Idiotie' by K. Schaffer. *Zentralbl Ges Neurol Psychiatr*, 63, 367–370.

Bielschowsky M (1936) Über eine bisher unbekannte Form von infantiler amaurotischer Idiotie. *Zentralbl Ges Neurol Psychiatr*, 155, 321–329 .

Biffi A, De Palma M, Quattrini A, Del Carro U, Amadio S, Visigalli I, Sessa M, Fasano S, Brambilla R, Marchesini S, Bordignon C, & Naldini L (2004) Correction of metachromatic leukodystrophy in the mouse model by transplantation of genetically modified hematopoietic stem cells. *J Clin Invest*, 113, 1118–1129.

Bildfell R, Matwichuk C, Mitchell S, & Ward P (1995) Neuronal ceroid-lipofuscinosis in a cat. *Vet Pathol*, 32, 485–488.

Binelli S, Canafoglia L, Panzica F, Pozzi A, & Franceschetti S (2000) Electroencephalographic features in a series of patients with neuronal ceroid lipofuscinoses. *Neurol Sci*, 21, S83–87.

Bischof G, Hammerstein W, & Goebel HH (1983) [Fundus dystrophy and ceroid-lipofuscinosis]. *Fortschr Ophthalmol*, 80, 97–99.

Blumenthal T & Gleason KS (2003) Caenorhabditis elegans operons: form and function. *Nat Rev Genet*, 4, 112–120.

Boehme DH, Cottrell JC, Leonberg SC, & Zeman W (1971) A dominant form of neuronal ceroid-lipofuscinosis. *Brain*, 94, 745–760.

Boellaard JW & Schlote W (1986) Ultrastructural heterogeneity of neuronal lipofuscin in the normal human cerebral cortex. *Acta Neuropathol*, 71, 285–294.

Bolivar VJ, Scott Ganus J, & Messer A (2002) The development of behavioral abnormalities in the motor neuron degeneration (mnd) mouse. *Brain Res*, 937, 74–82.

Bone N, Millar JB, Toda T, & Armstrong J (1998) Regulated vacuole fusion and fission in Schizosaccharomyces pombe: an osmotic response dependent on MAP kinases. *Curr Biol*, 8, 135–144.

Bonsignore M, Tessa A, Di Rosa G, Piemonte F, Dionisi-Vici C, Simonati A, Calamoneri F, Tortorella G, & Santorelli FM (2006) Novel CLN1 mutation in two Italian sibs with late infantile neuronal ceroid lipofuscinosis. *Eur J Paediatr Neurol*, 10, 154–156.

Boriack RL, Cortinas E, & Bennett MJ (1995) Mitochondrial damage results in a reversible increase in lysosomal storage material in lymphoblasts from patients with juvenile neuronal ceroid-lipofuscinosis (Batten Disease). *Am J Med Genet*, 57, 301–303.

Boulin T, Etchberger JF, & Hobert O (2006) Reporter gene fusions. *In The C. elegans Research Community (Eds.) WormBook*. doi/10.1895/wormbook.1.106.1, http://www.wormbook.org.

Boustany RM (1992) Neurology of the neuronal ceroid-lipofuscinoses: late infantile and juvenile types. *Am J Med Genet*, 42, 533–535.

Boustany RM & Zucker A (2006) Degenerative diseases primarily of gray matter. In Swaiman KF, Ashwal S, Ferriero DM (Eds.) *Pediatric Neurology: Principles and Practice*, 4th edn, pp. 1315–1344 Philadelphia, PA, Mosby.

Braak H & Braak E (1987) Projection neurons of basolateral amygdaloid nuclei develop meganeurites in juvenile and adult human neuronal ceroid lipofuscinosis. *Clin Neuropathol*, 6, 116–119.

Braak H & Braak E (1993) Pathoarchitectonic pattern of iso- and allocortical lesions in juvenile and adult neuronal ceroid-lipofuscinosis. *J Inherit Metab Dis*, 16, 259–262.

Braak H & Goebel HH (1978) Loss of pigment-laden stellate cells: a severe alteration of the isocortex in juvenile neuronal ceroid-lipofuscinosis. *Acta Neuropathol*, 42, 53–57.

Braak H & Goebel HH (1979) Pigmentoarchitectonic pathology of the isocortex in juvenile neuronal ceroid-lipofuscinosis: axonal enlargements in layer IIIab and cell loss in layer V. *Acta Neuropathol*, 46, 79–83.

Brand AH & Perrimon N (1993) Targeted gene expression as a means of altering cell fates and generating dominant phenotypes. *Development*, 118, 401–415.

Breen M, Hitte C, Lorentzen TD, Thomas R, Cadieu E, Sabacan L, Scott A, Evanno G, Parker HG, Kirkness EF, Hudson R, Guyon R, Mahairas GG, Gelfenbeyn B, Fraser CM, Andre C, Galibert F, & Ostrander EA (2004) An integrated 4249 marker FISH/RH map of the canine genome. *BMC Genomics*, 5, 65.

Brenner S (1974) The genetics of Caenorhabditis elegans. *Genetics*, 77, 71–94.

Brix K, Dunkhorst A, Mayer K, & Jordans S (2008) Cysteine cathepsins: cellular roadmap to different functions. *Biochimie*, 90, 194–207.

Brockmann K, Pouwels PJ, Christen HJ, Frahm J, & Hanefeld F (1996) Localized proton magnetic resonance spectroscopy of cerebral metabolic disturbances in children with neuronal ceroid lipofuscinosis. *Neuropediatrics*, 27, 242–248.

Bronson RT, Donahue LR, Johnson KR, Tanner A, Lane PW, & Faust JR (1998) Neuronal ceroid lipofuscinosis (nclf), a new disorder of the mouse linked to chromosome 9. *Am J Med Genet*, 77, 289–297.

Bronson RT, Lake BD, Cook S, Taylor S, & Davisson MT (1993) Motor neuron degeneration of mice is a model of neuronal ceroid lipofuscinosis (Batten's disease). *Ann Neurol*, 33, 381–385.

Brooks AI, Chattopadhyay S, Mitchison HM, Nussbaum RL, & Pearce DA (2003) Functional categorization of gene expression changes in the cerebellum of a Cln3-knockout mouse model for Batten disease. *Mol Genet Metab*, 78, 17–30.

Broom MF, Zhou C, Broom JE, Barwell KJ, Jolly RD, & Hill DF (1998) Ovine neuronal ceroid lipofuscinosis: a large animal model syntenic with the human neuronal ceroid lipofuscinosis variant CLN6. *J Med Genet*, 35, 717–721.

Brown NJ, Corner BD, & Dodgson MC (1954) A second case in the same family of congenital familial cerebral lipoidosis resembling amaurotic family idiocy. *Arch Dis Child*, 29, 48–54.

Broyer M, Tete MJ, Guest G, Bertheleme JP, Labrousse F, & Poisson M (1996) Clinical polymorphism of cystinosis encephalopathy. Results of treatment with cysteamine. *J Inherit Metab Dis*, 19, 65–75.

Brück W & Goebel HH (1998) Microglia activation in neuronal ceroid-lipofuscinosis. *Clin Neuropathol*, 5, 276 (poster P29).

Brunk UT & Terman A (2002) Lipofuscin: mechanisms of age-related accumulation and influence on cell function. *Free Radic Biol Med*, 33, 611–619.

Bruun I, Reske-Nielsen E, & Oster S (1991) Juvenile ceroid-lipofuscinosis and calcifications of the CNS. *Acta Neurol Scand*, 83, 1–8.

Buff H, Smith AC, & Korey CA (2007) Genetic modifiers of Drosophila palmitoyl-protein thioesterase 1-induced degeneration. *Genetics*, 176, 209–220.

Burneo JG, Arnold T, Palmer CA, Kuzniecky RI, Oh SJ, & Faught E (2003) Adult-onset neuronal ceroid lipofuscinosis (Kufs disease) with autosomal dominant inheritance in Alabama. *Epilepsia*, 44, 841–846.

Buzy A, Ryan EM, Jennings KR, Palmer DN, & Griffiths DE (1996) Use of electrospray ionization mass spectrometry and tandem mass spectrometry to study binding of F0 inhibitors to ceroid lipofuscinosis protein, a model system for subunit c of mitochondrial ATP synthase. *Rapid Commun Mass Spectrom*, 10, 790–796.

Cabrera-Salazar MA, Roskelley EM, Bu J, Hodges BL, Yew N, Dodge JC, Shihabuddin LS, Sohar I, Sleat DE, Scheule RK, Davidson BL, Cheng SH, Lobel P, & Passini MA (2007) Timing of therapeutic intervention determines functional and survival outcomes in a mouse model of late infantile Batten disease. *Mol Ther*, 15, 1782–1788.

Caillaud C, Manicom J, Puech JP, Lobel P, & Poenaru L (1999) Enzymatic and molecular pre and postnatal diagnosis of ceroid lipofuscinoses in France. *Am J Hum Genet*, 65 (Suppl), A232.

Calero G, Gupta P, Nonato MC, Tandel S, Biehl ER, Hofmann SL, & Clardy J (2003) The crystal structure of palmitoyl protein thioesterase-2 (PPT2) reveals the basis for divergent substrate specificities of the two lysosomal thioesterases, PPT1 and PPT2. *J Biol Chem*, 278, 37957–37964.

Callagy C, O'Neill G, Murphy SF, & Farrell MA (2000) Adult neuronal ceroid lipofuscinosis (Kufs' disease) in two siblings of an Irish family. *Clin Neuropathol*, 19, 109–118.

Camp LA & Hofmann SL (1993) Purification and properties of a palmitoyl-protein thioesterase that cleaves palmitate from H-Ras. *J Biol Chem*, 268, 22566–22574.

Camp LA & Hofmann SL (1995) Assay and isolation of palmitoyl-protein thioesterase from bovine brain using palmitoylated H-Ras as substrate. *Methods Enzymol*, 250, 336–347.

Camp LA, Verkruyse LA, Afendis SJ, Slaughter CA, & Hofmann SL (1994) Molecular cloning and expression of palmitoyl-protein thioesterase. *J Biol Chem*, 269, 23212–23219.

Cannelli N, Cassandrini D, Bertini E, Striano P, Fusco L, Gaggero R, Specchio N, Biancheri R, Vigevano F, Bruno C, Simonati A, Zara F, & Santorelli FM (2006) Novel mutations in CLN8 in Italian variant late infantile neuronal ceroid lipofuscinosis: Another genetic hit in the Mediterranean. *Neurogenetics*, 7, 111–117.

Cannelli N, Garavaglia B, Simonati A, Aiello C, Barzaghi C, Pezzini F, Cilio MR, Biancheri R, Morbin M, Dalla Bernardina B, Granata T, Tessa A, Invernizzi F, Pessagno A, Boldrini R, Zibordi F, Grazian L, Claps D, Carrozzo R, Mole SE, Nardocci N, & Santorelli FM (2009) Variant late infantile ceroid lipofuscinoses associated with novel mutations in CLN6. *Biochem Biophys Res Commun*, 379, 892–897.

Cannelli N, Nardocci N, Cassandrini D, Morbin M, Aiello C, Bugiani M, Criscuolo L, Zara F, Striano P, Granata T, Bertini E, Simonati A, & Santorelli FM (2007) Revelation of a novel CLN5 mutation in early juvenile neuronal ceroid lipofuscinosis. *Neuropediatrics*, 38, 46–49.

Canuel M, Libin Y, & Morales CR (2009) The interactomics of sortilin: an ancient lysosomal receptor evolving new functions. *Histol Histopathol*, 24, 481–492.

Cao Y, Espinola JA, Fossale E, Massey AC, Cuervo AM, MacDonald ME, & Cotman SL (2006) Autophagy is disrupted in a knock-in mouse model of juvenile neuronal ceroid lipofuscinosis. *J Biol Chem*, 281, 20483–20493.

Cardona F & Rosati E (1995) Neuronal ceroid-lipofuscinoses in Italy: an epidemiological study. *Am J Med Genet*, 57, 142–143.

Carpenter S (1988) Morphological diagnosis and misdiagnosis in Batten-Kufs disease. *Am J Med Genet*, 5 Suppl, 85–91.

Carpenter S, Karpati G, & Andermann F (1972) Specific involvement of muscle, nerve, and skin in late infantile and juvenile amaurotic idiocy. *Neurology*, 22, 170–186.

Carpenter S, Karpati G, Andermann F, Jacob JC, & Andermann E (1977) The ultrastructural characteristics of the abnormal cytosomes in Batten-Kufs' disease. *Brain*, 100, 137–156.

Cataldo AM, Barnett JL, Berman SA, Li J, Quarless S, Bursztajn S, Lippa C, & Nixon RA (1995) Gene expression and cellular content of cathepsin D in Alzheimer's disease brain: evidence for early upregulation of the endosomal-lysosomal system. *Neuron*, 14, 671–680.

Cataldo AM, Peterhoff CM, Troncoso JC, Gomez-Isla T, Hyman BT, & Nixon RA (2000) Endocytic pathway abnormalities precede amyloid beta deposition in sporadic Alzheimer's disease and Down syndrome: differential effects of APOE genotype and presenilin mutations. *Am J Pathol*, 157, 277–286.

Cearley CN & Wolfe JH (2006) Transduction characteristics of adeno-associated virus vectors expressing cap serotypes 7, 8, 9, and Rh10 in the mouse brain. *Mol Ther*, 13, 528–537.

Cesta MF, Mozzachio K, Little PB, Olby NJ, Sills RC, & Brown TT (2006) Neuronal ceroid lipofuscinosis in a Vietnamese pot-bellied pig (Sus scrofa). *Vet Pathol*, 43, 556–560.

Ceuterick C & Martin J-J (1998) Extracerebral biopsy in lysosomal and peroxisomal disorders: ultrastructural finding. *Brain Pathol*, 8, 121–132.

Ceuterick C, Martin JJ, Casaer P, & Edgar GW (1976) The diagnosis of infantile generalized ceroidlipofuscinosis (type Hagberg-Santavuori) using skin biopsy. *Neuropadiatrie*, 7, 250–260.

Chalhoub N, Benachenhou N, Rajapurohitam V, Pata M, Ferron M, Frattini A, Villa A, & Vacher J (2003) Grey-lethal mutation induces severe malignant autosomal recessive osteopetrosis in mouse and human. *Nat Med*, 9, 399–406.

Chan CH, Mitchison HM, & Pearce DA (2008) Transcript and in silico analysis of CLN3 in juvenile neuronal ceroid lipofuscinosis and associated mouse models. *Hum Mol Genet*, 17, 3332–3339.

Chan CH, Ramirez-Montealegre D, & Pearce DA (2009) Altered arginine metabolism in the central nervous system (CNS) of the $Cln3^{-/-}$ mouse model of juvenile Batten disease. *Neuropathol Appl Neurobiol*, 35, 189–207.

Chang B, Bronson RT, Hawes NL, Roderick TH, Peng C, Hageman GS, & Heckenlively JR (1994) Retinal degeneration in motor neuron degeneration: a mouse model of ceroid lipofuscinosis. *Invest Ophthalmol Vis Sci*, 35, 1071–1076.

Chang JW, Choi H, Kim HJ, Jo DG, Jeon YJ, Noh JY, Park WJ, & Jung YK (2007) Neuronal vulnerability of CLN3 deletion to calcium-induced cytotoxicity is mediated by calsenilin. *Hum Mol Genet*, 16, 317–326.

Chang M, Cooper JD, Sleat DE, Cheng SH, Dodge JC, Passini MA, Lobel P, & Davidson BL (2008) Intraventricular enzyme replacement improves disease phenotypes in a mouse model of late infantile neuronal ceroid lipofuscinosis. *Mol Ther*, 16, 649–656.

Charles N, Vighetto A, Pialat J, Confavreux C, & Aimard G (1990) [Dementia and psychiatric disorders in Kufs disease]. *Rev Neurol (Paris)*, 146, 752–756.

Chattopadhyay S, Ito M, Cooper JD, Brooks AI, Curran TM, Powers JM, & Pearce DA (2002a) An autoantibody inhibitory to glutamic acid decarboxylase in the neurodegenerative disorder Batten disease. *Hum Mol Genet*, 11, 1421–1431.

Chattopadhyay S, Kriscenski-Perry E, Wenger DA, & Pearce DA (2002b) An autoantibody to GAD65 in sera of patients with juvenile neuronal ceroid lipofuscinoses. *Neurology*, 59, 1816–1817.

Chattopadhyay S, Muzaffar NE, Sherman F, & Pearce DA (2000) The yeast model for Batten disease: mutations in BTN1, BTN2, and HSP30 alter pH homeostasis. *J Bacteriol*, 182, 6418–6423.

Chattopadhyay S & Pearce DA (2000) Neural and extraneural expression of the neuronal ceroid lipofuscinoses genes CLN1, CLN2, and CLN3: functional implications for CLN3. *Mol Genet Metab*, 71, 207–211.

Chattopadhyay S & Pearce DA (2002) Interaction with Btn2p is required for localization of Rsglp: Btn2p-mediated changes in arginine uptake in Saccharomyces cerevisiae. *Eukaryot Cell*, 1, 606–612.

Chattopadhyay S, Roberts PM, & Pearce DA (2003) The yeast model for Batten disease: a role for Btn2p in the trafficking of the Golgi-associated vesicular targeting protein, Yif1p. *Biochem Biophys Res Commun*, 302, 534–538.

Chen CS, Bach G, & Pagano RE (1998) Abnormal transport along the lysosomal pathway in mucolipidosis, type IV disease. *Proc Natl Acad Sci U S A*, 95, 6373–6378.

Chen R, Fearnley IM, Palmer DN, & Walker JE (2004) Lysine 43 is trimethylated in subunit C from bovine mitochondrial ATP synthase and in storage bodies associated with Batten disease. *J Biol Chem*, 279, 21883–21887.

Chen YH, Chang M, & Davidson BL (2009) Molecular signatures of disease brain endothelia provide new sites for CNS-directed enzyme therapy. *Nat Med*, 15, 1215–1218.

Chio KS & Tappel AL (1969a) Inactivation of ribonuclease and other enzymes by peroxidizing lipids and by malonaldehyde. *Biochemistry*, 8, 2827–2832.

Chio KS & Tappel AL (1969b) Synthesis and characterization of the fluorescent products derived from malonaldehyde and amino acids. *Biochemistry*, 8, 2821–2826.

Cho DY, Leipold HW, & Rudolph R (1986) Neuronal ceroidosis (ceroid-lipofuscinosis) in a Blue Heeler dog. *Acta Neuropathol*, 69, 161–164.

Cho S & Dawson G (2000) Palmitoyl protein thioesterase 1 protects against apoptosis mediated by Ras-Akt-caspase pathway in neuroblastoma cells. *J Neurochem*, 74, 1478–1488.

Cho S, Dawson PE, & Dawson G (2000) Antisense palmitoyl protein thioesterase 1 (PPT1) treatment inhibits PPT1 activity and increases cell death in LA-N-5 neuroblastoma cells. *J Neurosci Res*, 62, 234–240.

Cho S, Dawson PE, & Dawson G (2001) Role of palmitoyl-protein thioesterase in cell death: implications for infantile neuronal ceroid lipofuscinosis. *Eur J Paediatr Neurol*, 5 Suppl A, 53–55.

Cho SK & Hofmann SL (2004) pdf1, a palmitoyl protein thioesterase 1 Ortholog in Schizosaccharomyces pombe: a yeast model of infantile Batten disease. *Eukaryot Cell*, 3, 302–310.

Choi DW (1988) Glutamate neurotoxicity and diseases of the nervous system. *Neuron*, 1, 623–634.

Chow CW, Borg J, Billson VR, & Lake BD (1993) Fetal tissue involvement in the late infantile type of neuronal ceroid lipofuscinosis. *Prenat Diagn*, 13, 833–841.

Cismondi IA, Cannelli N, Aiello C, Santorelli FM, Kohan R, Ramírez AMO, & Halac IN (2008a) Novel human pathological mutations: Gene symbol: CLN5: Neuronal ceroid lipofuscinosis, Finnish variant. *Hum Genet*, 123, 537–555.

Cismondi IA, Kohan R, Ghio A, Ramirez AM, & Halac IN (2008b) Novel human pathological mutations: Gene symbol: CLN6. Disease: Neuronal ceroid lipofuscinosis, late infantile. *Hum Genet*, 124, 324.

Claussen M, Heim P, Knispel J, Goebel HH, & Kohlschutter A (1992) Incidence of neuronal ceroid-lipofuscinoses in West Germany: variation of a method for studying autosomal recessive disorders. *Am J Med Genet*, 42, 536–538.

Claussen M, Kubler B, Wendland M, Neifer K, Schmidt B, Zapf J, & Braulke T (1997) Proteolysis of insulin-like growth factors (IGF) and IGF binding proteins by cathepsin D. *Endocrinology*, 138, 3797–3803.

Codlin S, Haines RL, Burden JJ, & Mole SE (2008a) Btn1 affects cytokinesis and cell-wall deposition by independent mechanisms, one of which is linked to dysregulation of vacuole pH. *J Cell Sci*, 121, 2860–2870.

Codlin S, Haines RL, & Mole SE (2008b) btn1 affects endocytosis, polarization of sterol-rich membrane domains and polarized growth in Schizosaccharomyces pombe. *Traffic*, 9, 936–950.

Codlin S & Mole SE (2009) S. pombe btn1, the orthologue of the Batten disease gene CLN3, is required for vacuole protein sorting of Cpy1p and Golgi exit of Vps10p. *J Cell Sci*, 122, 1163–1173.

Collins J, Holder GE, Herbert H, & Adams GG (2006) Batten disease: features to facilitate early diagnosis. *Br J Ophthalmol*, 90, 1119–1124.

Comellas-Bigler M, Maskos K, Huber R, Oyama H, Oda K, & Bode W (2004) 1.2 A crystal structure of the serine carboxyl proteinase pro-kumamolisin; structure of an intact pro-subtilase. *Structure*, 12, 1313–1323.

Concha ML, Russell C, Regan JC, Tawk M, Sidi S, Gilmour DT, Kapsimali M, Sumoy L, Goldstone K, Amaya E, Kimelman D, Nicolson T, Grunder S, Gomperts M, Clarke JD, & Wilson SW (2003) Local tissue interactions across the dorsal midline of the forebrain establish CNS laterality. *Neuron*, 39, 423–438.

Constantinidis J, Wisniewski KE, & Wisniewski TM (1992) The adult and a new late adult forms of neuronal ceroid lipofuscinosis. *Acta Neuropathol*, 83, 461–468.

Cook RW, Jolly RD, Palmer DN, Tammen I, Broom MF, & McKinnon R (2002) Neuronal ceroid lipofuscinosis in Merino sheep. *Aust Vet J*, 80, 292–297.

Cooper JD (2008) Moving towards therapies for juvenile Batten disease? *Exp Neurol*, 211, 329–331.

Cooper JD, Messer A, Feng AK, Chua-Couzens J, & Mobley WC (1999) Apparent loss and hypertrophy of interneurons in a mouse model of neuronal ceroid lipofuscinosis: evidence for partial response to insulin-like growth factor-1 treatment. *J Neurosci*, 19, 2556–2567.

Cooper JD, Russell C, & Mitchison HM (2006) Progress towards understanding disease mechanisms in small vertebrate models of neuronal ceroid lipofuscinosis. *Biochim Biophys Acta*, 1762, 873–889.

Corpet F (1988) Multiple sequence alignment with hierarchical clustering. *Nucleic Acids Res*, 16, 10881–10890.

Cotman SL, Vrbanac V, Lebel LA, Lee RL, Johnson KA, Donahue LR, Teed AM, Antonellis K, Bronson RT, Lerner TJ, & MacDonald ME (2002) $Cln3^{\Delta ex7/8}$ knock-in mice with the common JNCL mutation exhibit progressive neurologic disease that begins before birth. *Hum Mol Genet*, 11, 2709–2721.

Cottone CD, Chattopadhyay S, & Pearce DA (2001) Searching for interacting partners of CLN1, CLN2 and Btn1p with the two-hybrid system. *Eur J Paediatr Neurol*, 5 Suppl A, 95–98.

Croopnick JB, Choi HC, & Mueller DM (1998) The subcellular location of the yeast Saccharomyces cerevisiae homologue of the protein defective in the juvenile form of Batten disease. *Biochem Biophys Res Commun*, 250, 335–341.

Crow YJ, Tolmie JL, Howatson AG, Patrick WJ, & Stephenson JB (1997) Batten disease in the west of Scotland 1974-1995 including five cases of the juvenile form with granular osmiophilic deposits. *Neuropediatrics*, 28, 140–144.

Cruts M, Gijselinck I, van der Zee J, Engelborghs S, Wils H, Pirici D, Rademakers R, Vandenberghe R, Dermaut B, Martin JJ, van Duijn C, Peeters K, Sciot R, Santens P, De Pooter T, Mattheijssens M, Van den Broeck M, Cuijt I, Vennekens K, De Deyn PP, Kumar-Singh S, & Van Broeckhoven C (2006) Null mutations in progranulin cause ubiquitin-positive frontotemporal dementia linked to chromosome 17q21. *Nature*, 442, 920–924.

Cruz-Sanchez FF, Rossi ML, Cardozo A, Picardo A, & Tolosa E (1992) Immunohistological study of grumose degeneration of the dentate nucleus in progressive supranuclear palsy. *J Neurol Sci*, 110, 228–231.

Crystal RG, Sondhi D, Hackett NR, Kaminsky SM, Worgall S, Stieg P, Souweidane M, Hosain S, Heier L, Ballon D, Dinner M, Wisniewski K, Kaplitt M, Greenwald BM, Howell JD, Strybing K, Dyke J, & Voss H (2004) Clinical protocol. Administration of a replication-deficient adeno-associated virus gene transfer vector expressing the human CLN2 cDNA to the brain of children with late infantile neuronal ceroid lipofuscinosis. *Hum Gene Ther*, 15, 1131–1154.

Culetto E & Sattelle DB (2000) A role for Caenorhabditis elegans in understanding the function and interactions of human disease genes. *Hum Mol Genet*, 9, 869–877.

Cullen V, Lindfors M, Ng J, Paetau A, Swinton E, Kolodziej P, Boston H, Saftig P, Woulfe J, Feany MB, Myllykangas L, Schlossmacher MG, & Tyynelä J (2009) Cathepsin D expression level affects alpha-synuclein processing, aggregation, and toxicity in vivo. *Mol Brain*, 2, 5.

Cummings BJ, Uchida N, Tamaki SJ, & Anderson AJ (2006) Human neural stem cell differentiation following transplantation into spinal cord injured mice: association with recovery of locomotor function. *Neurol Res*, 28, 474–481.

Cummings JF & de Lahunta A (1977) An adult case of canine neuronal ceroid-lipofuscinosis. *Acta Neuropathol*, 39, 43–51.

Das AK, Becerra CH, Yi W, Lu JY, Siakotos AN, Wisniewski KE, & Hofmann SL (1998) Molecular genetics of palmitoyl-protein thioesterase deficiency in the U.S. *J Clin Invest*, 102, 361–370.

Das AK, Bellizzi JJ, 3rd, Tandel S, Biehl E, Clardy J, & Hofmann SL (2000) Structural basis for the insensitivity of a serine enzyme (palmitoyl-protein thioesterase) to phenylmethylsulfonyl fluoride. *J Biol Chem*, 275, 23847–23851.

Das AK, Lu JY, & Hofmann SL (2001a) Biochemical analysis of mutations in palmitoyl-protein thioesterase causing infantile and late-onset forms of neuronal ceroid lipofuscinosis. *Hum Mol Genet*, 10, 1431–1439.

Das AM, Jolly RD, & Kohlschutter A (1999) Anomalies of mitochondrial ATP synthase regulation in four different types of neuronal ceroid lipofuscinosis. *Mol Genet Metab*, 66, 349–355.

Das AM, von Harlem R, Feist M, Lucke T, & Kohlschutter A (2001b) Altered levels of high-energy phosphate compounds in fibroblasts from different forms of neuronal ceroid lipofuscinoses: further evidence for mitochondrial involvement. *Eur J Paediatr Neurol*, 5 Suppl A, 143–146.

Dawson G, Kilkus J, Siakotos AN, & Singh I (1996) Mitochondrial abnormalities in CLN2 and CLN3 forms of Batten disease. *Mol Chem Neuropathol*, 29, 227–235.

Dawson G, Schroeder C, & Dawson PE (2010) Palmitoyl:protein thioesterase (PPT1) inhibitors can act as pharmacological chaperones in infantile Batten disease. *Biochem Biophys Res Commun*, 395, 66–69.

Dawson WW, Armstrong D, Greer M, Maida TM, & Samuelson DA (1985) Disease-specific electrophysiological findings in adult ceroid-lipofuscinosis (Kufs disease). *Doc Ophthalmol*, 60, 163–171.

de los Reyes E, Dyken PR, Phillips P, Brodsky M, Bates S, Glasier C, & Mrak RE (2004) Profound infantile neuroretinal dysfunction in a heterozygote for the CLN3 genetic defect. *J Child Neurol*, 19, 42–46.

de Voer G, der Bent P, Rodrigues AJ, van Ommen GJ, Peters DJ, & Taschner PE (2005) Deletion of the Caenorhabditis elegans homologues of the CLN3 gene, involved in human juvenile neuronal ceroid lipofuscinosis, causes a mild progeric phenotype. *J Inherit Metab Dis*, 28, 1065–1080.

de Voer G, Jansen G, van Ommen G-JB, Peters DJM, & Taschner PEM (2001) Caenorhabditis elegans homologues of the CLN3 gene, mutated in juvenile neuronal ceroid lipofuscinosis. *Eur J Paediat Neurol*, 5 SupplA, 115–120.

de Voer G, Peters D, & Taschner PE (2008) Caenorhabditis elegans as a model for lysosomal storage disorders. *Biochim Biophys Acta*, 1782, 433–446.

Defacque H, Egeberg M, Habermann A, Diakonova M, Roy C, Mangeat P, Voelter W, Marriott G, Pfannstiel J, Faulstich H, & Griffiths G (2000) Involvement of ezrin/moesin in de novo actin assembly on phagosomal membranes. *EMBO J*, 19, 199–212.

Dermaut B, Norga KK, Kania A, Verstreken P, Pan H, Zhou Y, Callaerts P, & Bellen HJ (2005) Aberrant lysosomal carbohydrate storage accompanies endocytic defects and neurodegeneration in Drosophila benchwarmer. *J Cell Biol*, 170, 127–139.

Desai UA, Pallos J, Ma AA, Stockwell BR, Thompson LM, Marsh JL, & Diamond MI (2006) Biologically active molecules that reduce polyglutamine aggregation and toxicity. *Hum Mol Genet*, 15, 2114–2124.

Dhar S, Bitting RL, Rylova SN, Jansen PJ, Lockhart E, Koeberl DD, Amalfitano A, & Boustany RM (2002) Flupirtine blocks apoptosis in Batten patient lymphoblasts and in human postmitotic CLN3- and CLN2-deficient neurons. *Ann Neurol*, 51, 448–466.

Dickerson LW, Bonthius DJ, Schutte BC, Yang B, Barna TJ, Bailey MC, Nehrke K, Williamson RA, & Lamb FS (2002) Altered GABAergic function accompanies hippocampal degeneration in mice lacking ClC-3 voltage-gated chloride channels. *Brain Res*, 958, 227–250.

Dickson LR, Dopfmer I, Dalefield RR, Graydon RJ, & Jolly RD (1989) A method of cerebro-cortical biopsy in lambs. *N Z Vet J*, 37, 21–22.

Dierks T, Dickmanns A, Preusser-Kunze A, Schmidt B, Mariappan M, von Figura K, Ficner R, & Rudolph MG (2005) Molecular basis for multiple sulfatase deficiency and mechanism for formylglycine generation of the human formylglycine-generating enzyme. *Cell*, 121, 541–552.

van Diggelen OP, Keulemans JL, Kleijer WJ, Thobois S, Tilikete C, & Voznyi YV (2001a) Pre- and postnatal enzyme analysis for infantile, late infantile and adult neuronal ceroid lipofuscinosis (CLN1 and CLN2). *Eur J Paediatr Neurol*, **5** Suppl A, 189–192.

van Diggelen OP, Keulemans JL, Winchester B, Hofman IL, Vanhanen SL, Santavuori P, & Voznyi YV (1999) A rapid fluorogenic palmitoyl-protein thioesterase assay: pre- and postnatal diagnosis of INCL. *Mol Genet Metab*, 66, 240–244.

van Diggelen OP, Thobois S, Tilikete C, Zabot MT, Keulemans JL, van Bunderen PA, Taschner PE, Losekoot M, & Voznyi YV (2001b) Adult neuronal ceroid lipofuscinosis with palmitoyl-protein thioesterase deficiency: first adult-onset patients of a childhood disease. *Ann Neurol*, 50, 269–272.

Diment S, Martin KJ, & Stahl PD (1989) Cleavage of parathyroid hormone in macrophage endosomes illustrates a novel pathway for intracellular processing of proteins. *J Biol Chem*, 264, 13403–13406.

Dittmer F, Ulbrich EJ, Hafner A, Schmahl W, Meister T, Pohlmann R, & von Figura K (1999) Alternative mechanisms for trafficking of lysosomal enzymes in mannose 6-phosphate receptor-deficient mice are cell type-specific. *J Cell Sci*, 112 (Pt 10), 1591–1597.

Dom R, Brucher JM, Ceuterick C, Carton H, & Martin JJ (1979) Adult ceroid-lipofuscinosis (Kufs' disease) in two brothers. Retinal and visceral storage in one; diagnostic muscle biopsy in the other. *Acta Neuropathol*, 45, 67–72.

Donnet A, Habib M, Pellissier JF, Regis H, Farnarier G, Pelletier J, Gosset A, Roger J, & Khalil R (1992) Kufs' disease presenting as progressive dementia with late-onset generalized seizures: a clinicopathological and electrophysiological study. *Epilepsia*, 33, 65–74.

Drach LM (1996) Meeting report: Dementia with Lewy bodies - Tower of Babel tumbled down? *Clin Neuropathol*, 15, 248.

Drögemüller C, Wohlke A, & Distl O (2005a) Characterization of candidate genes for neuronal ceroid lipofuscinosis in dog. *J Hered*, 96, 735–738.

Drögemüller C, Wohlke A, & Distl O (2005b) Evaluation of the canine TPP1 gene as a candidate for neuronal ceroid lipofuscinosis in Tibetan Terrier and Polish Owczarek Nizinny dogs. *Anim Genet*, 36, 178–179.

Duncan JA & Gilman AG (1998) A cytoplasmic acyl-protein thioesterase that removes palmitate from G protein alpha subunits and p21(RAS). *J Biol Chem*, 273, 15830–15837.

Dyken P & Wisniewski K (1995) Classification of the neuronal ceroid-lipofuscinoses: expansion of the atypical forms. *Am J Med Genet*, 57, 150–154.

Edwards JF, Storts RW, Joyce JR, Shelton JM, & Menzies CS (1994) Juvenile-onset neuronal ceroid-lipofuscinosis in Rambouillet sheep. *Vet Pathol*, 31, 48–54.

Eiberg H, Gardiner RM, & Mohr J (1989) Batten disease (Spielmeyer-Sjogren disease) and haptoglobins (HP): indication of linkage and assignment to chr. 16. *Clin Genet*, 36, 217–218.

Ekker SC & Larson JD (2001) Morphant technology in model developmental systems. *Genesis*, 30, 89–93.

Eksandh LB, Ponjavic VB, Munroe PB, Eiberg HE, Uvebrant PE, Ehinger BE, Mole SE, & Andreasson S (2000) Full-field ERG in patients with Batten/Spielmeyer-Vogt disease caused by mutations in the CLN3 gene. *Ophthalmic Genet*, 21, 69–77.

El-Husseini Ael D & Bredt DS (2002) Protein palmitoylation: a regulator of neuronal development and function. *Nat Rev Neurosci*, 3, 791–802.

Eliason SL, Stein CS, Mao Q, Tecedor L, Ding SL, Gaines DM, & Davidson BL (2007) A knock-in reporter model of Batten disease. *J Neurosci*, 27, 9826–9834.

Elleder M (1978) A histochemical and ultrastructural study of stored material in neuronal ceroid lipofuscinosis. *Virchows Arch B Cell Pathol*, 28, 167–178.

Elleder M (1981) *Chemical characterization of age pigments*. Amsterdam, New York, Elsevier North Holland Biomedical Press.

Elleder M (1989) Lectin histochemical study of lipopigments with special regard to neuronal ceroid-lipofuscinosis. Results with concanavalin A. *Histochemistry*, 93, 197–205.

Elleder M, Dvorakova L, Stolnaja L, Vlaskova H, Hulková H, Druga R, Poupetova H, Kostalova E, & Mikulastik J (2008) Atypical CLN2 with later onset and prolonged course: a neuropathologic study showing different sensitivity of neuronal subpopulations to TPP1 deficiency. *Acta Neuropathol*, 116, 119–124.

Elleder M, Franc J, Kraus J, Nevsimalova S, Sixtova K, & Zeman J (1997a) Neuronal ceroid lipofuscinosis in the Czech Republic: analysis of 57 cases. Report of the 'Prague NCL group'. *Eur J Paediatr Neurol*, 1, 109–114.

Elleder M, Goebel HH, & Koppang N (1989) Lectin histochemical study of lipopigments: results with concanavalin A. *Adv Exp Med Biol*, 266, 243–258.

Elleder M, Lake BD, Gobel HH, Rapola J, Haltia M, & Carpenter S (1999) Definitions of the ultrastructural patterns found in NCL. In Goebel HH, Mole SE, & Lake BD (Eds.) *The Neuronal Ceroid Lipofuscinoses (Batten Disease)*, pp. 5–15. Amsterdam, IOS Press.

Elleder M, Sokolova J, & Hrebicek M (1997b) Follow-up study of subunit c of mitochondrial ATP synthase (SCMAS) in Batten disease and in unrelated lysosomal disorders. *Acta Neuropathol*, 93, 379–390.

Elleder M & Tyynelä J (1998) Incidence of neuronal perikaryal spheroids in neuronal ceroid lipofuscinoses (Batten disease). *Clin Neuropathol*, 17, 184–189.

Elleder M, Voldrich L, Ulehlova L, Dimitt S, & Armstrong D (1988) Light and electron microscopic appearance of the inner ear in juvenile ceroid lipofuscinosis (CL). *Pathol Res Pract*, 183, 301–307.

Elshatory Y, Brooks AI, Chattopadhyay S, Curran TM, Gupta P, Ramalingam V, Hofmann SL, & Pearce DA (2003) Early changes in gene expression in two models of Batten disease. *FEBS Lett*, 538, 207–212.

Engel J (2006) *Multiaxial classification of child and adolescent psychiatric disorders: The ICD-10 classification of mental and behavioral disorders in children and adolescents*. Geneva, WHO.

Evans J, Katz ML, Levesque D, Shelton GD, A.Lahunta, & O'Brien D (2005) Neuronal ceroid lipofuscinosis in the American bulldog: a variant form of the storage disease in a related population. *J Vet Intern Med*, 19, 44–51.

Ezaki J, Takeda-Ezaki M, Koike M, Ohsawa Y, Taka H, Mineki R, Murayama K, Uchiyama Y, Ueno T, & Kominami E (2003) Characterization of Cln3p, the gene product responsible for juvenile neuronal ceroid lipofuscinosis, as a lysosomal integral membrane glycoprotein. *J Neurochem*, 87, 1296–1308.

Ezaki J, Takeda-Ezaki M, & Kominami E (2000a) Tripeptidyl peptidase I, the late infantile neuronal ceroid lipofuscinosis gene product, initiates the lysosomal degradation of subunit c of ATP synthase. *J Biochem*, 128, 509–516.

Ezaki J, Takeda-Ezaki M, Oda K, & Kominami E (2000b) Characterization of endopeptidase activity of tripeptidyl peptidase-I/CLN2 protein which is deficient in classical late infantile neuronal ceroid lipofuscinosis. *Biochem Biophys Res Commun*, 268, 904–908.

Ezaki J, Tanida I, Kanehagi N, & Kominami E (1999) A lysosomal proteinase, the late infantile neuronal ceroid lipofuscinosis gene (CLN2) product, is essential for degradation of a hydrophobic protein, the subunit c of ATP synthase. *J Neurochem*, 72, 2573–2582.

Ezaki J, Wolfe LS, & Kominami E (1997) Decreased lysosomal subunit c-degrading activity in fibroblasts from patients with late infantile neuronal ceroid lipofuscinosis. *Neuropediatrics*, 28, 53–55.

Fan JQ, Ishii S, Asano N, & Suzuki Y (1999) Accelerated transport and maturation of lysosomal alpha-galactosidase A in Fabry lymphoblasts by an enzyme inhibitor. *Nat Med*, 5, 112–115.

Fares H & Greenwald I (2001a) Genetic analysis of endocytosis in Caenorhabditis elegans: coelomocyte uptake defective mutants. *Genetics*, 159, 133–145.

Fares H & Greenwald I (2001b) Regulation of endocytosis by CUP-5, the Caenorhabditis elegans mucolipin-1 homolog. *Nat Genet*, 28, 64–68.

Farias FH, Zeng R; Johnson GS, Wininger FA, Taylor JF, Schnabel RD, McKay SD, Sanders DN; Lohi H, Seppälä EH, Wade CM, Lindblad-Toh K, O'Brien DP, Katz ML (2010) A truncating mutation in ATP13A2 is responsible for adult-onset neuronal ceroid lipofuscinosis in Tibetan Terriers. Submitted.

Faust JR, Rodman JS, Daniel PF, Dice JF, & Bronson RT (1994) Two related proteolipids and dolichol-linked oligosaccharides accumulate in motor neuron degeneration mice (mnd/mnd), a model for neuronal ceroid lipofuscinosis. *J Biol Chem*, 269, 10150–10155.

Fealey ME, Edwards WD, Grogan M, & Orszulak TA (2009) Neuronal ceroid lipofuscinosis in a 31-year-old woman presenting as biventricular heart failure with restrictive features. *Cardiovasc Pathol*, 18, 44–48.

Fearnley IM, Walker JE, Martinus RD, Jolly RD, Kirkland KB, Shaw GJ, & Palmer DN (1990) The sequence of the major protein stored in ovine ceroid lipofuscinosis is identical with that of the dicyclohexylcarbodiimide-reactive proteolipid of mitochondrial ATP synthase. *Biochem J*, 268, 751–758.

Felbor U, Kessler B, Mothes W, Goebel HH, Ploegh HL, Bronson RT, & Olsen BR (2002) Neuronal loss and brain atrophy in mice lacking cathepsins B and L. *Proc Natl Acad Sci U S A*, 99, 7883–7888.

Ferrer I, Arbizu T, Peña J, & Serra JP (1980) A golgi and ultrastructural study of a dominant form of Kufs' disease. *J Neurol*, 222, 183–190.

Finley KD, Edeen PT, Cumming RC, Mardahl-Dumesnil MD, Taylor BJ, Rodriguez MH, Hwang CE, Benedetti M, & McKeown M (2003) *Blue cheese* mutations define a novel, conserved gene involved in progressive neural degeneration. *J Neurosci*, 23, 1254–1264.

Fischer A, Carmichael KP, Munnell JF, Jhabvala P, Thompson JN, Matalon R, Jezyk PF, Wang P, & Giger U (1998) Sulfamidase deficiency in a family of Dachshunds: a canine model of mucopolysaccharidosis IIIA (Sanfilippo A). *Pediatr Res*, 44, 74–82.

Fiske RA & Storts RW (1988) Neuronal ceroid-lipofuscinosis in Nubian goats. *Vet Pathol*, 25, 171–173.

Fluegel ML, Parker TJ, & Pallanck LJ (2006) Mutations of a Drosophila NPC1 gene confer sterol and ecdysone metabolic defects. *Genetics*, 172, 185–196.

Fortini ME & Bonini NM (2000) Modeling human neurodegenerative diseases in Drosophila: on a wing and a prayer. *Trends Genet*, 16, 161–167.

Fossale E, Wolf P, Espinola JA, Lubicz-Nawrocka T, Teed AM, Gao H, Rigamonti D, Cattaneo E, MacDonald ME, & Cotman SL (2004) Membrane trafficking and mitochondrial abnormalities precede subunit c deposition in a cerebellar cell model of juvenile neuronal ceroid lipofuscinosis. *BMC Neurosci*, 5, 57.

Fowler DJ, Anderson G, Vellodi A, Malone M, & Sebire NJ (2007) Electron microscopy of chorionic villus samples for prenatal diagnosis of lysosomal storage disorders. *Ultrastruct Pathol*, 31, 15–21.

France M, Geraghty F, & Taylor R (1999) Ceroid lipofuscinosis in ferrets. *Annual Conference Australian Society Veterinary Pathology*, 1, 50.

Fratantoni JC, Hall CW, & Neufeld EF (1968) Hurler and Hunter syndromes: mutual correction of the defect in cultured fibroblasts. *Science*, 162, 570–572.

Frattini A, Pangrazio A, Susani L, Sobacchi C, Mirolo M, Abinun M, Andolina M, Flanagan A, Horwitz EM, Mihci E, Notarangelo LD, Ramenghi U, Teti A, Van Hove J, Vujic D, Young T, Albertini A, Orchard PJ, Vezzoni P, & Villa A (2003) Chloride channel ClCN7 mutations are responsible for severe recessive, dominant, and intermediate osteopetrosis. *J Bone Miner Res*, 18, 1740–1747.

Fritchie K, Siintola E, Armao D, Lehesjoki AE, Marino T, Powell C, Tennison M, Booker JM, Koch S, Partanen S, Suzuki K, Tyynelä J, & Thorne LB (2009) Novel mutation and the first prenatal screening of cathepsin D deficiency (CLN10). *Acta Neuropathol*, 117, 201–208.

Frugier T, Mitchell NL, Tammen I, Houweling PJ, Arthur DG, Kay GW, van Diggelen OP, Jolly RD, & Palmer DN (2008) A new large animal model of CLN5 neuronal ceroid lipofuscinosis in Borderdale sheep is caused by a nucleotide substitution at a consensus splice site (c.571+1G>>>A) leading to excision of exon 3. *Neurobiol Dis*, 29, 306–315.

Fujita K, Yamauchi M, Matsui T, Titani K, Takahashi H, Kato T, Isomura G, Ando M, & Nagata Y (1998) Increase of glial fibrillary acidic protein fragments in the spinal cord of motor neuron degeneration mutant mouse. *Brain Res*, 785, 31–40.

Fukushige T, Goszczynski B, Tian H, & McGhee JD (2003) The evolutionary duplication and probable demise of an endodermal GATA factor in Caenorhabditis elegans. *Genetics*, 165, 575–588.

Fusek M & Vetvicka V (1994) Mitogenic function of human procathepsin D: the role of the propeptide. *Biochem J*, 303 (Pt 3), 775–780.

Gachet Y, Codlin S, Hyams JS, & Mole SE (2005) btn1, the Schizosaccharomyces pombe homologue of the human

Batten disease gene CLN3, regulates vacuole homeostasis. *J Cell Sci*, 118, 5525–5536.

Galvin N, Vogler C, Levy B, Kovacs A, Griffey M, & Sands MS (2008) A murine model of infantile neuronal ceroid lipofuscinosis – ultrastructural evaluation of storage in the central nervous system and viscera. *Pediatr Dev Pathol*, 11, 185–192.

Gao H, Boustany RM, Espinola JA, Cotman SL, Srinidhi L, Antonellis KA, Gillis T, Qin X, Liu S, Donahue LR, Bronson RT, Faust JR, Stout D, Haines JL, Lerner TJ, & MacDonald ME (2002) Mutations in a novel CLN6-encoded transmembrane protein cause variant neuronal ceroid lipofuscinosis in man and mouse. *Am J Hum Genet*, 70, 324–335.

Garborg I, Torvik A, Hals J, Tangsrud SE, & Lindemann R (1987) Congenital neuronal ceroid lipofuscinosis. A case report. *Acta Pathol Microbiol Immunol Scand A*, 95, 119–125.

Gelot A, Maurage CA, Rodriguez D, Perrier-Pallisson D, Larmande P, & Ruchoux MM (1998) In vivo diagnosis of Kufs' disease by extracerebral biopsies. *Acta Neuropathol*, 96, 102–108.

Gille M Brucher JM, Indekeu P, Bis-teau M, & Kollmann P (1995) Maladie de Kufs avec leucoencéphalopathie. *Rev Neurol (Paris)*, 151, 392–397.

Glaser RL, Hickey AJ, Chotkowski HL, & Chu-LaGraff Q (2003) Characterization of Drosophila palmitoyl-protein thioesterase 1. *Gene*, 312, 271–279.

Glondu M, Coopman P, Laurent-Matha V, Garcia M, Rochefort H, & Liaudet-Coopman E (2001) A mutated cathepsin-D devoid of its catalytic activity stimulates the growth of cancer cells. *Oncogene*, 20, 6920–6929.

Glondu M, Liaudet-Coopman E, Derocq D, Platet N, Rochefort H, & Garcia M (2002) Down-regulation of cathepsin-D expression by antisense gene transfer inhibits tumor growth and experimental lung metastasis of human breast cancer cells. *Oncogene*, 21, 5127–5134.

Goebel HH (1997) Neurodegenerative diseases: Biopsy diagnosis in children. In Garcia JH, Budka H, McKeever PE, Sarnat HB, & Sima AAF (Eds.) *Neuropathology. The Diagnostic Approach*, pp. 581–635. St. Louis, MO, Mosby.

Goebel HH, Bilzer T, Dahme E, & Malkusch F (1988a) Morphological studies in canine (Dalmatian) neuronal ceroid-lipofuscinosis. *Am J Med Genet Suppl*, 5, 127–139.

Goebel HH & Braak H (1989) Adult neuronal ceroid-lipofuscinosis. *Clin Neuropathol*, 8, 109–119.

Goebel HH, Braak H, Seidel D, Doshi R, Marsden CD, & Gullotta F (1982) Morphologic studies on adult neuronal-ceroid lipofuscinosis (NCL). *Clin Neuropathol*, 1, 151–162.

Goebel HH & Dahme E (1985) Retinal ultrastructure of neuronal ceroid-lipofuscinosis in the dalmatian dog. *Acta Neuropathol*, 68, 224–229.

Goebel HH, Gerhard L, Kominami E, & Haltia M (1996) Neuronal ceroid-lipofuscinosis—late-infantile or Janský-Bielschowsky type—revisited. *Brain Pathol*, 6, 225–228.

Goebel HH, Gullotta F, Bajanowski T, Hansen FJ, & Braak H (1995a) Pigment variant of neuronal ceroid-lipofuscinosis. *Am J Med Genet*, 57, 155–159.

Goebel HH, Ikeda K, Schulz F, Burck U, & Kohlschutter A (1981) Fingerprint profiles in lymphocytic vacuoles of mucopolysaccharidoses I-H, II, III-A, and III-B. *Acta Neuropathol*, 55, 247–249.

Goebel HH, Jaynes M, Gutmann L, & Schochet S (1997) Diagnostic biopsy of extracerebral tissue in adult neuronal ceroid-lipofuscinosis. *Neuropathol Appl Neurobiol*, 23, 167–168.

Goebel HH, Klein H, Santavuori P, & Sainio K (1988b) Ultrastructural studies of the retina in infantile neuronal ceroid-lipofuscinosis. *Retina*, 8, 59–66.

Goebel HH, Kominami E, Neuen-Jacob E, & Wheeler RB (2001) Morphological studies on CLN2. *Eur J Paediatr Neurol*, 5 Suppl A, 203–207.

Goebel HH, Koppang N, & Zeman W (1979a) Ultrastructure of the retina in canine neuronal ceroid lipofuscinosis. *Ophthalmic Res*, 11, 65–72.

Goebel HH, Mole SE, & Lake BD (Eds.) (1999) *The Neuronal Ceroid Lipofuscinoses (Batten Disease)*. Amsterdam, IOS Press.

Goebel HH, Pilz H, & Gullotta F (1976) The protracted form of juvenile neuronal ceroid-lipofuscinosis. *Acta Neuropathol*, 36, 393–396.

Goebel HH, Schochet SS, Jaynes M, & Gutmann L (1998) Ultrastructure of the retina in adult neuronal ceroid lipofuscinosis. *Acta Anat (Basel)*, 162, 127–132.

Goebel HH, Warlo I, Klockgether T, & Harzer K (1995b) Significance of lipopigments with fingerprint profiles in eccrine sweat gland epithelial cells. *Am J Med Genet*, 57, 187–190.

Goebel HH, Zeman W, Patel VK, Pullarkat RK, & Lenard HG (1979b) On the ultrastructural diversity and essence of residual bodies in neuronal ceroid-lipofuscinosis. *Mech Ageing Dev*, 10, 53–70.

Golabek AA, Kaczmarski W, Kida E, Kaczmarski A, Michalewski MP, & Wisniewski KE (1999) Expression studies of CLN3 protein (battenin) in fusion with the green fluorescent protein in mammalian cells in vitro. *Mol Genet Metab*, 66, 277–282.

Golabek AA & Kida E (2006) Tripeptidyl-peptidase I in health and disease. *Biol Chem*, 387, 1091–1099.

Golabek AA, Kida E, Walus M, Kaczmarski W, Michalewski M, & Wisniewski KE (2000) CLN3 protein regulates lysosomal pH and alters intracellular processing of Alzheimer's amyloid-beta protein precursor and cathepsin D in human cells. *Mol Genet Metab*, 70, 203–213.

Golabek AA, Kida E, Walus M, Wujek P, Mehta P, & Wisniewski KE (2003) Biosynthesis, glycosylation, and enzymatic processing in vivo of human tripeptidyl-peptidase I. *J Biol Chem*, 278, 7135–7145.

Golabek AA, Walus M, Wisniewski KE, & Kida E (2005) Glycosaminoglycans modulate activation, activity, and stability of tripeptidyl-peptidase I in vitro and in vivo. *J Biol Chem*, 280, 7550–7561.

Golabek AA, Wujek P, Walus M, Bieler S, Soto C, Wisniewski KE, & Kida E (2004) Maturation of human tripeptidyl-peptidase I in vitro. *J Biol Chem*, 279, 31058–31067.

Goldberg-Stern H, Halevi A, Marom D, Straussberg R, & Mimouni-Bloch A (2009) Late infantile neuronal ceroid lipofuscinosis: a new mutation in Arabs. *Pediatr Neurol*, 41, 297–300.

Gorski SM, Chittaranjan S, Pleasance ED, Freeman JD, Anderson CL, Varhol RJ, Coughlin SM, Zuyderduyn SD, Jones SJ, & Marra MA (2003) A SAGE approach to discovery of genes involved in autophagic cell death. *Curr Biol*, 13, 358–363.

Gospe SM, Jr. & Jankovic J (1986) Drug-induced dystonia in neuronal ceroid-lipofuscinosis. *Pediatr Neurol*, 2, 236–237.

Gottlob I, Leipert KP, Kohlschutter A, & Goebel HH (1988) Electrophysiological findings of neuronal ceroid lipofuscinosis in heterozygotes. *Graefes Arch Clin Exp Ophthalmol*, 226, 516–521.

Granier LA, Langley K, Leray C, & Sarlieve LL (2000) Phospholipid composition in late infantile neuronal ceroid lipofuscinosis. *Eur J Clin Invest*, 30, 1011–1017.

Grasl-Kraupp B, Ruttkay-Nedecky B, Koudelka H, Bukowska K, Bursch W, & Schulte-Hermann R (1995) In situ detection of fragmented DNA (TUNEL assay) fails to discriminate among apoptosis, necrosis, and autolytic cell death: a cautionary note. *Hepatology*, 21, 1465–1468.

Gray F, Destee A, Bourre JM, Gherardi R, Krivosic I, Warot P, & Poirier J (1987) Pigmentary type of orthochromatic leukodystrophy (OLD): a new case with ultrastructural and biochemical study. *J Neuropathol Exp Neurol*, 46, 585–596.

Gray YH, Sved JA, Preston CR, & Engels WR (1998) Structure and associated mutational effects of the cysteine proteinase (CP1) gene of Drosophila melanogaster. *Insect Mol Biol*, 7, 291–293.

Graydon RJ & Jolly RD (1984) Ceroid-lipofuscinosis (Batten's disease). Sequential electrophysiologic and pathologic changes in the retina of the ovine model. *Invest Ophthalmol Vis Sci*, 25, 294–301.

Green PD & Little PB (1974) Neuronal ceroid-lipofuscin storage in Siamese cats. *Can J Comp Med*, 38, 207–212.

Gregory CY & Bird AC (1995) Cell loss in retinal dystrophies by apoptosis—death by informed consent! *Br J Ophthalmol*, 79, 186–190.

Griffey M, Bible E, Vogler C, Levy B, Gupta P, Cooper J, & Sands MS (2004) Adeno-associated virus 2-mediated gene therapy decreases autofluorescent storage material and increases brain mass in a murine model of infantile neuronal ceroid lipofuscinosis. *Neurobiol Dis*, 16, 360–369.

Griffey M, Macauley SL, Ogilvie JM, & Sands MS (2005) AAV2-mediated ocular gene therapy for infantile neuronal ceroid lipofuscinosis. *Mol Ther*, 12, 413–421.

Griffey MA, Wozniak D, Wong M, Bible E, Johnson K, Rothman SM, Wentz AE, Cooper JD, & Sands MS (2006) CNS-directed AAV2-mediated gene therapy ameliorates functional deficits in a murine model of infantile neuronal ceroid lipofuscinosis. *Mol Ther*, 13, 538–547.

Griffin JL, Muller D, Woograsingh R, Jowatt V, Hindmarsh A, Nicholson JK, & Martin JE (2002) Vitamin E deficiency and metabolic deficits in neuronal ceroid lipofuscinosis described by bioinformatics. *Physiol Genomics*, 11, 195–203.

Guarneri R, Russo D, Cascio C, D'Agostino S, Galizzi G, Bigini P, Mennini T, & Guarneri P (2004) Retinal oxidation, apoptosis and age- and sex-differences in the mnd mutant mouse, a model of neuronal ceroid lipofuscinosis. *Brain Res*, 1014, 209–220.

Guhaniyogi J, Sohar I, Das K, Stock AM & Lobel P (2009) Crystal structure and autoactivation pathway of the precursor form of human tripeptidyl-peptidase 1, the enzyme deficient in late infantile ceroid lipofuscinosis. *J Biol Chem*, 284: 3985–97.

Guo S (2004) Linking genes to brain, behavior and neurological diseases: what can we learn from zebrafish? *Genes Brain Behav*, 3, 63–74.

Guo WX, Mao C, Obeid LM, & Boustany RM (1999) A disrupted homologue of the human CLN3 or juvenile neuronal ceroid lipofuscinosis gene in Saccharomyces cerevisiae: a model to study Batten disease. *Cell Mol Neurobiol*, 19, 671–680.

Gupta P, Soyombo AA, Atashband A, Wisniewski KE, Shelton JM, Richardson JA, Hammer RE, & Hofmann SL (2001) Disruption of PPT1 or PPT2 causes neuronal ceroid lipofuscinosis in knockout mice. *Proc Natl Acad Sci U S A*, 98, 13566–13571.

Gupta P, Soyombo AA, Shelton JM, Wilkofsky IG, Wisniewski KE, Richardson JA, & Hofmann SL (2003) Disruption of PPT2 in mice causes an unusual lysosomal storage disorder with neurovisceral features. *Proc Natl Acad Sci U S A*, 100, 12325–12330.

Gutteridge JM (1985) Age pigments and free radicals: fluorescent lipid complexes formed by iron- and copper-containing proteins. *Biochim Biophys Acta*, 834, 144–148.

Gutteridge JM, Heys AD, & Lunec J (1977) Fluorescent malondialdehyde polymers from hydrolysed 1,1,3,3–tetramethoxypropane. *Anal Chim Acta*, 94, 209–211.

Gutteridge JM, Westermarck T, & Santavuori P (1983) Iron and oxygen radicals in tissue damage: implications for the neuronal ceroid lipofuscinoses. *Acta Neurol Scand*, 68, 365–370.

Guyon R, Lorentzen TD, Hitte C, Kim L, Cadieu E, Parker HG, Quignon P, Lowe JK, Renier C, Gelfenbeyn B, Vignaux F, DeFrance HB, Gloux S, Mahairas GG, Andre C, Galibert F, & Ostrander EA (2003) A 1-Mb resolution radiation hybrid map of the canine genome. *Proc Natl Acad Sci U S A*, 100, 5296–5301.

Haapanen A, Ramadan UA, Autti T, Joensuu R, & Tyynelä J (2007) In vivo MRI reveals the dynamics of pathological changes in the brains of cathepsin D-deficient mice and correlates changes in manganese-enhanced MRI with microglial activation. *Magn Reson Imaging*, 25, 1024–1031.

Hadaczek P, Kohutnicka M, Krauze MT, Bringas J, Pivirotto P, Cunningham J, & Bankiewicz K (2006) Convection-enhanced delivery of adeno-associated virus type 2 (AAV2) into the striatum and transport of AAV2 within monkey brain. *Hum Gene Ther*, 17, 291–302.

Hafner S, Flynn TE, Harmon BG, & Hill JE (2005) Neuronal ceroid-lipofuscinosis in a Holstein steer. *J Vet Diagn Invest*, 17, 194–197.

Hagen LO (1953) Lipid dystrophic changes in the central nervous system in dogs. *Acta Pathol Microbiol Scand*, 33, 22–35.

Haines RL, Codlin S, & Mole SE (2009) The fission yeast model for the lysosomal storage disorder Batten disease predicts disease severity caused by mutations in CLN3. *Dis Model Mech*, 2, 84–92.

Hainsworth DP, Liu GT, Hamm CW, & Katz ML (2009) Funduscopic and angiographic appearance in the neuronal ceroid lipofuscinoses. *Retina*, 29, 657–668.

Hall N, Lake B, Palmer D, Jolly R, & Patrick A (1990) Glycoconjugates in storage cytosomes from ceroid-lipofuscinosis (Batten's disease) and in lipofuscin from old age brain. In Porta AE (Ed.) *Lipofuscin and Ceroid Pigments*, pp. 225–241. New York, Plenum Press.

Hall NA, Jolly RD, Palmer DN, Lake BD, & Patrick AD (1989) Analysis of dolichyl pyrophosphoryl oligosaccharides in purified storage cytosomes from ovine ceroid-lipofuscinosis. *Biochim Biophys Acta*, 993, 245–251.

Hall NA, Lake BD, Dewji NN, & Patrick AD (1991) Lysosomal storage of subunit c of mitochondrial ATP synthase in Batten's disease (ceroid-lipofuscinosis). *Biochem J*, 275 (Pt 1), 269–272.

Halloran MC, Sato-Maeda M, Warren JT, Su F, Lele Z, Krone PH, Kuwada JY, & Shoji W (2000) Laser-induced gene expression in specific cells of transgenic zebrafish. *Development*, 127, 1953–1960.

Haltia M (1982) Infantile neuronal ceroid-lipofuscinosis: Neuropathological aspects. In Armstrong D, Koppang N, & Rider JA (Eds.) *Ceroid-lipofuscinosis (Batten's Disease)*, pp. 105–115. Amsterdam, Elsevier Biomedical Press.

Haltia M (2003) The neuronal ceroid-lipofuscinoses. *J Neuropathol Exp Neurol*, 62, 1–13.

Haltia M, Leivo I, Somer H, Pihko H, Paetau A, Kivela T, Tarkkanen A, Tome F, Engvall E, & Santavuori P (1997) Muscle-eye-brain disease: a neuropathological study. *Ann Neurol*, 41, 173–180.

Haltia M, Rapola J, & Santavuori P (1972) Neuronal ceroid-lipofuscinosis of early onset. A report of 6 cases. Acta Paediatr Scand, 61, 241–242.

Haltia M, Rapola J, & Santavuori P (1973a) Infantile type of so-called neuronal ceroid-lipofuscinosis. Histological and electron microscopic studies. *Acta Neuropathol*, 26, 157–170.

Haltia M, Rapola J, Santavuori P, & Keranen A (1973b) Infantile type of so-called neuronal ceroid-lipofuscinosis. 2. Morphological and biochemical studies. *J Neurol Sci*, 18, 269–285.

Haltia M, Tyynelä J, Hirvasniemi A, Herva R, Ranta US, & Lehesjoki AE (1999) CLN8 - Northern epilepsy. In Goebel HH, Mole SE, & Lake BD (Eds.) *The Neuronal Ceroid Lipofuscinoses (Batten Disease)*, pp. 117–124. Amsterdam, IOS Press.

Hannover A (1843) Mikroskopiske undersögelser af nervesystemet. *Det Kongelige Danske Videnskabernes Selskabs Naturvidenskabelige og Mathematiske Afhandlinger*, 10, 1–112.

Hansen E (1979) Familial cerebro-macular degeneration (the Stengel-Batten-Mayou-Spielmeyer-Vogt-Stock disease). Evaluation of the photoreceptors. *Acta Ophthalmol (Copenh)*, 57, 382–396.

Harden A, Pampiglione G, & Picton-Robinson N (1973) Electroretinogram and visual evoked response in a form of 'neuronal lipidosis' with diagnostic EEG features. *J Neurol Neurosurg Psychiatry*, 36, 61–67.

Harmatz P, Whitley CB, Waber L, Pais R, Steiner R, Plecko B, Kaplan P, Simon J, Butensky E, & Hopwood JJ (2004) Enzyme replacement therapy in mucopolysaccharidosis VI (Maroteaux-Lamy syndrome). *J Pediatr*, 144, 574–580.

Harper PA, Walker KH, Healy PJ, Hartley WJ, Gibson AJ, & Smith JS (1988) Neurovisceral ceroid-lipofuscinosis in blind Devon cattle. *Acta Neuropathol*, 75, 632–636.

Hartikainen JM, Ju W, Wisniewski KE, Moroziewicz DN, Kaczmarski AL, McLendon L, Zhong D, Suarez CT, Brown WT, & Zhong N (1999) Late infantile neuronal ceroid lipofuscinosis is due to splicing mutations in the CLN2 gene. *Mol Genet Metab*, 67, 162–168.

Hartley WJ, Kuberski T, LeGonidec G, & Daynes P (1982) The pathology of Gomen disease: a cerebellar disorder of horses in New Caledonia. *Vet Pathol*, 19, 399–405.

Hashmi S, Britton C, Liu J, Guiliano DB, Oksov Y, & Lustigman S (2002) Cathepsin L is essential for embryogenesis and development of Caenorhabditis elegans. *J Biol Chem*, 277, 3477–3486.

Hasilik A & Neufeld EF (1980a) Biosynthesis of lysosomal enzymes in fibroblasts. Synthesis as precursors of higher molecular weight. *J Biol Chem*, 255, 4937–4945.

Hasilik A & Neufeld EF (1980b) Biosynthesis of lysosomal enzymes in fibroblasts. Phosphorylation of mannose residues. *J Biol Chem*, 255, 4946–4950.

Haskell RE, Carr CJ, Pearce DA, Bennett MJ, & Davidson BL (2000) Batten disease: evaluation of CLN3 mutations on protein localization and function. *Hum Mol Genet*, 9, 735–744.

Haskell RE, Hughes SM, Chiorini JA, Alisky JM, & Davidson BL (2003) Viral-mediated delivery of the late-infantile neuronal ceroid lipofuscinosis gene, TPP-I to the mouse central nervous system. *Gene Ther*, 10, 34–42.

Hätönen T, Kirveskari E, Heiskala H, Sainio K, Laakso ML, & Santavuori P (1999) Melatonin ineffective in neuronal ceroid lipofuscinosis patients with fragmented or normal motor activity rhythms recorded by wrist actigraphy. *Mol Genet Metab*, 66, 401–406.

Hauswirth WW, Aleman TS, Kaushal S, Cideciyan AV, Schwartz SB, Wang L, Conlon TJ, Boye SL, Flotte TR, Byrne BJ, & Jacobson SG (2008) Treatment of leber congenital amaurosis due to RPE65 mutations by ocular subretinal injection of adeno-associated virus gene vector: short-term results of a phase I trial. *Hum Gene Ther*, 19, 979–990.

Haworth RS & Fliegel L (1993) Intracellular pH in Schizosaccharomyces pombe—comparison with Saccharomyces cerevisiae. *Mol Cell Biochem*, 124, 131–140.

Haynes ME, Manson JI, Carter RF, & Robertson E (1979) Electron microscopy of skin and peripheral blood lymphocytes in infantile (Santavuori) neuronal ceroid lipofuscinosis. *Neuropädiatrie*, 10, 245–263.

Heikkilä E, Hatonen TH, Telakivi T, Laakso ML, Heiskala H, Salmi T, Alila A, & Santavuori P (1995) Circadian rhythm studies in neuronal ceroid-lipofuscinosis (NCL). *Am J Med Genet*, 57, 229–234.

Heine C, Koch B, Storch S, Kohlschutter A, Palmer DN, & Braulke T (2004) Defective endoplasmic reticulum-resident membrane protein CLN6 affects lysosomal degradation of endocytosed arylsulfatase A. *J Biol Chem*, 279, 22347–22352.

Heine C, Quitsch A, Storch S, Martin Y, Lonka L, Lehesjoki AE, Mole SE, & Braulke T (2007) Topology and endoplasmic reticulum retention signals of the lysosomal storage disease-related membrane protein CLN6. *Mol Membr Biol*, 24, 74–87.

Heine C, Tyynelä J, Cooper JD, Palmer DN, Elleder M, Kohlschutter A, & Braulke T (2003) Enhanced expression of manganese-dependent superoxide dismutase in human and sheep CLN6 tissues. *Biochem J*, 376, 369–376.

Heinonen O, Kyttala A, Lehmus E, Paunio T, Peltonen L, & Jalanko A (2000a) Expression of palmitoyl protein thioesterase in neurons. *Mol Genet Metab*, 69, 123–129.

Heinonen O, Salonen T, Jalanko A, Peltonen L, & Copp A (2000b) CLN-1 and CLN-5, genes for infantile and variant late infantile neuronal ceroid lipofuscinoses, are expressed in the embryonic human brain. *J Comp Neurol*, 426, 406–412.

Heiskanen M, Kallioniemi O, & Palotie A (1996) Fiber-FISH: experiences and a refined protocol. *Genet Anal*, 12, 179–184.

Hellsten E, Vesa J, Olkkonen VM, Jalanko A, & Peltonen L (1996) Human palmitoyl protein thioesterase: evidence for lysosomal targeting of the enzyme and disturbed cellular routing in infantile neuronal ceroid lipofuscinosis. *EMBO J*, 15, 5240–5245.

Hendricks M & Jesuthasan S (2007) Electroporation-based methods for in vivo, whole mount and primary culture analysis of zebrafish brain development. *Neural Dev*, 2, 6.

Hermansson M, Kakela R, Berghall M, Lehesjoki AE, Somerharju P, & Lahtinen U (2005) Mass spectrometric analysis reveals changes in phospholipid, neutral sphingolipid and sulfatide molecular species in progressive epilepsy with mental retardation, EPMR, brain: a case study. *J Neurochem*, 95, 609–617.

Herrmann P, Druckrey-Fiskaaen C, Kouznetsova E, Heinitz K, Bigl M, Cotman SL, & Schliebs R (2008) Developmental impairments of select neurotransmitter systems in brains of Cln3(Deltaex7/8) knock-in mice, an animal model of juvenile neuronal ceroid lipofuscinosis. *J Neurosci Res*, 86, 1857–1870.

Hersh BM, Hartwieg E, & Horvitz HR (2002) The Caenorhabditis elegans mucolipin-like gene cup-5 is essential for viability and regulates lysosomes in multiple cell types. *Proc Natl Acad Sci U S A*, 99, 4355–4360.

Herva R, Tyynelä J, Hirvasniemi A, Syrjakallio-Ylitalo M, & Haltia M (2000) Northern epilepsy: a novel form of neuronal ceroid-lipofuscinosis. *Brain Pathol*, 10, 215–222.

Hickey AJ, Chotkowski HL, Singh N, Ault JG, Korey CA, MacDonald ME, & Glaser RL (2006) Palmitoyl-protein thioesterase 1 deficiency in Drosophila melanogaster causes accumulation of abnormal storage material and reduced life span. *Genetics*, 172, 2379–2390.

Hirawat S, Welch EM, Elfring GL, Northcutt VJ, Paushkin S, Hwang S, Leonard EM, Almstead NG, Ju W, Peltz SW, & Miller LL (2007) Safety, tolerability, and pharmacokinetics of PTC124, a nonaminoglycoside nonsense mutation suppressor, following single- and multiple-dose administration to healthy male and female adult volunteers. *J Clin Pharmacol*, 47, 430–444.

Hirvasniemi A, Herrala P, & Leisti J (1995) Northern epilepsy syndrome: clinical course and the effect of medication on seizures. *Epilepsia*, 36, 792–797.

Hirvasniemi A & Karumo J (1994) Neuroradiological findings in the northern epilepsy syndrome. *Acta Neurol Scand*, 90, 388–393.

Hirvasniemi A, Lang H, Lehesjoki AE, & Leisti J (1994) Northern epilepsy syndrome: an inherited childhood onset epilepsy with associated mental deterioration. *J Med Genet*, 31, 177–182.

Hobert JA & Dawson G (2007) A novel role of the Batten disease gene CLN3: association with BMP synthesis. *Biochem Biophys Res Commun*, 358, 111–116.

Hofman I (1990) *The Batten-Spielmeyer-Vogt Disease*. Doorn, Bartiméus Foundation.

Hofmann SL, Das AK, Yi W, Lu JY, & Wisniewski KE (1999) Genotype-phenotype correlations in neuronal ceroid lipofuscinosis due to palmitoyl-protein thioesterase deficiency. *Mol Genet Metab*, 66, 234–239.

Hofmann SL & Peltonen L (2001) The neuronal ceroid lipofuscinosis. In Scriver CR, Beaudet AL, Sly W, Valle D, Childs B, Kinzler KW, & Vogelstein B (Eds.) *The Metabolic and Molecular Bases of Inherited Disease*, 8th edn., pp. 3877–3894. New York, McGraw-Hill.

Holmberg V, Jalanko A, Isosomppi J, Fabritius AL, Peltonen L, & Kopra O (2004) The mouse ortholog of the neuronal ceroid lipofuscinosis CLN5 gene encodes a soluble lysosomal glycoprotein expressed in the developing brain. *Neurobiol Dis*, 16, 29–40.

Holmberg V, Lauronen L, Autti T, Santavuori P, Savukoski M, Uvebrant P, Hofman I, Peltonen L, & Jarvela I (2000) Phenotype-genotype correlation in eight patients with Finnish variant late infantile NCL (CLN5). *Neurology*, 55, 579–581.

Holopainen JM, Saarikoski J, Kinnunen PK, & Jarvela I (2001) Elevated lysosomal pH in neuronal ceroid lipofuscinoses (NCLs). *Eur J Biochem*, 268, 5851–5856.

Honing S, Ricotta D, Krauss M, Spate K, Spolaore B, Motley A, Robinson M, Robinson C, Haucke V, & Owen DJ (2005) Phosphatidylinositol-(4,5)-bisphosphate regulates sorting signal recognition by the clathrin-associated adaptor complex AP2. *Mol Cell*, 18, 519–531.

Hopwood JJ, Vellodi A, Scott HS, Morris CP, Litjens T, Clements PR, Brooks DA, Cooper A, & Wraith JE (1993) Long-term clinical progress in bone marrow transplanted mucopolysaccharidosis type I patients with a defined genotype. *J Inherit Metab Dis*, 16, 1024–1033.

Hosain S, Kaufmann WE, Negrin G, Watkins PA, Siakotos AN, Palmer DN, & Naidu S (1995) Diagnoses of neuronal ceroid-lipofuscinosis by immunochemical methods. *Am J Med Genet*, 57, 239–245.

Hoskins RA, Phan AC, Naeemuddin M, Mapa FA, Ruddy DA, Ryan JJ, Young LM, Wells T, Kopczynski C, & Ellis MC (2001) Single nucleotide polymorphism markers for genetic mapping in Drosophila melanogaster. *Genome Res*, 11, 1100–1113.

Houweling PJ, Cavanagh JA, Palmer DN, Frugier T, Mitchell NL, Windsor PA, Raadsma HW, & Tammen I (2006a) Neuronal ceroid lipofuscinosis in Devon cattle is caused by a single base duplication (c.662dupG) in the bovine CLN5 gene. *Biochim Biophys Acta*, 1762, 890–897.

Houweling PJ, Cavanagh JA, & Tammen I (2006b) Radiation hybrid mapping of three candidate genes for bovine Neuronal Ceroid Lipofuscinosis: CLN3, CLN5 and CLN6. *Cytogenet Genome Res*, 115, 5–6.

Huang K & El-Husseini A (2005) Modulation of neuronal protein trafficking and function by palmitoylation. *Curr Opin Neurobiol*, 15, 527–535.

Huang X, Suyama K, Buchanan J, Zhu AJ, & Scott MP (2005) A Drosophila model of the Niemann-Pick type C lysosome storage disease: dnpc1a is required for molting and sterol homeostasis. *Development*, 132, 5115–5124.

Hueck W (1912) Pigmentstudien. *Beitr Pathol Anat Allg Pathol*, 54, 68–232.

Hughes SM, Kay GW, Jordan TW, Rickards GK, & Palmer DN (1999) Disease-specific pathology in neurons cultured from sheep affected with ceroid lipofuscinosis. *Mol Genet Metab*, 66, 381–386.

Hulková H, Ledvinova J, Asfaw B, Koubek K, Kopriva K, & Elleder M (2005) Lactosylceramide in lysosomal storage disorders: a comparative immunohistochemical and biochemical study. *Virchows Arch*, 447, 31–44.

Humphrey W, Dalke A, & Schulten K (1996) VMD: visual molecular dynamics. *J Mol Graph*, 14, 33–38, 27–28.

Humphreys S, Lake BD, & Scholtz CL (1985) Congenital amaurotic idiocy—a pathological, histochemical, biochemical and ultrastructural study. *Neuropathol Appl Neurobiol*, 11, 475–484.

Hunot S & Hirsch EC (2003) Neuroinflammatory processes in Parkinson's disease. *Ann Neurol*, 53 Suppl 3, S49–58; discussion S58–60.

Huxtable CR, Chapman HM, Main DC, Vass D, Pearse BH, & Hilbert BJ (1987) Neurological disease and lipofuscinosis in horses and sheep grazing Trachyandra divaricata (branched onion weed) in south Western Australia. *Aust Vet J*, 64, 105–108.

Ikeda K & Goebel HH (1979) Ultrastructural pathology of lymphocytes in neuronal ceroid-lipofuscinoses. *Brain Dev*, 1, 285–292.

Ikeda K, Goebel HH, Burck U, & Kohlschutter A (1982) Ultrastructural pathology of human lymphocytes in lysosomal disorders: a contribution to their morphological diagnosis. *Eur J Pediatr*, 138, 179–185.

Ikeda K, Kosaka K, Oyanagi S, & Yamada K (1984) Adult type of neuronal ceroid-lipofuscinosis with retinal involvement. *Clin Neuropathol*, 3, 237–239.

Imai Y & Yamamoto M (1992) Schizosaccharomyces pombe sxa1+ and sxa2+ encode putative proteases involved in the mating response. *Mol Cell Biol*, 12, 1827–1834.

Isahara K, Ohsawa Y, Kanamori S, Shibata M, Waguri S, Sato N, Gotow T, Watanabe T, Momoi T, Urase K, Kominami E, & Uchiyama Y (1999) Regulation of a novel pathway for cell death by lysosomal aspartic and cysteine proteinases. *Neuroscience*, 91, 233–249.

Iseki E, Amano N, Yokoi S, Yamada Y, Suzuki K, & Yazaki M (1987) A case of adult neuronal ceroid-lipofuscinosis with the appearance of membranous cytoplasmic bodies localized in the spinal anterior horn. *Acta Neuropathol*, 72, 362–368.

Isosomppi J, Heinonen O, Hiltunen JO, Greene ND, Vesa J, Uusitalo A, Mitchison HM, Saarma M, Jalanko A, & Peltonen L (1999) Developmental expression of palmitoyl protein thioesterase in normal mice. *Brain Res Dev Brain Res*, 118, 1–11.

Isosomppi J, Vesa J, Jalanko A, & Peltonen L (2002) Lysosomal localization of the neuronal ceroid lipofuscinosis CLN5 protein. *Hum Mol Genet*, 11, 885–891.

Ivan CS, Saint-Hilaire MH, Christensen TG, & Milunsky JM (2005) Adult-onset neuronal ceroid lipofuscinosis type B in an African-American. *Mov Disord*, 20, 752–754.

Iwaki T, Goa T, Tanaka N, & Takegawa K (2004) Characterization of Schizosaccharomyces pombe mutants defective in vacuolar acidification and protein sorting. *Mol Genet Genomics*, 271, 197–207.

Jäättelä M, Cande C, & Kroemer G (2004) Lysosomes and mitochondria in the commitment to apoptosis: a potential role for cathepsin D and AIF. *Cell Death Differ*, 11, 135–136.

Jabs S, Quitsch A, Kakela R, Koch B, Tyynelä J, Brade H, Glatzel M, Walkley S, Saftig P, Vanier MT, & Braulke T (2008) Accumulation of bis(monoacylglycero) phosphate and gangliosides in mouse models of neuronal ceroid lipofuscinosis. *J Neurochem*, 106, 1415–1425.

Jakob H & Kolkmann FW (1973) [Pigment variant of the adult type of amaurotic idiocy (Kufs) (author's transl)]. *Acta Neuropathol*, 26, 225–236.

Jalanko A & Braulke T (2009) Neuronal ceroid lipofuscinoses. *Biochim Biophys Acta*, 1793, 697–709.

Jalanko A, Tyynelä J, & Peltonen L (2006) From genes to systems: new global strategies for the characterization of NCL biology. *Biochim Biophys Acta*, 1762, 934–944.

Jalanko A, Vesa J, Manninen T, von Schantz C, Minye H, Fabritius AL, Salonen T, Rapola J, Gentile M, Kopra O, & Peltonen L (2005) Mice with $Ppt1^{\Delta ex4}$ mutation replicate the INCL phenotype and show an inflammation-associated loss of interneurons. *Neurobiol Dis*, 18, 226–241.

Janes RW, Munroe PB, Mitchison HM, Gardiner RM, Mole SE, & Wallace BA (1996) A model for Batten disease protein CLN3: functional implications from homology and mutations. *FEBS Lett*, 399, 75–77.

Jansen G, Hazendonk E, Thijssen KL, & Plasterk RH (1997) Reverse genetics by chemical mutagenesis in Caenorhabditis elegans. *Nat Genet*, 17, 119–121.

Janský J (1907). Haematologick studie u. psychotiku. *Sborn Klinick*, 8, 85–139.

Janský J (1908) Dosud nepopsaný pripad familiárni amaurotické idiotie komplikované s hypoplasii mozeckovou. *Sborn Lék*, 13, 165–196.

Järplid B & Haltia M (1993) An animal model of the infantile type of neuronal ceroid-lipofuscinosis. *J Inherit Metab Dis*, 16, 274–277.

Järvelä I (1991) Infantile neuronal ceroid lipofuscinosis (CLN1): linkage disequilibrium in the Finnish population and evidence that variant late infantile form (variant CLN2) represents a nonallelic locus. *Genomics*, 10, 333–337.

Järvelä I, Autti T, Lamminranta S, Åberg L, Raininko R, & Santavuori P (1997) Clinical and magnetic resonance imaging findings in Batten disease: analysis of the major mutation (1.02-kb deletion). *Ann Neurol*, 42, 799–802.

Järvelä I, Lehtovirta M, Tikkanen R, Kyttala A, & Jalanko A (1999) Defective intracellular transport of CLN3 is the molecular basis of Batten disease (JNCL). *Hum Mol Genet*, 8, 1091–1098.

Järvelä I, Sainio M, Rantamaki T, Olkkonen VM, Carpen O, Peltonen L, & Jalanko A (1998) Biosynthesis and intracellular targeting of the CLN3 protein defective in Batten disease. *Hum Mol Genet*, 7, 85–90.

Järvelä IE, Mitchison HM, O'Rawe AM, Munroe PB, Taschner PE, de Vos N, Lerner TJ, D'Arigo KL, Callen DF, Thompson AD, Knight M, Marrone BL, Mund MO, Meincke L, Breuning MH, Gardiner RM, Doggett NA, Mole SE (1995) YAC and cosmid contigs spanning the Batten disease (CLN3) region at 16p12.1-p11.2. *Genomics*, 29, 478–489.

Jasty V, Kowalski RL, Fonseca EH, Porter MC, Clemens GR, Bare JJ, & Hartnagel RE (1984) An unusual case of generalized ceroid-lipofuscinosis in a cynomolgus monkey. *Vet Pathol*, 21, 46–50.

Jentsch TJ (2007) Chloride and the endosomal-lysosomal pathway: emerging roles of CLC chloride transporters. *J Physiol*, 578, 633–640.

Jeyakumar M, Dwek RA, Butters TD, & Platt FM (2005) Storage solutions: treating lysosomal disorders of the brain. *Nat Rev Neurosci*, 6, 713–725.

Johnstone D & Milward EA (2010) Genome-wide microarray analysis of brain gene expression in mice on a short-term high iron diet. *Neurochem Int*, 56, 856–863.

Jolly RD, Arthur DG, Kay GW, & Palmer DN (2002a) Neuronal ceroid-lipofuscinosis in Borderdale sheep. *N Z Vet J*, 50, 199–202.

Jolly RD, Brown S, Das AM, & Walkley SU (2002b) Mitochondrial dysfunction in the neuronal ceroid-lipofuscinoses (Batten disease). *Neurochem Int*, 40, 565–571.

Jolly RD, Charleston WA, & Hughes PL (2002) Disorders of New Zealand farm dogs. *N Z Vet J*, 50, 115–116.

Jolly RD, Gibson AJ, Healy PJ, Slack PM, & Birtles MJ (1992) Bovine ceroid-lipofuscinosis: pathology of blindness. *N Z Vet J*, 40, 107–111.

Jolly RD, Hartley WJ, Jones BR, Johnstone AC, Palmer AC, & Blakemore WF (1994a) Generalised ceroid-lipofuscinosis and brown bowel syndrome in Cocker spaniel dogs. *N Z Vet J*, 42, 236–239.

Jolly RD, Janmaat A, Graydon RJ, & Clemett RS (1982) *Ceroid-lipofuscinosis: The Ovine Model*. Amsterdam, Elsevier Biomedical Press.

Jolly RD, Janmaat A, West DM, & Morrison I (1980) Ovine ceroid-lipofuscinosis: a model of Batten's disease. *Neuropathol Appl Neurobiol*, 6, 195–209.

Jolly RD & Palmer DN (1995) The neuronal ceroid-lipofuscinoses (Batten disease): comparative aspects. *Neuropathol Appl Neurobiol*, 21, 50–60.

Jolly RD, Palmer DN, Studdert VP, Sutton RH, Kelly WR, Koppang N, Dahme G, Hartley WJ, Patterson JS, & Riis RC (1994b) Canine ceroid-lipofuscinoses: A review and classification. *J Small Anim Pract*, 35, 299–306.

Jolly RD, Shimada A, Craig AS, Kirkland KB, & Palmer DN (1988) Ovine ceroid-lipofuscinosis II: Pathologic changes interpreted in light of biochemical observations. *Am J Med Genet Suppl*, 5, 159–170.

Jolly RD, Shimada A, Dopfmer I, Slack PM, Birtles MJ, & Palmer DN (1989) Ceroid-lipofuscinosis (Batten's disease): pathogenesis and sequential neuropathological changes in the ovine model. *Neuropathol Appl Neurobiol*, 15, 371–383.

Jolly RD & Walkley SU (1997) Lysosomal storage diseases of animals: an essay in comparative pathology. *Vet Pathol*, 34, 527–548.

Jolly RD & Walkley SU (1999) Ovine ceroid lipofuscinosis (OCL6): postulated mechanism of neurodegeneration. *Mol Genet Metab*, 66, 376–380.

Jolly RD & West DM (1976) Blindness in South Hampshire sheep: a neuronal ceroidlipofuscinosis. *N Z Vet J*, 24, 123.

Jomary C, Vincent KA, Grist J, Neal MJ, & Jones SE (1997) Rescue of photoreceptor function by AAV-mediated gene transfer in a mouse model of inherited retinal degeneration. *Gene Ther*, 4, 683–690.

Jorgensen EM & Mango SE (2002) The art and design of genetic screens: Caenorhabditis elegans. *Nat Rev Genet*, 3, 356–369.

Josephson SA, Schmidt RE, Millsap P, McManus DQ, & Morris JC (2001) Autosomal dominant Kufs' disease: a cause of early onset dementia. *J Neurol Sci*, 188, 51–60.

Ju W, Zhong R, Moore S, Moroziewicz D, Currie JR, Parfrey P, Brown WT, & Zhong N (2002) Identification of novel CLN2 mutations shows Canadian specific NCL2 alleles. *J Med Genet*, 39, 822–825.

Junaid MA, Wu G, & Pullarkat RK (2000) Purification and characterization of bovine brain lysosomal pepstatin-insensitive proteinase, the gene product deficient in the human late-infantile neuronal ceroid lipofuscinosis. *J Neurochem*, 74, 287–294.

Kaczmarski W, Wisniewski KE, Golabek A, Kaczmarski A, Kida E, & Michalewski M (1999) Studies of membrane association of CLN3 protein. *Mol Genet Metab*, 66, 261–264.

Kaesgen U & Goebel HH (1989) Intraepidermal morphologic manifestations in lysosomal diseases. *Brain Dev*, 11, 338–341.

Kågedal K, Johansson U, & Ollinger K (2001) The lysosomal protease cathepsin D mediates apoptosis induced by oxidative stress. *FASEB J*, 15, 1592–1594.

Kakela R, Somerharju P, & Tyynelä J (2003) Analysis of phospholipid molecular species in brains from patients with infantile and juvenile neuronal-ceroid lipofuscinosis using liquid chromatography-electrospray ionization mass spectrometry. *J Neurochem*, 84, 1051–1065.

Kakkis E, McEntee M, Vogler C, Le S, Levy B, Belichenko P, Mobley W, Dickson P, Hanson S, & Passage M (2004) Intrathecal enzyme replacement therapy reduces lysosomal storage in the brain and meninges of the canine model of MPS I. *Mol Genet Metab*, 83, 163–174.

Kakkis ED, Muenzer J, Tiller GE, Waber L, Belmont J, Passage M, Izykowski B, Phillips J, Doroshow R, Walot I, Hoft R, & Neufeld EF (2001) Enzyme-replacement therapy in mucopolysaccharidosis I. *N Engl J Med*, 344, 182–188.

Kaletta T & Hengartner MO (2006) Finding function in novel targets: C. elegans as a model organism. *Nat Rev Drug Discov*, 5, 387–398.

Kalviainen R, Eriksson K, Losekoot M, Sorri I, Harvima I, Santavuori P, Jarvela I, Autti T, Vanninen R, Salmenpera T, & van Diggelen OP (2007) Juvenile-onset neuronal ceroid lipofuscinosis with infantile CLN1 mutation and palmitoyl-protein thioesterase deficiency. *Eur J Neurol*, 14, 369–372.

Kama R, Robinson M, & Gerst JE (2007) Btn2, a Hook1 ortholog and potential Batten disease-related protein, mediates late endosome-Golgi protein sorting in yeast. *Mol Cell Biol*, 27, 605–621.

Kang Y, Moressi CJ, Scheetz TE, Xie L, Tran DT, Casavant TL, Ak P, Benham CJ, Davidson BL, & McCray PB, Jr. (2006) Integration site choice of a feline immunodeficiency virus vector. *J Virol*, 80, 8820–8823.

Kang Y, Stein CS, Heth JA, Sinn PL, Penisten AK, Staber PD, Ratliff KL, Shen H, Barker CK, Martins I, Sharkey CM, Sanders DA, McCray PB, Jr., & Davidson BL (2002) In vivo gene transfer using a nonprimate lentiviral vector pseudotyped with Ross River Virus glycoproteins. *J Virol*, 76, 9378–9388.

Karagiannis J & Young PG (2001) Intracellular pH homeostasis during cell-cycle progression and growth state transition in Schizosaccharomyces pombe. *J Cell Sci*, 114, 2929–2941.

Karlsson EK, Baranowska I, Wade CM, Salmon Hillbertz NH, Zody MC, Anderson N, Biagi TM, Patterson N, Pielberg GR, Kulbokas EJ, 3rd, Comstock KE, Keller ET, Mesirov JP, von Euler H, Kampe O, Hedhammar A, Lander ES, Andersson G, Andersson L, & Lindblad-Toh K (2007) Efficient mapping of mendelian traits in dogs through genome-wide association. *Nat Genet*, 39, 1321–1328.

Kasper D, Planells-Cases R, Fuhrmann JC, Scheel O, Zeitz O, Ruether K, Schmitt A, Poet M, Steinfeld R, Schweizer M, Kornak U, & Jentsch TJ (2005) Loss of the chloride channel ClC-7 leads to lysosomal storage disease and neurodegeneration. *EMBO J*, 24, 1079–1091.

Katz ML, Christianson JS, Norbury NE, Gao CL, Siakotos AN, & Koppang N (1994) Lysine methylation of mitochondrial ATP synthase subunit c stored in tissues of dogs with hereditary ceroid lipofuscinosis. *J Biol Chem*, 269, 9906–9911.

Katz ML, Coates JR, Cooper JJ, O'Brien DP, Jeong M, & Narfstrom K (2008) Retinal pathology in a canine model of late infantile neuronal ceroid lipofuscinosis. *Invest Ophthalmol Vis Sci*, 49, 2686–2695.

Katz ML, Farias FH, Sanders DN, Zeng R, Khan S, Johnson GS, & O'Brien DP (2010) A missense mutation in CLN6 in an Australian Shepherd with neuronal ceroid lipofuscinosis. *J Biomed Biotech*, in press.

Katz ML, Gao CL, Tompkins JA, Bronson RT, & Chin DT (1995) Mitochondrial ATP synthase subunit c stored in hereditary ceroid-lipofuscinosis contains trimethyllysine. *Biochem J*, 310 (Pt 3), 887–892.

Katz ML, Khan S, Awano T, Shahid SA, Siakotos AN, & Johnson GS (2005a) A mutation in the CLN8 gene in English Setter dogs with neuronal ceroid-lipofuscinosis. *Biochem Biophys Res Commun*, 327, 541–547.

Katz ML, Narfstrom K, Johnson GS, & O'Brien DP (2005b) Assessment of retinal function and characterization of lysosomal storage body accumulation in the retinas and brains of Tibetan Terriers with ceroid-lipofuscinosis. *Am J Vet Res*, 66, 67–76.

Katz ML, Shibuya H, Liu PC, Kaur S, Gao CL, & Johnson GS (1999) A mouse gene knockout model for juvenile ceroid-lipofuscinosis (Batten disease). *J Neurosci Res*, 57, 551–556.

Katz ML & Siakotos AN (1995) Canine hereditary ceroid-lipofuscinosis: evidence for a defect in the carnitine biosynthetic pathway. *Am J Med Genet*, 57, 266–271.

Kay GW, Hughes SM, & Palmer DN (1999) In vitro culture of neurons from sheep with Batten disease. *Mol Genet Metab*, 67, 83–88.

Kay GW, Oswald MJ, & Palmer DN (2006a) The development and characterisation of complex ovine neuron cultures from fresh and frozen foetal neurons. *J Neurosci Methods*, 155, 98–108.

Kay GW, Palmer DN, Rezaie P, & Cooper JD (2006b) Activation of non-neuronal cells within the prenatal developing brain of sheep with neuronal ceroid lipofuscinosis. *Brain Pathol*, 16, 110–116.

Kay GW, Verbeek MM, Furlong JM, Willemsen MA, & Palmer DN (2009) Neuropeptide changes and neuroactive amino acids in CSF from humans and sheep with neuronal ceroid lipofuscinoses (NCLs, Batten disease). *Neurochem Int*, 55, 783–788.

Keeling KM, Brooks DA, Hopwood JJ, Li P, Thompson JN, & Bedwell DM (2001) Gentamicin-mediated suppression of Hurler syndrome stop mutations restores a low level of alpha-L-iduronidase activity and reduces lysosomal glycosaminoglycan accumulation. *Hum Mol Genet*, 10, 291–299.

Keller RK, Armstrong D, Crum FC, & Koppang N (1984) Dolichol and dolichyl phosphate levels in brain tissue from English setters with ceroid lipofuscinosis. *J Neurochem*, 42, 1040–1047.

Kida E, Golabek AA, Walus M, Wujek P, Kaczmarski W, & Wisniewski KE (2001) Distribution of tripeptidyl peptidase I in human tissues under normal and pathological conditions. *J Neuropathol Exp Neurol*, 60, 280–292.

Kida E, Kaczmarski W, Golabek AA, Kaczmarski A, Michalewski M, & Wisniewski KE (1999) Analysis of intracellular distribution and trafficking of the CLN3 protein in fusion with the green fluorescent protein in vitro. *Mol Genet Metab*, 66, 265–271.

Kida E, Wisniewski KE, & Golabek AA (1993) Increased expression of subunit c of mitochondrial ATP synthase in brain tissue from neuronal ceroid lipofuscinoses and mucopolysaccharidosis cases but not in long-term fibroblast cultures. *Neurosci Lett*, 164, 121–124.

Kielar C, Maddox L, Bible E, Pontikis CC, Macauley SL, Griffey MA, Wong M, Sands MS, & Cooper JD (2007) Successive neuron loss in the thalamus and cortex in a mouse model of infantile neuronal ceroid lipofuscinosis. *Neurobiol Dis*, 25, 150–162.

Kielar C, Wishart TM, Palmer A, Dihanich S, Wong AM, Macauley SL, Chan CH, Sands MS, Pearce DA, Cooper JD, & Gillingwater TH (2009) Molecular correlates of axonal and synaptic pathology in mouse models of Batten disease. *Hum Mol Genet*, 18, 4066–4080.

Kim KH, Sleat DE, Bernard O & Lobel P (2009) Genetic modulation of apoptotic pathways fails to alter disease course in tripeptidyl-peptidase 1 deficient mice. *Neurosci Lett*, 453, 27-30.

Kim KH, Pham CT, Sleat DE & Lobel P (2008) Dipeptidyl-peptidase I does not functionally compensate for the loss of tripeptidyl-peptidase I in the neurodegenerative disease late-infantile neuronal ceroid lipofuscinosis. *Biochem J*, 415, 225-32.

Kim SJ, Zhang Z, Hitomi E, Lee YC, & Mukherjee AB (2006) Endoplasmic reticulum stress-induced caspase-4 activation mediates apoptosis and neurodegeneration in INCL. *Hum Mol Genet*, 15, 1826–1834.

Kim SJ, Zhang Z, Sarkar C, Tsai PC, Lee YC, Dye L, & Mukherjee AB (2008) Palmitoyl protein thioesterase-1 deficiency impairs synaptic vesicle recycling at nerve terminals, contributing to neuropathology in humans and mice. *J Clin Invest*, 118, 3075–3086.

Kim Y, Chattopadhyay S, Locke S, & Pearce DA (2005) Interaction among Btn1p, Btn2p, and Ist2p reveals potential interplay among the vacuole, amino acid levels, and ion homeostasis in the yeast Saccharomyces cerevisiae. *Eukaryot Cell*, 4, 281–288.

Kim Y, Ramirez-Montealegre D, & Pearce DA (2003) A role in vacuolar arginine transport for yeast Btn1p and for human CLN3, the protein defective in Batten disease. *Proc Natl Acad Sci U S A*, 100, 15458–15462.

Kimura S & Goebel HH (1988) Light and electron microscopic study of juvenile neuronal ceroid-lipofuscinosis lymphocytes. *Pediatr Neurol*, 4, 148–152.

Kimura S, Sasaki Y, Warlo I, & Goebel HH (1987) Axonal pathology of the skin in infantile neuroaxonal dystrophy. *Acta Neuropathol*, 75, 212–215.

Kirkness EF, Bafna V, Halpern AL, Levy S, Remington K, Rusch DB, Delcher AL, Pop M, Wang W, Fraser CM, & Venter JC (2003) The dog genome: survey sequencing and comparative analysis. *Science*, 301, 1898–1903.

Kirveskari E, Partinen M, Salmi T, Sainio K, Telakivi T, Hamalainen M, Larsen A, & Santavuori P (2000) Sleep alterations in juvenile neuronal ceroid-lipofuscinosis. *Pediatr Neurol*, 22, 347–354.

Kitamoto K, Yoshizawa K, Ohsumi Y, & Anraku Y (1988) Dynamic aspects of vacuolar and cytosolic amino acid pools of Saccharomyces cerevisiae. *J Bacteriol*, 170, 2683–2686.

Kitzmüller C, Haines RL, Codlin S, Cutler DF, & Mole SE (2008) A function retained by the common mutant CLN3 protein is responsible for the late onset of juvenile neuronal ceroid lipofuscinosis. *Hum Mol Genet*, 17, 303–312.

Klenk E (1939) Beiträge zur Chemie der Lipidosen, Niemann–Pickschen Krankheit und amaurotischen Idiotie. *Hoppe-Seyler Z Physiol Chem*, 262, 128–143.

Klockars T, Savukoski M, Isosomppi J, Laan M, Jarvela I, Petrukhin K, Palotie A, & Peltonen L (1996) Efficient construction of a physical map by fiber-FISH of the CLN5 region: refined assignment and long-range contig covering the critical region on 13q22. *Genomics*, 35, 71–78.

Kohan R, Cannelli N, Aiello C, Santorelli FM, Cismondi AI, Milà M, Ramírez AMO, & Halac IN (2008) Novel human pathological mutations: Gene symbol: CLN5: Neuronal Ceroid Lipofuscinosis, Finnish Variant. *Hum Genet*, 123, 537–555 (552).

Kohan R, Cismondi IA, Kremer RD, Muller VJ, Guelbert N, Anzolini VT, Fietz MJ, Ramirez AM, & Halac IN (2009) An integrated strategy for the diagnosis of neuronal ceroid lipofuscinosis types 1 (CLN1) and 2 (CLN2) in eleven Latin American patients. *Clin Genet*, 76, 372–382.

Kohan R, de Halac IN, Tapia Anzolini V, Cismondi A, Oller Ramirez AM, Paschini Capra A, & de Kremer RD (2005) Palmitoyl Protein Thioesterase1 (PPT1) and Tripeptidyl Peptidase-I (TPP-I) are expressed in the human saliva. A reliable and non-invasive source for the diagnosis of infantile (CLN1) and late infantile (CLN2) neuronal ceroid lipofuscinoses. *Clin Biochem*, 38, 492–494.

Koike M, Nakanishi H, Saftig P, Ezaki J, Isahara K, Ohsawa Y, Schulz-Schaeffer W, Watanabe T, Waguri S, Kametaka S, Shibata M, Yamamoto K, Kominami E, Peters C, von Figura K, & Uchiyama Y (2000) Cathepsin D deficiency induces lysosomal storage with ceroid lipofuscin in mouse CNS neurons. *J Neurosci*, 20, 6898–6906.

Koike M, Shibata M, Ohsawa Y, Kametaka S, Waguri S, Kominami E, & Uchiyama Y (2002) The expression of tripeptidyl peptidase I in various tissues of rats and mice. *Arch Histol Cytol*, 65, 219–232.

Koike M, Shibata M, Ohsawa Y, Nakanishi H, Koga T, Kametaka S, Waguri S, Momoi T, Kominami E, Peters C, Figura K, Saftig P, & Uchiyama Y (2003) Involvement of two different cell death pathways in retinal atrophy of cathepsin D-deficient mice. *Mol Cell Neurosci*, 22, 146–161.

Koike M, Shibata M, Waguri S, Yoshimura K, Tanida I, Kominami E, Gotow T, Peters C, von Figura K, Mizushima N, Saftig P, & Uchiyama Y (2005) Participation of autophagy in storage of lysosomes in neurons from mouse models of neuronal ceroid-lipofuscinoses (Batten disease). *Am J Pathol*, 167, 1713–1728.

Kominami E, Ezaki J, Muno D, Ishido K, Ueno T, & Wolfe LS (1992) Specific storage of subunit c of mitochondrial ATP synthase in lysosomes of neuronal ceroid lipofuscinosis (Batten's disease). *J Biochem*, 111, 278–282.

Koneff H (1886) *Beiträge zur Kenntniss der Nervenzellen in den peripheren Ganglien*. Inaugural-Dissertation zur Erlangung der Doctorwürde. Bern, Buchdruckerei Paul Haller.

Kopan S, Sivasubramaniam U, & Warburton MJ (2004) The lysosomal degradation of neuromedin B is dependent on tripeptidyl peptidase-I: evidence for the impairment of neuropeptide degradation in late-infantile neuronal ceroid lipofuscinosis. *Biochem Biophys Res Commun*, 319, 58–65.

Koppang N (1966) Familiäre Glykosphingolipoidose des Hundes (Juvenile Amaurotische Idiotie). *Erg Pathol*, 47, 1–43.

Koppang N (1970) Neuronal ceroid-lipofuscinosis in English setters. *J Small Anim Pract*, 10, 639–644.

Koppang N (1973) Canine ceroid-lipofuscinosis-a model for human neuronal ceroid-lipofuscinosis and aging. *Mech Ageing Dev*, 2, 421–445.

Koppang N (1988) The English setter with ceroid-lipofuscinosis: a suitable model for the juvenile type of ceroid-lipofuscinosis in humans. *Am J Med Genet Suppl*, 5, 117–125.

Koppang N (1992) English setter model and juvenile ceroid-lipofuscinosis in man. *Am J Med Genet*, 42, 599–604.

Kopra O, Vesa J, von Schantz C, Manninen T, Minye H, Fabritius AL, Rapola J, van Diggelen OP, Saarela J, Jalanko A, & Peltonen L (2004) A mouse model for Finnish variant late infantile neuronal ceroid lipofuscinosis, CLN5, reveals neuropathology associated with early aging. *Hum Mol Genet*, 13, 2893–2906.

Korey CA & MacDonald ME (2003) An over-expression system for characterizing Ppt1 function in Drosophila. *BMC Neurosci*, 4, 30.

Kornak U, Kasper D, Bosl MR, Kaiser E, Schweizer M, Schulz A, Friedrich W, Delling G, & Jentsch TJ (2001) Loss of the ClC-7 chloride channel leads to osteopetrosis in mice and man. *Cell*, 104, 205–215.

Kornak U, Ostertag A, Branger S, Benichou O, & de Vernejoul MC (2006) Polymorphisms in the CLCN7 gene modulate bone density in postmenopausal women and in patients with autosomal dominant osteopetrosis type II. *J Clin Endocrinol Metab*, 91, 995–1000.

Kostich M, Fire A, & Fambrough DM (2000) Identification and molecular-genetic characterization of a LAMP/CD68-like protein from Caenorhabditis elegans. *J Cell Sci*, 113 (Pt 14), 2595–2606.

Koul R, Al-Futaisi A, Ganesh A, & Rangnath Bushnarmuth S (2007) Late-infantile neuronal ceroid lipofuscinosis (CLN2/Janský-Bielschowsky type) in Oman. *J Child Neurol*, 22, 555–559.

Kousi M, Siintola E, Dvorakova L, Vlaskova H, Turnbull J, Topcu M, Yuksel D, Gokben S, Minassian BA, Elleder M, Mole SE, & Lehesjoki AE (2009) Mutations in CLN7/MFSD8 are a common cause of variant late-infantile neuronal ceroid lipofuscinosis. *Brain*, 132, 810–819.

Kovács AD & Pearce DA (2008) Attenuation of AMPA receptor activity improves motor skills in a mouse model of juvenile Batten disease. *Exp Neurol*, 209, 288–291.

Kovács AD, Saje A, Wong A, Szénási G, Kiricsi P, Szabó E, Cooper JD, Pearce DA (2010). Temporary inhibition of AMPA receptors induces a prolonged improvement of motor performance in a mouse model of juvenile Batten disease. Neuropharmacology. 2010 Oct 28. [Epub ahead of print] PMID: 20971125 [PubMed - as supplied by publisher]

Kovács AD, Weimer JM, & Pearce DA (2006) Selectively increased sensitivity of cerebellar granule cells to AMPA receptor-mediated excitotoxicity in a mouse model of Batten disease. *Neurobiol Dis*, 22, 575–585.

Kremmidiotis G, Lensink IL, Bilton RL, Woollatt E, Chataway TK, Sutherland GR, & Callen DF (1999) The Batten disease gene product (CLN3p) is a Golgi integral membrane protein. *Hum Mol Genet*, 8, 523–531.

Kriscenski-Perry E, Applegate CD, Serour A, Mhyre TR, Leonardo CC, & Pearce DA (2002) Altered flurothyl seizure induction latency, phenotype, and subsequent mortality in a mouse model of juvenile neuronal ceroid lipofuscinosis/Batten disease. *Epilepsia*, 43, 1137–1140.

Kufs H (1925) Über eine Spätform der amaurotischen Idiotie und ihre heredofamiliären Grundlagen. *Z Ges Neurol Psychiatr*, 95, 168–188.

Kufs H (1927) Über die Bedeutung der optischen Komponente der amaurotischen Idiotie in diagnostischer und erbbiologischer Beziehung und über die

Existenz 'spätester' Fälle bei dieser Krankheit. Z *Ges Neurol Psychiatr*, 109, 453–487.

Kufs H (1929) Über einen Fall von Spätform der amaurotischen Idiotie mit atypischem Verlauf und mit terminalen schweren Störungen des Fettstoffwechsels im Gesamtorganismus. *Z Ges Neurol Psychiatr*, 122, 395–415.

Kufs H (1931) Über einen Fall von spätester Form der amaurotische Idiotie mit dem Beginn im 42 und Tod im 59. Lebensjahre in klinischer, histologischer und vererbungspathologischer Beziehung. *Z Ges Neurol Psychiatr*, 137, 432–448.

Kurachi Y, Oka A, Itoh M, Mizuguchi M, Hayashi M, & Takashima S (2001) Distribution and development of CLN2 protein, the late-infantile neuronal ceroid lipofuscinosis gene product. *Acta Neuropathol*, 102, 20–26.

Kurachi Y, Oka A, Mizuguchi M, Ohkoshi Y, Sasaki M, Itoh M, Hayashi M, Goto Y, & Takashima S (2000) Rapid immunologic diagnosis of classic late infantile neuronal ceroid lipofuscinosis. *Neurology*, 54, 1676–1680.

Kuronen M, Talvitie M, Lehesjoki AE, & Myllykangas L (2009) Genetic modifiers of degeneration in the cathepsin D deficient Drosophila model for neuronal ceroid lipofuscinosis. *Neurobiol Dis*, 36, 488–493.

Kurze AK, Galliciotti G, Heine C, Mole SE, Quitsch A, & Braulke T (2010) Pathogenic mutations cause rapid degradation of lysosomal storage disease-related membrane protein CLN6. *Hum Mutat*, 31, E1163–1174.

Kuwamura M, Hattori R, Yamate J, Kotani T, & Sasai K (2003) Neuronal ceroid-lipofuscinosis and hydrocephalus in a chihuahua. *J Small Anim Pract*, 44, 227–230.

Kwon JM, Rothberg PG, Leman AR, Weimer JM, Mink JW, & Pearce DA (2005) Novel CLN3 mutation predicted to cause complete loss of protein function does not modify the classical JNCL phenotype. *Neurosci Lett*, 387, 111–114.

Kyttälä A, Ihrke G, Vesa J, Schell MJ, & Luzio JP (2004) Two motifs target Batten disease protein CLN3 to lysosomes in transfected nonneuronal and neuronal cells. *Mol Biol Cell*, 15, 1313–1323.

Kyttälä A, Lahtinen U, Braulke T, & Hofmann SL (2006) Functional biology of the neuronal ceroid lipofuscinoses (NCL) proteins. *Biochim Biophys Acta*, 1762, 920–933.

Kyttalä A, Yliannala K, Schu P, Jalanko A, & Luzio JP (2005) AP-1 and AP-3 facilitate lysosomal targeting of Batten disease protein CLN3 via its dileucine motif. *J Biol Chem*, 280, 10277–10283.

Lacorazza HD, Flax JD, Snyder EY, & Jendoubi M (1996) Expression of human beta-hexosaminidase alpha-subunit gene (the gene defect of Tay-Sachs disease) in mouse brains upon engraftment of transduced progenitor cells. *Nat Med*, 2, 424–429.

Lake BD, Brett EM, & Boyd SG (1996) A form of juvenile Batten disease with granular osmiophilic deposits. *Neuropediatrics*, 27, 265–269.

Lake BD & Cavanagh NP (1978) Early-juvenile Batten's disease—a recognisable sub-group distinct from other forms of Batten's disease. Analysis of 5 patients. *J Neurol Sci*, 36, 265–271.

Lake BD & Hall NA (1993) Immunolocalization studies of subunit c in late-infantile and juvenile Batten disease. *J Inherit Metab Dis*, 16, 263–266.

Lake BD & Rowan SA (1997) Light and electron microscopic studies on subunit c in cultured fibroblasts in late infantile and juvenile Batten disease. *Neuropediatrics*, 28, 56–59.

Lake BD, Steward CG, Oakhill A, Wilson J, & Perham TG (1997) Bone marrow transplantation in late infantile Batten disease and juvenile Batten disease. *Neuropediatrics*, 28, 80–81.

Lake BD, Young EP, & Winchester BG (1998) Prenatal diagnosis of lysosomal storage diseases. *Brain Pathol*, 8, 133–149.

Lam CW, Poon PM, Tong SF, & Ko CH (2001) Two novel CLN2 gene mutations in a Chinese patient with classical late-infantile neuronal ceroid lipofuscinosis. *Am J Med Genet*, 99, 161–163.

Lamminranta S, Åberg LE, Autti T, Moren R, Laine T, Kaukoranta J, & Santavuori P (2001) Neuropsychological test battery in the follow-up of patients with juvenile neuronal ceroid lipofuscinosis. *J Intellect Disabil Res*, 45, 8–17.

Lane SC, Jolly RD, Schmechel DE, Alroy J, & Boustany RM (1996) Apoptosis as the mechanism of neurodegeneration in Batten's disease. *J Neurochem*, 67, 677–683.

Lange PF, Wartosch L, Jentsch TJ, & Fuhrmann JC (2006) ClC-7 requires Ostm1 as a beta-subunit to support bone resorption and lysosomal function. *Nature*, 440, 220–223.

Larnaout A, Belal S, Zouari M, Fki M, Ben Hamida C, Goebel HH, Ben Hamida M, & Hentati F (1997) Friedreich's ataxia with isolated vitamin E deficiency: a neuropathological study of a Tunisian patient. *Acta Neuropathol*, 93, 633–637.

Larsen A, Sainio K, Åberg L, & Santavuori P (2001) Electroencephalography in juvenile neuronal ceroid lipofuscinosis: visual and quantitative analysis. *Eur J Paediatr Neurol*, 5 Suppl A, 179–183.

Lauronen L, Heikkila E, Autti T, Sainio K, Huttunen J, Aronen HJ, Korvenoja A, Ilmoniemi RJ, & Santavuori P (1997) Somatosensory evoked magnetic fields from primary sensorimotor cortex in juvenile neuronal ceroid lipofuscinosis. *J Child Neurol*, 12, 355–360.

Lauronen L, Munroe PB, Jarvela I, Autti T, Mitchison HM, O'Rawe AM, Gardiner RM, Mole SE, Puranen J, Hakkinen AM, Kirveskari E, & Santavuori P (1999) Delayed classic and protracted phenotypes of compound heterozygous juvenile neuronal ceroid lipofuscinosis. *Neurology*, 52, 360–365.

Lavrov AY, Ilyna ES, Zakharova EY, Boukina AM, & Tishkanina SV (2002) The first three Russian cases of classical, late-infantile, neuronal ceroid lipofuscinosis. *Eur J Paediatr Neurol*, 6, 161–164.

Le Meur G, Stieger K, Smith AJ, Weber M, Deschamps JY, Nivard D, Mendes-Madeira A, Provost N, Pereon Y, Cherel Y, Ali RR, Hamel C, Moullier P, & Rolling F (2007) Restoration of vision in RPE65-deficient Briard dogs using an AAV serotype 4 vector that specifically targets the retinal pigmented epithelium. *Gene Ther*, 14, 292–303.

Lebrun AH, Storch S, Ruschendorf F, Schmiedt ML, Kyttala A, Mole SE, Kitzmuller C, Saar K, Mewasingh LD, Boda V, Kohlschutter A, Ullrich K, Braulke T, & Schulz A (2009) Retention of lysosomal protein CLN5 in the endoplasmic reticulum causes neuronal ceroid lipofuscinosis in Asian sibship. *Hum Mutat*, 30, E651–661.

Lee TS, Poon SH, & Chang P (2010) Dissimilar neuropsychiatric presentations of two siblings with juvenile neuronal ceroid lipofuscinosis (Batten disease). *J Neuropsychiatry Clin Neurosci*, 22, 123.E14–15.

Lehtovirta M, Kyttala A, Eskelinen EL, Hess M, Heinonen O, & Jalanko A (2001) Palmitoyl protein thioesterase (PPT) localizes into synaptosomes and synaptic vesicles in neurons: implications for infantile neuronal ceroid lipofuscinosis (INCL). *Hum Mol Genet*, 10, 69–75.

Lei B, Tullis GE, Kirk MD, Zhang K, & Katz ML (2006) Ocular phenotype in a mouse gene knockout model for infantile neuronal ceroid lipofuscinosis. *J Neurosci Res*, 84, 1139–1149.

Leman AR, Pearce DA, & Rothberg PG (2005) Gene symbol: CLN3. Disease: Juvenile neuronal ceroid lipofuscinosis (Batten disease). *Hum Genet*, 116, 544.

Leonberg SCJ, Armstrong D, & Boehme D (1982) A century of Kufs disease in an American family. In Armstrong, D., Koppang, N., Rider, J.A. (Eds) *Ceroid-lipofuscinosis (Batten disease)*, pp87–93. Amsterdam, Elsevier Biomedical Press.

Lercher MJ, Blumenthal T, & Hurst LD (2003) Coexpression of neighboring genes in Caenorhabditis elegans is mostly due to operons and duplicate genes. *Genome Res*, 13, 238–243.

Lerner TJ, Boustany RM, MacCormack K, Gleitsman J, Schlumpf K, Breakefield XO, Gusella JF, & Haines JL (1994) Linkage disequilibrium between the juvenile neuronal ceroid lipofuscinosis gene and marker loci on chromosome 16p 12.1. *Am J Hum Genet*, 54, 88–94.

Li J, Brown G, Ailion M, Lee S, & Thomas JH (2004) NCR-1 and NCR-2, the C. elegans homologs of the human Niemann-Pick type C1 disease protein, function upstream of DAF-9 in the dauer formation pathways. *Development*, 131, 5741–5752.

Libert J (1980) Diagnosis of lysosomal storage diseases by the ultrastructural study of conjunctival biopsies. *Pathol Annu*, 15, 37–66.

Lim MJ, Alexander N, Benedict JW, Chattopadhyay S, Shemilt SJ, Guerin CJ, Cooper JD, & Pearce DA (2007) IgG entry and deposition are components of the neuroimmune response in Batten disease. *Neurobiol Dis*, 25, 239–251.

Lim MJ, Beake J, Bible E, Curran TM, Ramirez-Montealegre D, Pearce DA, & Cooper JD (2006) Distinct patterns of serum immunoreactivity as evidence for multiple brain-directed autoantibodies in juvenile neuronal ceroid lipofuscinosis. *Neuropathol Appl Neurobiol*, 32, 469–482.

Lin L & Lobel P (2001a) Expression and analysis of CLN2 variants in CHO cells: Q100R represents a polymorphism, and G389E and R447H represent loss-of-function mutations. *Hum Mutat*, 18, 165.

Lin L & Lobel P (2001b) Production and characterization of recombinant human CLN2 protein for enzyme-replacement therapy in late infantile neuronal ceroid lipofuscinosis. *Biochem J*, 357, 49–55.

Lin L, Sohar I, Lackland H, & Lobel P (2001) The human CLN2 protein/tripeptidyl-peptidase I is a serine protease that autoactivates at acidic pH. *J Biol Chem*, 276, 2249–2255.

Lindblad-Toh K, Wade CM, Mikkelsen TS, Karlsson EK, Jaffe DB, Kamal M, Clamp M, Chang JL, Kulbokas EJ, 3rd, Zody MC, et al. (2005) Genome sequence, comparative analysis and haplotype structure of the domestic dog. *Nature*, 438, 803–819.

Linder ME & Deschenes RJ (2007) Palmitoylation: policing protein stability and traffic. *Nat Rev Mol Cell Biol*, 8, 74–84.

Lindstedt L, Lee M, Oorni K, Bromme D, & Kovanen PT (2003) Cathepsins F and S block HDL3-induced cholesterol efflux from macrophage foam cells. *Biochem Biophys Res Commun*, 312, 1019–1024.

Lingaas F, Aarskaug T, Sletten M, Bjerkas I, Grimholt U, Moe L, Juneja RK, Wilton AN, Galibert F, Holmes NG, & Dolf G (1998) Genetic markers linked to neuronal ceroid lipofuscinosis in English setter dogs. *Anim Genet*, 29, 371–376.

Lingaas F, Sorensen A, Juneja RK, Johansson S, Fredholm M, Wintero AK, Sampson J, Mellersh C, Curzon A, Holmes NG, Binns MM, Dickens HF, Ryder EJ, Gerlach J, Baumle E, & Dolf G (1997) Towards construction of a canine linkage map: establishment of 16 linkage groups. *Mamm Genome*, 8, 218–221.

Linthorst GE, Hollak CE, Donker-Koopman WE, Strijland A, & Aerts JM (2004) Enzyme therapy for Fabry disease: neutralizing antibodies toward agalsidase alpha and beta. *Kidney Int*, 66, 1589–1595.

Liu CG, Sleat DE, Donnelly RJ, & Lobel P (1998) Structural organization and sequence of CLN2, the defective gene in classical late infantile neuronal ceroid lipofuscinosis. *Genomics*, 50, 206–212.

Liu G, Martins I, Wemmie JA, Chiorini JA, & Davidson BL (2005) Functional correction of CNS phenotypes in a lysosomal storage disease model using adeno-associated virus type 4 vectors. *J Neurosci*, 25, 9321–9327.

Loiseau P, Chedru F, Habib M, & Pellissier JF (1990) [Conference at the Salpetriere. November 1988. Progressive dementia and generalized epilepsy in a young woman]. *Rev Neurol (Paris)*, 146, 383–389.

Lonka L, Aalto A, Kopra O, Kuronen M, Kokaia Z, Saarma M, & Lehesjoki AE (2005) The neuronal ceroid lipofuscinosis Cln8 gene expression is developmentally regulated in mouse brain and up-regulated in the hippocampal kindling model of epilepsy. *BMC Neurosci*, 6, 27.

Lonka L, Kyttala A, Ranta S, Jalanko A, & Lehesjoki AE (2000) The neuronal ceroid lipofuscinosis CLN8 membrane protein is a resident of the endoplasmic reticulum. *Hum Mol Genet*, 9, 1691–1697.

Lonka L, Salonen T, Siintola E, Kopra O, Lehesjoki AE, & Jalanko A (2004) Localization of wild-type and mutant neuronal ceroid lipofuscinosis CLN8 proteins in non-neuronal and neuronal cells. *J Neurosci Res*, 76, 862–871.

Lonnqvist T, Vanhanen SL, Vettenranta K, Autti T, Rapola J, Santavuori P, & Saarinen-Pihkala UM (2001) Hematopoietic stem cell transplantation in infantile neuronal ceroid lipofuscinosis. *Neurology*, 57, 1411–1416.

Lonser RR, Walbridge S, Murray GJ, Aizenberg MR, Vortmeyer AO, Aerts JM, Brady RO, & Oldfield EH (2005) Convection perfusion of glucocerebrosidase for neuronopathic Gaucher's disease. *Ann Neurol*, 57, 542–548.

Lorenz R (2002) A casuistic rationale for the treatment of spastic and myocloni in a childhood neurodegenerative disease: neuronal ceroid lipofuscinosis of the type Janský-Bielschowsky. *Neuro Endocrinol Lett*, 23, 387–390.

Lou HC & Kristensen K (1973) A clinical and psychological investigation into juvenile amaurotic idiocy in Denmark. *Dev Med Child Neurol*, 15, 313–323.

Louvet-Vallee S (2000) ERM proteins: from cellular architecture to cell signaling. *Biol Cell*, 92, 305–316.

Lowery LA & Sive H (2004) Strategies of vertebrate neurulation and a re-evaluation of teleost neural tube formation. *Mech Dev*, 121, 1189–1197.

Lu JY, Hu J, & Hofmann SL (2010) Human recombinant palmitoyl-protein thioesterase-1 (PPT1) for preclinical evaluation of enzyme replacement therapy for infantile neuronal ceroid lipofuscinosis. *Mol Genet Metab*, 99, 374–378.

Lu JY, Verkruyse LA, & Hofmann SL (2002) The effects of lysosomotropic agents on normal and INCL cells provide further evidence for the lysosomal nature of palmitoyl-protein thioesterase function. *Biochim Biophys Acta*, 1583, 35–44.

Luiro K, Kopra O, Blom T, Gentile M, Mitchison HM, Hovatta I, Tornquist K, & Jalanko A (2006) Batten disease (JNCL) is linked to disturbances in mitochondrial, cytoskeletal, and synaptic compartments. *J Neurosci Res*, 84, 1124–1138.

Luiro K, Kopra O, Lehtovirta M, & Jalanko A (2001) CLN3 protein is targeted to neuronal synapses but excluded from synaptic vesicles: new clues to Batten disease. *Hum Mol Genet*, 10, 2123–2131.

Luiro K, Yliannala K, Ahtiainen L, Maunu H, Jarvela I, Kyttala A, & Jalanko A (2004) Interconnections of CLN3, Hook1 and Rab proteins link Batten disease to defects in the endocytic pathway. *Hum Mol Genet*, 13, 3017–3027.

Lukacs Z, Santavuori P, Keil A, Steinfeld R, & Kohlschutter A (2003) Rapid and simple assay for the determination of tripeptidyl peptidase and palmitoyl protein thioesterase activities in dried blood spots. *Clin Chem*, 49, 509–511.

Lyly A, Marjavaara SK, Kyttala A, Uusi-Rauva K, Luiro K, Kopra O, Martinez LO, Tanhuanpaa K, Kalkkinen N, Suomalainen A, Jauhiainen M, & Jalanko A (2008) Deficiency of the INCL protein Ppt1 results in changes in ectopic F1-ATP synthase and altered cholesterol metabolism. *Hum Mol Genet*, 17, 1406–1417.

Lyly A, von Schantz C, Heine C, Schmiedt ML, Sipila T, Jalanko A, & Kyttala A (2009) Novel interactions of CLN5 support molecular networking between neuronal ceroid lipofuscinosis proteins. *BMC Cell Biol*, 10, 83.

Macauley SL, Wozniak DF, Kielar C, Tan Y, Cooper JD, & Sands MS (2009) Cerebellar pathology and motor deficits in the palmitoyl protein thioesterase 1-deficient mouse. *Exp Neurol*, 217, 124–135.

MacLeod PM, Dolman CL, Chang E, Applegarth DA, & Bryant B (1976) The neuronal ceroid lipofuscinoses in British Columbia: a clinical epidemiologic and ultrastructural study. *Birth Defects Orig Artic Ser*, 12, 289–296.

Maguire AM, Simonelli F, Pierce EA, Pugh EN, Jr., Mingozzi F, Bennicelli J, Banfi S, Marshall KA, Testa F, Surace EM, Rossi S, Lyubarsky A, Arruda VR, Konkle B, Stone E, Sun J, Jacobs J, Dell'Osso L, Hertle R, Ma JX, Redmond TM, Zhu X, Hauck B, Zelenaia O, Shindler KS, Maguire MG, Wright JF, Volpe NJ, McDonnell JW, Auricchio A, High KA, & Bennett J (2008) Safety and efficacy of gene transfer for Leber's congenital amaurosis. *N Engl J Med*, 358, 2240–2248.

Majander A, Pihko H, & Santavuori P (1995) Palmitate oxidation in muscle mitochondria of patients with the juvenile form of neuronal ceroid-lipofuscinosis. *Am J Med Genet*, 57, 298–300.

Mannerkoski MK, Heiskala HJ, Santavuori PR, & Pouttu JA (2001) Transdermal fentanyl therapy for pains in children with infantile neuronal ceroid lipofuscinosis. *Eur J Paediatr Neurol*, 5 Suppl A, 175–177.

Mao Q, Foster BJ, Xia H, & Davidson BL (2003) Membrane topology of CLN3, the protein underlying Batten disease. *FEBS Lett*, 541, 40–46.

March PA, Wurzelmann S, & Walkley SU (1995) Morphological alterations in neocortical and cerebellar GABAergic neurons in a canine model of juvenile Batten disease. *Am J Med Genet*, 57, 204–212.

Markova M, Barker JN, Miller JS, Arora M, Wagner JE, Burns LJ, MacMillan ML, Douek D, DeFor T, Tan Y, Repka T, Blazar BR, & Weisdorf DJ (2007) Fludarabine vs cladribine plus busulfan and low-dose TBI as reduced intensity conditioning for allogeneic hematopoietic stem cell transplantation: a prospective randomized trial. *Bone Marrow Transplant*, 39, 193–199.

Marshall FJ, de Blieck EA, Mink JW, Dure L, Adams H, Messing S, Rothberg PG, Levy E, McDonough T, DeYoung J, Wang M, Ramirez-Montealegre D, Kwon JM, & Pearce DA (2005) A clinical rating scale for Batten disease: reliable and relevant for clinical trials. *Neurology*, 65, 275–279.

Martin JJ (1991) Adult type of neuronal ceroid lipofuscinosis. *Dev Neurosci*, 13, 331–338.

Martin JJ (1993) Adult type of neuronal ceroid-lipofuscinosis. *J Inherit Metab Dis*, 16, 237–240.

Martin JJ & Ceuterick C (1997) Adult neuronal ceroid-lipofuscinosis—personal observations. *Acta Neurol Belg*, 97, 85–92.

Martin JJ, Libert J, & Ceuterick C (1987) Ultrastructure of brain and retina in Kufs' disease (adult type-ceroid-lipofuscinosis). *Clin Neuropathol*, 6, 231–235.

Martinus RD, Harper PA, Jolly RD, Bayliss SL, Midwinter GG, Shaw GJ, & Palmer DN (1991) Bovine ceroid-lipofuscinosis (Batten's disease): the major component stored is the DCCD-reactive proteolipid, subunit C, of mitochondrial ATP synthase. *Vet Res Commun*, 15, 85–94.

Mastakov MY, Baer K, Symes CW, Leichtlein CB, Kotin RM, & During MJ (2002) Immunological aspects of recombinant adeno-associated virus delivery to the mammalian brain. *J Virol*, 76, 8446–8454.

Mayhew IG, Jolly RD, Pickett BT, & Slack PM (1985) Ceroid-lipofuscinosis (Batten's disease): pathogenesis of blindness in the ovine model. *Neuropathol Appl Neurobiol*, 11, 273–290.

Mazzei R, Conforti FL, Magariello A, Bravaccio C, Militerni R, Gabriele AL, Sampaolo S, Patitucci A, Di Iorio G, Muglia M, & Quattrone A (2002) A novel mutation in the CLN1 gene in a patient with juvenile neuronal ceroid lipofuscinosis. *J Neurol*, 249, 1398–1400.

McCaughan KK, Brown CM, Dalphin ME, Berry MJ, & Tate WP (1995) Translational termination efficiency in mammals is influenced by the base following the stop codon. *Proc Natl Acad Sci U S A*, 92, 5431–5435.

McDonald JK (1998) Dipeptidyl peptidase II. In Barrett AJ, Rawlings ND, & Woessner JF (Eds.) *Handbook of Proteolytic Enzymes*, pp. 408–411. London, Academic Press.

McDonald JK, Hoisington AR, & Eisenhauer DA (1985) Partial purification and characterization of an ovarian tripeptidyl peptidase: a lysosomal exopeptidase that sequentially releases collagen-related (Gly-Pro-X) triplets. *Biochem Biophys Res Commun*, 126, 63–71.

McDonald JK & Schwabe C (1980) Dipeptidyl peptidase II of bovine dental pulp. Initial demonstration and characterization as a fibroblastic, lysosomal peptidase of the serine class active on collagen-related peptides. *Biochim Biophys Acta*, 616, 68–81.

McGeoch JE & Palmer DN (1999) Ion pores made of mitochondrial ATP synthase subunit c in the neuronal plasma membrane and Batten disease. *Mol Genet Metab*, 66, 387–392.

Mellersh CS, Langston AA, Acland GM, Fleming MA, Ray K, Wiegand NA, Francisco LV, Gibbs M, Aguirre GD, & Ostrander EA (1997) A linkage map of the canine genome. *Genomics*, 46, 326–336.

Melville SA, Wilson CL, Chiang CS, Studdert VP, Lingaas F, & Wilton AN (2005) A mutation in canine CLN5 causes neuronal ceroid lipofuscinosis in Border collie dogs. *Genomics*, 86, 287–294.

Mennini T, Bigini P, Cagnotto A, Carvelli L, Di Nunno P, Fumagalli E, Tortarolo M, Buurman WA, Ghezzi P, & Bendotti C (2004) Glial activation and TNFR-I upregulation precedes motor dysfunction in the spinal cord of mnd mice. *Cytokine*, 25, 127–135.

Mennini T, Bigini P, Ravizza T, Vezzani A, Calvaresi N, Tortarolo M, & Bendotti C (2002) Expression of glutamate receptor subtypes in the spinal cord of control and mnd mice, a model of motor neuron disorder. *J Neurosci Res*, 70, 553–560.

Messer A & Flaherty L (1986) Autosomal dominance in a late-onset motor neuron disease in the mouse. *J Neurogenet*, 3, 345–355.

Messer A, Plummer J, MacMillen MC, & Frankel WN (1995) Genetics of primary and timing effects in the mnd mouse. *Am J Med Genet*, 57, 361–364.

Messer A, Strominger NL, & Mazurkiewicz JE (1987) Histopathology of the late-onset motor neuron degeneration (Mnd) mutant in the mouse. *J Neurogenet*, 4, 201–213.

Metcalf P & Fusek M (1993) Two crystal structures for cathepsin D: the lysosomal targeting signal and active site. *EMBO J*, 12, 1293–1302.

Metcalfe DJ, Calvi AA, Seamann MNJ, Mitchison HM, & Cutler DF (2008) Loss of the Batten disease gene CLN3 prevents exit from the TGN of the mannose 6-phosphate receptor. *Traffic*, 11, 1905–1914.

Metzler M, Legendre-Guillemin V, Gan L, Chopra V, Kwok A, McPherson PS, & Hayden MR (2001) HIP1 functions in clathrin-mediated endocytosis through binding to clathrin and adaptor protein 2. *J Biol Chem*, 276, 39271–39276.

Michalewski MP, Kaczmarski W, Golabek AA, Kida E, Kaczmarski A, & Wisniewski KE (1998) Evidence for phosphorylation of CLN3 protein associated with Batten disease. *Biochem Biophys Res Commun*, 253, 458–462.

Michalewski MP, Kaczmarski W, Golabek AA, Kida E, Kaczmarski A, & Wisniewski KE (1999) Posttranslational modification of CLN3 protein and its possible functional implication. *Mol Genet Metab*, 66, 272–276.

Millichamp NJ, Curtis R, & Barnett KC (1988) Progressive retinal atrophy in Tibetan terriers. *J Am Vet Med Assoc*, 192, 769–776.

Minagar A, Shapshak P, Fujimura R, Ownby R, Heyes M, & Eisdorfer C (2002) The role of macrophage/microglia and astrocytes in the pathogenesis of three neurologic disorders: HIV-associated dementia, Alzheimer disease, and multiple sclerosis. *J Neurol Sci*, 202, 13–23.

Minatel L, Underwood SC, & Carfagnini JC (2000) Ceroid-lipofuscinosis in a Cocker Spaniel dog. *Vet Pathol*, 37, 488–490.

Mitchell DA, Vasudevan A, Linder ME, & Deschenes RJ (2006) Protein palmitoylation by a family of DHHC protein S-acyltransferases. *J Lipid Res*, 47, 1118–1127.

Mitchell WA, Porter M, Kuwabara P, & Mole SE (2001) Genomic structure of three CLN3-like genes in Caenorhabditis elegans. *Eur J Paediatr Neurol*, 5 Suppl A, 121–125.

Mitchison HM, Bernard DJ, Greene ND, Cooper JD, Junaid MA, Pullarkat RK, de Vos N, Breuning MH, Owens JW, Mobley WC, Gardiner RM, Lake BD, Taschner PE, & Nussbaum RL (1999) Targeted disruption of the Cln3 gene provides a mouse model for Batten disease. The Batten Mouse Model Consortium [corrected]. *Neurobiol Dis*, 6, 321–334.

Mitchison HM, Hofmann SL, Becerra CH, Munroe PB, Lake BD, Crow YJ, Stephenson JB, Williams RE, Hofman IL, Taschner PE, Martin JJ, Philippart M, Andermann E, Andermann F, Mole SE, Gardiner RM, & O'Rawe AM (1998) Mutations in the palmitoyl-protein thioesterase gene (PPT; CLN1) causing juvenile neuronal ceroid lipofuscinosis with granular osmiophilic deposits. *Hum Mol Genet*, 7, 291–297.

Mitchison HM, Lim MJ, & Cooper JD (2004) Selectivity and types of cell death in the neuronal ceroid lipofuscinoses. *Brain Pathol*, 14, 86–96.

Mitchison HM, Munroe PB, O'Rawe AM, Taschner PE, de Vos N, Kremmidiotis G, Lensink I, Munk AC, D'Arigo KL, Anderson JW, Lerner TJ, Moyzis RK, Callen DF, Breuning MH, Doggett NA, Gardiner RM, & Mole SE (1997a) Genomic structure and complete nucleotide sequence of the Batten disease gene, CLN3. *Genomics*, 40, 346–350.

Mitchison HM, O'Rawe AM, Taschner PE, Sandkuijl LA, Santavuori P, de Vos N, Breuning MH, Mole SE, Gardiner RM, & Jarvela IE (1995) Batten disease gene, CLN3: linkage disequilibrium mapping in the Finnish population, and analysis of European haplotypes. *Am J Hum Genet*, 56, 654–662.

Mitchison HM, Taschner PE, Kremmidiotis G, Callen DF, Doggett NA, Lerner TJ, Janes RB, Wallace BA, Munroe PB, O'Rawe AM, Gardiner RM, & Mole SE (1997b) Structure of the CLN3 gene and predicted structure, location and function of CLN3 protein. *Neuropediatrics*, 28, 12–14.

Mitchison HM, Thompson AD, Mulley JC, Kozman HM, Richards RI, Callen DF, Stallings RL, Doggett NA, Attwood J, McKay TR, et al. (1993) Fine genetic mapping of the Batten disease locus (CLN3) by haplotype analysis and demonstration of allelic association with chromosome 16p microsatellite loci. *Genomics*, 16, 455–460.

Miyahara A, Saito Y, Sugai K, Nakagawa E, Sakuma H, Komaki H, & Sasaki M (2009) Reassessment of phenytoin for treatment of late stage progressive myoclonus epilepsy complicated with status epilepticus. *Epilepsy Res*, 84, 201–209.

Mizutani Y, Kihara A, & Igarashi Y (2005) Mammalian Lass6 and its related family members regulate synthesis of specific ceramides. *Biochem J*, 390, 263–271.

Mole SE (2004) The genetic spectrum of human neuronal ceroid-lipofuscinoses. *Brain Pathol*, 14, 70–76.

Mole SE, Michaux G, Codlin S, Wheeler RB, Sharp JD, & Cutler DF (2004) CLN6, which is associated with a lysosomal storage disease, is an endoplasmic reticulum protein. *Exp Cell Res*, 298, 399–406.

Mole SE, Williams RE, & Goebel HH (2005) Correlations between genotype, ultrastructural morphology and clinical phenotype in the neuronal ceroid lipofuscinoses. *Neurogenetics*, 6, 107–126.

Mole SE, Zhong NA, Sarpong A, Logan WP, Hofmann S, Yi W, Franken PF, van Diggelen OP, Breuning MH, Moroziewicz D, Ju W, Salonen T, Holmberg V, Jarvela I, & Taschner PE (2001) New mutations in the neuronal ceroid lipofuscinosis genes. *Eur J Paediatr Neurol*, 5 Suppl A, 7–10.

Moore SJ, Buckley DJ, MacMillan A, Marshall HD, Steele L, Ray PN, Nawaz Z, Baskin B, Frecker M, Carr SM, Ives E, & Parfrey PS (2008) The clinical and genetic epidemiology of neuronal ceroid lipofuscinosis in Newfoundland. *Clin Genet*, 74, 213–222.

Mueller T & Wulliman MF (2005) *Atlas of Early Zebrafish Brain Development: A Tool for Molecular Neurogeneticists*. Amsterdam, Elsevier.

Munroe PB, Greene ND, Leung KY, Mole SE, Gardiner RM, Mitchison HM, Stephenson JB, & Crow YJ (1998) Sharing of PPT mutations between distinct clinical forms of neuronal ceroid lipofuscinoses in patients from Scotland. *J Med Genet*, 35, 790.

Munroe PB, Mitchison HM, O'Rawe AM, Anderson JW, Boustany RM, Lerner TJ, Taschner PE, de Vos N, Breuning MH, Gardiner RM, & Mole SE (1997) Spectrum of mutations in the Batten disease gene, CLN3. *Am J Hum Genet*, 61, 310–316.

Munroe PB, Rapola J, Mitchison HM, Mustonen A, Mole SE, Gardiner RM, & Jarvela I (1996) Prenatal diagnosis of Batten's disease. *Lancet*, 347, 1014–1015.

Muqit MM, & Feany MB (2002) Modelling neurodegenerative diseases in Drosophila: a fruitful approach? *Nat Rev Neurosci*, 3, 237–243.

Mutka AL, Haapanen A, Kakela R, Lindfors M, Wright AK, Inkinen T, Hermansson M, Rokka A, Corthals G, Jauhiainen M, Gillingwater TH, Ikonen E, & Tyynelä J (2010) Murine cathepsin D deficiency is associated with dysmyelination/myelin disruption and accumulation of cholesteryl esters in the brain. *J Neurochem*, 112, 193–203.

Myllykangas L, Tyynelä J, Page-McCaw A, Rubin GM, Haltia MJ, & Feany MB (2005) Cathepsin D-deficient Drosophila recapitulate the key features of neuronal ceroid lipofuscinoses. *Neurobiol Dis*, 19, 194–199.

Nakanishi H, Amano T, Sastradipura DF, Yoshimine Y, Tsukuba T, Tanabe K, Hirotsu I, Ohono T, & Yamamoto K (1997) Increased expression of cathepsins E and D in neurons of the aged rat brain and their colocalization with lipofuscin and carboxy-terminal fragments of Alzheimer amyloid precursor protein. *J Neurochem*, 68, 739–749.

Nakanishi H, Tominaga K, Amano T, Hirotsu I, Inoue T, & Yamamoto K (1994) Age-related changes in activities and localizations of cathepsins D, E, B, and L in the rat brain tissues. *Exp Neurol*, 126, 119–128.

Nakanishi H, Zhang J, Koike M, Nishioku T, Okamoto Y, Kominami E, von Figura K, Peters C, Yamamoto K, Saftig P, & Uchiyama Y (2001) Involvement of nitric oxide released from microglia-macrophages in pathological changes of cathepsin D-deficient mice. *J Neurosci*, 21, 7526–7533.

Nakano Y, Fujitani K, Kurihara J, Ragan J, Usui-Aoki K, Shimoda L, Lukacsovich T, Suzuki K, Sezaki M, Sano Y, Ueda R, Awano W, Kaneda M, Umeda M, & Yamamoto D (2001) Mutations in the novel membrane protein spinster interfere with programmed cell death and cause neural degeneration in Drosophila melanogaster. *Mol Cell Biol*, 21, 3775–3788.

Nakayama H, Uchida K, Shouda T, Uetsuka K, Sasaki N, & Goto N (1993) Systemic ceroid-lipofuscinosis in a Japanese domestic cat. *J Vet Med Sci*, 55, 829–831.

Narayan SB, Rakheja D, Pastor JV, Rosenblatt K, Greene SR, Yang J, Wolf BA, & Bennett MJ (2006) Over-expression of CLN3P, the Batten disease protein, inhibits PANDER-induced apoptosis in neuroblastoma cells: further evidence that CLN3P has anti-apoptotic properties. *Mol Genet Metab*, 88, 178–183.

Narayan SB, Tan L, & Bennett MJ (2008) Intermediate levels of neuronal palmitoyl-protein Delta-9 desaturase in heterozygotes for murine Batten disease. *Mol Genet Metab*, 93, 89–91.

Nardocci N, Verga ML, Binelli S, Zorzi G, Angelini L, & Bugiani O (1995) Neuronal ceroid-lipofuscinosis: a clinical and morphological study of 19 patients. *Am J Med Genet*, 57, 137–141.

Narfstrom K & Wrigstad A (1995) Clinical, electrophysiological, and morphological findings in a case of neuronal ceroid lipofuscinosis in the Polish Owczarek Nizinny (PON) dog. *Vet Q*, 17 Suppl 1, S46.

Narfstrom K, Wrigstad A, Ekesten B, & Berg AL (2007) Neuronal ceroid lipofuscinosis: clinical and morphologic findings in nine affected Polish Owczarek Nizinny (PON) dogs. *Vet Ophthalmol*, 10, 111–120.

Nehrke K, Begenisich T, Pilato J, & Melvin JE (2000) Into ion channel and transporter function. Caenorhabditis elegans ClC-type chloride channels: novel variants and functional expression. *Am J Physiol Cell Physiol*, 279, C2052–2066.

Neumann H (2001) Control of glial immune function by neurons. *Glia*, 36, 191–199.

Ng Ying Kin NM, Palo J, Haltia M, & Wolfe LS (1983) High levels of brain dolichols in neuronal ceroid-lipofuscinosis and senescence. *J Neurochem*, 40, 1465–1473.

Nicholas KB, Nicholas HB, Jr, & Deerfield DW, II (1997) GeneDoc: analysis and visualization of genetic variation. *EMBNEW.NEWS*, 4, 14.

Nijssen PC, Brekelmans GJ, & Roos RA (2009) Electroencephalography in autosomal dominant adult neuronal ceroid lipofuscinosis. *Clin Neurophysiol*, 120, 1782–1786.

Nijssen PC, Brusse E, Leyten AC, Martin JJ, Teepen JL, & Roos RA (2002) Autosomal dominant adult neuronal ceroid lipofuscinosis: parkinsonism due to both striatal and nigral dysfunction. *Mov Disord*, 17, 482–487.

Nijssen PC, Ceuterick C, van Diggelen OP, Elleder M, Martin JJ, Teepen JL, Tyynelä J, & Roos RA (2003) Autosomal dominant adult neuronal ceroid lipofuscinosis: a novel form of NCL with granular osmiophilic deposits without palmitoyl protein thioesterase 1 deficiency. *Brain Pathol*, 13, 574–581.

Nilsson I (2003) Karl Gustaf Torsten Sjögren. In Nilzén G (Ed.) *Svenskt Biografiskt Lexikon*, pp. 381–384. Stockholm.

Nissen AJ (1954) Juvenil amaurotisk idioti I Norge (Juvenile amaurotic idiocy in Norway). *Nord Med*, 52, 1542–1546.

Noher de Halac I, Dodelson de Kremer R, Kohan RN et al. (2005) *Clinical, morphological, biochemical and molecular study of atypical forms of neuronal ceroid lipofuscinoses in Argentina*. pp. 103–116, Cordoba, Publicaciones Universitarias.

Norman RM & Wood N (1941) Congenital form of amaurotic family idiocy. *J Neurol Psych*, 4, 175–190.

Nugent T, Mole SE, & Jones D (2008) The transmembrane topology of Batten disease protein CLN3 determined by consensus computational prediction constrained by experimental data. *FEBS Letters*, 582, 1019–1024.

Nüsslein-Volhard C & Dahm R (2002) *Zebrafish (A Practical Approach)*. Oxford, Oxford University Press.

O'Brien DP & Katz ML (2008) Neuronal ceroid lipofuscinosis in 3 Australian shepherd littermates. *J Vet Intern Med*, 22, 472–475.

O'Neill G, Murphy SF, Moran H, Burke H, & Farrell MA (1993) Kufs disease - a clinicopathologic study in two siblings. *J Neuropathol Exp Neurol*, 52, 300.

Ohno K, Saito S, Sugawara K, Suzuki T, Togawa T, & Sakuraba H (2010) Structural basis of neuronal ceroid lipofuscinosis 1. *Brain Dev*, 32, 524–530.

Oorni K, Sneck M, Bromme D, Pentikainen MO, Lindstedt KA, Mayranpaa M, Aitio H, & Kovanen PT (2004) Cysteine protease cathepsin F is expressed in human atherosclerotic lesions, is secreted by cultured macrophages, and modifies low density lipoprotein particles in vitro. *J Biol Chem*, 279, 34776–34784.

Oresic K, Mueller B, & Tortorella D (2009) Cln6 mutants associated with neuronal ceroid lipofuscinosis are degraded in a proteasome-dependent manner. *Biosci Rep*, 29, 173–181.

Osório NS, Carvalho A, Almeida AJ, Padilla-Lopez S, Leao C, Laranjinha J, Ludovico P, Pearce DA, & Rodrigues F (2007) Nitric oxide signaling is disrupted in the yeast model for Batten disease. *Mol Biol Cell*, 18, 2755–2767.

Osório NS, Sampaio-Marques B, Chan CH, Oliveira P, Pearce DA, Sousa N, & Rodrigues F (2009) Neurodevelopmental delay in the Cln3Deltaex7/8 mouse model for Batten disease. *Genes Brain Behav*, 8, 337–345.

Østergaard JR, Egeblad H, & Molgaard H (2005) *The evolution of cardiac involvement in juvenile neuronal ceroid lipofuscinoses. NCL-2005: The 10th International Congress on Neuronal Ceroid Lipofuscinoses*, p.28.

Ostrander EA, Galibert F, & Patterson DF (2000) Canine genetics comes of age. *Trends Genet*, 16, 117–124.

Oswald MJ, Kay GW, & Palmer DN (2001) Changes in GABAergic neuron distribution in situ and in neuron cultures in ovine (OCL6) Batten disease. *Eur J Paediatr Neurol*, 5 Suppl A, 135–142.

Oswald MJ, Palmer DN, Kay GW, Barwell KJ, & Cooper JD (2008) Location and connectivity determine GABAergic interneuron survival in the brains of South Hampshire sheep with CLN6 neuronal ceroid lipofuscinosis. *Neurobiol Dis*, 32, 50–65.

Oswald MJ, Palmer DN, Kay GW, Shemilt SJ, Rezaie P, & Cooper JD (2005) Glial activation spreads from specific cerebral foci and precedes neurodegeneration in presymptomatic ovine neuronal ceroid lipofuscinosis (CLN6). *Neurobiol Dis*, 20, 49–63.

Oyama H, Fujisawa T, Suzuki T, Dunn BM, Wlodawer A, & Oda K (2005) Catalytic residues and substrate specificity of recombinant human tripeptidyl peptidase I (CLN2). *J Biochem*, 138, 127–134.

Padilla-Lopez S & Pearce DA (2006) Saccharomyces cerevisiae lacking Btn1p modulate vacuolar ATPase activity to regulate pH imbalance in the vacuole. *J Biol Chem*, 281, 10273–10280.

Page AE, Fuller K, Chambers TJ, & Warburton MJ (1993) Purification and characterization of a tripeptidyl peptidase I from human osteoclastomas: evidence for its role in bone resorption. *Arch Biochem Biophys*, 306, 354–359.

Pal C, Papp B, & Lercher MJ (2006) An integrated view of protein evolution. *Nat Rev Genet*, 7, 337–348.

Pal A, Kraetzner R, Gruene T, Grapp M, Schreiber K, Grønborg M, Urlaub H, Becker S, Asif AR, Gärtner J, Sheldrick GM, & Steinfeld R (2009) Structure of tripeptidyl-peptidase I provides insight into the molecular basis of late infantile neuronal ceroid lipofuscinosis. *J Biol Chem*, 284, 3976–84.

Palmer DN, Barns G, Husbands DR, & Jolly RD (1986a) Ceroid lipofuscinosis in sheep. II. The major component of the lipopigment in liver, kidney, pancreas, and brain is low molecular weight protein. *J Biol Chem*, 261, 1773–1777.

Palmer DN, Bayliss SL, Clifton PA, & Grant VJ (1993) Storage bodies in the ceroid-lipofuscinoses (Batten disease): low-molecular-weight components, unusual amino acids and reconstitution of fluorescent bodies from non-fluorescent components. *J Inherit Metab Dis*, 16, 292–295.

Palmer DN, Bayliss SL, & Westlake VJ (1995) Batten disease and the ATP synthase subunit c turnover pathway: raising antibodies to subunit c. *Am J Med Genet*, 57, 260–265.

Palmer DN, Fearnley IM, Medd SM, Walker JE, Martinus RD, Bayliss SL, Hall NA, Lake BD, Wolfe LS, & Jolly RD (1989a) Lysosomal storage of the DCCD reactive proteolipid subunit of mitochondrial ATP synthase in human and ovine ceroid lipofuscinoses. *Adv Exp Med Biol*, 266, 211–222; discussion 223.

Palmer DN, Fearnley IM, Walker JE, Hall NA, Lake BD, Wolfe LS, Haltia M, Martinus RD, & Jolly RD (1992) Mitochondrial ATP synthase subunit c storage in the ceroid-lipofuscinoses (Batten disease). *Am J Med Genet*, 42, 561–567.

Palmer DN, Husbands DR, & Jolly RD (1985) Phospholipid fatty acids in brains of normal sheep and sheep with ceroid-lipofuscinosis. *Biochim Biophys Acta*, 834, 159–163.

Palmer DN, Husbands DR, Winter PJ, Blunt JW, & Jolly RD (1986b) Ceroid lipofuscinosis in sheep. I. Bis(monoacylglycero)phosphate, dolichol, ubiquinone, phospholipids, fatty acids, and fluorescence in liver lipopigment lipids. *J Biol Chem*, 261, 1766–1772.

Palmer DN, Jolly RD, van Mil HC, Tyynelä J, & Westlake VJ (1997a) Different patterns of hydrophobic protein storage in different forms of neuronal ceroid lipofuscinosis (NCL, Batten disease). *Neuropediatrics*, 28, 45–48.

Palmer DN, Martinus RD, Barns G, Reeves RD, & Jolly RD (1988) Ovine ceroid-lipofuscinosis. I: Lipopigment composition is indicative of a lysosomal proteinosis. *Am J Med Genet Suppl*, 5, 141–158.

Palmer DN, Martinus RD, Cooper SM, Midwinter GG, Reid JC, & Jolly RD (1989b) Ovine ceroid lipofuscinosis. The major lipopigment protein and the lipid-binding subunit of mitochondrial ATP synthase have the same NH2-terminal sequence. *J Biol Chem*, 264, 5736–5740.

Palmer DN, Oswald MJ, Westlake VJ, & Kay GW (2002) The origin of fluorescence in the neuronal ceroid lipofuscinoses (Batten disease) and neuron cultures from affected sheep for studies of neurodegeneration. *Arch Gerontol Geriatr*, 34, 343–357.

Palmer DN, Tyynelä J, van Mil HC, Westlake VJ, & Jolly RD (1997b) Accumulation of sphingolipid activator proteins (SAPs) A and D in granular osmiophilic deposits in miniature Schnauzer dogs with ceroid-lipofuscinosis. *J Inherit Metab Dis*, 20, 74–84.

Pampiglione G & Harden A (1977) So-called neuronal ceroid lipofuscinosis. Neurophysiological studies in 60 children. *J Neurol Neurosurg Psychiatry*, 40, 323–330.

Pane MA, Puranam KL, & Boustany RM (1999) Expression of cln3 in human NT2 neuronal precursor cells and neonatal rat brain. *Pediatr Res*, 46, 367–374.

Pao SS, Paulsen IT, & Saier MH, Jr. (1998) Major facilitator superfamily. *Microbiol Mol Biol Rev*, 62, 1–34.

Pardo CA, Rabin BA, Palmer DN, & Price DL (1994) Accumulation of the adenosine triphosphate synthase subunit C in the mnd mutant mouse. A model for neuronal ceroid lipofuscinosis. *Am J Pathol*, 144, 829–835.

Partanen S, Haapanen A, Kielar C, Pontikis C, Alexander N, Inkinen T, Saftig P, Gillingwater TH, Cooper JD, & Tyynelä J (2008) Synaptic changes in the thalamocortical system of cathepsin D-deficient mice: a model of human congenital neuronal ceroid-lipofuscinosis. *J Neuropathol Exp Neurol*, 67, 16–29.

Partanen S, Storch S, Loffler HG, Hasilik A, Tyynelä J, & Braulke T (2003) A replacement of the active-site aspartic acid residue 293 in mouse cathepsin D affects its intracellular stability, processing and transport in HEK-293 cells. *Biochem J*, 369, 55–62.

Pasquinelli G, Cenacchi G, Piane EL, Russo C, & Aguglia U (2004) The problematic issue of Kufs disease diagnosis as performed on rectal biopsies: a case report. *Ultrastruct Pathol*, 28, 43–48.

Passini MA, Dodge JC, Bu J, Yang W, Zhao Q, Sondhi D, Hackett NR, Kaminsky SM, Mao Q, Shihabuddin LS, Cheng SH, Sleat DE, Stewart GR, Davidson BL, Lobel P, & Crystal RG (2006) Intracranial delivery of CLN2 reduces brain pathology in a mouse model of classical late infantile neuronal ceroid lipofuscinosis. *J Neurosci*, 26, 1334–1342.

Pearce DA, Carr CJ, Das B, & Sherman F (1999a) Phenotypic reversal of the btn1 defects in yeast by chloroquine: a yeast model for Batten disease. *Proc Natl Acad Sci U S A*, 96, 11341–11345.

Pearce DA, Ferea T, Nosel SA, Das B, & Sherman F (1999b) Action of BTN1, the yeast orthologue of the gene mutated in Batten disease. *Nat Genet*, 22, 55–58.

Pearce DA, McCall K, Mooney RA, Chattopadhyay S, & Curran TM (2003) Altered amino acid levels in sera of a mouse model for juvenile neuronal ceroid lipofuscinoses. *Clin Chim Acta*, 332, 145–148.

Pearce DA, Nosel SA, & Sherman F (1999c) Studies of pH regulation by Btn1p, the yeast homolog of human Cln3p. *Mol Genet Metab*, 66, 320–323.

Pearce DA & Sherman F (1997) BTN1, a yeast gene corresponding to the human gene responsible for Batten's disease, is not essential for viability, mitochondrial function, or degradation of mitochondrial ATP synthase. *Yeast*, 13, 691–697.

Pearce DA & Sherman F (1998) A yeast model for the study of Batten disease. *Proc Natl Acad Sci U S A*, 95, 6915–6918.

Pears MR, Codlin S, Haines RL, White IJ, Mortishire-Smith RJ, Mole SE, & Griffin JL (2010) Deletion of btn1, an orthologue of CLN3, increases glycolysis and perturbs amino acid metabolism in the fission yeast model of Batten disease. *Mol Biosyst*, 6, 1093–1102.

Pears MR, Cooper JD, Mitchison HM, Mortishire-Smith RJ, Pearce DA, & Griffin JL (2005) High resolution 1H NMR-based metabolomics indicates a neurotransmitter cycling deficit in cerebral tissue from a mouse model of Batten disease. *J Biol Chem*, 280, 42508–42514.

Pears MR, Salek RM, Palmer DN, Kay GW, Mortishire-Smith RJ, & Griffin JL (2007) Metabolomic investigation of CLN6 neuronal ceroid lipofuscinosis in affected South Hampshire sheep. *J Neurosci Res*, 85, 3494–3504.

Peña JA, Cardozo JJ, Montiel CM, Molina OM, & Boustany R (2001) Serial MRI findings in the Costa Rican variant of neuronal ceroid-lipofuscinosis. *Pediatr Neurol*, 25, 78–80.

Persaud-Sawin DA & Boustany RM (2005) Cell death pathways in juvenile Batten disease. *Apoptosis*, 10, 973–985.

Persaud-Sawin DA, McNamara JO, 2nd, Rylova S, Vandongen A, & Boustany RM (2004) A galactosylceramide binding domain is involved in trafficking of CLN3 from Golgi to rafts via recycling endosomes. *Pediatr Res*, 56, 449–463.

Petersen B, Handwerker M, & Huppertz HI (1996) Neuroradiological findings in classical late infantile neuronal ceroid-lipofuscinosis. *Pediatr Neurol*, 15, 344–347.

Pham CT, Armstrong RJ, Zimonjic DB, Popescu NC, Payan DG, & Ley TJ (1997) Molecular cloning, chromosomal localization, and expression of murine dipeptidyl peptidase I. *J Biol Chem*, 272, 10695–10703.

Phillips SN, Muzaffar N, Codlin S, Korey CA, Taschner PE, de Voer G, Mole SE, & Pearce DA (2006) Characterizing pathogenic processes in Batten disease: use of small eukaryotic model systems. *Biochim Biophys Acta*, 1762, 906–919.

Pineda-Trujillo N, Cornejo W, Carrizosa J, Wheeler RB, Munera S, Valencia A, Agudelo-Arango J, Cogollo A, Anderson G, Bedoya G, Mole SE, & Ruiz-Linares A (2005) A CLN5 mutation causing an atypical neuronal ceroid lipofuscinosis of juvenile onset. *Neurology*, 64, 740–742.

Piomelli D (2005) The challenge of brain lipidomics. *Prostaglandins Other Lipid Mediat*, 77, 23–34.

Piper PW, Ortiz-Calderon C, Holyoak C, Coote P, & Cole M (1997) Hsp30, the integral plasma membrane heat shock protein of Saccharomyces cerevisiae, is a stress-inducible regulator of plasma membrane $H(^{+})$-ATPase. *Cell Stress Chaperones*, 2, 12–24.

Pisoni RL, Flickinger KS, Thoene JG, & Christensen HN (1987a) Characterization of carrier-mediated transport systems for small neutral amino acids in human fibroblast lysosomes. *J Biol Chem*, 262, 6010–6017.

Pisoni RL, Thoene JG, Lemons RM, & Christensen HN (1987b) Important differences in cationic amino acid transport by lysosomal system c and system y+ of the human fibroblast. *J Biol Chem*, 262, 15011–15018.

Poët M, Kornak U, Schweizer M, Zdebik AA, Scheel O, Hoelter S, Wurst W, Schmitt A, Fuhrmann JC, Planells-Cases R, Mole SE, Hubner CA, & Jentsch TJ (2006) Lysosomal storage disease upon disruption of the neuronal chloride transport protein ClC-6. *Proc Natl Acad Sci U S A*, 103, 13854–13859.

Pohl S, Mitchison HM, Kohlschutter A, van Diggelen O, Braulke T, & Storch S (2007) Increased expression of lysosomal acid phosphatase in CLN3-defective cells and mouse brain tissue. *J Neurochem*, 103, 2177–2188.

Pontikis CC, Cella CV, Parihar N, Lim MJ, Chakrabarti S, Mitchison HM, Mobley WC, Rezaie P, Pearce DA, & Cooper JD (2004) Late onset neurodegeneration in the $Cln3^{-/-}$ mouse model of juvenile neuronal ceroid lipofuscinosis is preceded by low level glial activation. *Brain Res*, 1023, 231–242.

Pontikis CC, Cotman SL, MacDonald ME, & Cooper JD (2005) Thalamocortical neuron loss and localized astrocytosis in the Cln3$^{\Delta ex7/8}$ knock-in mouse model of Batten disease. *Neurobiol Dis*, 20, 823–836.

Porta EA (2002) Pigments in aging: an overview. *Ann N Y Acad Sci*, 959, 57–65.

Porter MY, Turmaine M, & Mole SE (2005) Identification and characterization of Caenorhabditis elegans palmitoyl protein thioesterase1. *J Neurosci Res*, 79, 836–848.

Portera-Cailliau C, Sung CH, Nathans J, & Adler R (1994) Apoptotic photoreceptor cell death in mouse models of retinitis pigmentosa. *Proc Natl Acad Sci U S A*, 91, 974–978.

Poupetova H, Ledvinova J, Berna L, Dvorakova L, Kozich V, Elleder M (2010) The birth prevalence of lysosomal storage disorders in the Czech Republic: comparison with data in different populations. *J Inherit Metab Dis*, 33, 387–396.

Press EM, Porter RR, & Cebra J (1960) The isolation and properties of a proteolytic enzyme, cathepsin D, from bovine spleen. *Biochem J*, 74, 501–514.

Pujic Z & Malicki J (2004) Retinal pattern and the genetic basis of its formation in zebrafish. *Semin Cell Dev Biol*, 15, 105–114.

Pullarkat RK & Morris GN (1997) Farnesylation of Batten disease CLN3 protein. *Neuropediatrics*, 28, 42–44.

Puranam K, Qian WH, Nikbakht K, Venable M, Obeid L, Hannun Y, & Boustany RM (1997) Upregulation of Bcl-2 and elevation of ceramide in Batten disease. *Neuropediatrics*, 28, 37–41.

Puranam KL, Guo WX, Qian WH, Nikbakht K, & Boustany RM (1999) CLN3 defines a novel antiapoptotic pathway operative in neurodegeneration and mediated by ceramide. *Mol Genet Metab*, 66, 294–308.

Qiao L, Hamamichi S, Caldwell KA, Caldwell GA, Yacoubian TA, Wilson S, Xie ZL, Speake LD, Parks R, Crabtree D, Liang Q, Crimmins S, Schneider L, Uchiyama Y, Iwatsubo T, Zhou Y, Peng L, Lu Y, Standaert DG, Walls KC, Shacka JJ, Roth KA, & Zhang J (2008) Lysosomal enzyme cathepsin D protects against alpha-synuclein aggregation and toxicity. *Mol Brain*, 1, 17.

Qiao X, Lu JY, & Hofmann SL (2007) Gene expression profiling in a mouse model of infantile neuronal ceroid lipofuscinosis reveals upregulation of immediate early genes and mediators of the inflammatory response. *BMC Neurosci*, 8, 95.

Raben N, Nagaraju K, Lee A, Lu N, Rivera Y, Jatkar T, Hopwood JJ, & Plotz PH (2003) Induction of tolerance to a recombinant human enzyme, acid alpha-glucosidase, in enzyme deficient knockout mice. *Transgenic Res*, 12, 171–178.

Raitta C & Santavuori P (1973) Ophthalmological findings in infantile type of so-called neuronal ceroid lipofuscinosis. *Acta Ophthalmol (Copenh)*, 51, 755–763.

Raitta K & Santavuori P (1981) *Ophthalmological Findings and Main Clinical Characteristics in Childhood Types of Neuronal Ceroid Lipofuscinoses*. Amsterdam, Elsevier North Holland Biomedical Press.

Rajan I, Read R, Small DL, Perrard J, & Vogel P (2010) An alternative splicing variant in Clcn7$^{-/-}$ mice prevents osteopetrosis but not neural and retinal degeneration. *Vet Pathol*. May 13. [Epub].

Rakheja D, Narayan SB, Pastor JV, & Bennett MJ (2004) CLN3P, the Batten disease protein, localizes to membrane lipid rafts (detergent-resistant membranes). *Biochem Biophys Res Commun*, 317, 988–991.

Ramadan H, Al-Din AS, Ismail A, Balen F, Varma A, Twomey A, Watts R, Jackson M, Anderson G, Green E, & Mole SE (2007) Adult neuronal ceroid lipofuscinosis caused by deficiency in palmitoyl protein thioesterase 1. *Neurology*, 68, 387–388.

Ramirez-Montealegre D & Pearce DA (2005) Defective lysosomal arginine transport in juvenile Batten disease. *Hum Mol Genet*, 14, 3759–3773.

Ranta S, Lehesjoki AE, Hirvasniemi A, Weissenbach J, Ross B, Leal SM, de la Chapelle A, & Gilliam TC (1996) Genetic and physical mapping of the progressive epilepsy with mental retardation (EPMR) locus on chromosome 8p. *Genome Res*, 6, 351–360.

Ranta S, Topcu M, Tegelberg S, Tan H, Ustübütün A, Saatci I, Dufke A, Enders H, Pohl K, Alembik Y, Mitchell WA, Mole SE, & Lehesjoki AE (2004) Variant late infantile neuronal ceroid lipofuscinosis in a subset of Turkish patients is allelic to Northern epilepsy. *Hum Mutat*, 23, 300–305.

Ranta S, Zhang Y, Ross B, Lonka L, Takkunen E, Messer A, Sharp J, Wheeler R, Kusumi K, Mole S, Liu W, Soares MB, Bonaldo MF, Hirvasniemi A, de la Chapelle A, Gilliam TC, & Lehesjoki AE (1999) The neuronal ceroid lipofuscinoses in human EPMR and mnd mutant mice are associated with mutations in CLN8. *Nat Genet*, 23, 233–236.

Rao NV, Rao GV, & Hoidal JR (1997) Human dipeptidyl-peptidase I. Gene characterization, localization, and expression. *J Biol Chem*, 272, 10260–10265.

Rapola J & Haltia M (1973) Cytoplasmic inclusions in the vermiform appendix and skeletal muscle in two types of so-called neuronal ceroid-lipofuscinosis. *Brain*, 96, 833–840.

Rapola J, Lahdetie J, Isosomppi J, Helminen P, Penttinen M, & Jarvela I (1999) Prenatal diagnosis of variant late infantile neuronal ceroid lipofuscinosis (vLINCL[Finnish]; CLN5). *Prenat Diagn*, 19, 685–688.

Rapola J & Lake BD (2000) Lymphocyte inclusions in Finnish-variant late infantile neuronal ceroid lipofuscinosis (CLN5). *Neuropediatrics*, 31, 33–34.

Rapola J, Salonen R, Ammala P, & Santavuori P (1990) Prenatal diagnosis of the infantile type of neuronal ceroid lipofuscinosis by electron microscopic investigation of human chorionic villi. *Prenat Diagn*, 10, 553–559.

Rapola J, Santavuori P, & Savilahti E (1984) Suction biopsy of rectal mucosa in the diagnosis of infantile and juvenile types of neuronal ceroid lipofuscinoses. *Hum Pathol*, 15, 352–360.

Rawlings ND & Barrett AJ (1995) Families of aspartic peptidases, and those of unknown catalytic mechanism. *Methods Enzymol*, 248, 105–120.

Read WK & Bridges CH (1969) Neuronal lipodystrophy. Occurrence in an inbred strain of cattle. *Pathol Vet*, 6, 235–243.

Reece RL & MacWhirter P (1988) Neuronal ceroid lipofuscinosis in a lovebird. *Vet Rec*, 122, 187.

Reichard U, Lechenne B, Asif AR, Streit F, Grouzmann E, Jousson O, & Monod M (2006) Sedolisins, a new class of secreted proteases from Aspergillus fumigatus with endoprotease or tripeptidyl-peptidase activity at acidic pHs. *Appl Environ Microbiol*, 72, 1739–1748.

Reif A, Schneider MF, Hoyer A, Schneider-Gold C, Fallgatter AJ, Roggendorf W, & Pfuhlmann B (2003)

Neuroleptic malignant syndrome in Kufs' disease. *J Neurol Neurosurg Psychiatry*, 74, 385–387.
Reinhardt K, Grapp M, Schlachter K, Bruck W, Gartner J, & Steinfeld R (2010) Novel CLN8 mutations confirm the clinical and ethnic diversity of late infantile neuronal ceroid lipofuscinosis. *Clin Genet*, 77, 79–85.
Reske-Nielsen E, Baandrup U, Bjerregaard P, & Bruun I (1981) Cardiac involvement in juvenile amaurotic idiocy—a specific heart muscle disorder. Histological findings in 13 autopsied patients. *Acta Pathol Microbiol Scand A*, 89, 357–365.
Reugels AM, Boggetti B, Scheer N, & Campos-Ortega JA (2006) Asymmetric localization of Numb:EGFP in dividing neuroepithelial cells during neurulation in Danio rerio. *Dev Dyn*, 235, 934–948.
Reznik M, Arrese-Estrada J, Sadzot B, & Franck G (1995) Un cas anatomo-clinique de la maladie de Kufs familiale. *Rev Neurol (Paris)*, 151, 597.
Richards SM, Olson TA, & McPherson JM (1993) Antibody response in patients with Gaucher disease after repeated infusion with macrophage-targeted glucocerebrosidase. *Blood*, 82, 1402–1409.
Richardson SC, Winistorfer SC, Poupon V, Luzio JP, & Piper RC (2004) Mammalian late vacuole protein sorting orthologues participate in early endosomal fusion and interact with the cytoskeleton. *Mol Biol Cell*, 15, 1197–1210.
Riis RC, Cummings JF, Loew ER, & de Lahunta A (1992) Tibetan terrier model of canine ceroid lipofuscinosis. *Am J Med Genet*, 42, 615–621.
Rinne JO, Ruottinen HM, Nagren K, Åberg LE, & Santavuori P (2002) Positron emission tomography shows reduced striatal dopamine D1 but not D2 receptors in juvenile neuronal ceroid lipofuscinosis. *Neuropediatrics*, 33, 138–141.
Robertson T, Tannenberg AE, Hiu J, & Reimers J (2008) 53-year-old man with rapid cognitive decline. *Brain Pathol*, 18, 292–294.
Rodman JS, Lipman R, Brown A, Bronson RT, & Dice JF (1998) Rate of accumulation of Luxol Fast Blue staining material and mitochondrial ATP synthase subunit 9 in motor neuron degeneration mice. *Neurochem Res*, 23, 1291–1296.
Rohrbough J & Broadie K (2005) Lipid regulation of the synaptic vesicle cycle. *Nat Rev Neurosci*, 6, 139–150.
Rorth P, Szabo K, Bailey A, Laverty T, Rehm J, Rubin GM, Weigmann K, Milan M, Benes V, Ansorge W, & Cohen SM (1998) Systematic gain-of-function genetics in Drosophila. *Development*, 125, 1049–1057.
Rose C, Vargas F, Facchinetti P, Bourgeat P, Bambal RB, Bishop PB, Chan SM, Moore AN, Ganellin CR, & Schwartz JC (1996) Characterization and inhibition of a cholecystokinin-inactivating serine peptidase. *Nature*, 380, 403–409.
Rossmeisl JH, Jr., Duncan R, Fox J, Herring ES, & Inzana KD (2003) Neuronal ceroid-lipofuscinosis in a Labrador Retriever. *J Vet Diagn Invest*, 15, 457–460.
Rowan SA & Lake BD (1995) Tissue and cellular distribution of subunit c of ATP synthase in Batten disease (neuronal ceroid-lipofuscinosis). *Am J Med Genet*, 57, 172–176.
Ruchoux MM, Gelot A, Perrier D, Larmande P (1996) Two families with Kufs disease, contribution of extracerebral biopsies for diagnosis. *Neuropathol Appl Neurobiol*, 22, 118.
Rumbach L, Warter JM, Coquillat G, Marescaux C, Collard M, Rohmer F, Bieth R, & Zawislak R (1983) [Anomalies in fatty acids distribution and superoxide dismutase activity in lymphocytes of an adult with atypical ceroid lipofuscinosis]. *Rev Neurol (Paris)*, 139, 269–276.
Russell C (2003) The roles of Hedgehogs and Fibroblast Growth Factors in eye development and retinal cell rescue. *Vision Res*, 43, 899–912.
Rusyn E, Mousallem T, Persaud-Sawin DA, Miller S, & Boustany RM (2008) CLN3p impacts galactosylceramide transport, raft morphology, and lipid content. *Pediatr Res*, 63, 625–631.
Ryan EM, Buzy A, Griffiths DE, Jennings KR, & Palmer DN (1996) Electrospray ionisation mass spectrometry (ESI/MS) of ceroid lipofuscin protein; a model system for the study of F0 inhibitor interactions with mitochondrial subunit C. *Biochem Soc Trans*, 24, 289S.
Sachs B (1896) A family form of idiocy, generally fatal and associated with early blindness (amaurotic family idiocy). *NY Med J*, 63, 697–703.
Sadzot B, Reznik M, Arrese-Estrada JE, & Franck G (2000) Familial Kufs' disease presenting as a progressive myoclonic epilepsy. *J Neurol*, 247, 447–454.
Saftig P, Hetman M, Schmahl W, Weber K, Heine L, Mossmann H, Koster A, Hess B, Evers M, von Figura K, et al. (1995) Mice deficient for the lysosomal proteinase cathepsin D exhibit progressive atrophy of the intestinal mucosa and profound destruction of lymphoid cells. *EMBO J*, 14, 3599–3608.
Saha A, Kim SJ, Zhang Z, Lee YC, Sarkar C, Tsai PC, & Mukherjee AB (2008) RAGE signaling contributes to neuroinflammation in infantile neuronal ceroid lipofuscinosis. *FEBS Lett*, 582, 3823–3831.
Saja S, Buff H, Smith AC, Williams TS, & Korey CA (2010) Identifying cellular pathways modulated by Drosophila palmitoyl-protein thioesterase 1 function. *Neurobiol Dis*, 40, 135–145.
Sakajiri K, Matsubara N, Nakajima T, Fukuhara N, Makifuchi T, Wakabayashi M, Oyanagi S, & Kominami E (1995) A family with adult type ceroid lipofuscinosis (Kufs' disease) and heart muscle disease: report of two autopsy cases. *Intern Med*, 34, 1158–1163.
Sakurai K, Iizuka S, Shen JS, Meng XL, Mori T, Umezawa A, Ohashi T, & Eto Y (2004) Brain transplantation of genetically modified bone marrow stromal cells corrects CNS pathology and cognitive function in MPS VII mice. *Gene Ther*, 11, 1475–1481.
Salonen T, Hellsten E, Horelli-Kuitunen N, Peltonen L, & Jalanko A (1998) Mouse palmitoyl protein thioesterase: gene structure and expression of cDNA. *Genome Res*, 8, 724–730.
Salonen T, Jarvela I, Peltonen L, & Jalanko A (2000) Detection of eight novel palmitoyl protein thioesterase (PPT) mutations underlying infantile neuronal ceroid lipofuscinosis (INCL;CLN1). *Hum Mutat*, 15, 273–279.
Sandbank U (1968) Congenital amaurotic idiocy. *Pathol Eur*, 3, 226–229.
Sanders DN, Farias FH, Johnson GS, Chiang V, Cook JR, O'Brien DP, Hofmann SL, Lu JY, & Katz ML (2010) A mutation in canine PPT1 causes early onset neuronal ceroid lipofuscinosis in a Dachshund. *Mol Genet Metab*, 100, 349–56.
Santavuori P (1982) Clinical findings in 69 patients with infantile neuronal ceroid lipofuscinosis. In Armstrong D, Koppang N, & Rider A (Eds.) *Ceroid Lipofuscinoses (Batten disease)*, pp. 23–34. Amsterdam, Elsevier.
Santavuori P, Gottlob I, Haltia M, Rapola J, Lake BD, Tyynelä J, & Peltonen L (1999) CLN1, infantile and

other types of NCL with GROD. In Goebel HH, Lake BD, & Mole SE (Eds.) *The Neuronal Ceroid Lipofuscinoses (Batten Disease)*, pp. 16–36, Amsterdam, IOS Press.

Santavuori P, Haltia M, & Rapola J (1974) Infantile type of so-called neuronal ceroid-lipofuscinosis. *Dev Med Child Neurol*, 16, 644–653.

Santavuori P, Haltia M, Rapola J, & Raitta C (1973) Infantile type of so-called neuronal ceroid-lipofuscinosis. 1. A clinical study of 15 patients. *J Neurol Sci*, 18, 257–267.

Santavuori P, Heiskala H, Autti T, Johansson E, & Westermarck T (1989a) Comparison of the clinical courses in patients with juvenile neuronal ceroid lipofuscinosis receiving antioxidant treatment and those without antioxidant treatment. *Adv Exp Med Biol*, 266, 273–282.

Santavuori P, Rapola J, Nuutila A, Raininko R, Lappi M, Launes J, Herva R, & Sainio K (1991) The spectrum of Janský-Bielschowsky disease. *Neuropediatrics*, 22, 92–96.

Santavuori P, Rapola J, Sainio K, & Raitta C (1982) A variant of Janský-Bielschowsky disease. *Neuropediatrics*, 13, 135–141.

Santavuori P, Somer H, Sainio K, Rapola J, Kruus S, Nikitin T, Ketonen L, & Leisti J (1989b) Muscle-eye-brain disease (MEB). *Brain Dev*, 11, 147–153.

Santavuori P, Vanhanen SL, Sainio K, Nieminen M, Wallden T, Launes J, & Raininko R (1993) Infantile neuronal ceroid-lipofuscinosis (INCL): diagnostic criteria. *J Inherit Metab Dis*, 16, 227–229.

Santorelli FM, Bertini E, Petruzzella V, Di Capua M, Calvieri S, Gasparini P, & Zeviani M (1998) A novel insertion mutation (A169i) in the CLN1 gene is associated with infantile neuronal ceroid lipofuscinosis in an Italian patient. *Biochem Biophys Res Commun*, 245, 519–522.

Sappington RM, Pearce DA, & Calkins DJ (2003) Optic nerve degeneration in a murine model of juvenile ceroid lipofuscinosis. *Invest Ophthalmol Vis Sci*, 44, 3725–3731.

Sarpong A, Schottmann G, Ruther K, Stoltenburg G, Kohlschutter A, Hubner C, & Schuelke M (2009) Protracted course of juvenile ceroid lipofuscinosis associated with a novel CLN3 mutation (p.Y199X). *Clin Genet*, 76, 38–45.

Savukoski M, Kestila M, Williams R, Jarvela I, Sharp J, Harris J, Santavuori P, Gardiner M, & Peltonen L (1994) Defined chromosomal assignment of CLN5 demonstrates that at least four genetic loci are involved in the pathogenesis of human ceroid lipofuscinoses. *Am J Hum Genet*, 55, 695–701.

Savukoski M, Klockars T, Holmberg V, Santavuori P, Lander ES, & Peltonen L (1998) CLN5, a novel gene encoding a putative transmembrane protein mutated in Finnish variant late infantile neuronal ceroid lipofuscinosis. *Nat Genet*, 19, 286–288.

Sawkar AR, Adamski-Werner SL, Cheng WC, Wong CH, Beutler E, Zimmer KP, & Kelly JW (2005) Gaucher disease-associated glucocerebrosidases show mutation-dependent chemical chaperoning profiles. *Chem Biol*, 12, 1235–1244.

Schaffer K (1906) Beiträge zur Nosographie und Histopathologie der amaurotisch-paralytischen Idiotieformen. *Arch Psychiatr Nervenkr*, 42, 127–160.

Schaffer K (1910) Über die Anatomie und Klinik der Tay–Sachs'schen amaurotisch-familiären Idiotie mit Rücksicht auf verwandte Formen. *Z. Erforsch. Behandl Jugendl Schwachsinns*, 19–73, 147–186.

Schaffer K (1931) Revision in der Pathohistologie und Pathogenese der infantil-amaurotischen Idiotie. *Arch Psychiatr*, 95, 714–722.

Schaffer K (1932) Grundsätzliche Bemerkungen zur Pathogenese der amaurotischen Idiotie. *Mschr Psychiat*, 84, 117–129.

Schiffmann R, Kopp JB, Austin HA, 3rd, Sabnis S, Moore DF, Weibel T, Balow JE, & Brady RO (2001) Enzyme replacement therapy in Fabry disease: a randomized controlled trial. *JAMA*, 285, 2743–2749.

Schmiedt ML, Bessa C, Heine C, Ribeiro MG, Jalanko A, & Kyttala A (2010) The neuronal ceroid lipofuscinosis protein CLN5: new insights into cellular maturation, transport, and consequences of mutations. *Hum Mutat*, 31, 356–365.

Schreiner R, Becker I, & Wiegand MH (2000) [Kufs-disease; a rare cause of early-onset dementia]. *Nervenarzt*, 71, 411–415.

Schriner JE, Yi W, & Hofmann SL (1996) cDNA and genomic cloning of human palmitoyl-protein thioesterase (PPT), the enzyme defective in infantile neuronal ceroid lipofuscinosis. *Genomics*, 34, 317–322.

Schulz A, Dhar S, Rylova S, Dbaibo G, Alroy J, Hagel C, Artacho I, Kohlschutter A, Lin S, & Boustany RM (2004) Impaired cell adhesion and apoptosis in a novel CLN9 Batten disease variant. *Ann Neurol*, 56, 342–350.

Schulz A, Mousallem T, Venkataramani M, Persaud-Sawin DA, Zucker A, Luberto C, Bielawska A, Bielawski J, Holthuis JC, Jazwinski SM, Kozhaya L, Dbaibo GS, & Boustany RM (2006) The CLN9 protein, a regulator of dihydroceramide synthase. *J Biol Chem*, 281, 2784–2794.

Schuur M, Ikram MA, van Swieten JC, Isaacs A, Vergeer-Drop JM, Hofman A, Oostra BA, Breteler MM, & van Duijn CM (2010) Cathepsin D gene and the risk of Alzheimer's disease: A population-based study and meta-analysis. *Neurobiol Aging*, doi:10.1016/j.neurobiolaging.2009.10.011.

Seehafer SS, Ramirez-Montealegre D, Wong AM, Chan CH, Castaneda J, Horak M, Ahmadi SM, Lim MJ, Cooper JD, Pearce DA (2010). Immunosuppression alters disease severity in juvenile Batten disease mice. *J Neuroimmunol*. 2010 Oct 9. [Epub ahead of print] PMID: 20937531 [PubMed - as supplied by publisher]

Seigel GM, Lotery A, Kummer A, Bernard DJ, Greene ND, Turmaine M, Derksen T, Nussbaum RL, Davidson B, Wagner J, & Mitchison HM (2002) Retinal pathology and function in a Cln3 knockout mouse model of juvenile Neuronal Ceroid Lipofuscinosis (Batten disease). *Mol Cell Neurosci*, 19, 515–527.

Seigel GM, Wagner J, Wronska A, Campbell L, Ju W, & Zhong N (2005) Progression of early postnatal retinal pathology in a mouse model of neuronal ceroid lipofuscinosis. *Eye (Lond)*, 19, 1306–1312.

Seitz D, Grodd W, Schwab A, Seeger U, Klose U, & Nagele T (1998) MR imaging and localized proton MR spectroscopy in late infantile neuronal ceroid lipofuscinosis. *Am J Neuroradiol*, 19, 1373–1377.

Seto ES, Bellen HJ, & Lloyd TE (2002) When cell biology meets development: endocytic regulation of signaling pathways. *Genes Dev*, 16, 1314–1336.

Shacka JJ, Klocke BJ, Young C, Shibata M, Olney JW, Uchiyama Y, Saftig P, & Roth KA (2007) Cathepsin D deficiency induces persistent neurodegeneration in the absence of Bax-dependent apoptosis. *J Neurosci*, 27, 2081–2090.

Sharifi A, Kousi M, Sagné C, Bellenchi GC, Morel L, Darmon M, Hulková H, Ruivo R, Debacker C, El Mestikawy S, Elleder M, Lehesjoki AE, Jalanko A, Gasnier B, Kyttälä A (2010) Expression and lysosomal targeting of CLN7, a major facilitator superfamily transporter associated with variant late-infantile neuronal ceroid lipofuscinosis. *Hum Mol Genet*, 19, 4497–4514.

Sharp JD, Wheeler RB, Lake BD, Fox M, Gardiner RM, & Williams RE (1999) Genetic and physical mapping of the CLN6 gene on chromosome 15q21-23. *Mol Genet Metab*, 66, 329–331.

Sharp JD, Wheeler RB, Lake BD, Savukoski M, Jarvela IE, Peltonen L, Gardiner RM, & Williams RE (1997) Loci for classical and a variant late infantile neuronal ceroid lipofuscinosis map to chromosomes 11p15 and 15q21-23. *Hum Mol Genet*, 6, 591–595.

Sharp JD, Wheeler RB, Parker KA, Gardiner RM, Williams RE, & Mole SE (2003) Spectrum of CLN6 mutations in variant late infantile neuronal ceroid lipofuscinosis. *Hum Mutat*, 22, 35–42.

Sharp JD, Wheeler RB, Schultz RA, Joslin JM, Mole SE, Williams RE, & Gardiner RM (2001) Analysis of candidate genes in the CLN6 critical region using in silico cloning. *Eur J Paediatr Neurol*, 5 Suppl A, 29–31.

Shelton M, Willingham T, Menzine TC, Storts R, & Wood PR (1993) Neuronal ceroid lipofuscinosis, an inherited form of blindness in sheep. *Sheep Res J*, 9, 105–108.

Shevtsova Z, Garrido M, Weishaupt J, Saftig P, Bahr M, Luhder F, & Kugler S (2010) CNS-expressed cathepsin D prevents lymphopenia in a murine model of congenital neuronal ceroid lipofuscinosis. *Am J Pathol*, 177, 271–279.

Shi GP, Bryant RA, Riese R, Verhelst S, Driessen C, Li Z, Bromme D, Ploegh HL, & Chapman HA (2000) Role for cathepsin F in invariant chain processing and major histocompatibility complex class II peptide loading by macrophages. *J Exp Med*, 191, 1177–1186.

Shihabuddin LS, Numan S, Huff MR, Dodge JC, Clarke J, Macauley SL, Yang W, Taksir TV, Parsons G, Passini MA, Gage FH, & Stewart GR (2004) Intracerebral transplantation of adult mouse neural progenitor cells into the Niemann-Pick-A mouse leads to a marked decrease in lysosomal storage pathology. *J Neurosci*, 24, 10642–10651.

Siakotos AN, Goebel H, Patel V, Watanabe I, & Zeman W (1972) The morphogenesis and biochemical characteristics of ceroid isolated from cases of neuronal ceroid lipofuscinosis. In Volk BW & Aronson SM (Eds.) *Sphingolipids, Sphingolipodoses and Allied Disorders*, pp. 53–61. New York, Plenum Press.

Siakotos AN, Blair PS, Savill JD, & Katz ML (1998) Altered mitochondrial function in canine ceroid-lipofuscinosis. *Neurochem Res*, 23, 983–989.

Siakotos AN, & Koppang N (1973) Procedures for the isolation of lipopigments from brain, heart and liver, and their properties: a review. *Mech Ageing Dev*, 2, 177–200.

Siintola E, Lehesjoki AE, & Mole SE (2006a) Molecular genetics of the NCLs—status and perspectives. *Biochim Biophys Acta*, 1762, 857–864.

Siintola E, Partanen S, Stromme P, Haapanen A, Haltia M, Maehlen J, Lehesjoki AE, & Tyynelä J (2006b) Cathepsin D deficiency underlies congenital human neuronal ceroid-lipofuscinosis. *Brain*, 129, 1438–1445.

Siintola E, Topcu M, Aula N, Lohi H, Minassian BA, Paterson AD, Liu XQ, Wilson C, Lahtinen U, Anttonen AK, & Lehesjoki AE (2007) The novel neuronal ceroid lipofuscinosis gene MFSD8 encodes a putative lysosomal transporter. *Am J Hum Genet*, 81, 136–146.

Siintola E, Topcu M, Kohlschutter A, Salonen T, Joensuu T, Anttonen AK, & Lehesjoki AE (2005) Two novel CLN6 mutations in variant late-infantile neuronal ceroid lipofuscinosis patients of Turkish origin. *Clin Genet*, 68, 167–173.

Sikora J, Dvorakova L, Vlaskova H, Stolnaja L, Betlach J, Spacek J, & Elleder M (2007) A case of excessive autophagocytosis with multiorgan involvement and low clinical penetrance. *Cesk Patol*, 43, 93–103.

Simmer F, Moorman C, van der Linden AM, Kuijk E, van den Berghe PV, Kamath RS, Fraser AG, Ahringer J, Plasterk RH (2003) Genome-wide RNAi of C. elegans using the hypersensitive rrf-3 strain reveals novel gene functions. *PLoS Biology*, 1, 77–84.

Simonati A, Santorum E, Tessa A, Polo A, Simonetti F, Bernardina BD, Santorelli FM, & Rizzuto N (2000) A CLN2 gene nonsense mutation is associated with severe caudate atrophy and dystonia in LINCL. *Neuropediatrics*, 31, 199–201.

Simonati A, Tessa A, Bernardina BD, Biancheri R, Veneselli E, Tozzi G, Bonsignore M, Grosso S, Piemonte F, & Santorelli FM (2009) Variant late infantile neuronal ceroid lipofuscinosis because of CLN1 mutations. *Pediatr Neurol*, 40, 271–276.

Sinha S, Satishchandra P, Santosh V, Gayatri N, & Shankar SK (2004) Neuronal ceroid lipofuscinosis: a clinicopathological study. *Seizure*, 13, 235–240.

Sisk DB, Levesque DC, Wood PA, & Styer EL (1990) Clinical and pathologic features of ceroid lipofuscinosis in two Australian cattle dogs. *J Am Vet Med Assoc*, 197, 361–364.

Siso S, Navarro C, Hanzlicek D, & Vandevelde M (2004) Adult onset thalamocerebellar degeneration in dogs associated to neuronal storage of ceroid lipopigment. *Acta Neuropathol*, 108, 386–392.

Sjögren T (1931) Die juvenile amaurotische Idiotie. Klinische und erblichkeitsmedizinische Untersuchungen. *Hereditas (Lund)*, 14, 197–426.

Sjögren T (1947) Hereditary congenital spinocerebellar ataxia combined with congenital cataract and oligophrenia. *Acta Psychiat Neurol Scand*, 46 (suppl), 286–289.

Sjögren T (1950) Hereditary congenital spinocerebellar ataxia accompanied by congenital cataract and oligophrenia. A genetic and clinical investigation. *Confin Neurol*, 10, 293–308.

Sjögren T & Larsson T (1957) Oligophrenia in combination with congenital ichthyosis and spastic disorders; a clinical and genetic study. *Acta Psychiat Neurol Scand*, 32 (suppl 113), 1–112.

Slater AF (1993) Chloroquine: mechanism of drug action and resistance in Plasmodium falciparum. *Pharmacol Ther*, 57, 203–235.

Sleat DE, Ding L, Wang S, Zhao C, Wang Y, Xin W, Zheng H, Moore DF, Sims KB, & Lobel P (2009) Mass spectrometry-based protein profiling to determine the cause of lysosomal storage diseases of unknown etiology. *Mol Cell Proteomics*, 8, 1708–1718.

Sleat DE, Donnelly RJ, Lackland H, Liu CG, Sohar I, Pullarkat RK, & Lobel P (1997) Association of mutations in a lysosomal protein with classical late-infantile neuronal ceroid lipofuscinosis. *Science*, 277, 1802–1805.

Sleat DE, Gin RM, Sohar I, Wisniewski K, Sklower-Brooks S, Pullarkat RK, Palmer DN, Lerner TJ, Boustany RM, Uldall P, Siakotos AN, Donnelly RJ, & Lobel P (1999) Mutational analysis of the defective protease in classic late-infantile neuronal ceroid lipofuscinosis, a neurodegenerative lysosomal storage disorder. *Am J Hum Genet*, 64, 1511–1523.

Sleat DE, Lackland H, Wang Y, Sohar I, Xiao G, Li H, & Lobel P (2005) The human brain mannose 6-phosphate glycoproteome: a complex mixture composed of multiple isoforms of many soluble lysosomal proteins. *Proteomics*, 5, 1520–1532.

Sleat DE, Sohar I, Gin RM, & Lobel P (2001) Aminoglycoside-mediated suppression of nonsense mutations in late infantile neuronal ceroid lipofuscinosis. *Eur J Paediatr Neurol*, 5 Suppl A, 57–62.

Sleat DE, Sohar I, Pullarkat PS, Lobel P, & Pullarkat RK (1998) Specific alterations in levels of mannose 6-phosphorylated glycoproteins in different neuronal ceroid lipofuscinoses. *Biochem J*, 334 (Pt 3), 547–551.

Sleat DE, Wiseman JA, El-Banna M, Kim KH, Mao Q, Price S, Macauley SL, Sidman RL, Shen MM, Zhao Q, Passini MA, Davidson BL, Stewart GR, & Lobel P (2004) A mouse model of classical late-infantile neuronal ceroid lipofuscinosis based on targeted disruption of the CLN2 gene results in a loss of tripeptidyl-peptidase I activity and progressive neurodegeneration. *J Neurosci*, 24, 9117–9126.

Smith AJ, Bainbridge JW, & Ali RR (2009) Prospects for retinal gene replacement therapy. *Trends Genet*, 25, 156–165.

Smotrys JE & Linder ME (2004) Palmitoylation of intracellular signaling proteins: regulation and function. *Annu Rev Biochem*, 73, 559–587.

Snyder CK, Ho K-C, & Antuono PG (1998) Comparison of neuronal lipofuscin deposition and neuronal size in the hippocampus of normal aging and Alzheimer's disease population. *J Neuropathol Exp Neurol*, 57, 471.

Snyder DS & Whitaker JN (1983) Postnatal changes in cathepsin D in rat neural tissue. *J Neurochem*, 40, 1161–1170.

Snyder EY, Taylor RM, & Wolfe JH (1995) Neural progenitor cell engraftment corrects lysosomal storage throughout the MPS VII mouse brain. *Nature*, 374, 367–370.

Sohar I, Lin L, & Lobel P (2000) Enzyme-based diagnosis of classical late infantile neuronal ceroid lipofuscinosis: comparison of tripeptidyl peptidase I and pepstatin-insensitive protease assays. *Clin Chem*, 46, 1005–1008.

Sondhi D, Hackett NR, Apblett RL, Kaminsky SM, Pergolizzi RG, & Crystal RG (2001) Feasibility of gene therapy for late neuronal ceroid lipofuscinosis. *Arch Neurol*, 58, 1793–1798.

Sondhi D, Hackett NR, Peterson DA, Stratton J, Baad M, Travis KM, Wilson JM, & Crystal RG (2007) Enhanced survival of the LINCL mouse following CLN2 gene transfer using the rh.10 rhesus macaque-derived adeno-associated virus vector. *Mol Ther*, 15, 481–491.

Sondhi D, Peterson DA, Edelstein AM, del Fierro K, Hackett NR, & Crystal RG (2008) Survival advantage of neonatal CNS gene transfer for late infantile neuronal ceroid lipofuscinosis. *Exp Neurol*, 213, 18–27.

Sondhi D, Peterson DA, Giannaris EL, Sanders CT, Mendez BS, De B, Rostkowski AB, Blanchard B, Bjugstad K, Sladek JR, Jr., Redmond DE, Jr., Leopold PL, Kaminsky SM, Hackett NR, & Crystal RG (2005) AAV2-mediated CLN2 gene transfer to rodent and non-human primate brain results in long-term TPP-I expression compatible with therapy for LINCL. *Gene Ther*, 12, 1618–1632.

Song JW, Misgeld T, Kang H, Knecht S, Lu J, Cao Y, Cotman SL, Bishop DL, & Lichtman JW (2008) Lysosomal activity associated with developmental axon pruning. *J Neurosci*, 28, 8993–9001.

Soyombo AA & Hofmann SL (1997) Molecular cloning and expression of palmitoyl-protein thioesterase 2 (PPT2), a homolog of lysosomal palmitoyl-protein thioesterase with a distinct substrate specificity. *J Biol Chem*, 272, 27456–27463.

Spalton DJ, Taylor DS, & Sanders MD (1980) Juvenile Batten's disease: an ophthalmological assessment of 26 patients. *Br J Ophthalmol*, 64, 726–732.

Spielmeyer W (1905a) Über familiäre amaurotische Idiotien. *Neurol Cbl*, 24, 620–621.

Spielmeyer W (1905b) Weitere Mitteilungen über eine besondere Form von familiärer amaurotischer Idiotie. *Neurol Cbl*, 24, 1131–1132.

Spielmeyer W (1906) Über eine besondere Form von familiärer amaurotischer Idiotie. *Neurol Cbl*, 25, 51–55.

Spielmeyer W (1908) Klinische und amaurotische Untersuchungen über eine besondere Form von familiärer amaurotischer Idiotie. *Histol und Histopathol*, 2, 193–251.

Spielmeyer W (1923) Familiäre amaurotische Idiotie. *Zentralbl Ges Ophthalmol*, 10, 161–208.

Spielmeyer W (1929) Vom Wesen des anatomischen Prozesses bei der familiären amaurotischen Idiotie. *J Psychol Neurol (Leipzig)*, 38, 120–133.

Spielmeyer W (1933) Review on 'Grundsätzliche Bemerkungen zur Pathogenese der amaurotischen Idiotie' by K. Schaffer. *Zentralbl Ges Neurol Psychiatr*, 67, 76–79.

Steenhuis P, Herder S, Gelis S, Braulke T, & Storch S (2010) Lysosomal targeting of the CLN7 membrane glycoprotein and transport via the plasma membrane require a dileucine motif. *Traffic*, 11, 987–1000.

Stein CS, Martins I, & Davidson BL (2005) The lymphocytic choriomeningitis virus envelope glycoprotein targets lentiviral gene transfer vector to neural progenitors in the murine brain. *Mol Ther*, 11, 382–389.

Stein CS, Yancey PH, Martins I, Sigmund RD, Stokes JB, & Davidson BL (2010) Osmoregulation of ceroid neuronal lipofuscinosis type 3 (CLN3) in the renal medulla. *Am J Physiol Cell Physiol*, 298, C1388–C1400.

Stein LD, Bao Z, Blasiar D, Blumenthal T, Brent MR, Chen N, Chinwalla A, Clarke L, Clee C, Coghlan A, Coulson A, D'Eustachio P, Fitch DH, Fulton LA, Fulton RE, Griffiths-Jones S, Harris TW, Hillier LW, Kamath R, Kuwabara PE, Mardis ER, Marra MA, Miner TL, Minx P, Mullikin JC, Plumb RW, Rogers J, Schein JE, Sohrmann M, Spieth J, Stajich JE, Wei C, Willey D, Wilson RK, Durbin R, & Waterston RH (2003) The genome sequence of Caenorhabditis briggsae: a platform for comparative genomics. *PLoS Biol*, 1, E45.

Steinfeld R, Heim P, von Gregory H, Meyer K, Ullrich K, Goebel HH, & Kohlschutter A (2002) Late infantile neuronal ceroid lipofuscinosis: quantitative description of the clinical course in patients with CLN2 mutations. *Am J Med Genet*, 112, 347–354.

Steinfeld R, Reinhardt K, Schreiber K, Hillebrand M, Kraetzner R, Bruck W, Saftig P, & Gartner J (2006)

Cathepsin D deficiency is associated with a human neurodegenerative disorder. *Am J Hum Genet*, 78, 988–998.

Steinfeld R, Steinke HB, Isbrandt D, Kohlschutter A, & Gartner J (2004) Mutations in classical late infantile neuronal ceroid lipofuscinosis disrupt transport of tripeptidyl-peptidase I to lysosomes. *Hum Mol Genet*, 13, 2483–2491.

Stemple DL (2004) TILLING—a high-throughput harvest for functional genomics. *Nat Rev Genet*, 5, 145–150.

Stengel OC (1826a) Beretning om et mærkeligt Sygdomstilfælde hos fire Sødskende I Nærheden af Röraas. *Eyr*, 1, 347–352.

Stengel OC (1826b/1982) Account of a singular illness among four siblings in the vicinity of Røraas. Reprinted in Armstrong D, Koppang N, & Rider JA (Eds.) *Ceroid-lipofuscinosis (Batten's Disease)*, pp. 17–19. Amsterdam, Elsevier/North Holland Biomedical Press.

Stephan L, Pichavant C, Bouchentouf M, Mills P, Camirand G, Tagmouti S, Rothstein D, & Tremblay JP (2006) Induction of tolerance across fully mismatched barriers by a nonmyeloablative treatment excluding antibodies or irradiation use. *Cell Transplant*, 15, 835–846.

Stephenson JB, Greene ND, Leung KY, Munroe PB, Mole SE, Gardiner RM, Taschner PE, O'Regan M, Naismith K, Crow YJ, & Mitchison HM (1999) The molecular basis of GROD-storing neuronal ceroid lipofuscinoses in Scotland. *Mol Genet Metab*, 66, 245–247.

Steward CG (2003) Neurological aspects of osteopetrosis. *Neuropathol Appl Neurobiol*, 29, 87–97.

Stobrawa SM, Breiderhoff T, Takamori S, Engel D, Schweizer M, Zdebik AA, Bosl MR, Ruether K, Jahn H, Draguhn A, Jahn R, & Jentsch TJ (2001) Disruption of ClC-3, a chloride channel expressed on synaptic vesicles, leads to a loss of the hippocampus. *Neuron*, 29, 185–196.

Stock W (1908) Über eine bis jetzt noch nicht beschriebene Form der familiär auftretenden Netzhautdegeneration bei gleichzeitiger Verblödung und über Pigmentdegeneration der Netzhaut. *Klin Mbl Augenheilk*, 5, 225–244.

Stogmann E, El Tawil S, Wagenstaller J, Gaber A, Edris S, Abdelhady A, Assem-Hilger E, Leutmezer F, Bonelli S, Baumgartner C, Zimprich F, Strom TM, & Zimprich A (2009) A novel mutation in the MFSD8 gene in late infantile neuronal ceroid lipofuscinosis. *Neurogenetics*, 10, 73–77.

Stoll G & Jander S (1999) The role of microglia and macrophages in the pathophysiology of the CNS. *Prog Neurobiol*, 58, 233–247.

Storch S, Pohl S, & Braulke T (2004) A dileucine motif and a cluster of acidic amino acids in the second cytoplasmic domain of the Batten disease-related CLN3 protein are required for efficient lysosomal targeting. *J Biol Chem*, 279, 53625–53634.

Storch S, Pohl S, Quitsch A, Falley K, & Braulke T (2007) C-terminal prenylation of the CLN3 membrane glycoprotein is required for efficient endosomal sorting to lysosomes. *Traffic*, 8, 431–444.

Striano P, Specchio N, Biancheri R, Cannelli N, Simonati A, Cassandrini D, Rossi A, Bruno C, Fusco L, Gaggero R, Vigevano F, Bertini E, Zara F, Santorelli FM, & Striano S (2007) Clinical and electrophysiological features of epilepsy in Italian patients with CLN8 mutations. *Epilepsy Behav*, 10, 187–191.

Studdert VP & Mitten RW (1991) Clinical features of ceroid lipofuscinosis in border collie dogs. *Aust Vet J*, 68, 137–140.

Sugimoto H, Hayashi H, & Yamashita S (1996) Purification, cDNA cloning, and regulation of lysophospholipase from rat liver. *J Biol Chem*, 271, 7705–7711.

Sulston JE, Schierenberg E, White JG, & Thomson JN (1983) The embryonic cell lineage of the nematode Caenorhabditis elegans. *Dev Biol*, 100, 64–119.

Sun X, Marks DL, Park WD, Wheatley CL, Puri V, O'Brien JF, Kraft DL, Lundquist PA, Patterson MC, Pagano RE, & Snow K (2001) Niemann-Pick C variant detection by altered sphingolipid trafficking and correlation with mutations within a specific domain of NPC1. *Am J Hum Genet*, 68, 1361–1372.

Suopanki J, Lintunen M, Lahtinen H, Haltia M, Panula P, Baumann M, & Tyynelä J (2002) Status epilepticus induces changes in the expression and localization of endogenous palmitoyl-protein thioesterase 1. *Neurobiol Dis*, 10, 247–257.

Suopanki J, Partanen S, Ezaki J, Baumann M, Kominami E, & Tyynelä J (2000) Developmental changes in the expression of neuronal ceroid lipofuscinoses-linked proteins. *Mol Genet Metab*, 71, 190–194.

Suopanki J, Tyynelä J, Baumann M, & Haltia M (1999a) Palmitoyl-protein thioesterase, an enzyme implicated in neurodegeneration, is localized in neurons and is developmentally regulated in rat brain. *Neurosci Lett*, 265, 53–56.

Suopanki J, Tyynelä J, Baumann M, & Haltia M (1999b) The expression of palmitoyl-protein thioesterase is developmentally regulated in neural tissues but not in nonneural tissues. *Mol Genet Metab*, 66, 290–293.

Svennerholm L (1962) The chemical structure of normal human brain and Tay-Sachs gangliosides. *Biochem Biophys Res Commun*, 9, 436–441.

Sweeney ST & Davis GW (2002) Unrestricted synaptic growth in spinster-a late endosomal protein implicated in TGF-beta-mediated synaptic growth regulation. *Neuron*, 36, 403–416.

Sym M, Basson M, & Johnson C (2000) A model for niemann-pick type C disease in the nematode Caenorhabditis elegans. *Curr Biol*, 10, 527–530.

Syntichaki P, Xu K, Driscoll M, & Tavernarakis N (2002) Specific aspartyl and calpain proteases are required for neurodegeneration in C. elegans. *Nature*, 419, 939–944.

Tahvanainen E, Ranta S, Hirvasniemi A, Karila E, Leisti J, Sistonen P, Weissenbach J, Lehesjoki AE, & de la Chapelle A (1994) The gene for a recessively inherited human childhood progressive epilepsy with mental retardation maps to the distal short arm of chromosome 8. *Proc Natl Acad Sci U S A*, 91, 7267–7270.

Tamaki SJ, Jacobs Y, Dohse M, Capela A, Cooper JD, Reitsma M, He D, Tushinski R, Belichenko PV, Salehi A, Mobley W, Gage FH, Huhn S, Tsukamoto AS, Weissman IL, & Uchida N (2009) Neuroprotection of host cells by human central nervous system stem cells in a mouse model of infantile neuronal ceroid lipofuscinosis. *Cell Stem Cell*, 5, 310–319.

Tammen I, Cook RW, Nicholas FW, & Raadsma HW (2001) Neuronal ceroid lipofuscinosis in Australian Merino sheep: a new animal model. *Eur J Paediatr Neurol*, 5 Suppl A, 37–41.

Tammen I, Houweling PJ, Frugier T, Mitchell NL, Kay GW, Cavanagh JA, Cook RW, Raadsma HW, & Palmer

DN (2006) A missense mutation (c.184C>T) in ovine CLN6 causes neuronal ceroid lipofuscinosis in Merino sheep whereas affected South Hampshire sheep have reduced levels of CLN6 mRNA. *Biochim Biophys Acta*, 1762, 898–905.

Tang CH, Lee JW, Galvez MG, Robillard L, Mole SE, & Chapman HA (2006) Murine cathepsin F deficiency causes neuronal lipofuscinosis and late-onset neurological disease. *Mol Cell Biol*, 26, 2309–2316.

Tardy C, Sabourdy F, Garcia V, Jalanko A, Therville N, Levade T, & Andrieu-Abadie N (2009) Palmitoyl protein thioesterase 1 modulates tumor necrosis factor alpha-induced apoptosis. *Biochim Biophys Acta*, 1793, 1250–1258.

Tarkkanen A, Haltia M, & Merenmies L (1977) Ocular pathology in infantile type of neuronal ceroid-lipofuscinosis. *J Pediatr Ophthalmol*, 14, 235–241.

Taschner PE, de Vos N, & Breuning MH (1997) Cross-species homology of the CLN3 gene. *Neuropediatrics*, 28, 18–20.

Taschner PE, de Vos N, Thompson AD, Callen DF, Doggett N, Mole SE, Dooley TP, Barth PG, & Breuning MH (1995) Chromosome 16 microdeletion in a patient with juvenile neuronal ceroid lipofuscinosis (Batten disease). *Am J Hum Genet*, 56, 663–668.

Taylor CR & Levenson RM (2006) Quantification of immunohistochemistry—issues concerning methods, utility and semiquantitative assessment II. *Histopathology*, 49, 411–424.

Taylor RM & Farrow BR (1988) Ceroid-lipofuscinosis in border collie dogs. *Acta Neuropathol*, 75, 627–631.

Taylor RM & Farrow BR (1992) Ceroid lipofuscinosis in the border collie dog: retinal lesions in an animal model of juvenile Batten disease. *Am J Med Genet*, 42, 622–627.

Taylor RM & Wolfe JH (1997) Decreased lysosomal storage in the adult MPS VII mouse brain in the vicinity of grafts of retroviral vector-corrected fibroblasts secreting high levels of beta-glucuronidase. *Nat Med*, 3, 771–774.

Tcherepanova I, Bhattacharyya L, Rubin CS, & Freedman JH (2000) Aspartic proteases from the nematode Caenorhabditis elegans. Structural organization and developmental and cell-specific expression of asp-1. *J Biol Chem*, 275, 26359–26369.

Teixeira C, Guimaraes A, Bessa C, Ferreira MJ, Lopes L, Pinto E, Pinto R, Boustany RM, Sa Miranda MC, & Ribeiro MG (2003) Clinicopathological and molecular characterization of neuronal ceroid lipofuscinosis in the Portuguese population. *J Neurol*, 250, 661–667.

Teixeira CA, Lin S, Mangas M, Quinta R, Bessa CJ, Ferreira C, Sa Miranda MC, Boustany RM, & Ribeiro MG (2006) Gene expression profiling in vLINCL CLN6-deficient fibroblasts: Insights into pathobiology. *Biochim Biophys Acta*, 1762, 637–646.

Telakivi T, Partinen M, & Salmi T (1985) Sleep disturbance in patients with juvenile neuronal ceroid lipofuscinosis: a new application of the SCSB-method. *J Ment Defic Res*, 29 (Pt 1), 29–35.

Terry RD & Korey SR (1960) Membranous cytoplasmic granules in infantile amaurotic idiocy. *Nature*, 188, 1000–1002.

Tessa A, Simonati A, Tavoni A, Bertini E, & Santorelli FM (2000) A novel nonsense mutation (Q509X) in three Italian late-infantile neuronal ceroid-lipofuscinosis children. *Hum Mutat*, 15, 577.

The International Batten Disease Consortium (1995) Isolation of a novel gene underlying Batten disease, CLN3. *Cell*, 82, 949–957.

Tian Y, Sohar I, Taylor JW, & Lobel P (2006) Determination of the substrate specificity of tripeptidyl-peptidase I using combinatorial peptide libraries and development of improved fluorogenic substrates. *J Biol Chem*, 281, 6559–6572.

Tobo M, Mitsuyama Y, Ikari K, & Itoi K (1984) Familial occurrence of adult-type neuronal ceroid lipofuscinosis. *Arch Neurol*, 41, 1091–1094.

Tominaga I, Hattori M, Kaihou M, Takazawa H, Kato Y, Kasahara M, Onaya M, Nojima T, Kashima H, & Iwabuchi K (1994) [Dementia and amyotrophy in Kufs disease. The adult type of neuronal ceroid lipofuscinosis]. *Rev Neurol (Paris)*, 150, 413–417.

Tomkinson B (1999) Tripeptidyl peptidases: enzymes that count. *Trends Biochem Sci*, 24, 355–359.

Topçu M, Tan H, Yalnizoglu D, Usubütün A, Saatci I, Aynaci M, Anlar B, Topaloglu H, Turanli G, Kose G, & Aysun S (2004) Evaluation of 36 patients from Turkey with neuronal ceroid lipofuscinosis: clinical, neurophysiological, neuroradiological and histopathologic studies. *Turk J Pediatr*, 46, 1–10.

Traboulsi EI, Green WR, Luckenbach MW, & de la Cruz ZC (1987) Neuronal ceroid lipofuscinosis. Ocular histopathologic and electron microscopic studies in the late infantile, juvenile, and adult forms. *Graefes Arch Clin Exp Ophthalmol*, 225, 391–402.

Trillet M, Bady B, Kopp N, & Girard PF (1973) [Neuronal ceroid-lipofuscinosis. Apropos of 3 familial cases, one with pathological examination]. *Rev Neurol (Paris)*, 129, 233–250.

Tryselius Y & Hultmark D (1997) Cysteine proteinase 1 (CP1), a cathepsin L-like enzyme expressed in the Drosophila melanogaster haemocyte cell line mbn-2. *Insect Mol Biol*, 6, 173–181.

Tsiakas K, Steinfeld R, Storch S, Ezaki J, Lukacs Z, Kominami E, Kohlschutter A, Ullrich K, & Braulke T (2004) Mutation of the glycosylated asparagine residue 286 in human CLN2 protein results in loss of enzymatic activity. *Glycobiology*, 14, 1C–5C.

Turk B, Dolenc I, & Turk V (1998) Dipeptidyl peptidase I. In Barrett AJ, Rawlings ND, & Woessner JF (Eds.) *Handbook of Proteolytic Enzymes*, pp. 631–34. London, Academic Press.

Tuxworth RI, Vivancos V, O'Hare MB, & Tear G (2009) Interactions between the juvenile Batten disease gene, CLN3, and the Notch and JNK signalling pathways. *Hum Mol Genet*, 18, 667–678.

Tyynelä J, Baumann M, Henseler M, Sandhoff K, & Haltia M (1995) Sphingolipid activator proteins (SAPs) are stored together with glycosphingolipids in the infantile neuronal ceroid-lipofuscinosis (INCL). *Am J Med Genet*, 57, 294–297.

Tyynelä J, Cooper JD, Khan MN, Shemilts SJ, & Haltia M (2004) Hippocampal pathology in the human neuronal ceroid-lipofuscinoses: distinct patterns of storage deposition, neurodegeneration and glial activation. *Brain Pathol*, 14, 349–357.

Tyynelä J, Palmer DN, Baumann M, & Haltia M (1993) Storage of saposins A and D in infantile neuronal ceroid-lipofuscinosis. *FEBS Lett*, 330, 8–12.

Tyynelä J, Sohar I, Sleat DE, Gin RM, Donnelly RJ, Baumann M, Haltia M, & Lobel P (2000) A mutation in the ovine cathepsin D gene causes a congenital lysosomal storage disease with profound neurodegeneration. *EMBO J*, 19, 2786–2792.

Tyynelä J, Suopanki J, Baumann M, & Haltia M (1997a) Sphingolipid activator proteins (SAPs) in neuronal ceroid lipofuscinoses (NCL). *Neuropediatrics*, 28, 49–52.

Tyynelä J, Suopanki J, Santavuori P, Baumann M, & Haltia M (1997b) Variant late infantile neuronal ceroid-lipofuscinosis: pathology and biochemistry. *J Neuropathol Exp Neurol*, 56, 369–375.

Udvadia AJ & Linney E (2003) Windows into development: historic, current, and future perspectives on transgenic zebrafish. *Dev Biol*, 256, 1–17.

Umemura T, Sato H, Goryo M, & Itakura C (1985) Generalized lipofuscinosis in a dog. *Nippon Juigaku Zasshi*, 47, 673–677.

Url A, Bauder B, Thalhammer J, Nowotny N, Kolodziejek J, Herout N, Furst S, & Weissenbock H (2001) Equine neuronal ceroid lipofuscinosis. *Acta Neuropathol*, 101, 410–414.

Uusi-Rauva K, Luiro K, Tanhuanpaa K, Kopra O, Martin-Vasallo P, Kyttala A, & Jalanko A (2008) Novel interactions of CLN3 protein link Batten disease to dysregulation of fodrin-Na^+, K^+ ATPase complex. *Exp Cell Res*, 314, 2895–2905.

Uvebrant P & Hagberg B (1997) Neuronal ceroid lipofuscinoses in Scandinavia. Epidemiology and clinical pictures. *Neuropediatrics*, 28, 6–8.

Vadlamudi L, Westmoreland BF, Klass DW, & Parisi JE (2003) Electroencephalographic findings in Kufs disease. *Clin Neurophysiol*, 114, 1738–1743.

Van Den Hazel HB, Kielland-Brandt MC, & Winther JR (1996) Review: biosynthesis and function of yeast vacuolar proteases. *Yeast*, 12, 1–16.

Van Furden D, Johnson K, Segbert C, & Bossinger O (2004) The C. elegans ezrin-radixin-moesin protein ERM-1 is necessary for apical junction remodelling and tubulogenesis in the intestine. *Dev Biol*, 272, 262–276.

Vandevelde M & Fatzer R (1980) Neuronal ceroid-lipofuscinosis in older dachshunds. *Vet Pathol*, 17, 686–692.

Vanhanen SL, Puranen J, Autti T, Raininko R, Liewendahl K, Nikkinen P, Santavuori P, Suominen P, Vuori K, & Hakkinen AM (2004) Neuroradiological findings (MRS, MRI, SPECT) in infantile neuronal ceroid-lipofuscinosis (infantile CLN1) at different stages of the disease. *Neuropediatrics*, 35, 27–35.

Vanhanen SL, Raininko R, Autti T, & Santavuori P (1995a) MRI evaluation of the brain in infantile neuronal ceroid-lipofuscinosis. Part 2: MRI findings in 21 patients. *J Child Neurol*, 10, 444–450.

Vanhanen SL, Raininko R, Santavuori P, Autti T, & Haltia M (1995b) MRI evaluation of the brain in infantile neuronal ceroid-lipofuscinosis. Part 1: Postmortem MRI with histopathologic correlation. *J Child Neurol*, 10, 438–443.

Vanhanen SL, Sainio K, Lappi M, & Santavuori P (1997) EEG and evoked potentials in infantile neuronal ceroid-lipofuscinosis. *Dev Med Child Neurol*, 39, 456–463.

Vantaggiato C, Redaelli F, Falcone S, Perrotta C, Tonelli A, Bondioni S, Morbin M, Riva D, Saletti V, Bonaglia MC, Giorda R, Bresolin N, Clementi E, & Bassi MT (2009) A novel CLN8 mutation in late-infantile-onset neuronal ceroid lipofuscinosis (LINCL) reveals aspects of CLN8 neurobiological function. *Hum Mutat*, 30, 1104–1116.

Varilo T, Savukoski M, Norio R, Santavuori P, Peltonen L, & Jarvela I (1996) The age of human mutation: genealogical and linkage disequilibrium analysis of the CLN5 mutation in the Finnish population. *Am J Hum Genet*, 58, 506–512.

Vercammen L, Buyse GM, Proost JE, & Van Hove JL (2003) Neuroleptic malignant syndrome in juvenile neuronal ceroid lipofuscinosis associated with low-dose risperidone therapy. *J Inherit Metab Dis*, 26, 611–612.

Vercruyssen A, Martin JJ, Ceuterick C, Jacobs K, & Swerts L (1982) Adult ceroid-lipofuscinosis: diagnostic value of biopsies and of neurophysiological investigations. *J Neurol Neurosurg Psychiatry*, 45, 1056–1059.

Verity C, Winstone AM, Stellitano L, Will R, & Nicoll A (2010) The epidemiology of progressive intellectual and neurological deterioration in childhood. *Arch Dis Child*, 95, 361–364.

Verkruyse LA & Hofmann SL (1996) Lysosomal targeting of palmitoyl-protein thioesterase. *J Biol Chem*, 271, 15831–15836.

Vesa J, Chin MH, Oelgeschlager K, Isosomppi J, DellAngelica EC, Jalanko A, & Peltonen L (2002) Neuronal ceroid lipofuscinoses are connected at molecular level: interaction of CLN5 protein with CLN2 and CLN3. *Mol Biol Cell*, 13, 2410–2420.

Vesa J, Hellsten E, Verkruyse LA, Camp LA, Rapola J, Santavuori P, Hofmann SL, & Peltonen L (1995) Mutations in the palmitoyl protein thioesterase gene causing infantile neuronal ceroid lipofuscinosis. *Nature*, 376, 584–587.

Vetvicka V (2009) Pleiotropic effects of cathepsin D. *Endocr Metab Immune Disord Drug Targets*, 9, 385–391.

Vines D & Warburton MJ (1998) Purification and characterisation of a tripeptidyl aminopeptidase I from rat spleen. *Biochim Biophys Acta*, 1384, 233–242.

Vines DJ & Warburton MJ (1999) Classical late infantile neuronal ceroid lipofuscinosis fibroblasts are deficient in lysosomal tripeptidyl peptidase I. *FEBS Lett*, 443, 131–135.

Virmani T, Gupta P, Liu X, Kavalali ET, & Hofmann SL (2005) Progressively reduced synaptic vesicle pool size in cultured neurons derived from neuronal ceroid lipofuscinosis-1 knockout mice. *Neurobiol Dis*, 20, 314–323.

Vital A, Vital C, Orgogozo JM, Mazeaux JM, Pautrizel B, & Lariviere JM (1991) Adult dementia due to intraneuronal accumulation of ceroidlipofuscinosis (Kufs' disease): ultrastructural study of two cases. *J Geriatr Psychiatry Neurol*, 4, 110–115.

Vitiello SP, Benedict JW, Padilla-Lopez S, & Pearce DA (2010) Interaction between Sdo1p and Btn1p in the Saccharomyces cerevisiae model for Batten disease. *Hum Mol Genet*, 19, 931–942.

Vitiello SP, Wolfe DM, & Pearce DA (2007) Absence of Btn1p in the yeast model for juvenile Batten disease may cause arginine to become toxic to yeast cells. *Hum Mol Genet*, 16, 1007–1016.

Vogt H (1905) Über familiäre amaurotische Idiotie und verwandte Krankheitsbilder. *Mschr Psychiatr Neurol*, 18, 161–171.

Vogt H (1907) Zur Pathologie und pathologischen Anatomie der verschiedenen Idiotie-Formen. *Mschr Psychiatr Neurol*, 22, 403–418.

Vogt H (1909) Familiäre amaurotische Idiotie, Histologische und histopathologische Studien. *Arch Kinderheilkd*, 51, 1–35.

von Schantz C, Kielar C, Hansen SN, Pontikis CC, Alexander NA, Kopra O, Jalanko A, & Cooper JD (2009) Progressive thalamocortical neuron loss in Cln5 deficient mice: Distinct effects in Finnish variant late infantile NCL. *Neurobiol Dis*, 34, 308–319.

von Schantz C, Saharinen J, Kopra O, Cooper JD, Gentile M, Hovatta I, Peltonen L, & Jalanko A (2008) Brain gene expression profiles of Cln1 and Cln5 deficient mice unravels common molecular pathways underlying neuronal degeneration in NCL diseases. *BMC Genomics*, 9, 146.

Voznyi YV, Keulemans JL, Mancini GM, Catsman-Berrevoets CE, Young E, Winchester B, Kleijer WJ, & van Diggelen OP (1999) A new simple enzyme assay for pre- and postnatal diagnosis of infantile neuronal ceroid lipofuscinosis (INCL) and its variants. *J Med Genet*, 36, 471–474.

Wada R, Tifft CJ, & Proia RL (2000) Microglial activation precedes acute neurodegeneration in Sandhoff disease and is suppressed by bone marrow transplantation. *Proc Natl Acad Sci U S A*, 97, 10954–10959.

Walenta JH, Didier AJ, Liu X, & Kramer H (2001) The Golgi-associated hook3 protein is a member of a novel family of microtubule-binding proteins. *J Cell Biol*, 152, 923–934.

Waliany S, Das AK, Gaben A, Wisniewski KE, & Hofmann SL (2000) Identification of three novel mutations of the palmitoyl-protein thioesterase-1 (PPT1) gene in children with neuronal ceroid-lipofuscinosis. *Hum Mutat*, 15, 206–207.

Walkley SU (1998) Cellular pathology of lysosomal storage disorders. *Brain Pathol*, 8, 175–193.

Walkley SU, March PA, Schroeder CE, Wurzelmann S, & Jolly RD (1995) Pathogenesis of brain dysfunction in Batten disease. *Am J Med Genet*, 57, 196–203.

Walter S & Goebel HH (1988) Ultrastructural pathology of dermal axons and Schwann cells in lysosomal diseases. *Acta Neuropathol*, 76, 489–495.

Walus M, Kida E, & Golabek AA (2010) Functional consequences and rescue potential of pathogenic missense mutations in tripeptidyl peptidase I. *Hum Mutat*, 31, 710–721.

Walus M, Kida E, Wisniewski KE, & Golabek AA (2005) Ser475, Glu272, Asp276, Asp327, and Asp360 are involved in catalytic activity of human tripeptidyl-peptidase I. *FEBS Lett*, 579, 1383–1388.

Wang B, Shi GP, Yao PM, Li Z, Chapman HA, & Bromme D (1998) Human cathepsin F. Molecular cloning, functional expression, tissue localization, and enzymatic characterization. *J Biol Chem*, 273, 32000–32008.

Warburton MJ & Bernardini F (2001) The specificity of lysosomal tripeptidyl peptidase-I determined by its action on angiotensin-II analogues. *FEBS Lett*, 500, 145–148.

Warburton MJ & Bernardini F (2002) Tripeptidyl peptidase-I is essential for the degradation of sulphated cholecystokinin-8 (CCK-8S) by mouse brain lysosomes. *Neurosci Lett*, 331, 99–102.

Wartosch L, Fuhrmann JC, Schweizer M, Stauber T, & Jentsch TJ (2009) Lysosomal degradation of endocytosed proteins depends on the chloride transport protein ClC-7. *FASEB J*, 23, 4056–4068.

Waterston R & Sulston J (1995) The genome of Caenorhabditis elegans. *Proc Natl Acad Sci U S A*, 92, 10836–10840.

Wei H, Kim SJ, Zhang Z, Tsai PC, Wisniewski KE, & Mukherjee AB (2008) ER and oxidative stresses are common mediators of apoptosis in both neurodegenerative and non-neurodegenerative lysosomal storage disorders and are alleviated by chemical chaperones. *Hum Mol Genet*, 17, 469–477.

Weimer JM, Benedict JW, Elshatory YM, Short DW, Ramirez-Montealegre D, Ryan DA, Alexander NA, Federoff HJ, Cooper JD, & Pearce DA (2007) Alterations in striatal dopamine catabolism precede loss of substantia nigra neurons in a mouse model of juvenile neuronal ceroid lipofuscinosis. *Brain Res*, 1162, 98–112.

Weimer JM, Benedict JW, Getty AL, Pontikis CC, Lim MJ, Cooper JD, & Pearce DA (2009) Cerebellar defects in a mouse model of juvenile neuronal ceroid lipofuscinosis. *Brain Res*, 1266, 93–107.

Weimer JM, Chattopadhyay S, Custer AW, & Pearce DA (2005) Elevation of Hook1 in a disease model of Batten disease does not affect a novel interaction between Ankyrin G and Hook1. *Biochem Biophys Res Commun*, 330, 1176–1181.

Weimer JM, Custer AW, Benedict JW, Alexander NA, Kingsley E, Federoff HJ, Cooper JD, & Pearce DA (2006) Visual deficits in a mouse model of Batten disease are the result of optic nerve degeneration and loss of dorsal lateral geniculate thalamic neurons. *Neurobiol Dis*, 22, 284–293.

Weimken A & Dürr M (1974) Characterization of amino acid pools in the vacuolar compartment of Saccharomyces cerevisiae. *Arch Microbiol*, 101, 45–57.

Weissenbock H & Rossel C (1997) Neuronal ceroid-lipofuscinosis in a domestic cat: clinical, morphological and immunohistochemical findings. *J Comp Pathol*, 117, 17–24.

Welch EM, Barton ER, Zhuo J, Tomizawa Y, Friesen WJ, Trifillis P, Paushkin S, Patel M, Trotta CR, Hwang S, Wilde RG, Karp G, Takasugi J, Chen G, Jones S, Ren H, Moon YC, Corson D, Turpoff AA, Campbell JA, Conn MM, Khan A, Almstead NG, Hedrick J, Mollin A, Risher N, Weetall M, Yeh S, Branstrom AA, Colacino JM, Babiak J, Ju WD, Hirawat S, Northcutt VJ, Miller LL, Spatrick P, He F, Kawana M, Feng H, Jacobson A, Peltz SW, & Sweeney HL (2007) PTC124 targets genetic disorders caused by nonsense mutations. *Nature*, 447, 87–91.

Weleber RG, Gupta N, Trzupek KM, Wepner MS, Kurz DE, & Milam AH (2004) Electroretinographic and clinicopathologic correlations of retinal dysfunction in infantile neuronal ceroid lipofuscinosis (infantile Batten disease). *Mol Genet Metab*, 83, 128–137.

Wendt KD, Lei B, Schachtman TR, Tullis GE, Ibe ME, & Katz ML (2005) Behavioral assessment in mouse models of neuronal ceroid lipofuscinosis using a light-cued T-maze. *Behav Brain Res*, 161, 175–182.

Westermarck T, Åberg L, Santavuori P, Antila E, Edlund P, & Atroshi F (1997) Evaluation of the possible role of coenzyme Q10 and vitamin E in juvenile neuronal ceroid-lipofuscinosis (JNCL). *Mol Aspects Med*, 18 Suppl, S259–262.

Westlake VJ, Jolly RD, Bayliss SL, & Palmer DN (1995a) Immunocytochemical studies in the ceroid-lipofuscinoses

(Batten disease) using antibodies to subunit c of mitochondrial ATP synthase. *Am J Med Genet*, 57, 177–181.

Westlake VJ, Jolly RD, Jones BR, Mellor DJ, Machon R, Zanjani ED, & Krivit W (1995b) Hematopoietic cell transplantation in fetal lambs with ceroid-lipofuscinosis. *Am J Med Genet*, 57, 365–368.

Wheeler RB, Schlie M, Kominami E, Gerhard L, & Goebel HH (2001) Neuronal ceroid lipofuscinosis: late infantile or Janský Bielschowsky type—re-revisited. *Acta Neuropathol*, 102, 485–488.

Wheeler RB, Sharp JD, Schultz RA, Joslin JM, Williams RE, & Mole SE (2002) The gene mutated in variant late-infantile neuronal ceroid lipofuscinosis (CLN6) and in nclf mutant mice encodes a novel predicted transmembrane protein. *Am J Hum Genet*, 70, 537–542.

Whitaker JN & Rhodes RH (1983) The distribution of cathepsin D in rat tissues determined by immunocytochemistry. *Am J Anat*, 166, 417–428.

Wienholds E, van Eeden F, Kosters M, Mudde J, Plasterk RH, & Cuppen E (2003) Efficient target-selected mutagenesis in zebrafish. *Genome Res*, 13, 2700–2707.

Williams R, Vesa J, Jarvela I, McKay T, Mitchison H, Hellsten E, Thompson A, Callen D, Sutherland G, Luna-Battadano D, Stallings R, Peltonen L, & Gardiner M (1993) Genetic heterogeneity in neuronal ceroid lipofuscinosis (NCL): evidence that the late-infantile subtype (Janský-Bielschowsky disease; CLN2) is not an allelic form of the juvenile or infantile subtypes. *Am J Hum Genet*, 53, 931–935.

Williams RE, Åberg L, Autti T, Goebel HH, Kohlschutter A, & Lonnqvist T (2006) Diagnosis of the neuronal ceroid lipofuscinoses: an update. *Biochim Biophys Acta*, 1762, 865–872.

Williams RE, Topçu M, Lake BD, Mitchell W, & Mole SE (1999) Turkish variant late infantile NCL. In Goebel HH, Mole S, & Lake BD (Eds.) *The Neuronal Ceroid Lipofuscinoses (Batten Disease)*, pp. 114–116. Amsterdam, IOS Press.

Williams RS, Lott IT, Ferrante RJ, & Caviness VS, Jr. (1977) The cellular pathology of neuronal ceroid-lipofuscinosis. A Golgi-electronmicroscopic study. *Arch Neurol*, 34, 298–305.

Wilschanski M, Yahav Y, Yaacov Y, Blau H, Bentur L, Rivlin J, Aviram M, Bdolah-Abram T, Bebok Z, Shushi L, Kerem B, & Kerem E (2003) Gentamicin-induced correction of CFTR function in patients with cystic fibrosis and CFTR stop mutations. *N Engl J Med*, 349, 1433–1441.

Winter E & Ponting CP (2002) TRAM, LAG1 and CLN8: members of a novel family of lipid-sensing domains? *Trends Biochem Sci*, 27, 381–383.

Wisniewski KE, Becerra CR, & Hofmann SL (1997) A novel granular variant (GROD) form of late infantile neuronal ceroid lipofuscinosis (CLN2) is an infantile form of NCL (CLN1) when biochemically studied. *J Neuropathol Exp Neurol*, 56, 594.

Wisniewski KE, Connell F, Kaczmarski W, Kaczmarski A, Siakotos A, Becerra CR, & Hofmann SL (1998a) Palmitoyl-protein thioesterase deficiency in a novel granular variant of LINCL. *Pediatr Neurol*, 18, 119–123.

Wisniewski KE, Gordon-Krajcer W, & Kida E (1993) Abnormal processing of carboxy-terminal fragment of beta precursor protein (beta PP) in neuronal ceroid-lipofuscinosis (NCL) cases. *J Inherit Metab Dis*, 16, 312–316.

Wisniewski KE, Kaczmarski A, Kida E, Connell F, Kaczmarski W, Michalewski MP, Moroziewicz DN, & Zhong N (1999) Reevaluation of neuronal ceroid lipofuscinoses: atypical juvenile onset may be the result of CLN2 mutations. *Mol Genet Metab*, 66, 248–252.

Wisniewski KE, Kida E, Gordon-Majszak W, & Saitoh T (1990a) Altered amyloid beta-protein precursor processing in brains of patients with neuronal ceroid lipofuscinosis. *Neurosci Lett*, 120, 94–96.

Wisniewski KE, Kida E, Patxot OF, & Connell F (1992) Variability in the clinical and pathological findings in the neuronal ceroid lipofuscinoses: review of data and observations. *Am J Med Genet*, 42, 525–532.

Wisniewski KE, Kida E, Walus M, Wujek P, Kaczmarski W, & Golabek AA (2001) Tripeptidyl-peptidase I in neuronal ceroid lipofuscinoses and other lysosomal storage disorders. *Eur J Paediatr Neurol*, 5 Suppl A, 73–79.

Wisniewski KE & Maslinska D (1990) Lectin histochemistry in brains with juvenile form of neuronal ceroid-lipofuscinosis (Batten disease). *Acta Neuropathol*, 80, 274–279.

Wisniewski KE, Maslinska D, Kitaguchi T, Kim KS, Goebel HH, & Haltia M (1990b) Topographic heterogeneity of amyloid B-protein epitopes in brains with various forms of neuronal ceroid lipofuscinoses suggesting defective processing of amyloid precursor protein. *Acta Neuropathol*, 80, 26–34.

Wisniewski KE & Zhong N (2001) *Batten Disease: Diagnosis, Treatment and Research*. San Diego, CA, Academic Press.

Wisniewski KE, Zhong N, Kaczmarski W, Kaczmarski A, Kida E, Brown WT, Schwarz KO, Lazzarini AM, Rubin AJ, Stenroos ES, Johnson WG, & Wisniewski TM (1998b) Compound heterozygous genotype is associated with protracted juvenile neuronal ceroid lipofuscinosis. *Ann Neurol*, 43, 106–110.

Wisniewski KE, Zhong N, Kaczmarski W, Kaczmarski A, Sklower-Brooks S, & Brown WT (1998c) Studies of atypical JNCL suggest overlapping with other NCL forms. *Pediatr Neurol*, 18, 36–40.

Wlodawer A, Durell SR, Li M, Oyama H, Oda K, & Dunn BM (2003) A model of tripeptidyl-peptidase I (CLN2), a ubiquitous and highly conserved member of the sedolisin family of serine-carboxyl peptidases. *BMC Struct Biol*, 3, 8.

Wlodawer A, Li M, Dauter Z, Gustchina A, Uchida K, Oyama H, Dunn BM, & Oda K (2001) Carboxyl proteinase from Pseudomonas defines a novel family of subtilisin-like enzymes. *Nat Struct Biol*, 8, 442–446.

Wlodawer A, Li M, Gustchina A, Oyama H, Dunn BM, & Oda K (2003b) Structural and enzymatic properties of the sedolisin family of serine-carboxyl peptidases. *Acta Biochim Pol*, 50, 81–102.

Wlodawer A, Li M, Gustchina A, Tsuruoka N, Ashida M, Minakata H, Oyama H, Oda K, Nishino T, & Nakayama T (2004) Crystallographic and biochemical investigations of kumamolisin-As, a serine-carboxyl peptidase with collagenase activity. *J Biol Chem*, 279, 21500–21510.

Wohlke A, Distl O, & Drogemuller C (2005) The canine CTSD gene as a candidate for late-onset neuronal ceroid lipofuscinosis. *Anim Genet*, 36, 530–532.

Wohlke A, Distl O, & Drogemuller C (2006) Characterization of the canine CLCN3 gene and evaluation as candidate for late-onset NCL. *BMC Genet*, 7, 13.

Wolfe LS, Kin NM, Baker RR, Carpenter S, & Andermann F (1977) Identification of retinoyl complexes as the autofluorescent component of the neuronal storage material in Batten disease. *Science*, 195, 1360–1362.

Wolfe LS & Ng Ying Kin NM (1982) Batten disease: new research findings on the biochemical defect. *Birth Defects Orig Artic Ser*, 18, 233–239.

Wong LF, Azzouz M, Walmsley LE, Askham Z, Wilkes FJ, Mitrophanous KA, Kingsman SM, & Mazarakis ND (2004) Transduction patterns of pseudotyped lentiviral vectors in the nervous system. *Mol Ther*, 9, 101–111.

Woods PR, Storts RW, Shelton M, & Menzies C (1994) Neuronal ceroid lipofuscinosis in Rambouillet sheep: characterization of the clinical disease. *J Vet Intern Med*, 8, 370–375.

Woods PR, Walker MA, Weir VA, Storts RW, Menzies C, & Shelton M (1993) Computed tomography of Rambouillet sheep affected with neuronal ceroid lipofuscinosis. *Vet Radiol Ultrasound*, 34, 259–262.

Worgall S, Kekatpure MV, Heier L, Ballon D, Dyke JP, Shungu D, Mao X, Kosofsky B, Kaplitt MG, Souweidane MM, Sondhi D, Hackett NR, Hollmann C, & Crystal RG (2007) Neurological deterioration in late infantile neuronal ceroid lipofuscinosis. *Neurology*, 69, 521–535.

Worgall S, Sondhi D, Hackett NR, Kosofsky B, Kekatpure MV, Neyzi N, Dyke JP, Ballon D, Heier L, Greenwald BM, Christos P, Mazumdar M, Souweidane MM, Kaplitt MG, & Crystal RG (2008) Treatment of late infantile neuronal ceroid lipofuscinosis by CNS administration of a serotype 2 adeno-associated virus expressing CLN2 cDNA. *Hum Gene Ther*, 19, 463–474.

Wraith JE, Clarke LA, Beck M, Kolodny EH, Pastores GM, Muenzer J, Rapoport DM, Berger KI, Swiedler SJ, Kakkis ED, Braakman T, Chadbourne E, Walton-Bowen K, & Cox GF (2004) Enzyme replacement therapy for mucopolysaccharidosis I: a randomized, double-blinded, placebo-controlled, multinational study of recombinant human alpha-L-iduronidase (laronidase). *J Pediatr*, 144, 581–588.

Wrigstad A, Nilsson SE, Dubielzig R, & Narfstrom K (1995) Neuronal ceroid lipofuscinosis in the Polish Owczarek Nizinny (PON) dog. A retinal study. *Doc Ophthalmol*, 91, 33–47.

Wu YP & Proia RL (2004) Deletion of macrophage-inflammatory protein 1 alpha retards neurodegeneration in Sandhoff disease mice. *Proc Natl Acad Sci U S A*, 101, 8425–8430.

Wujek P, Kida E, Walus M, Wisniewski KE, & Golabek AA (2004) N-glycosylation is crucial for folding, trafficking, and stability of human tripeptidyl-peptidase I. *J Biol Chem*, 279, 12827–12839.

Wulliman MF, Rupp B, & Reichart H (1996) *Neuroanatomy of the Zebrafish Brain: A Topological Atlas*. Basel, Birkhauser Verlag.

Xin W, Mullen TE, Kiely R, Min J, Feng X, Cao Y, O'Malley L, Shen Y, Chu-Shore C, Mole SE, Goebel HH, & Sims K (2010) CLN5 mutations are frequent in juvenile and late-onset non-Finnish patients with NCL. *Neurology*, 74, 565–571.

Xu S, Sleat DE, Jadot M, & Lobel P (2010) Glial fibrillary acidic protein is elevated in the lysosomal storage disease classical late-infantile neuronal ceroid lipofuscinosis, but is not a component of the storage material. *Biochem J*, 428, 355–362.

Yan W, Boustany RM, Konradi C, Ozelius L, Lerner T, Trofatter JA, Julier C, Breakefield XO, Gusella JF, & Haines JL (1993) Localization of juvenile, but not late-infantile, neuronal ceroid lipofuscinosis on chromosome 16. *Am J Hum Genet*, 52, 89–95.

Yeh DC, Duncan JA, Yamashita S, & Michel T (1999) Depalmitoylation of endothelial nitric-oxide synthase by acyl-protein thioesterase 1 is potentiated by Ca(2+)-calmodulin. *J Biol Chem*, 274, 33148–33154.

Yoshikawa M, Uchida S, Ezaki J, Rai T, Hayama A, Kobayashi K, Kida Y, Noda M, Koike M, Uchiyama Y, Marumo F, Kominami E, & Sasaki S (2002) CLC-3 deficiency leads to phenotypes similar to human neuronal ceroid lipofuscinosis. *Genes Cells*, 7, 597–605.

Young EP, Worthington VC, Jackson M, & Winchester BG (2001) Pre- and postnatal diagnosis of patients with CLN1 and CLN2 by assay of palmitoyl-protein thioesterase and tripeptidyl-peptidase I activities. *Eur J Paediatr Neurol*, 5 Suppl A, 193–196.

Yuza Y, Yokoi K, Sakurai K, Ariga M, Yanagisawa T, Ohashi T, Hoshi Y, & Eto Y (2005) Allogenic bone marrow transplantation for late-infantile neuronal ceroid lipofuscinosis. *Pediatr Int*, 47, 681–683.

Zaiss AK & Muruve DA (2005) Immune responses to adeno-associated virus vectors. *Curr Gene Ther*, 5, 323–331.

Zelnik N, Mahajna M, Iancu TC, Sharony R, & Zeigler M (2007) A novel mutation of the CLN8 gene: is there a Mediterranean phenotype? *Pediatr Neurol*, 36, 411–413.

Zeman W (1974) Presidential address: Studies in the neuronal ceroid-lipofuscinoses. *J Neuropathol Exp Neurol*, 33, 1–12.

Zeman W (1976) The neuronal ceroid lipofuscinoses. In Zimmerman HM (Ed.) *Progress in Neuropathology*, pp. 207–223. New York, Grune and Stratton.

Zeman W & Donahue S (1963) Fine structure of the lipid bodies in juvenile amaurotic idiocy. *Acta Neuropathol*, 3, 144–149.

Zeman W, Donahue S, Dyken P, & Green J (1970) The neuronal ceroid-lipofuscinoses (Batten–Vogt syndrome). In Vinken PJ, & Bruyn GW (Eds.) *Handbook of Clinical Neurology*, pp. 588–679. Amsterdam, North Holland Publ Co.

Zeman W & Dyken P (1969) Neuronal ceroid-lipofuscinosis (Batten's disease): relationship to amaurotic family idiocy? *Pediatrics*, 44, 570–583.

Zeman W & Rider JA (Eds.) (1975) *The dissection of a degenerative disease. Proceedings of four round-table conferences on the pathogenesis of Batten's disease (neuroronal ceroid-lipofuscinosis)*, p393, Amsterdam, Excerpta Medica.

Zeng J, Racicott J, & Morales CR (2009) The inactivation of the sortilin gene leads to a partial disruption of prosaposin trafficking to the lysosomes. *Exp Cell Res*, 315, 3112–3124.

Zhang Z, Butler JD, Levin SW, Wisniewski KE, Brooks SS, & Mukherjee AB (2001) Lysosomal ceroid depletion by drugs: therapeutic implications for a hereditary neurodegenerative disease of childhood. *Nat Med*, 7, 478–484.

Zhang Z, Lee YC, Kim SJ, Choi MS, Tsai PC, Saha A, Wei H, Xu Y, Xiao YJ, Zhang P, Heffer A, & Mukherjee AB (2007) Production of lysophosphatidylcholine by cPLA2 in the brain of mice lacking PPT1 is a signal for phagocyte infiltration. *Hum Mol Genet*, 16, 837–847.

Zhang Z, Lee YC, Kim SJ, Choi MS, Tsai PC, Xu Y, Xiao YJ, Zhang P, Heffer A, & Mukherjee AB (2006) Palmitoyl-protein thioesterase-1 deficiency mediates the activation of the unfolded protein response and neuronal apoptosis in INCL. *Hum Mol Genet*, 15, 337–346.

Zheng Y, Rozengurt N, Ryazantsev S, Kohn DB, Satake N, & Neufeld EF (2003) Treatment of the mouse model of mucopolysaccharidosis I with retrovirally transduced bone marrow. *Mol Genet Metab*, 79, 233–244.

Zhong N, Moroziewicz DN, Ju W, Jurkiewicz A, Johnston L, Wisniewski KE, & Brown WT (2000) Heterogeneity of late-infantile neuronal ceroid lipofuscinosis. *Genet Med*, 2, 312–318.

Zhong N, Wisniewski KE, Hartikainen J, Ju W, Moroziewicz DN, McLendon L, Sklower Brooks SS, & Brown WT (1998a) Two common mutations in the CLN2 gene underlie late infantile neuronal ceroid lipofuscinosis. *Clin Genet*, 54, 234–238.

Zhong N, Wisniewski KE, Kaczmarski AL, Ju W, Xu WM, Xu WW, McLendon L, Liu B, Kaczmarski W, Sklower Brooks SS, & Brown WT (1998b) Molecular screening of Batten disease: identification of a missense mutation (E295K) in the CLN3 gene. *Hum Genet*, 102, 57–62.

Zini A, Cenacchi G, Nichelli P, Zunarelli E, Todeschini A, & Meletti S (2008) Early-onset dementia with prolonged occipital seizures: an atypical case of Kufs disease. *Neurology*, 71, 1709–1712.

Zon LI & Peterson RT (2005) In vivo drug discovery in the zebrafish. *Nat Rev Drug Discov*, 4, 35–44.

Author Index

Subject Index